PSYCHOLOGICAL AND MEDICAL PERSPECTIVES ON FERTILITY CARE AND SEXUAL HEALTH

PSYCHOLOGICAL AND MEDICAL PERSPECTIVES ON FERTILITY CARE AND SEXUAL HEALTH

Edited by

KIM BERGMAN
Growing Generations, Los Angeles, CA, United States

WILLIAM D. PETOK
Department of Obstetrics and Gynecology, Sidney Kimmel Medical College, Thomas Jefferson University,
Philadelphia, PA, United States

ELSEVIER

Elsevier
Radarweg 29, PO Box 211, 1000 AE Amsterdam, Netherlands
The Boulevard, Langford Lane, Kidlington, Oxford OX5 1GB, United Kingdom
50 Hampshire Street, 5th Floor, Cambridge, MA 02139, United States

Copyright © 2022 Elsevier Inc. All rights reserved.

No part of this publication may be reproduced or transmitted in any form or by any means, electronic or mechanical, including photocopying, recording, or any information storage and retrieval system, without permission in writing from the publisher. Details on how to seek permission, further information about the Publisher's permissions policies and our arrangements with organizations such as the Copyright Clearance Center and the Copyright Licensing Agency, can be found at our website: www.elsevier.com/permissions.

This book and the individual contributions contained in it are protected under copyright by the Publisher (other than as may be noted herein).

Notices
Knowledge and best practice in this field are constantly changing. As new research and experience broaden our understanding, changes in research methods, professional practices, or medical treatment may become necessary.

Practitioners and researchers must always rely on their own experience and knowledge in evaluating and using any information, methods, compounds, or experiments described herein. In using such information or methods they should be mindful of their own safety and the safety of others, including parties for whom they have a professional responsibility.

To the fullest extent of the law, neither the Publisher nor the authors, contributors, or editors, assume any liability for any injury and/or damage to persons or property as a matter of products liability, negligence or otherwise, or from any use or operation of any methods, products, instructions, or ideas contained in the material herein.

British Library Cataloguing-in-Publication Data
A catalogue record for this book is available from the British Library

Library of Congress Cataloging-in-Publication Data
A catalog record for this book is available from the Library of Congress

ISBN: 978-0-12-822288-1

For Information on all Elsevier publications
visit our website at https://www.elsevier.com/books-and-journals

Publisher: Stacy Masucci
Acquisitions Editor: Ana Claudia A. Garcia
Editorial Project Manager: Sara Pianavilla
Production Project Manager: Swapna Srinivasan
Cover Designer: Miles Hitchen

Typeset by MPS Limited, Chennai, India

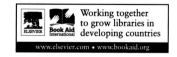

Dedication

This book is dedicated to all of my students and teachers: to the families I have had the privilege of helping throughout my career, I will always listen to you, to my mom, Joan Bergman, everyone I have helped is your legacy, and to my daughters, Abby and Jenna, the future is all yours.

—Kim Bergman

To the patients I have counseled over the years who gave me the privilege of working with them so I could practically apply the knowledge I acquired from my teachers and mentors; to the professionals who entrusted their referrals to my care; and to my parents Dorothy and Ted Petok, who valued both learning and a sense of humor, qualities I consider essential to my goal of helping others create families.

—William D. Petok

Contents

List of contributors   xiii
Preface: The intimate interface of sexuality and fertility   xv
Acknowledgments   xxi

I
Reproductive health

1. The acquisition of sexual and reproductive health knowledge   3
WILLIAM D. PETOK AND ARIK V. MARCELL

Introduction   3
Prehistory of sexual and reproductive knowledge   3
Early historical evidence   4
Recorded history   5
Science and fertility   6
The evolution of modern reproductive health and sex education in the United States   9
Fertility awareness and its acquisition   14
Interventions to improve fertility awareness, knowledge, and access to care   17
Summary   17
References   18

II
Sexual dysfunctions and infertility

2. Emotional consequences of male infertility   23
VASSILI GLAZYRINE, DANE STEPHENS, EMILY WENTZELL, KIMBERLY WALLACE-YOUNG AND AJAY K. NANGIA

Introduction   23
    Conceptualizing male infertility   23
    Patient and partner perceptions of reproductive health and conception   24
    Perception of duration of trying/infertility   25
    The financial burden   25
Specific conditions   26
    Hormonal   26
    Medications   28
    Genetic   29
    Anatomic   31
Some specific medical conditions   33
    Diabetes mellitus   33
    Spinal cord injury   34
    Cancer   35
    Pediatric conditions and transitional care   35
    Transgender fertility issues   36
Lifestyle issues   36
Conclusion   37
References   38

3. Female sexual function and fertility   45
ELIZABETH A. GRILL, ALISON J. MEYERS AND ALICE D. DOMAR

Highlights   45
Case   45
Introduction   46
Psychological effects of infertility in women   46
Psychological distress and female sexual function   48
Infertility leading to female sexual dysfunction   48
Female sexual function disorders leading to infertility   49
Treatment outcomes   50
Referral, consultation, and treatment   50
    Sex therapy   51
    Infertility counseling   52
    Pharmacological and medical treatment   53
Conclusion   54
References   54

4. The impact of erectile dysfunction on infertility and its treatment   57
AMIR ISHAQ KHAN, JENNIFER LINDELOF AND STANTON HONIG

Historical and anatomical overview of erectile dysfunction   57
    Introduction   57
    History, prevalence, and incidence   57
    Anatomy   58
Infertility and its relationship with erectile dysfunction   59

Causes of erectile dysfunction	60	Sexual health	100
Vascular	60	Emotional health	101
Neurologic	60	Looking toward the future of POI treatment	101
Medication-induced	61	Conclusion	102
Hormonal	61	References	102
Psychological or situational anxiety−related	63		
Lifestyle	63	7. Reproductive and sexual health concerns for cancer survivors	105
Treatment of erectile dysfunction: effects on infertility	63	JESSICA R. GORMAN AND ELIZABETH K. ARTHUR	
Treatment options	64		
Treatment of infertility when erectile dysfunction is an issue	68	Introduction	105
Treat the underlying problem	68	The reproductive and sexual health consequences of cancer and cancer treatment	105
Move the sperm closer to the eggs via assisted reproductive techniques	69	The impact of cancer treatment on fertility	105
Natural cycle intrauterine insemination with ejaculated sperm	69	Reproductive concerns after cancer	106
Sperm retrieval/ICSI (more for ejaculatory dysfunction)	69	Cancer's impact on sexual health	106
Conclusions	71	Managing reproductive and sexual health concerns after cancer	107
References	71	Improving patient-provider communication about reproductive and sexual health	108
		Clinical guidelines for fertility consultation and preservation	109
5. Ejaculatory dysfunction and infertility	77	Management of infertility risk	109
DANIEL N. WATTER AND KATHRYN S.K. HALL		Clinical guidelines for sexual health after cancer	110
Introduction	77	Management of women's sexual health problems	111
Retrograde ejaculation and anejaculation	77	Management of men's sexual health problems	111
Premature or rapid ejaculation	78	Improving partner communication about reproductive and sexual health concerns	111
Premature ejaculation and infertility	80	Special considerations	112
Treatment for premature or rapid ejaculation	80	Assumptions about sexual health	112
The case of Joan and Maxwell	82	LGBTQ+ cancer survivors	112
Delayed ejaculation	83	Black, indigenous, and people of color (BIPOC) cancer survivors	113
Etiological factors in delayed ejaculation	85	Older adult cancer survivors	113
Treatment of delayed ejaculation	86	Key points and recommendations	113
The case of Philip and Yolanda: lifelong, situational delayed ejaculation	88	References	114
The case of Desmond and Mollie: acquired situational delayed ejaculation	89		
Conclusions	90		
References	90		

III

Additional considerations

6. Early menopause: diagnosis and management	93	
TANYA GLENN AND AMANDA KALLEN		
		8. Lesbians pursuing parenthood: pathways, challenges, and best practices	123
Introduction	93	MARIE HAYES AND JULIA T. WOODWARD
Etiologies of primary ovarian insufficiency	93	
Diagnosis of primary ovarian insufficiency and early menopause	95	Case example	123
Comorbidities associated with early menopause	96	Introduction	125
Treatment of early menopause	97	Historical context	125
HT: a changing landscape	97	Decisions, decisions: preparing for pregnancy	127
Choice of HT	98	Pathways to parenthood	128
Contraceptive needs	99	Adoption	128
Fertility	99		

At-home insemination	128	Ovarian tissue cryopreservation	157
Assisted reproductive technology	129	Oocyte cryopreservation	159
Psychological consultation for patients using donor sperm	131	Embryo cryopreservation	159
Psychological preparation for lesbians working with a known sperm donor	132	Fertility preservation outcomes for transgender men	159
Understanding the fertility clinic experience or lesbians seeking parenthood	133	Fertility preservation options for transgender women	160
Pregnancy and childbirth	134	Sperm cryopreservation	161
Postpartum phase: benefits and challenges	135	Embryo cryopreservation	162
Legal considerations	136	Testicular tissue cryopreservation	162
Policies, procedures, and practices to support lesbians pursuing parenthood	137	Fertility preservation outcomes for transgender women	163
Recommendations for individual providers	137	Fertility care	164
Recommendations for clinics and programs	138	Pregnancy	166
Conclusion	138	Preconception and antepartum experience	166
Key takeaways	138	Experience of pregnancy loss	166
References	139	Intrapartum care	167
		Postpartum experience	167
		Impact of parenting on children	168
		Impact of parenting on gender identity and quality of life	169
9. Gay men, as individuals and as a community, overcoming reproductive challenges to have children	**141**	Conclusions	169
GUY RINGLER AND CYD ZEIGLER		References	170
Article	141	**11. Trauma and its impact on reproduction and sexuality**	**173**
Progress in acceptance and law for gay men	141	LAURA COVINGTON	
Emerging assisted reproductive technologies give gay men hope of a family	142		
The evolving landscape of fertility treatments for gay men	143	Introduction	173
		Trauma and the sexual relationship	173
The process of gestational surrogacy pregnancy in five steps	144	Grief at the core of trauma and infertility	174
Sexualizing the gestational-surrogacy process for gay men	146	Psychological trauma theory	174
		How trauma impacts attachment	175
Broader societal implications of gay men having children	146	Trauma response theory	175
References	147	Trauma and relationships	176
		Providing a foundation for growth	177
		Assessment	178
10. Parenting in transgender and nonbinary individuals	**149**	Understanding the problem	178
AMANDA R. SCHWARTZ AND MOLLY B. MORAVEK		Partner 1 history gathering	180
		Partner 2 history gathering	181
		Feedback	182
Introduction	149	Special considerations	184
Demographics of transgender parenting	150	Clinical considerations	184
Transgender parenting desires	151	Conclusion and takeaways	185
Healthcare barriers	151	References	186
Barriers to parenting	152		
Impact of gender-affirming care on reproductive function	153	**12. How the medicalization of reproduction takes the fun out of the process**	**189**
Masculinizing hormones and fertility	153	ALICE D. DOMAR, ALISON J. MEYERS AND ELIZABETH A. GRILL	
Feminizing hormones and fertility	155		
Fertility preservation	155	Highlights	189
Fertility preservation options for transgender men	157	Introduction	189
		Case study	190
		Background	191

General stress and sexual dysfunction in men and women 191
Infertility—prevalence, etiology, and diagnosis 192
Psychological impact of infertility 192
The impacts of infertility-related stress on sexuality 193
Infertility and sexuality in men—clinical implications 194
Infertility and sexuality in men—psychosocial implications 194
Infertility and sexuality in women—clinical implications 195
Infertility and sexuality in women—psychosocial implications 196
Infertility and sexuality in the couple—marital implications 196
Infertility-related stress on sexuality and pregnancy—treatment outcomes 197
Consultation, referral, and treatment options 198
Marital intervention—the couple 198
Sex therapy 199
Psychosocial intervention 199
Clinical intervention 200
Prevention of sexual dysfunction in infertile couples 200
Conclusion 200
Key points 201
References 202

13. Unintended infertility: labor markets, software workers, and fertility decision-making 205
SHARMILA RUDRAPPA

Introduction 205
Defining unintended infertility 206
Meeting with couples undergoing fertility assistance 207
Workplace demands and relationship needs 208
Marriage counselors who work with IT couples in Bangalore 210
Emergent modes of reproduction 210
Conclusions 211
References 211

14. Traditional Chinese Medicine, infertility, and sexuality dysfunction 213
DENISE WIESNER

The Three Treasures: Jing, Qi, and Shen 214
Jing 214
Qi 215
Shen 216

TCM texts on gynecology, sexuality, and fertility 216
Diagnosing according to Traditional Chinese Medicine 217
The five elements, fertility, and sexuality 217
The Eight Extraordinary vessels, fertility, and sexuality 218
Modalities used in Traditional Chinese Medicine 219
Acupuncture 219
Electroacupuncture 219
Cupping 220
Moxabustion 220
Herbal medicine 220
Eastern medicine: an alternative perspective on sexual dysfunction and fertility care 220
Sex drive and reproduction in Traditional Chinese Medicine 220
Case study: low sex drive and trauma 222
Microcosmic orbit breathing 222
Stress, fertility, sexuality, and Traditional Chinese Medicine 222
Case: stress, infertility, and sexuality 223
Male sexual problems and Traditional Chinese Medicine 223
Erectile dysfunction 223
Diagnosis of erectile dysfunction in Traditional Chinese Medicine 223
Traditional Chinese Medicine treatment of erectile dysfunction 224
Case Study 1—erectile dysfunction 225
Case Study 2— erectile dysfunction 225
The male deer exercise 225
Herbal medicine and erectile dysfunction 225
Ejaculatory dysfunction 226
A case on intravaginal ejaculatory dysfunction 226
Premature ejaculation and Traditional Chinese Medicine 227
Edging practice for early ejaculators 227
Female sexual issues 227
Traditional Chinese Medicine for sexual dysfunctions; dyspareunia, vulvodynia, vaginismus 227
Research on Traditional Chinese Medicine and female sexual pain 228
Chinese medical theory and female sexual pain 229
Lichen sclerosus and Traditional Chinese Medicine 230
Traditional Chinese Medicine treatment plans for female problems 230
Vaginal steaming 231
Case study: vaginismus 231
Conclusion 232
References 232
Addendum 233
Herbal medicine 233

15. Sex, religion, and infertility: the complications of G-d in the bedroom	237
JULIE BINDEMAN	
Historical overview of sex, religion, and assisted reproductive technology	237
Sex	237
Origin of Judaism	238
Origin of Christianity	238
Origin of Islam	239
Assisted reproductive technology	239
Judeo-Christian views on sexuality and sex	239
Judeo-Christian views of homosexuality and status	242
Judeo-Christian perspectives on infertility and assisted reproduction	244
Infertility in the Old Testament	244
Navigating Jewish infertility	246
Infertility in the New Testament	249
Navigating Christian infertility	250
Infertility in the Qur'an	251
Navigating Muslim infertility (Sunni Muslims)	252
Navigating Muslim infertility (Shi'a Muslims)	253
Implications and recommendations	254
Toward the collaboration of religion with treatment	256
Summary	258
References	258

IV
Looking forward

16. Thoughts on education, reproduction, and sexual function. Futures directions and obstacles	265
ANGELA K. LAWSON	
A brief history of reproductive education	265
The example of the US education system	265
Reproductive education in the United States	266
The disparate effects of sex/reproductive education	267
The dangers of poor sex/reproductive education	268
Reproductive knowledge	268
Violence/discrimination/harassment/hostility toward women, racial/ethnic minority group members, gender nonconforming, nonheterosexual, and/or differently abled individuals	269
Sexual dysfunction, the forgotten education	270
Future directions	270
References	271

Index 275

List of contributors

Elizabeth K. Arthur College of Nursing and Comprehensive Cancer Center – Arthur G. James Cancer Hospital, Richard. J. Solove Research Institute, The Ohio State University, Columbus, OH, United States

Julie Bindeman Integrative Therapy of Greater Washington, Rockville, MD, United States

Laura Covington Shady Grove Fertility, Covington & Hafkin and Associates, Washington, DC, United States

Alice D. Domar Domar Centers for Mind/Body Health, Waltham, MA, United States

Vassili Glazyrine Department of Urology, University of Kansas Medical Center, Kansas City, KS, United States

Tanya Glenn Division of Reproductive Endocrinology and Infertility, Department of Obstetrics, Gynecology and Reproductive Sciences, Yale School of Medicine, New Haven, CT, United States

Jessica R. Gorman College of Public Health and Human Sciences, Oregon State University, Corvallis, OR, United States

Elizabeth A. Grill Center for Reproductive Medicine, Weill Cornell Medical College, New York, NY, United States

Kathryn S.K. Hall Private Practice, Princeton, NJ, United States

Marie Hayes Departments of Psychiatry and Behavioral Sciences, Department of Obstetrics and Gynecology, Duke University Health System, Durham, NC, United States

Stanton Honig Department of Urology, Yale School of Medicine, Yale University, New Haven, CT, United States

Amanda Kallen Division of Reproductive Endocrinology and Infertility, Department of Obstetrics, Gynecology and Reproductive Sciences, Yale School of Medicine, New Haven, CT, United States

Amir Ishaq Khan Department of Urology, Yale School of Medicine, Yale University, New Haven, CT, United States

Angela K. Lawson Northwestern University, Evanston, IL, United States

Jennifer Lindelof Division of Urology, UConn Health, Farmington, CT, United States

Arik V. Marcell Departments of Pediatrics and Population, Family & Reproductive Health, The Johns Hopkins University, Baltimore, MD, United States

Alison J. Meyers Domar Centers for Mind/Body Health, Waltham, MA, United States

Molly B. Moravek Division of Reproductive Endocrinology and Infertility, Department of Obstetrics and Gynecology, University of Michigan, Ann Arbor, MI, United States

Ajay K. Nangia University of Kansas Medical Center, Kansas City, KS, United States

William D. Petok Department of Obstetrics and Gynecology, Sidney Kimmel Medical College, Thomas Jefferson University, Philadelphia, PA, United States; Independent Practice, Baltimore, MD, United States

Guy Ringler California Fertility Partners, Los Angeles, CA, United States

Sharmila Rudrappa Department of Sociology, University of Texas at Austin, Austin, TX, United States

Amanda R. Schwartz Division of Reproductive Endocrinology and Infertility, Department of Obstetrics and Gynecology, University of Michigan, Ann Arbor, MI, United States

Dane Stephens Department of Urology, University of Kansas Medical Center, Kansas City, KS, United States

Kimberly Wallace-Young Department of Psychiatry and Behavioral Sciences, University of Kansas Medical Center, Kansas City, KS, United States

Daniel N. Watter Morris Psychological Group, P.A., Parsippany, NJ, United States

Emily Wentzell Department of Anthropology, University of Iowa, Iowa City, IA, United States

Denise Wiesner Yo San University of Traditional Chinese Medicine, Los Angeles, CA, United States

Julia T. Woodward Departments of Psychiatry and Behavioral Sciences, Department of Obstetrics and Gynecology, Duke University Health System, Durham, NC, United States

Cyd Zeigler Department of Journalism and Communication, University of Florida, Gainesville, FL, United States

Preface: The intimate interface of sexuality and fertility

Fertility and sexuality are two of the most natural and ubiquitous human processes and yet both are also associated with shame and secretiveness, even when things go right, all the more so when things go wrong. Sexual dysfunction and infertility are two highly stigmatized and taboo subjects often not spoken of openly (by people and parallel in a lack of literature) [1–10].

According to *Encyclopedia Britannica*,

> "Taboo is the prohibition of an action based on the belief that such behaviour is either too sacred and consecrated or too dangerous and accursed for ordinary individuals to undertake." [11]

And yet, infertility and sexual dysfunction each affect millions of people [12] and often go hand in hand, staying as silent and forbidden topics for those who suffer. This book attempts to bring these topics into the forefront and provide a reference for clinicians of all disciplines to be able to provide much needed help for their patients.

Before we provide an overview of the chapters some brief notes about fertility, infertility, sex, sexuality, and sexual health.

Fertility or problems with fertility have been a subject worth discussion since Abraham prayed about Sarah's inability to conceive in biblical times [13]. There are references to remedies for reproductive failure in Greek writings of the late fifth and early fourth centuries BCE [10] and Aristotle was fascinated by understanding reproduction [14]. In "modern" times, King Henry the IV was said to use artificial insemination to impregnate his wife (claims later refuted but a topic of discussion in that era nonetheless) [15]. Harvey crossed the line from myth to science in looking at the actual role of the egg in reproduction in 1651 [14] and Leeuwenhoek first observed human spermatozoa in 1678–9 [14–16]. Almost 100 years later in 1770, Hunter reported the first case of artificial insemination in a human [15]. Next, von Baer and van Beneden reported discovering the mammalian oocyte in 1827 and observed and wrote about mammalian fertilization in 1875 [14,17]. Fully 100 years later we would hear about Baby Louise, the world's first "test-tube" baby [18] and with that the advent of in vitro fertilization (IVF) and the field of fertility care burst forth. This milestone paved the way for the more than 8 million babies that have been born through IVF since 1978 [19]. These millions of babies represent the millions of parents and would be parents struggling with infertility or undergoing fertility care—a significant portion of the population.

Infertility rates are soaring:

- One in eight couples have difficulty conceiving and sustaining pregnancy [20].
- About 12%–18% of women aged 15–44 years and 7% of men experience infertility [21,22].
- Global infertility rates between 1990 and 2010 in 190 countries equal 48.5 million couples, 19.2 million with primary infertility, and 29.3 million from secondary infertility [23,24].

These numbers are significant and speak to the impact of infertility on individuals and couples throughout the world.

Infertility is inextricably linked to sexuality by its very definition. The American Society for Reproductive Medicine describes infertility thus:

> "For women under the age of 35 years, infertility is defined as the inability to conceive a child after 1 year of unprotected sexual intercourse. For women aged 35–40 years, it is defined as inability to conceive after 6 months of unprotected intercourse. For women over the age of 40 years, it is the inability to conceive after 3 months of unprotected intercourse." [25]

In addition, infertile couples report a higher risk of sexual dysfunction than fertile couples and the rates of sexual dysfunction in infertile couples is significant [23,26–33], is associated with many layers of distress [34–38], and the longer couples experience infertility the higher the rate of sexual difficulty [30].

We offer the following descriptive and explanatory comments regarding sexual health to clarify our thought on its importance and impact on humans worldwide.

The World Health Organization (WHO) defines sexual health as

> "...a state of physical, emotional, mental and social well-being in relation to sexuality; it is not merely the absence of disease, dysfunction or infirmity. Sexual health requires a positive and respectful approach to sexuality and sexual relationships, as well as the possibility of having pleasurable and safe sexual experiences, free of coercion, discrimination and violence. For sexual health to be attained and maintained, the sexual rights of all persons must be respected, protected and fulfilled." [39]

Note well that there is no hint of reproduction included in this definition. Sexual health has nothing to do with conception or family building from this point of view. However, as our authors will describe, reproduction can be severely compromised without a functioning sexual relationship. Conversely, reproduction without a healthy sexual relationship is possible, though not as enjoyable! And the failure to conceive can have a wide range of impacts on sexual function.

Most would agree that there are some conditions which enhance or contribute to positive sexual relations. They would include but are not limited to:

- A feeling of connection to a partner, preferably in a positive way;
- The absence of strong anxiety about sexual performance;
- A sense that your partner can provide a positive experience with respect to attitude, response, and stimulation;
- A sense of well-being with regard to health and rest;
- A positive sense about the encounter before it starts;
- A feeling of arousal or sexual excitement;
- Absence of emotional conditions which interfere with the above;
- No adverse influence from alcohol or other drugs; and
- Environmental conditions such as temperature, light, sound, and privacy conducive to a positive experience (adapted from Zilbergeld) [40].

In our experience, no book comprehensively addresses the topics of sexual function and fertility together. Clearly, the interface of sexuality and fertility, sexual and reproductive health, is a complex one. Our authors have been chosen to highlight the various threads that run through this rich tapestry. The issues cross between personal and public health. As a result, the chapters touch on sexuality and reproduction for the individual and society. And, in an effort to work with a broad brush we have included chapters that are nonheteronormative because the pursuit of parenthood cuts across lines of sexual orientation and gender identity.

Some of the chapters deal with the absence of these optimal conditions and how they impact family building. Others describe how reproductive health issues can compromise the sexual relationship both when reproduction is the goal, and when pleasure or relationship enhancement is the primary aim. We hope that readers will have a greater appreciation for the nuanced nature of our overall topic, the interface of sex and fertility.

This book seeks to dispel myths, look at current research, and bring this topic out of the shadows.

Organization of the book

This book is devoted to providing a broad range of topics dealing with sex, sexuality, and fertility/family building. We first provide a perspective on how knowledge about sex and reproduction has been acquired by humans to set the stage for what follows. The second section deals with the medical intricacies and psychological consequences of sexual function/dysfunction and their impact on fertility as well as the reverse relationship of infertility on sexual function. Health, culture, and religion all play a role in both sex and family building and the next section is devoted to additional considerations. In this section, we have included chapters on the reproductive and family building complexities faced by the LGBTQ+ community. Finally, a look to the future with regard to research and this intimate interface.

Reproductive health

Chapter 1, The Acquisition of Sexual and Reproductive Health Knowledge by William D. Petok and Arik V. Marcell, provides a deep historical backdrop as well as a look at the more contemporary scene for this topic. They note the initial slow growth of information and understanding of how humans conceive followed by a relative explosion of information in the last two centuries, with the most expansive developments taking place in the last 50 years. They also describe the obstacles to a reliable understanding of sexual function that existed prior to 1966. That year saw the publication of research by William Masters and Virginia Johnson, opening the door to better understanding of the human sexual response and advances made by researchers who followed them. A discussion of the impediments to a greater awareness of the fragility of fertility that exist today concludes the chapter.

Sexual dysfunctions, medical and social conditions, and infertility

Chapter 2, The Emotional Consequences of Male Infertility by Vassili Glazyrine, Dane Stephens, Emily Wentzell, Kimberly Wallace-Young, and Ajay K. Nanja, examines the diversity of medical issues that can lead to male factor infertility and some of the emotional sequelae that men can face. Often overlooked in texts for mental health clinicians, male factor infertility is essential because, as the authors note, it accounts for 40% of infertility. When taken in conjunction with combined male and female, the figure jumps to 50%. Anyone seeking a well-rounded understanding of the field must take it into account.

Breaking down the causes of male infertility into hormonal, anatomic, genetic, medical, and idiopathic variants, the authors provide readers with an atlas of conditions that impair reproduction on the male side of the equation. Practitioners who work with anyone coping with a male component infertility will have a more complete understanding of these issues and the challenges they present. The use of anabolic steroids by men seeking to improve muscle mass and physical performance receives attention. Since a group of men are attracted to cultural stereotypes of masculinity, this section is significant and highlights the misunderstood impact of these agents. And for those working with men who have had a reproductive "change of mind/heart" after vasectomy, there is a section addressing this issue as well.

Chapter 3, Female Sexual Function and Fertility by Elizabeth A. Grill, Alison J. Meyers, and Alice D. Domar, tackles the problem of female factor infertility, the stress created by a diagnosis of such, and its treatment and the potential impact the stressful process has on female sexual function. They discuss how desire, satisfaction, and self-esteem can suffer during infertility treatment, noting that gender identity, femininity, and sexuality can become linked with negative consequences. They note that sex as a relationship enhancer can take a "leave of absence" when fertility treatments become the sole focus of a woman and her partner. Looking at opposite sides of the same coin, infertility leading to sexual dysfunction and the reverse, they offer guidance for referral, consultation, and treatment of these problems.

Chapter 4, The Impact of Erectile Dysfunction on Infertility and Its Treatment by Amir Ishaq Khan, Jennifer Lindelof, and Stanton Honig, discusses erectile dysfunction and the interplay of sexuality, virility, and fertility. Erectile dysfunction (ED), a sexual dysfunction with a significant incidence rate in the population in general, is known to affect men who are infertile at rates as high as double that found in fertile men. The combination of ED and infertility can lead to multiple psychological consequences. After describing the anatomy and physiology of erection, the authors provide an etiological overview of the causes of ED and offer treatment suggestions. Finally, they provide a helpful overview of infertility treatment options when male factor is a contributor to the problem.

Chapter 5, Ejaculatory Dysfunction and Infertility by Daniel N. Watter and Kathryn S.K. Hall, examines the other significant set of male sexual dysfunctions with an impact on fertility. Some suggest that it is the most common set of sexual disorders and clearly contributes to dissatisfaction for men and their partners. They highlight the importance of both medical and psychosocial issues critical for therapists to understand to best help couples dealing with these distressing problems. Their chapter utilizes both literature review and case examples, providing a robust set of tools for clinicians.

Chapter 6, Early Menopause: Diagnosis and Management by Tanya Glenn and Amanda Kallen, discusses the impact of reproductive aging on women, hormonally, psychologically, and physiologically. Fertility is severely compromised by primary ovarian insufficiency and they provide a detailed look at the problem, taking care to correct earlier, misinformed definitions and descriptions of the issue. Their section on comorbidities associated with early menopause is essential for both medical and mental health clinicians working with this population as it details a range of complications that can affect the lives of these women in addition to compromised fertility. The connection between reproductive and sexual health described addresses the need for multidimensional treatment and clear opportunities for collaboration between medical and mental health providers.

Chapter 7, Reproductive and Sexual Health Concerns for Cancer Survivors by Jessica R. Gorman and Elizabeth K. Arthur, offers a view of the impact of cancer and its treatment on reproductive and sexual health. Cancer treatments can threaten future fertility, and have a distressing impact on the lives of patients. While these health concerns are real for most patients of reproductive age and younger, care for this issue is often inadequate. Younger cancer survivors talk about feeling they have been robbed of something important due to changes in their ability to have children. They further feel additional losses because cancer and its treatment has disrupted their sexual function and their ability to have the type of sexual satisfaction, they presumed would be theirs. Certainly, breast and reproductive system cancers have the most significant impact, but as the authors note, these concerns can affect all cancer survivors. Included in this chapter is a discussion of the implications for older adult, BIPOC (black, indigenous, and people of Color), and LGBTQ+ (lesbian, gay, bisexual, transgender, queer/questioning) survivors. Providers working in the field of reproductive healthcare will treat patients concerned about fertility preservation or the resumption of sexual activity postcancer treatment. This chapter provides guidance on how to improve therapist–patient communication regarding reproductive and sexual health as well as strategies for facilitating conversations about sexual health in general.

Additional considerations

Chapter 8, Lesbians Pursuing Parenthood: Pathways, Challenges, and Best Practices by Marie Hayes and Julia T. Woodward, discusses the issues faced when lesbians decide to create a family. They outline the unique experiences and needs of lesbians becoming parents from finding a sperm donor to obtaining proper legal advice and documents. Barriers to care faced by this demographic are financial, starting with the cost of using donor sperm, and can include subtle and overt discrimination from providers. The authors highlight strategies that lesbians use to deal with these barriers. Readers are introduced to many of the issues via a case study which offers real-life examples. Finally, public policy suggestions and recommendations for clinics and programs are offered. This chapter and the next make it clear that any professional practicing in reproductive healthcare must be aware of the issues facing LGBTQ+ folks wishing to create families.

Chapter 9, Gay Men, as Individuals and as a Community, Overcoming Reproductive Challenges to Have Children by Guy Ringler and Cyd Zeigler, looks at the experiences of gay men. Describing similar and different barriers to care that lesbians face, they note that "…young men who feel a desire to have children but who do not have a sexual attraction to women can experience distress and anxiety as they come to terms with their sexuality." The history of male only parenting has evolved from adoption to the use of egg donors and gestational carriers. The social and political obstacles form a backdrop for understanding the challenges men in same sex relationships have faced. Included in this chapter is a detailed look at the process male couples undertake with themselves, their donors and their carriers. Finally, we get a look at the broader social implications of gay men having children.

Chapter 10, Parenting in Transgender and Nonbinary Individuals by Amanda R. Schwartz and Molly B. Moravek, offers a comprehensive look at the issues faced by transgender and nonbinary individuals when considering family building. While comprising a small percentage of the world's population—an estimated 25 million—professionals working in reproductive healthcare need to be prepared to properly help them. The authors provide a comprehensive discussion of gender identity and sexual orientation as a stepping off point for the ensuing description of transgender and nonbinary parenting. While similar yet more powerful barriers to care exist in the social arena, transgender parenting involves many decisions that are hormonally based. Notably, gender affirming care can have a significant impact on a person's reproductive function necessitating complex discussions about becoming a parent at a time when many individuals in this community are not thinking in those terms, often due to their young age, or other more pressing challenges. Additional sections discuss fertility preservation options as well as fertility care. As with any pregnancy, pregnancy loss is a real and present possibility. The emotional impact is different due to the impact of pregnancy on gender identity and the authors provide a context for understanding these issues. As society struggles with issues of diversity and inclusion, this chapter is essential for reproductive healthcare professionals who want to ensure proper care for all who seek it.

Chapter 11, Trauma and Its Impact on Reproduction and Sexuality by Laura Covington, gives readers an opportunity to explore and understand trauma informed care for patients coping with the intersection of reproductive and sexual health problems. Utilizing a case study model, she provides a thorough overview of the theoretical and practical matters clinicians should take into account when working in this arena. Her examination of the impact of trauma on both relationship and sexuality dynamics will be useful to clinicians from both medical and mental health perspectives. This chapter discusses common issues present in both infertility and trauma; grief, relationships, and sexuality, and provides clinicians with a framework for treating patients coping with them. Tools provided include an assessment strategy and detailed guidance on taking a history for these cases. The case study deals with trauma acquired during military service and provides the reader with a look into some of the issues that some veterans face.

Chapter 12, How the "Medicalization" of Reproduction Takes the Fun Out of the Process by Alice D. Domar, Alison J. Meyers, and Elizabeth A. Grill, addresses the way in which a diagnosis of infertility and the accompanying stressors of that diagnosis can have psychosocial repercussions, as well as clinical implications contributing to changes in sexuality within a couple. Patients often report that sex for intimacy or fun has become the work of sex, or more often, sex equating with failure. Employing stress as a focal point, they explore the impact of infertility and its treatment on hormonal components of sexual function for men and women. They note that relationship satisfaction and personal well-being can be compromised when one or both partners have a sexual dysfunction. The chapter discusses clinical, psychosocial, and marital implications for the combination of sexual dysfunction and infertility in both men and women. An overview of treatment options including marital, sex therapy, and medical interventions is included.

Chapter 13, Unintended Infertility: Labor Markets, Software Workers, and Fertility Decision-Making by Sharmila Rudrappa, examines the dual action of culture and economics on the forces that drive some to delay family building and can impact the sexual lives of those employed in those environments. As the world has grown smaller due to technological and transportation advances clinicians are more likely to see individuals and couples raised in circumstances other than which they present for treatment. While this chapter provides a look into high wage technology workers in Indian cities the astute clinician will readily understand the broader implications for the professional providing reproductive and sexual health services almost anywhere. The author discusses the interplay between workplace demands and relationship needs that are important considerations in most instances. In addition to interviewing patients coping with the stresses of both culture and economics, interviews with counselors treating these individuals and couples are described.

Chapter 14, Traditional Chinese Medicine, Infertility, and Sexuality Dysfunction by Denise Wiesner, is included in recognition of the contributions of traditional Chinese medicine (TCM). The discussion of treatments for infertility and sexual problems with acupuncture, cupping, moxibustion, and herbal medicine is thorough and will leave the reader with a better understanding of them. As patients seek a wider range of therapies for their reproductive and sexual health, it behooves clinicians to have a basic understanding of these modalities. Woven along with a discussion of the basic concepts of TCM the author has provided a historical overview of its practice. Through a series of case studies, the reader is given a view of how TCM practice might be employed with various sexual problems that could impact fertility.

Chapter 15, Sex, Religion, and Infertility: The Complications of G-d in the Bedroom by Julie Bindeman, outlines the role of religion in the life of many patients and discusses each religions, guidance about sex and procreation. She provides a chapter that focuses on these concepts from the perspective of the "Abrahamic" religions, Judaism, Christianity, and Islam. Starting with an historical overview of sex, religion, and assisted reproductive technology, we get a look at how these three monotheistic faiths treat sex and sexuality. Also addressed are the way they have dealt with assisted reproductive technologies which alter the way families can be created. Both advances in the understanding of fertility and humanity's appreciation for the complexities of sex have changed since the foundational texts for the three faiths were created. Accordingly, this chapter reviews those changes, giving the clinician a background for understanding the challenges that some patients may face when their religious beliefs and family creation desires come into conflict. Above all, this chapter provides the clinician with tools for sensitively helping patients for whom faith is a guiding force in their sexual and reproductive lives.

Looking forward

Chapter 16, Thoughts on Education, Reproduction, and Sexual Function. Future Directions and Obstacles by Angela K. Lawson. As her title notes, Angela Lawson provides suggestions about future research on the interface of sexuality and reproduction. She notes that the current lack of structured education regarding reproduction/fertility results in increased risks of infertility (and associated psychological distress) with significant and disproportionate risk to specific populations. Briefly reprising some themes from Chapter 1, The Acquisition of Sexual and Reproductive Health Knowledge, she highlights gaps in educational opportunities that exist for the LGBTQ + community, those facing racial, ethnic, and socioeconomic disparities, differently abled groups, and sex disparities in current sex education models. Also discussed are the consequences of the failure to improve both fertility awareness and sexual function knowledge. Also highlighted is the often-overlooked fact that the combined stressors of infertility and infertility treatment can contribute to intimate partner violence. Finally, suggestions for future research and methods to improve education models in both human sexuality and reproductive health wrap up this chapter and our text.

Kim Bergman and William Petok

References

[1] Smith S, Gillam T. Sexual dysfunction-the forgotten taboo. Ment Health Nurs 2003;25:6−9.

[2] Bos G, van Dijk JG, Lambers KJ. The big secret: male infertility. In: Prill H-J, Stauber M, Pechatschek P-G, editors. Advances in psychosomatic obstetrics and gynecology. Berlin, Heidelberg: Springer; 1982. p. 234−6.

[3] Cook RJ, Dickens BM. Reducing stigma in reproductive health. Int J Gynecol Obstet 2014;125(1):89−92.

[4] Donkor ES, Sandall J. The impact of perceived stigma and mediating social factors on infertility-related stress among women seeking infertility treatment in Southern Ghana. Soc Sci Med 2007;65(8):1683−94.

[5] Ergin RN, Polat A, Kars B, Öztekin D, Sofuoğlu K, Çalışkan E. Social stigma and familial attitudes related to infertility. Turk J Obstet Gynecol 2018;15(1):46−9.

[6] Gannon K, Glover L, Abel P. Masculinity, infertility, stigma and media reports. Soc Sci Med 2004;59(6):1169−75.

[7] Miall CE. The stigma of involuntary childlessness*. Soc Probl 1986;33(4):268−82.

[8] Slade P, O'Neill C, Simpson AJ, Lashen H. The relationship between perceived stigma, disclosure patterns, support and distress in new attendees at an infertility clinic. Hum Reprod 2007;22(8):2309−17.

[9] Sternke EA, Abrahamson K. Perceptions of women with infertility on stigma and disability. Sex Disabil 2015;33(1):3−17.

[10] Flemming R. The invention of infertility in the classical Greek world: medicine, divinity, and gender. Bull Hist Med 2013;87(4):565−90.

[11] Taboo | sociology | Britannica [Internet]. [cited 11.05.21]. Available from: https://www.britannica.com/topic/taboo-sociology

[12] NSFG—National Survey of Family Growth Homepage [Internet]; 2020 [cited 11.05.21]. Available from: https://www.cdc.gov/nchs/nsfg/index.htm

[13] Official King James Bible online [Internet]. [cited 11.05.21]. Available from: https://www.kingjamesbibleonline.org

[14] Clarke GN. A.R.T. and history, 1678−1978. Hum Reprod 2006;21(7):1645−50.

[15] Ombelet W, Van Robays J. Artificial insemination history: hurdles and milestones. Facts Views Vis ObGyn 2015;7(2):137−43.

[16] Mortimer ST. Essentials of sperm biology In: Patton PE, Battaglia DE, editors. Office andrology. Totowa, NJ: Humana Press; 2005. p. 1−9(Contemporary Endocrinology). Available from. Available from: https://doi.org/10.1007/978-1-59259-876-2_1.

[17] Altmäe S, Acharya G, Salumets A. Celebrating Baer—a Nordic scientist who discovered the mammalian oocyte. Acta Obstet Gynecol Scand 2017;96(11):1281−2.

[18] Editors H com. World's first "test tube" baby born [Internet]. History. [cited 12.05.21]. Available from: https://www.history.com/this-day-in-history/worlds-first-test-tube-baby-born

[19] Eight million IVF babies since the birth of the world's first in 1978 [Internet]. [cited 12.05.21]. Available from: https://www.focusonreproduction.eu/article/ESHRE-News-GlobalIVF18

[20] Domar AD, Zuttermeister PC, Friedman R. The psychological impact of infertility: a comparison with patients with other medical conditions. J Psychosom Obstet Gynaecol 1993;14(Suppl):45−52.

[21] Vander Borght M, Wyns C. Fertility and infertility: definition and epidemiology. Clin Biochem 2018;62:2−10.

[22] Lotti F, Maggi M. Ultrasound of the male genital tract in relation to male reproductive health. Hum Reprod Update 2015;21(1):56−83.

[23] Starc A, Trampuš M, Pavan Jukić D, Grgas-Bile C, Jukić T, Polona Mivšek A. Infertility and sexual dysfunctions: a systematic literature review. Acta Clin Croat 2019;58(3):508−15.

[24] Mascarenhas MN, Flaxman SR, Boerma T, Vanderpoel S, Stevens GA. National, regional, and global trends in infertility prevalence since 1990: a systematic analysis of 277 health surveys. PLoS Med 2012;9(12):e1001356.

[25] Practice Committee of the American Society for Reproductive Medicine. Definitions of infertility and recurrent pregnancy loss: a committee opinion. Fertil Steril 2020;113(3):533−5.

[26] Zayed AA, El-Hadidy MA. Sexual satisfaction and self-esteem in women with primary infertility. Middle East Fertil Soc J. 2020;25(1):13.

[27] Sany RF, Lucia ASL, Marcos FS, de S, Rosana MR, Ana CJSReS. Current research on how infertility affects the sexuality of men and women. Recent Pat Endocr Metab Immune Drug Discov 2013;7(3):198−202.

[28] Khademi A, Alleyassin A, Amini M, Ghaemi M. Evaluation of sexual dysfunction prevalence in infertile couples. J Sex Med 2008;5(6):1402−10.

[29] Monga M, Alexandrescu B, Katz SE, Stein M, Ganiats T. Impact of infertility on quality of life, marital adjustment, and sexual function. Urology 2004;63(1):126−30.

[30] Gabr AA, Omran EF, Abdallah AA, Kotb MM, Farid EZ, Dieb AS, et al. Prevalence of sexual dysfunction in infertile versus fertile couples. Eur J Obstet Gynecol Reprod Biol 2017;217:38−43.

[31] Nelson CJ, Shindel AW, Naughton CK, Ohebshalom M, Mulhall JP. Prevalence and predictors of sexual problems, relationship stress, and depression in female partners of infertile couples. J Sex Med 2008;5(8):1907−14.

[32] Agustus P, Munivenkatappa M, Prasad P. Sexual functioning, beliefs about sexual functioning and quality of life of women with infertility problems. J Hum Reprod Sci 2017;10(3):213−20.

[33] Ferraresi SR, Lara LAS, de Sá MFS, Reis RM, Rosa e Silva ACJS. Current research on how infertility affects the sexuality of men and women. Recent Pat Endocr Metab Immune Drug Discov 2013;7(3):198−202.

[34] Ezzell W. The impact of infertility on women's mental health. N C Med J 2016;77(6):427−8.

[35] Anderson KM, Sharpe M, Rattray A, Irvine DS. Distress and concerns in couples referred to a specialist infertility clinic. J Psychosom Res 2003;54(4):353−5.

[36] Benazon N, Wright J, Sabourin S. Stress, sexual satisfaction, and marital adjustment in infertile couples. J Sex Marital Ther 1992;18(4):273−84.

[37] Connolly KJ, Edelmann RJ, Cooke ID, Robson J. The impact of infertility on psychological functioning. J Psychosom Res 1992;36(5):459−68.

[38] Dunkel-Schetter C, Lobel M. Psychological reactions to infertility. In: Stanton AL, Dunkel-Schetter C, editors. Infertility: perspectives from stress and coping research, The Springer series on stress and coping. Boston, MA: Springer US; 1991. p. 29−57. Available from: https://doi.org/10.1007/978-1-4899-0753-0_3.

[39] WHO | Gender and human rights [Internet]. World Health Organization; [cited 11.05.21]. Available from: https://www.who.int/reproductivehealth/topics/gender_rights/sexual_health/en/

[40] Zilbergeld B. The new male sexuality: the truth about men, sex, and pleasure. New York: Bantam; 1999. Available from: https://www.penguinrandomhouse.com/books/195905/the-new-male-sexuality-by-bernie-zilbergeld/.

Acknowledgments

When I was asked to create this text, I immediately knew that I wanted to do it with a partner, and not just any partner, Dr. Bill Petok in particular. Bill Petok is a rare soul who is unendingly loyal, dependable, wise, funny, and positive. It has been an absolute joy to take on this project with Bill and I cannot thank him enough.

I could not do what I do without my business partners Stuart Bell, Erica Horton, and Teo Martinez who always encourage me and give me the space to take on all kinds of "side projects" like this book. I also want to thank my dedicated staff at Growing Generations who make it all look easy. I could not ask for a better team.

Thank you to all of the incredible authors who put their faith in me and Bill, trusting that would showcase their work in a meaningful and important way. I know how hard it is to let go of your creative babies, and I appreciate you entrusting your chapters to us. This book is all about you and your important work.

Thank you from the bottom of my heart to all the parents, gestational carriers, egg donors, and sperm donors, whom I have had the pleasure to work with all of these years. You have taught me everything I know about family building and fertility care. I promise to always listen to you.

I also want to thank my colleagues and friends in the Mental Health Professional Group of the American Society for Reproductive Medicine: you continue to challenge, teach, and support me, and your mentorship is invaluable.

To all of the other professionals I have had the pleasure to work with, it takes a village to do what we do and I am honored to work side by side with you to create families.

Thank you to our editorial team at Elsevier: you saw a gap in the literature and sought to provide something that would have a long-lasting impact on professionals. Thank you for giving us the space to create this meaningful and important text.

Finally, to my amazing family—I am in awe of the unconditional love and support that I have always felt from you. To my wife Natalie who has an honorary degree in family building from all of our discussions and my asking her to read my ramblings, and my daughters, Abby and Jenna, who have had to put up with my divided attention but do so with pride in what I am up to, I am eternally grateful.

Kim Bergman

The creation of this text has a been both challenging and rewarding. I owe a great deal to those who inspired me professionally and those who opened the doors that allowed me to work in the field of reproductive health care. Without their support and the occasional shove, I would not have walked through them.

First, I acknowledge my teachers and mentors who both invited me to become a clinician and pushed me to explore what shape that might take. My graduate advisor, Donald K. Pumroy, encouraged me to follow research and clinical interests that piqued my imagination rather than serve his benefit. He introduced me to the field of sex therapy early in my graduate education and sparked my interest in helping others with these most human of problems. Don taught me that it was always useful to look on the positive side when seeking to help others change, and he taught me how to teach by allowing me to sit in on countless presentations of his to professionals and lay people and then providing me with opportunities to teach them myself.

Jay Haley taught me about the dynamics of interpersonal communication in my postdoctoral studies. With him I learned that the family/couple is an important unit to understand. As I moved into the world of reproductive health care, this became essential. He emphasized the value that symptoms can hold in relationships, a critical understanding when sex is the presenting problem. His teaching also emphasized helping individuals and couples build from their strengths.

Bill Schlaff opened several important doors for me. He gave me my first opportunity to teach medical residents about human sexuality in 1984. Without it I doubt I would have entered that arena on my own. Bill also encouraged me to work with fertility patients while he was in his REI fellowship, noting that he could help those patients with their reproductive struggles but had only a rudimentary understanding of the psychological issues they faced. He knew that infertility was more than a failure to conceive, and he knew that patients' mental health was an important contributor to their physical wellbeing. He continues to support the mental health of fertility patients to this day by ensuring the Jefferson Infertility Counseling Conference has his and his institution's backing.

My colleagues in the Mental Health Professional Group of the American Society for Reproductive Medicine have taught me much about our field. MHPG has provided me with a professional "home" and nurtured my interest in male reproductive health. The organization has provided a platform for my advocacy for this inadequately represented demographic. Colleagues too numerous to name have shared their knowledge and insight into the struggles couples face and how best to work with them. I am indebted to them for this.

Kim Bergman, my coeditor, has been a valued companion on this journey. Her perseverance, ability to juggle multiple balls at one time, and maintain a positive attitude throughout it all are immeasurable in their value.

Finally, I must acknowledge my family, particularly my wife, Barbara Schlaff, who has supported me during this project and encouraged me when a pandemic created obstacles for our contributors and editorial staff. She understood that for years I had wanted to create a collection that dealt with the intersection of sexuality and fertility. I also want to acknowledge my children, Ben and Alison, who must have endured unending ribbing from their friends for having a dad who is a sex therapist. Along with Barbara they comprise the family I only wish my patients could have.

William D. Petok

PART I

Reproductive health

CHAPTER

1

The acquisition of sexual and reproductive health knowledge

William D. Petok[1,2] and Arik V. Marcell[3]

[1]Department of Obstetrics and Gynecology, Sidney Kimmel Medical College, Thomas Jefferson University, Philadelphia, PA, United States [2]Independent Practice, Baltimore, MD, United States [3]Departments of Pediatrics and Population, Family & Reproductive Health, The Johns Hopkins University, Baltimore, MD, United States

Introduction

Humanity continues to struggle to understand basic concepts related to conception. While the biology of human reproduction is well known today, it was not always so. Humankind speculated for millennia on the acts and actors that create life, each discovery part of a slowly unfolding drama. Now, with the play almost complete, it has become clear that sexual and reproductive health (SRH) is important and related to overall health [1] as well as quality of life [2].

Even with the advanced state of our knowledge, significant numbers of men and women struggle to build families. Some have difficulty with the biological components of conception whereas others have problems with the sexual side of the equation. A lack of success with either can lead to great emotional distress and interpersonal challenges. When the two collide, it can create difficulties that are more than additive. If knowledge is power, then a good understanding of SRH can lead to substantial improvements in personal and interpersonal wellbeing.

This chapter will review the history of our comprehension of sex and fertility and explore the current status of how that knowledge is acquired.

Prehistory of sexual and reproductive knowledge

Two critical evolutionary changes are important in our understanding part of the connection between sex and fertility. The first point, for the purposes of this discussion, is the prehuman development of *Ramapethicus*, and bipedal locomotion, walking on two feet. From *Ramapethicus* came *Homo Erectus*, the oldest known early humans with modern human-like body proportions. This evolutionary milestone changed the mating position of our ancestors to face to face. Quite different from rear entry mating of many primates, the possibility of a different sensual experience exists that most nonhuman primates do not have. Some have theorized that this evolutionary change led to the female orgasm [3]. Sex, which other animal species instinctively have for procreation, now becomes something that provides pleasure as well [4] (p. 16). As Komisaruk et al. state, "...women and men derive pleasure from orgasm and it is the pleasure of orgasm that helps reinforce the performance of sexual intercourse, thereby promoting procreation" [5] (p. 12).

The other significant human development is that of menstruation. The vast majority of sexually reproducing animals have an estrous cycle. For these species, pheromones, behavioral or visual cues indicate to males that a female is in a fertile state. Males, in return, become interested in mating. These species generally copulate for reproductive purposes alone. Sex for pleasure is not part of their scheme. Humans and a small number of other mammals have a menstrual cycle in which the lining of the uterus is shed on a regular basis. The mechanism by which human females may provide pheromonal information to potential male partners indicating they are in a fertile state is only recently being understood [6,7]. However, it has been demonstrated that human female subjective arousal levels are stable across the phases of the menstrual cycle [5], suggesting that pleasure is a significant reason for sexual activity. And so, sexual intercourse is possible at all times, rather than during a specific hormonally determined period. Sex for pleasure and relationship enhancement become additional reasons for humans to engage in the acts and setting us apart from other animals [8]. We aren't in it just for the babies!

Humans are not "just like" other animals as some would opine. One way we are different is that we know where babies come from. While all animals have a powerful sex drive, otherwise they become extinct, humans have a "baby drive." During the course of history, we have created veneration of virgins, marriage, castration, assisted reproductive technologies (ARTs), and genetic manipulation. All allow humans to experience sex differently than any other animal and imbue it with cultural and emotional meaning. We have reproductive consciousness [9].

The anthropologist, Holly Dunsworth, asks the questions "do animals know where babies come from?" After evaluating the data, she concludes:

> No matter how passionate or nurturing it is, nothing about the sexual, social and parental behavior of animals requires knowledge of reproduction. In contrast, much about *Homo sapiens* behavior does. Somewhere along the line, our species developed cultures rich in beliefs about procreation, family and connectedness—beliefs that in many ways set us apart from our ape cousins and indeed every other creature on the planet [10] (p. 69).

Dunsworth, in discussing reproductive consciousness, says that sex is not something that just happens with humans. Rather, we know what can happen when we have it. We understand that the act can create relatedness and kinship. "And this knowledge—sex equals babies, and babies equals kinship—marks one of the turning points of the history of life." She dates reproductive consciousness to approximately 100,000 years ago with the development of abstract thinking in *Homo sapiens* [9].

Humans moved from hunter–gatherers to farmers about 10,000–12,000 years ago at the end of the last Ice Age. Breeding of plants and animals for specific traits, such as better crop yields or more milk, was only possible if the farmers knew about events like pollination or mating. They knew about sex and reproduction and this allowed for the transition to agricultural societies which require improved output. With this evolution these cultures developed stories and myths about fertility [9]. A glimpse into these societies and their view of sex and fertility is contained in the archeological record.

Early historical evidence

Rene' Neuville, a French prehistorian, published an article in 1933 describing what has become known as the Ain Sakhri Figurine or sometimes, the Lovers of Ain Sakhri [11]. It is the oldest known representation of two humans copulating and is dated at approximately 9000 BCE. It currently resides in the British Museum (https://www.bmimages.com/preview.asp?image = M0000000028&itemw = 0&itemf = 0002&itemstep = 1&itemx = 8). Believed to be associated with fertility rites, it strongly suggests that the peoples of the Natufian period were concerned with fertility and knew something about where babies come from.

The archaeologic record reveals earlier symbols redolent of sex. The best known are the Venus figures, the most notable being the Venus of Willendorf, dating to the time period 30,000–25,000 BCE. Historians often describe her as a fertility goddess because she has pendulous breasts, a rounded belly, and a prominent mons pubis. Approximately 60 similar artifacts have been discovered, primarily in Central Europe [4]. Whether she was a human fertility goddess is questionable and the assignment of her as such is speculative at best. Regardless, contemporary authors see her as symbolic of female sexuality [12] (Fig. 1.1).

Symbols of male sexuality from a similar time period are available as well. A 28,000-year-old phallus with an obvious glans penis was found in the Hohle Fels cave in southwest Germany [12]. It was likely used as a tool for working with flint blades and is clearly an erect penis. Once again, a definitive understanding of the object's meaning with regard to sex or fertility is unknown. Other European Paleolithic art contains images of erections, circumcision, and tattooed penises [13,14] (Fig. 1.2).

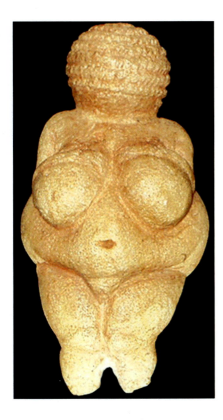

FIGURE 1.1 Venus von Willendorf, Naturhistorisches Museum Wien, Public Domain.

Fertility images from the early Chalcolithic or Copper Age (5000 BCE), most famously the "Lemba Lady" from Cyprus, are similar to the older Venuses in that they have emphasized breast, hips, and pubic regions [15]. There is debate about this categorization, with some suggesting that just because she has breasts and genitalia fertility is not the only interpretation of her meaning. In other words, Lemba Lady could be "sexy" and therefore a goddess of sexuality not associated with fertility [16] (Fig. 1.3).

Recorded history

Human fertility was important to most ancient cultures. Fertility gods and goddesses are present in story and myth, presumably to help understand fertility and cope with infertility via offerings and ritual observances. Female fertility and pregnancy was better understood, while male infertility was an afterthought at best. The Egyptian Kahun papyrus (c.1825 BCE) offers gynecologic advice that deals with female infertility. The Egyptians understood the relationship between sexual intercourse and pregnancy. Man planted his seed into the fertile ground of the uterus where it grew into a fetus. Osiris was the god of fertility [17]. According to the myth, the birth of new crops each year signified his resurrection after his dismemberment (Figs. 1.4 and 1.5).

Sumerian texts and seals describe the sexual act and relate it to fertility. Simple drawings of male and female sexual organs showed a marriage bond by juxtaposing them. A translation of several Sumerian literary texts dated 1900–1600 BCE describe intercourse consummated by a priest and priestess as a means of gaining fertility for the community. These texts also describe seduction and lovemaking. From them we see that the purpose of marriage was procreation and not necessarily a pair bond for life. Pictorial representations exist from the same time period of couples having intercourse. Other scholars have suggested that the depiction of nude female forms in Mesopotamian art from the second and third millennia BCE are more linked to sexuality than fertility [18]. Some of these artifacts display sexual acts between two men, indicative of homosexual intercourse [19] (p. 22).

Male fertility and virility have been associated with Min, the son of Isis and Osiris, an ancient Egyptian god. Worship of Min dates to the fourth millennium BCE. Men who sought fertility and virility would offer sacrifices to Min and eat a type of lettuce, *Lactua serriola*, probably because of its phallic shape and the semen-like substance it releases when rubbed. Priapus, the Greek god with an oversized permanent erection, was considered the protector of fertility, sexuality, male genitalia as well as agriculture. The Lingam, linked to Shiva the Hindu destroyer god, is

I. Reproductive health

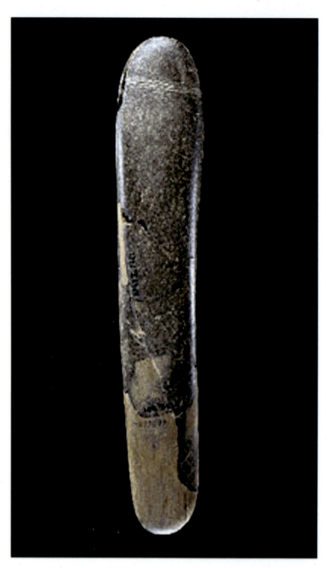

FIGURE 1.2 Hohle Fels phallus. Reproduced with permission of Senckenberg Centre for Human Evolution and Palaeoenvironment (HEP), University of Tübingen.

sometimes represented phallically and considered a symbol of Shiva's creative power. Representations of Kokopelli, the fertility god worshiped by some southwestern Native American communities date to CE 200. Once again, an erect phallus represents fertility and virility. In these and other representations of fertility/virility gods an erect penis capable of ejaculation indicates the communities that worshiped them knew that semen was crucial to reproduction [20].

Similar art, artifacts, and writings occur in ancient cultures around the world. They visualize sexual and fertility gods and goddesses as well as rituals and speak to the interest humankind has in reproduction since reproductive consciousness could be recorded in a lasting form.

"Modern" religious writings, beginning with the Hebrew Bible, are aware of fertility and sexuality. They begin to address the psychological impact of infertility, most notably on women, and will be discussed more thoroughly in a subsequent chapter. With the advent of these monotheistic religions, sexuality is reserved for matrimonial bonds. These writings, which include the Christian Bible and Islamic Fiqh [21], have a decided view on sexual intercourse and its role in human relations and seek to bring it under control for procreation within marriage only.

Science and fertility

Aristotle was among the first to give a scientific explanation to conception. For those animals who were observed to mate, he thought each brought specific matter to the process. The female, her menstrual blood, and

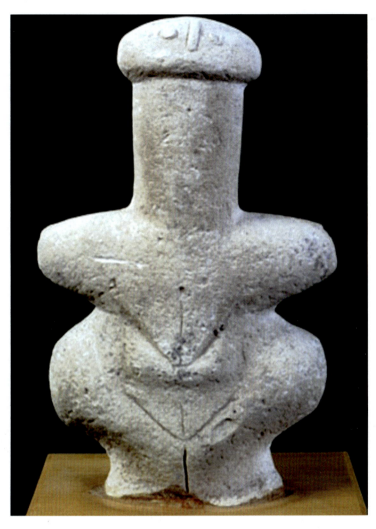

FIGURE 1.3 Lemba Lady. Reproduced with permission of Department of Antiquities, Republic of Cyprus.

the male his semen. Those two combined, blood given form by semen, with the outcome being a baby. Following Hippocrates' opinion, Galen, the Roman physician, thought there were two semens, male and female, but the female semen could not be seen. Aristotle's view prevailed before the turn of the millennium [22].

Monotheistic religious thinkers believed semen was the primary component of conception. Chinese thinkers talked about the generative capacity of the energy created in organ networks in both sexes, referred to as "generative vitality." World science views, such as they were then, were decidedly not in agreement [22].

These early views predominated for 1500 years. In 1651 William Harvey became convinced that the egg had something to do with conception, but his animal dissections failed to reveal the "it" or "how" of this process. He decided that new life was produced in the uterus following intercourse similar to how imagination and appetite are produced in the brain. The female's "testicles," as he termed the ovaries, played no role at all [23]. Within 25 years scientific thinking had changed and egg theory was being embraced for the female contribution to all animal reproduction, including humans [24].

The work of Swammerdam, Stenson, Van Horne, and eventually de Graaf confirmed that female eggs, from ovarian follicles, were the elusive other side of the equation. The observation, by de Graaf, that ruptured rabbit follicles released spheres into the fallopian tubes and the number of spheres was most often the same as the number of ruptured follicles was decisive. However, his notion of a seminal vapor reaching the egg and fertilizing it missed the mark. But the specific female contribution to conception had been proven [22]. In 1679 the French Journal des Sçavans wrote: "The view that man, as well as all other animals, are formed from eggs is something that is now so widespread that there are hardly any new philosophers who do not now accept it" [22] (p. 4). How the egg's contribution took place was as yet unclear. In fact, it was not until the human egg was first seen by Karl Ernst von Baer in 1827 that its existence was proven [25] (Fig. 1.6).

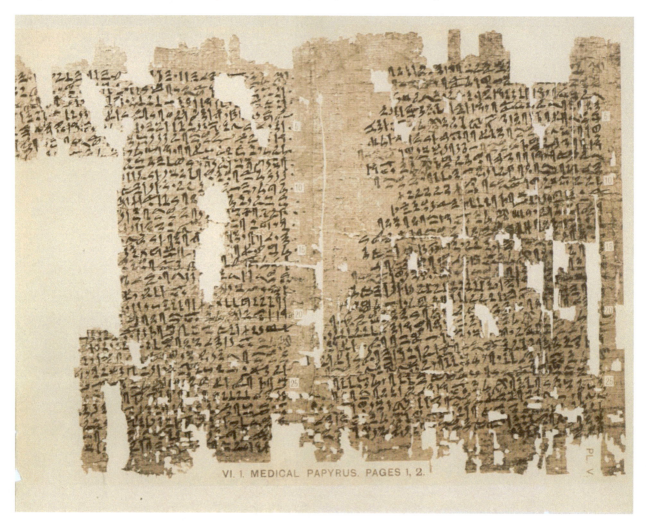

FIGURE 1.4 Papyrus Kahun VI. 1, pages 1 and 2; medical papyrus 12th Dynasty. Public domain.

In the fall of 1677 Leeuwenhoek, a microscope enthusiast who made a career of examining "animalcules" with his devices, discovered millions of those creatures in his own semen. He gave them the name they carry to this day, spermatozoa, or semen animals. But he did not connect them to fertilization. That discovery fell to a collection of biologists, including Réeamur and Nollett and eventually Spallanzani, about 1736. Spallanzani, using the first artificial insemination process, was able to fertilize a variety of amphibians and demonstrate that the sperm he obtained fertilized an egg and allowed it to develop [25]. Unlike Reamur, Spallanzani was able to fit "drawers" over the hind quarter of green toads and have them tolerate the process long enough to collect sperm. He also did experiments with sperm obtained directly from the testis or vas deferens. How the fertilization process worked was again unclear as neither he nor von Harbke, who accomplished the same feat with trout and salmon, saw a sperm penetrate an egg, resulting in the development of a fetus (Figs. 1.7 and 1.8).

Over the 150 years after Leeuwenhoek's discovery two camps emerged, the "ovist" and "spermist." Each thought that only one component provided the source of life and the other was merely food or a force that "woke" the other, causing life. Not until the cell theory of Schleiden and Schwann and the selective breeding programs for agricultural means as well as research on family trees to study the inheritance of disease did a final focus become clear. In the late 1870s Hertwig and Fol observed the first fusion of egg and sperm and finally the knowledge of how humans are created was complete [22]. Finally, the knowledge that both male and female made equal contributions was fact.

The journey of hundreds of thousands of years had now reached a new junction. With the understanding of conception, accurate teaching of how pregnancy occurs could take place. And the way had been paved for a host of ARTs that would eventually allow previously infertile individuals and couples to create the children of their dreams.

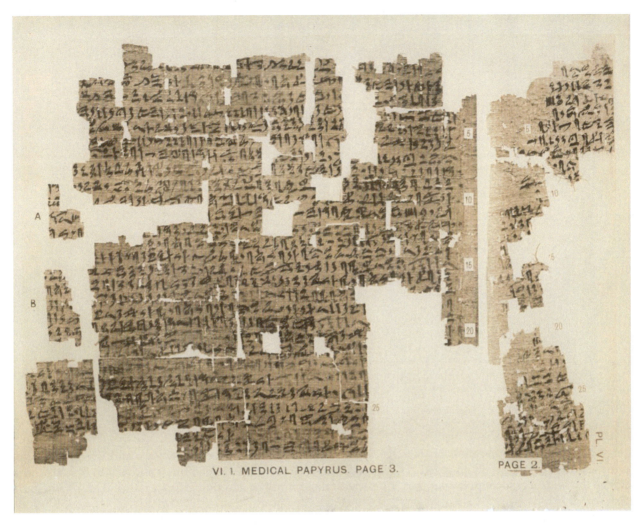

FIGURE 1.5 Papyrus Kahun VI. 1, pages 2 and 3; medical papyrus 12th Dynasty. Public domain.

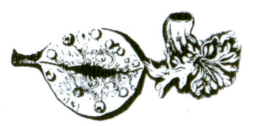

FIGURE 1.6 The Ovary by Regnier de Graaf. Public domain.

But human sexual interaction, as we have seen, is not solely about creating offspring. Sex can be more than baby making and disseminating that information has a history of its own.

The evolution of modern reproductive health and sex education in the United States

Sex education, as with other types of education, is generally agreed to involve three components: *knowledge, attitudes/values*, and *skills* [26]. As noted before, until late in the 19th century, accurate *knowledge* about conception was missing. Equally missing was accurate *knowledge* of the human sexual response. It wasn't until 1966 with

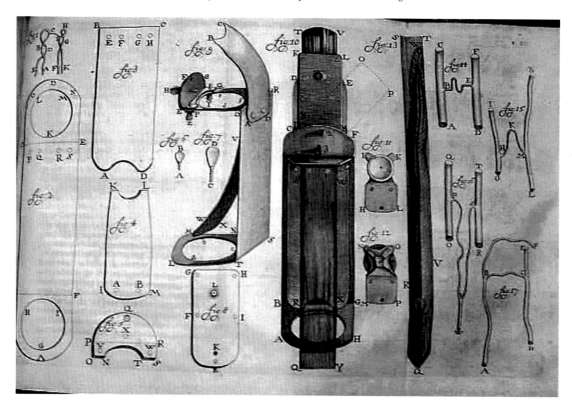

FIGURE 1.7 Van_Leeuwenhoek's_microscopes_by_Henry_Baker. Public domain.

Masters and Johnsons' publication of their research that a clear idea of the physiology and anatomy of sexual behavior leading to conception emerged. They wryly noted "If the current tentative approach to sex education is to achieve the widespread popular support it deserves, there must be physiologic fact rather than phallic fantasy to teach (p. vi)" [27].

An impediment to accurate education was the prevailing Victorian *attitudes* about sex which appear repressive and repressed. William Acton (1813–75), well known during the Victorian period for his marriage manual, noted "As a general rule, a modest woman seldom desires any sexual gratification for herself..." [28] (p. 625). The Victorians seemed obsessed with sexual behavior, and its control for women and homosexuals. These attitudes have cast a long shadow over 20th-century sex education. *Values* often derived from religious or philosophical beliefs are critical as well. Until recently, sex positive values were not considered in sex education.

And then there is the challenge of teaching *skills* when it comes to sex.

> The correct use of a condom during sexual intercourse is an example of a "sexual skill." Obviously, knowing nothing at all about condoms will result in their not being used.
>
> However, having knowledge of condoms but believing their use to be sinful or thinking that they interfere with sexual pleasure may also result in nonuse. Further, it is possible to know all about condoms, have no attitude or value conflicts regarding their use, but still not use them (or misuse them), based upon behavioral deficits resulting from experiential unfamiliarity [26] (p. 93).

It is easy to see how attitudes and values can obstruct the teaching of relevant skills with regard to sex.

The discovery of sexually transmitted diseases and concerns about preventing pregnancy became focal points for the fledgling field of sex education at the turn of the 20th century. Fertility and reproductive health are a different story.

Before sexual transmission of infection was understood syphilis was thought to be spread via a wide range of methods, including writing utensils, toothbrushes, and doorknobs as well as medical procedures. Concerns in the early 20th century about the spread of the disease created a desire for education regarding both syphilis and gonorrhea among physicians, public health officials, and social reformers. These professionals were working against the Victorian sexual ethic that respectable society does not discuss sexual matters, regardless of the risk posed by infection to the population at large [29].

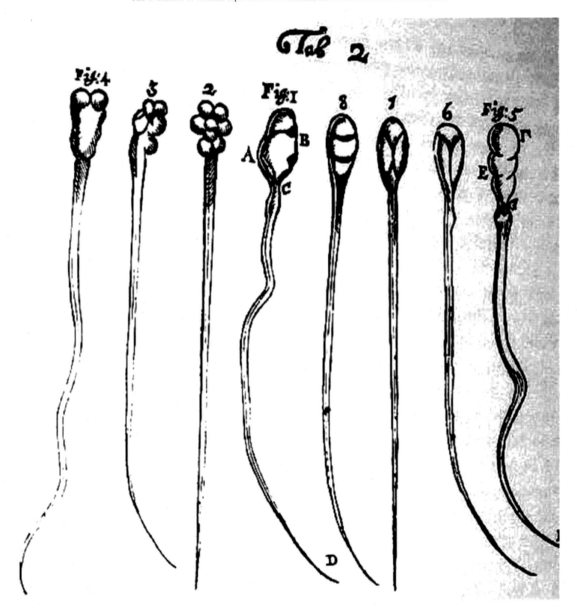

FIGURE 1.8 Van-Leeuwenhoeks-drawings-of-spermatozoa. RightsLink.License number 5012650321385.

The Comstock Act of 1873 and subsequent state laws outlawed interstate commerce with regard to information about and devices used "for the prevention of conception," because they were deemed obscene and immoral [30]. The state laws which grew out of Comstock banned distribution of information or advertising about articles, instruments, and medicine for the prevention of conception. Notably, these laws prevented the dissemination of information about pregnancy prevention but in some states not the devices themselves. Nevertheless, many pharmacists and physicians were prohibited from fitting diaphragms, selling condoms, and prescribing birth control pills, once they too were available. The 1965 United States Supreme Court decision in *Griswold v. Connecticut* opened the door for these laws to be overturned and by 1971 most states removed their prohibition on contraceptive sales to married persons [30]. In 1972 sale of contraceptives became legal to nonmarried people [31].

Early sex educational programs would be considered antisex education today. They focused on disease and emphasized fear of infection rather than protective actions that could be taken. Not surprisingly, these programs did not reduce infection rates. At the same time, concern regarding widespread transmission of venereal disease created a discussion about the need for sexual knowledge. The age old debate that sexual knowledge would lead to sexual activity, especially with adolescents, was considered a dangerous outcome of improved sex education [31].

Sex education in public schools of the United States began about 1910 and its focal message could be boiled down to "Just Say No [31]." It appears the primary goal was to discourage individuals from having sex outside the bonds of marriage. World War I and the upsurge in military activities brought increased attention on sex education to protect soldiers from venereal disease. The goal was to reduce the incidence of disease via abstinence [31]. A secondary goal was to protect "the family" and children who might be born with birth defects such as blindness. Apparently missing from the discussion was the potential of infertility for the man involved. Comparable educational materials for women did hint at the impact on reproductive capacity of wives [31].

Issues of morality, concerns about family structure, and stereotypes regarding masculinity and femininity were driving concerns of sex education during the first half of the 20th century.

> Between 1910 and 1940, sex educators faced the problem of how to teach young people about sex without encouraging licentiousness—in other words, how to educate them in a way that would guarantee premarital chastity and marital monogamy... For fear of encouraging licentiousness by giving people too much information about sex, educators frequently sacrificed the "scientific truth" in favor of whatever kind of information or teaching strategy was most likely to encourage premarital chastity and marital monogamy [31] (p. 248).

It was not until World War II that education programs prescribed prevention rather than fear [29]. United States military personnel now received information that condom use prevented disease transmission. Condoms were widely distributed because it was clear that abstinence would be unpopular. Pragmatism took precedence over contemporary notions of morality and even legislative mandate from laws derived from the Comstock Act.

At about the same time or shortly after several events began to change thought about sex education in the United States. Margaret Sanger and other proponents of the birth control movement made a case for women having sex without fear of pregnancy. This influenced the notion that sexual and reproductive self-determination were important. Sanger believed that the sexual freedom men had, at least tacitly, should be given to women as well. She also helped fund the development of the first birth control pill by Gregory Pincus which was made available in 1959. Sanger's efforts clearly changed views about sex and influenced how sex education evolved [32].

At about the same time, Alfred Kinsey, a University of Indiana zoologist, published his two volumes on sex. *Sexual Behavior in the Human Male* (1948) and *Sexual Behavior in the Human Female* (1953) were based on thousands of detailed interviews. Kinsey and his team reported that masturbation, oral sex, and marital infidelity were common for both men and women. The books' reports on the incidence of homosexual behavior were controversial but opened the door for discussion of sexual orientation that would follow in later decades. The work led to the establishment of the Kinsey Institute for Sex Research [32].

The 1960s and 1970s, labeled the era of the sexual revolution, brought in more relaxed community standards about sexual behavior. A rising counterculture experimented with sexual behavior outside of traditional constraints on sex within marriage, in part due to the availability of oral contraceptive birth control that prevented pregnancy without requiring action to do so in the "heat of the moment," at least on the part of men. Women had the burden of remembering to take the pill and still bore the major responsibility for pregnancy prevention.

During this period, Hugh Hefner's Playboy Foundation established some of the funding for the Sexuality Information and Education Council of the United States (SIECUS). The organization supported "values neutral" sex education. Founded in 1964 with the help of Mary Calderone, a former medical director of Planned Parenthood, it fostered an approach that encouraged students to make personal decisions about when to engage in sex, what do about contraception or the termination of an unwanted pregnancy. An offshoot of SIECUS was the formation of the American Association of Sex Educators, Counselors and Therapists (AASECT) in 1967. AASECT created standards and training for sex education providers [32] (p. 37). Both organizations favored Comprehensive Sex Education (CSE) over abstinence only curricula and have been termed by some as "Pro-Sex" [32] (p. 37).

Eventually, the United States Federal Government became involved in promoting sex education. The United States Office of Education provided funding to 645 agencies to assist the development of sex education programs across the country as early as 1964. In 1971 the White House held a Conference on Youth that supported sex education programs for all secondary and elementary schools. And the focus of these programs was shifting from preventing sexual activity to preventing pregnancy from adolescent sexual activity [32] (p. 39).

One of the main barriers to "controlling" content of comprehensive sex education (as per SEICUS guidelines described further) is the health education and, specifically, sex education is not mandated in the United States at the Federal level. Decisions about sex education are made at the state and local level—no federal laws dictate what sex education should look like or how it should be taught in schools. This lack of guidance creates a patchwork of variable and sometimes contradictory curricula from state to state [33].

Still, there was little or no discussion of fertility issues in these curricula.

In 1970 Congress passed the Title X Public Health Service Act (Public Law 91-572) with bipartisan support with House of Representative sponsors Republican George H.W. Bush from Texas and Democrat James Scheuer from New York and Senate sponsors Democrat Joseph Tydings from Maryland and Republican Charles Percy from Illinois. A key purpose of the Title X program is "to assist in making comprehensive voluntary family planning services readily available to all persons desiring such services." Today, this is the only Federal program that is dedicated to providing men and women with comprehensive family planning and related preventive health services [34]. However, men represent a small but increasing percentage of all clients served; the percentage of male clients was 3% in 1999 and 8% in 2011 [35].

There was opposition to the change in focus. Proponents of abstinence until marriage were vocal and many objected to publicly funded sex education that taught otherwise. By the 1980s a counterrevolution sought to reverse the impact of the sexual revolution. Abstinence only education began to receive federal funding in 1983 [36]. And the discovery of HIV, a sexually transmitted virus that could kill and was without cure, increased efforts at abstinence only education. Battle lines were drawn, and sex education evolved into two camps.

> Two sides of the debate advocated two very different solutions to modern problems related to teen sex. Sex education advocates of the 1960s called for "safe sex" or so-called comprehensive sex education, which permitted a continuation of sexual freedom, as long as contraception was used. Abstinence proponents sought to equip teens with the skills to avoid any of the potential risks of sex, physical and emotional ... The issue of sex education became increasingly volatile during the modern sex education era, as indicated by the emergence of two oppositional efforts: the first designated funding for abstinence education and the increased strength of pro-sex organizations [32] (p. 40).

Throughout all these changes, fertility knowledge has been the stepchild. It has been noted that in the majority of sex education curricula "Inordinate amounts of time are spent on reproductive anatomy and physiology, contraception, and STDs, compared with minimal effort affirming the pleasures of touch, the requirements for orgasmic release, or the importance of trust and open communication in specific sexual interactions" [26] (p. 94). Said another way, plumbing, disease, and pregnancy prevention form the bulk of what is taught.

In the last 20 years some educational efforts have adopted what is termed "sex positive" approaches. Proponents of this approach call for a more holistic view of sexual health, placing the emotional and physical aspects of sex and relationships in the foreground. The supposition is that young people will derive more favorable and equitable outcomes. Advocates for sex positive education note that desire and pleasure have been absent in prior efforts, that they employ heteronormativity and fear and that they ignore a profeminist point of view [37].

Pleasure as a component of sexuality education has been cited as contributing to several desirable outcomes: more open communication about sexuality, increased awareness of diverse sexual communities, increased use of condoms, more effective family planning, increased knowledge of sexual responses, and empowerment for young women [37]. Contrary values and beliefs present barriers to its inclusion in many publicly funded programs.

Sex positive approaches avoid moralistic value statements and promote diversity of sexuality worldwide as well as the ability to make personal choices. Sex is seen to be valence free and depends on the context in which it occurs. An additional aim is to reduce stigma surrounding sex.

On an international level, the World Health Organization (WHO) prefers a well-rounded approach to SRH that speaks to physical health, mental health, personal choice, and self-efficacy as important factors. The WHO advocates education that highlights "... a state of complete physical, mental and social wellbeing and not merely the absence of disease or infirmity, in all matters relating to the reproductive system and to its functions and processes. Reproductive health therefore implies that people are able to have a satisfying and safe sex life ..." [38] (p. 622). It further states that "...Sexual health requires a positive and respectful approach to sexuality and sexual relationships, as well as the possibility of having pleasurable and safe sexual experiences, free of coercion, discrimination, and violence. For sexual health to be attained and maintained, the sexual rights of all persons must be respected, protected, and fulfilled" [39] (p. 206).

The ineffectiveness of abstinence only programs is well documented. For example, one review of 13 studies found that abstinence only education did not reduce or exacerbate risk for youths in high-income countries [40]. Outcomes such as this have led some to see sex positive education as more useful to achieve the goals of decreasing sexually transmitted infection (STI) transmission and pregnancy through improved use of barrier contraceptives.

Abstinence only programs typically offer sex negative messaging. They employ language that is value laden and is often based on their religious origins. A review of United States programs found they reinforce gender stereotypes, ignore the fact that for some youth sexual behavior is the result of intimate partner violence, sexual abuse or molestation, and they tend to be heteronormative, ignoring the sexual health needs of sexual minority youth [41].

In 2012 SIECUS published the first National Sexuality Education Standards (NSES) for content and skills for grades K–12 [42]. The document offers a rationale for sexuality education in public schools, noting that the average student receives 17.2 hours of sexuality education during their journey through the public education system. The content of most programs is focused on HIV, pregnancy, and STI prevention, with a little more than 50% of that education taking place in high school. Further noted are the incidence of teenagers who either have unwanted pregnancies (600,000) or STIs (9,500,000) and disproportionate number of annual HIV infections in the same group (50,000) [43].

Citing the interrelationship of health status and academic outcomes in a range of areas the NSES further notes

> Evaluations of comprehensive sexuality education programs show that many of these programs can help youth delay the onset of sexual activity, reduce the frequency of sexual activity, reduce the number of sexual partners, and increase condom and contraceptive use.... Researchers recently examined the National Survey of Family Growth to determine the impact of sexuality education on sexual risk-taking for young people ages 15–19, and found that teens who received comprehensive sexuality education were 50 percent less likely to report a pregnancy than those who received abstinence-only education [43] (p. 7).

NSES recommends minimum essential content and skills for K–12 education programs.

- Anatomy and physiology
- Puberty and adolescent development
- Identity
- Pregnancy and reproduction
- Sexually transmitted diseases and HIV
- Healthy relationships
- Personal safety

The section on pregnancy and reproduction addresses information about how pregnancy happens and decision making to avoid pregnancy. The minimum topics do not specifically mention fertility awareness (FA). Early research on 10 programs employing the standards finds that they overwhelmingly focused on risk prevention and delaying sexual activity by teens. In addition, the focus is on current behavior and does not prepare teens for lifelong sexual decision making, necessary for understanding and preserving future fertility, among other things [44].

If a significant focus of past and present sex education is pregnancy prevention, it is not surprising that reproductive health and positive thinking about pregnancy creation would not be high on the educational spectrum. Yet, as we will see, this deficit in knowledge, or FA, has real consequences for people wanting to build families.

Guidance for grades K–12 were updated in 2020 by the Future of Sex Education (FOSE) Initiative that include standards by topic strand, including Consent and Healthy Relationships (CHR), Anatomy and Physiology (AP), Puberty and Adolescent Sexual Development (PD), Gender Identity and Expression (GI), Sexual Orientation and Identity (SO), Sexual Health (SH), and Interpersonal Violence (IV), but still does not capture any content related to reproductive life planning or problems with fertility or infertility concerns. The Blueprint for Sexual and Reproductive Health, Rights, and Justice, published in 2019, outlines as part of its five principles to promote comprehensive access to SRH services domestically, including requiring all plans to cover infertility treatment and services, including in vitro fertilization and artificial insemination even when infertility is not indicated and for LGBTQ+ couples [45].

Fertility awareness and its acquisition

FA is "...the understanding of reproduction, fecundity, fecundability, and related individual risk factors (e.g., advanced age), sexual health factors such as STIs, and life-style factors such as smoking and obesity and nonindividual risk factors (e.g., environmental and work place factors); including the awareness of societal and cultural factors affecting options to meet reproductive family planning, as well as family building needs [46]."

FA can be tied to the use of SRH services. SRH care use has risen but disparities do exist [47,48]. For both women and men, racial and ethnic minorities are at a disadvantage. General economics also play a role in SRH care access and availability and are subject to fluctuations in national fiscal factors which can include such issues as recessions and most recently, the COVID19 pandemic [49].

In general, while reproductive aged young adults desire having children, the majority lack information about infertility risk factors. In addition, this group typically has low to moderate FA. A literature review of 71 articles, with subjects in 24 countries, found that there is greater awareness among women, more educated individuals, people reporting difficulty conceiving and those who planned their pregnancies [50]. Other studies demonstrate that knowledge about fertility is limited regardless of age, gender, or educational background [51,52].

One recent qualitative study with British adolescents (ages 16–18) and emerging adults (ages 21–24) demonstrated that these age groups wanted the knowledge but had a hard time integrating it without worrying about the implication for them in the present or future. While these young people had knowledge, its breadth and depth were not enough for them to make informed decisions. The subjects reported that they saw no point to the knowledge at a stage of life when family building was not on their minds. The researchers speculated that the content, amount, and timing of FA information needs to be tailored to the developmental stage of the learners. They conclude "Young people welcome fertility information but qualitative data illustrate the need for it to be tailored to specific age groups to maximize its benefits and ensure young people can integrate the information they need to maintain reproductive health and make informed decisions about future parenthood [53]." While the sample size was small ($n = 33$), the findings hint at the complexity of providing useful and meaningful FA information.

Important sex discrepancies do exist. One study found that Canadian men aged 18–50 have poor knowledge regarding male infertility [54]. About half of men (51%) correctly identified male infertility-related risk factors and 45% could identify health-related issues. Of the men studied, 58% reported wanting more information about male infertility and reproductive health and they preferred two sources for that information, medical professionals and online sources [54]. It is not a surprise that men have low knowledge about infertility or infertility risk factors; young men's awareness and knowledge about issues such as female birth control methods is not much better—they have low awareness of highly effective female contraception methods as compared to condoms and shorter-acting female birth control methods (pills, patch) and have very poor knowledge about any form of female contraception methods other than condoms [55].

A recent United States study found that about 60% of men are in need of preconception care. In general, male preconception care focuses on conception prevention. As the authors note, preconception care requires reproductive aged persons to have "high reproductive awareness." In other words, a plan that includes what is necessary to prevent an unintended pregnancy as well as create optimal health conditions prior to a desired pregnancy. They note that women have been the primary focus of such improvement efforts [56]. The men in that study varied on multiple factors, including age, locale, ethnicity, and poverty level, among other variables. A significant number of men in the study had health risks that could impair reproductive capacity. Poor health status, overweight or obesity, daily marijuana use, binge drinking, addictive drug use, and high STI risk were some of the factors found in this study. Significant numbers of these men had usual sources of care (71%), health insurance (76%), and a yearly physical exam (49%). At the same time, among all men in the study, healthcare provider counseling in the preceding year was reported by 11% for STIs; 10% for HIV; and 10% for contraception, highlighting the gap between observed need for care and actual delivery of the services.

Women had greater FA in 12 of the studies reviewed before. At the same time 10 studies found no difference between women's and men's FA. Some studies reported mixed results [50]. There are probably good reasons for women's greater awareness that will be discussed later. One of the significant findings from the review is that while people are aware of the risk age plays in reduced fertility, they overestimate the age at which declines begin. They also overestimate the probability of becoming pregnant either spontaneously or via fertility treatment. The authors suggest that the focus on pregnancy prevention in school-based sexuality education is a contributing factor to this finding.

When it comes to men's help seeking for infertility concerns, help seeking was quite low, especially for younger men. For example, although infertility prevalence was slightly lower for males aged 16–24 (4%) and 25–24 (9%) as compared to older aged men, only 14% of men aged 16–24 sought help as compared to 50% of men aged 24–34 and 57% of men aged 35–44 [57].

Although many conditions place children and youth at risk for infertility, including males, many youth may not be aware of conditions that occurred earlier in childhood (e.g., anorchia, testicular torsion) or conditions that may not present until adolescence (Klinefelter syndrome, Kallman syndrome) [58]. Even among males with cancer, the prevalence of help seeking for men with infertility is low. For example, the prevalence of male infertility prevalence in the Childhood Cancer Survivor Study was 46% among cancer survivors as compared to 18% in the sibling comparison group, but only 54% went for infertility care as compared to 21% of the sibling comparison group [59]. Another study that conducted a medical record review of males aged 13 with a new cancer diagnosis found that only 29% received fertility counseling and only 11% attempted sperm banking [60].

In 2006 the CDC published recommendation guidance to improve both preconception health and care with the goal to improve the health of women and couples, before conception of a first or subsequent pregnancy [61]. One of the key recommendations is that individuals take responsibility across the lifespan, and, specifically, each woman, man, and couple should be encouraged to have a reproductive life plan and use a lifespan approach to focus individual attention on reproductive health to reduce unintended pregnancies, age-related infertility, fetal exposures to teratogens, and to improve women's health and pregnancy outcomes. In 2014 updates to the nation's Title X guidelines by the Office of Population Affairs and the CDC incorporated these guidelines along with additional guidance to make comprehensive clinical care guidelines for women and men related to family planning and SRH care, including need for basic infertility counseling as an important component [62]. These guidelines are separate but parallel to women's health guidance that was implemented as part of the Patient Protection and Affordable Care Act (ACA) [63] A similar emphasis on the SRH needs of men had not existed. Between 2011 and 2014 several agencies collaborated to create them for the first time for the United States. It has been noted that development of guidelines for men is critical for a variety of reasons, including the health of their partners, including men in family planning, and improving the fathering capacity of men. An additional desired outcome is the need to integrate men's healthcare into reproductive health programs nationwide [64]. As documented elsewhere, public awareness as well as research about male infertility is substantially missing [65,66].

More recent guidelines published in 2018 by the American Academy of Pediatrics (AAP) promote counseling at-risk pediatric populations about fertility and sexual function beginning in infancy with parents or at earliest time point a patient may be affected [67]. This guidance contributes to other condition-specific guidance in 2008 by the AAP (referring patients at risk for fertility loss primarily focused on childhood cancer for fertility preservation (FP) before gonadotoxic therapy) and in 2006 by the Pediatric Endocrine Society (disclosing to youth with disorders of sex development about their condition and counseling about fertility and sexual function, using "collaborative, ongoing" approach) [68,69].

Despite the guidelines aforementioned, FA among women of reproductive age in the United States, including medical trainees, is low. The data, collected with a validated measure, indicate that even trainees in obstetrics and gynecology have gaps in their knowledge of natural fertility and infertility treatment [70]. Others have noted that fertility knowledge in groups likely to delay childbearing is lacking [71]. Participants in these studies typically overestimate pregnancy probability with increasing age as well as the success rate of ARTs. Multiple studies report similar findings [52,72]. Many of these studies have surveyed populations that are overwhelmingly white and primarily female.

Several studies have specifically evaluated college students of Latin origins or those living in Mexico [73,74]. One study of Latino college students at a midwestern United States university found that cultural issues, including shame and privacy regarding matters related to sex kept them from considering or talking about infertility [74]. This group did not see infertility as a medical problem that could be resolved, in part due to the high cost of ART. The authors surmise that some help seeking for fertility problems takes place outside customary Western medical models due to infertility's suggestion of traditional gender role failure for both sexes.

The second study, conducted in Mexico, demonstrated poor FA for both men and women. Most participants believed it would be easy to become pregnant at a later age. For example, the great majority thought a woman's fertility did not significantly decline until age 40. The authors note that this misinformation places young people at risk for involuntary childlessness due to delaying childbearing. They also were surprised at the high percentages of both men and women who had no intention to have children, 48% for women and 59% for men [73].

Barriers in providing fertility care have been described among care providers who are seeing patients most at risk. For example, despite most oncologists agreeing that pubertal cancer patients be offered fertility referral (84%), only 46% referred their male patients to fertility specialist before treatment more than 50% of the time [75]. Despite most oncologists demonstrating knowledge of FP and discussing and describing they feel comfortable discussing FP, only half (55%) referred their patients to an infertility specialist. Barriers to discussing FP identified by clinicians in this study included the perception that patients were too ill to delay care, patients were already infertile from prior therapy, time constraints, and inadequate access to infertility specialists [76].

One recent literature synthesis identified five themes influencing providers' FP discussions with young cancer patients: lack of knowledge about guidelines, costs, where to refer, conducting informed consent with minors and parents, how to have these discussions; lack of comfort and being embarrassed to talk about sex and masturbation; patient-related factors such as being less likely to talk with young patients, beliefs that patients cannot afford procedures, who should be involved in conversation, and being more likely to discuss it if the patient brings it up; parent-related factors, including ethical concerns about parent involvement; and the lack of educational materials to share with patients and families [77].

Development of more age and sex developmentally appropriate materials are also needed. For example, one program in Canada used an evidence-based approach to develop informational brochures in plain language with patients and families for understanding the process of sperm banking for teens with cancer [60]. Similar approaches can also be developed for engaging parents of at-risk youth, partners of at-risk individuals, and gatekeeper clinicians. Finally, for some populations strategies may be needed to account for the lack of socialization around healthcare use, especially among men, that require healthcare system modifications that can better meet needs of boys and men throughout the life course [78,79].

Interventions to improve fertility awareness, knowledge, and access to care

Interventions to engage populations in fertility care have had mixed results. One randomized control trial that examined the effects of fertility education using a brochure on participants' knowledge and use of consultative services 2 years later demonstrated that intervention versus control men aged 20–39 had 11% increased change in fertility knowledge, as compared to no change in the control groups and 12% increased new medical consult/treatment for fertility versus 8% in the control group that received information about healthy prepregnancy and 1% in the control group that received information about family policies [80].

A study that examined an online education about knowledge of fertility and ARTs, and beliefs about parenthood timing using a pre/posttest design found that all childless participants read 10 online posts and that knowledge and beliefs increased immediately after the training, but this was not sustained at 6-month follow-up [81]. Another web-based intervention that targeted young cancer patients with sexual problems and fertility distress was found to be feasible and acceptable by participants, but this study did not examine linkages to fertility care [82]. One innovative direct-to-consumer strategy to increase young people's knowledge about factors that could lead to infertility was developed by the UK Fertility Education Initiative (FEI). Released on YouTube on January 3, 2019, the created video has had more than 4450 views [83].

Structural interventions have also been utilized to assist in improving referrals for infertility care within institutional care programs. For example, one report that evaluated a hospital-wide FP service after developing a centralized team for standard referral and active scanning of inpatient and clinic lists for newly diagnosed patients demonstrated that referral patterns 20-month pre versus postinitiative increased by 70% and doubled from divisions outside oncology from 15% preinitiative versus 34% postinitiative [84]. Another program described their guidance for developing pediatric FP programs and recommended that overcoming barriers, such as low referral rates, required institutional commitment, multidisciplinary meetings to train staff across institution, fertility referral as part of checklists/order sets or use of "opt out" approach, easily accessible and educational website, and social work/patient navigator to assist families in financial need [85].

Summary

Both fertility and sexuality are important components of human life and are represented in various forms throughout the archeological and historical record. Importantly, a variety of evolutionary factors created a human capacity to engage in sexual activity without reproducing. However, misconception and misunderstanding about how babies are created were impediments to our understanding of the process. At the same time, humanity has been intrigued, driven by, and been enthralled with sexual activity. Human sexuality is a complex process and experience and is often considered one of the three important drives. When either the sexual drive goes awry or the drive to reproduce is impeded it can lead to distinct emotional and relational difficulties. When these two drives encounter problems at the same time it can be devastating.

Knowledge about both sex and fertility can be seen as critical to a more satisfying human experience. Competing values have at times made the acquisition of comprehensive sexual knowledge a challenge. However, recent research suggests that a more thorough understanding of "how sex works" can have a positive impact on both personal satisfaction and the process of family building. Advances in the science of conception and the advent of ARTs have made it possible for families to be created under conditions that were prohibitive less than 50 years ago. But deficits in FA may prevent some from having the families they want. We believe that society has an obligation to provide more than adequate knowledge about both sex and fertility so that individuals can lead more satisfying and productive lives.

Recommendations for education, training, and research

- Education.
  - Greater education is needed about FA, knowledge, and care resources as well as integrating infertility education as part of current comprehensive sexual educational curriculum that incorporates promotion of gender inclusiveness and gender equity as appropriate by age.
  - Access to comprehensive evidence-based sexual educational programs should be available to all young people regardless of socioeconomic status, race, ethnicity, intellectual or physical ability, gender, sex, or geographic location. One of the goals of these programs should be to help young people communicate about and make informed decisions about their SRH and understand where to seek help, as needed.
  - An increase in education about male factors with regard to fertility and infertility bringing it up to par with that provided for women.
- Training and improved structural linkages to care.
  - Greater education about fertility and infertility is needed as part of standard education for practitioners, including physicians, nurse practitioners, and physician assistants, in training as well as part of postgraduate training. Other healthcare providers, including psychologists, social workers, professional counselors, and marriage and family therapists would also benefit from similar education.
  - There is a need to better incorporate content about reproductive life plan, preconception care, and screening for individuals at risk for fertility concerns and counseling about infertility and referral resources into educational curriculum, routine primary care, and subspecialty care, including oncology, endocrinology, urology, etc.
  - There is also a need to facilitate improved connectivity between primary care providers and subspecialists providing fertility care as well as for developing institutional structural changes with active monitoring for new patients and use of gonadotoxic agents.
- Research.
  - Greater investment is needed to understand FA among more diverse populations than have been studied in the past as well as best mechanism approaches to engage men and women in need of fertility services.

References

[1] Dean J, Shechter A, Vertkin A, Weiss P, Yaman O, Hodik M, et al. Sexual health and overall wellness (show) survey in men and women in selected European and middle eastern countries. J Int Med Res 2013;41(2):482–92. Available from: https://doi.org/10.1177/0300060513476429.

[2] Flynn KE, Lin L, Bruner DW, Cyranowski JM, Hahn EA, Jeffery DD, et al. Sexual satisfaction and the importance of sexual health to quality of life throughout the life course of United States adults. J Sex Med 2016;13(11):1642–50. Available from: https://doi.org/10.1016/j.jsxm.2016.08.011.

[3] Cartmill M. Primate classification and diversity. In: Ghazanfar AA, Platt ML, editors. Primate neuroethol. Oxford: Oxford University Press; 2010.

[4] Tannahil R. Sex in history. Briarcliff Manor, NY: Stein and Day; 1980.

[5] Komisaruk B, Beyer-Flores C, Whipple B. The science of orgasm. Baltimore, MD: Johns Hopkins Press; 2006. p. 358.

[6] Mostafa T, Khouly G El, Hassan A. Pheromones in sex and reproduction: do they have a role in humans? J Adv Res 2012;3(1):1–9. Available from: https://doi.org/10.1016/j.jare.2011.03.003.

[7] Lübke KT, Pause BM. Always follow your nose: the functional significance of social chemosignals in human reproduction and survival. Horm Behav 2015;68:134–44. Available from: http://doi.org/10.1016/j.yhbeh.2014.10.001.

[8] Emera D, Romero R, Wagner G. The evolution of menstruation: a new model for genetic assimilation: explaining molecular origins of maternal responses to fetal invasiveness. BioEssays 2012;34(1):26–35.

[9] Dunsworth H, Buchanan A. Sex makes babies. Psyche. 2017. Available from: https://aeon.co/essays/i-think-i-know-where-babies-come-from-therefore-i-am-human, [cited January 9, 2020].

[10] Dunsworth H. Do animals know where babies come from? Sci Am 2015;314(1):66–9. Available from: http://doi.org/10.1038/scientificamerican0116-66.

[11] Boyd B, Cook J. A reconsideration of the 'Ain Sakhri' figurine. Proc Prehist Soc 1993;59:399–405.

[12] Taylor T. The origins of human sexual culture the origins of human sexual culture: sex, gender and social control. J Psychol Human Sex 2006;18(2/3):69–105.

[13] Angulo JC, García-Díez M. Male genital representation in Paleolithic art: erection and circumcision before history. Urology 2009;74(1):10–14. Available from: https://doi.org/10.1016/j.urology.2009.01.010.

[14] Angulo JC, García-Díez M, Martínez M. Phallic decoration in Paleolithic art: genital scarification, piercing and tattoos. J Urol 2011;186(6):2498–503. Available from: https://doi.org/10.1016/j.juro.2011.07.077.

[15] Bolger D. Figurines, fertility, and the emergence of complex society in prehistoric Cyprus. Curr Anthropol 2008;37(2):365–73. Available from: http://www.jstor.org.

[16] Budin S. Creating a goddess of sex. In: Bolger D, Serwint N, editors. Engendering Aphrodite women and society in ancient Cyprus, CAARI monographs, Vol. 3. Boston, MA: American School of Oriental Research; 2002. p. 315–24. Available from: https://www.jstor.org/stable/10.5615/j.ctt2jc9sc.26.

References

[17] Haimov-Kochman R, Sciaky-Tamir Y, Hurwitz A. Reproduction concepts and practices in ancient Egypt mirrored by modern medicine. Eur J Obstet Gynecol Reprod Biol 2005;123(1):3–8.

[18] Graff SB. Sexuality, reproduction and gender in terracotta plaques from the late third-early second millennia BCE. In: Feldman MH, Brown BB, editors. Critical approaches to ancient near eastern art. Boston, MA: De Gruyter; 2014. p. 371–90.

[19] Bullough VL. Sex, society & history. New York: Science History Publications; 1976. p. 185.

[20] Neto FTL, Bach PV, Lyra RJL, Borges Junior JC, Maia GTDS, Araujo LCN, et al. Gods associated with male fertility and virility. Andrology 2019;7(3):267–72.

[21] Bilikisu Yusuf H. Sexuality and the marriage institution in Islam: an appraisal. Semin Ser 2005;4:1–19.

[22] Cobb M. An amazing 10 years: the discovery of egg and sperm in the 17th century. Reprod Domest Anim 2012;47((Suppl. 4):2–6.

[23] Short RV. Harvey's conception: 'de generatione animalium', 1651. In: Dickinson CJMJ, editor. Developments in cardiovascular medicine. Lancaster: MTP; 1978. p. 353–63.

[24] Short RV. The discovery of the ovaries. In: Zuckerman S, Weir BJ, editors. The ovary, volume 1: general aspects. New York: Academic Press; 1977. p. 1–39.

[25] Capanna E. Lazzaro Spallanzani: at the roots of modern biology. J Exp Zool 1999;285(3):178–96.

[26] Dailey D. The failure of sexuality education: meeting the challenge of behavioral change in a sex-positive context. J Psychol Human Sex 1997;9(3–4):87–97.

[27] Masters WH, Johnson VE. Human sexual response. Oxford: Little, Brown; 1966.

[28] CZ S, PN S. Victorian sexuality: can historians do it better? J Soc Hist 1985;18(4):625–34.

[29] Brandt AM. AIDS in historical perspective: four lessons from the history of sexually transmitted diseases. Am J Public Health 1988;78(4):367–71.

[30] Bailey MJ. "Momma's got the pill": how Anthony Comstock and Griswold v. Connecticut shaped United States childbearing. Am Econ Rev 2010;100(1):98–129.

[31] Carter J. Birds, bees, and venereal disease: toward an intellectual history of sex education. J Hist Sex 2001;10(2):213–49.

[32] Huber VJ, Firmin MW. A history of sex education in the United States since 1900. Int J Educ Reform 2014;23(1):25–51. Available from: https://doi.org/10.1177/105678791402300102.

[33] Planned Parenthood. Sex education laws and state attacks. Available from: https://www.plannedparenthoodaction.org/issues/sex-education/sex-education-laws-and-state-attacks, [cited January 17, 2021].

[34] Gavin L, Moskosky S, Carter M, Curtis K, Glass E, Godfrey E, et al. Providing quality family planning services: recommendations of CDC and the U.S. Office of Population Affairs. MMWR Recomm Rep 2014;63(4):1–54. Available from: http://www.jstor.org/stable/24832591.

[35] Fowler CI, Lloyd SW, Gable J. Family planning annual report: 2009 national summary. Research Triangle Park, NC: RTI International; 2010. revised 2011.

[36] Pear RS. Treating the nation's epidemic of teen-age pregnancy. NY Times. Available from: http://www.nytimes.com/1984/06/03/weekinreview/treating-the-nation-s-epidemic-of-teen-age-pregnancy.html?&pagewanted = 1, [cited June 3, 1984].

[37] McGeeney E, Kehily MJ. Young people and sexual pleasure—where are we now? Sex Educ 2016;16(3):235–9.

[38] Brickman J, Willoughby JF. 'You shouldn't be making people feel bad about having sex': exploring young adults' perceptions of a sex-positive sexual health text message intervention. Sex Educ 2017;17(6):621–34.

[39] Koepsel ER. The power in pleasure: practical implementation of pleasure in sex education classrooms. Am J Sex Educ 2016;11(3):205–65. Available from: https://doi.org/10.1080/15546128.2016.1209451.

[40] Underhill K, Montgomery P, Operario D. Sexual abstinence only programmes to prevent HIV infection in high income countries: systematic review. Br Med J 2007;335(7613):248–52.

[41] Santelli JS, Kantor LM, Grilo SA, Speizer IS, Lindberg LD, Heitel J, et al. Abstinence-only-until-marriage: an updated review of United States policies and programs and their impact. J Adolesc Health 2017;61(3):273–80. Available from: https://doi.org/10.1016/j.jadohealth.2017.05.031.

[42] Wiley D, Cory A. National sexuality education standards. Encyclopedia of school health. Thousand Oaks, CA: Sage Publications; 2013.

[43] Future of Sex Education Initiative. National Sexuality Education Standards: core content and skills, K-12 [a special publication of the Journal of School Health], 2012. Retrieved from: http://www.futureofsexeducation.org/documents/josh-fose-standards-web.pdf.

[44] Schmidt SC, Wandersman A, Hills KJ. Evidence-based sexuality education programs in schools: do they align with the National Sexuality Education Standards? Am J Sex Educ 2015;10(2):177–95.

[45] Blueprint for Sexual and Reproductive Health, Rights, and Justice, 2019. Available from: https://reproblueprint.org/wp-content/uploads/2019/07/BlueprintPolicyAgenda-v14-PR-All-1.pdf.

[46] Zegers-Hochschild F, Adamson GD, Dyer S, Racowsky C, de Mouzon J, Sokol R, et al. The International Glossary on Infertility and Fertility Care, 2017. Fertil Steril 2017;108(3):393–406. Available from: http://doi.org/10.1016/j.fertnstert.2017.06.005.

[47] Hall KS, Moreau C, Trussell J. Continuing social disparities despite upward trends in sexual and reproductive health service use among young women in the United States. Contraception 2012;86(6):681–6. Available from: https://doi.org/10.1016/j.contraception.2012.05.013.

[48] Gavin L, MacKay AP, Brown K, Harrier S, Ventura SJ, Kann L, et al. Sexual and reproductive health of persons aged 10–24 years—United States, 2002–2007. MMWR Surveill Summ 2009;58(SS06):1–58.

[49] Lindberg LD, Bell DL, Kantor LM. The sexual and reproductive health of adolescents and young adults during the COVID-19 pandemic. Perspect Sex Reprod Health 2020;52(2):75–9.

[50] Pedro J, Brandão T, Schmidt L, Costa ME, Martins MV. What do people know about fertility? A systematic review on fertility awareness and its associated factors. Ups J Med Sci 2018;123(2):71–81. Available from: https://doi.org/10.1080/03009734.2018.1480186.

[51] Kudesia R, Talib HJ, Pollack SE. Fertility awareness counseling for adolescent girls; guiding conception: the tight time, right weight, and right way. J Pediatr Adolesc Gynecol 2017;30(1):9–17. Available from: https://doi.org/10.1016/j.jpag.2016.07.004.

[52] Ekelin M, Åkesson C, Ångerud M, Kvist LJ. Swedish high school students' knowledge and attitudes regarding fertility and family building. Reprod Health 2012;9(1):6. Available from: http://www.reproductive-health-journal.com/content/9/1/6.

[53] Boivin J, Sandhu A, Brian K, Harrison C. Fertility-related knowledge and perceptions of fertility education among adolescents and emerging adults: a qualitative study. Hum Fertil (Camb) 2019;22(4):291–9. Available from: https://doi.org/10.1080/14647273.2018.1486514.

[54] Daumler D, Chan P, Lo KC, Takefman J, Zelkowitz P. Men's knowledge of their own fertility: a population-based survey examining the awareness of factors that are associated with male infertility. Hum Reprod 2016;31(12):2781–90.

[55] Borrero S, Farkas A, Dehlendorf C, Rocca CH. Racial and ethnic differences in men's knowledge and attitudes about contraception. Contraception 2013;88(4):532–8. Available from: https://doi.org/10.1016/j.contraception.2013.04.002.

[56] Choiriyyah I, Sonenstein FL, Astone NM, Pleck JH, Dariotis JK, Marcell AV. Men aged 15–44 in need of preconception care. Matern Child Health J 2015;19(11):2358–65.

[57] Datta J, Palmer MJ, Tanton C, Gibson LJ, Jones KG, Macdowall W, et al. Prevalence of infertility and help seeking among 15,000 women and men. Hum Reprod 2016;31(9):2108–18.

[58] Dy GW, Rust M, Ellsworth P. Detection and management of pediatric conditions that may affect male fertility. Urol Nurs 2012;32(5):237–48.

[59] Wasilewski-Masker K, Seidel KD, Leisenring W, Mertens AC, Shnorhavorian M, Ritenour CW, et al. Male infertility in long-term survivors of pediatric cancer: a report from the childhood cancer survivor study. J Cancer Surviv 2014;8(3):437–47.

[60] Grover NS, Deal AM, Wood WA, Mersereau JE. Young men with cancer experience low referral rates for fertility counseling and sperm banking. J Oncol Pract 2016;12(5):465–71.

[61] Johnson K, Posner SF, Biermann J, Cordero JF, Atrash HK, Parker CS, et al. Recommendations to improve preconception health and health care—United States. MMWR Recomm Rep 2006;55(6):1–4. Available from: http://www.jstor.org/stable/24842326.

[62] Godfrey EM, Tepper NK, Curtis KM, Moskosky SB, Gavin LE. Developing federal clinical care recommendations for women. Am J Prev Med 2015;49(2):S6–13. Available from: https://doi.org/10.1016/j.amepre.2015.02.023.

[63] Women C on PS for, Medicine I of, Practice B on PH and PH. Clinical preventive services for women: closing the gaps. Washington, D.C.: National Academies Press; 2011. Available from: http://ebookcentral.proquest.com/lib/philau/detail.action?docID=3378923.

[64] Marcell AV, Gavin LE, Moskosky SB, McKenna R, Rompalo AM. Developing federal clinical care recommendations for men. Am J Prev Med 2015;49(2):S14–22. Available from: https://doi.org/10.1016/j.amepre.2015.03.006.

[65] Petok WD. Infertility counseling (or the lack thereof) of the forgotten male partner. Fertil Steril 2015;104(2):260–6. Available from: https://doi.org/10.1016/j.fertnstert.2015.04.040.

[66] Wischmann T. Your count is zero'—counselling the infertile man. Hum Fertil (Camb) 2013;16(1):35–9.

[67] Nahata L, Quinn GP, Tishelman AC. Counseling in pediatric populations at risk for infertility and/or sexual function concerns. Pediatrics 2018;142(2):e20181435.

[68] Fallat ME, Hutter J. Preservation of fertility in pediatric and adolescent patients with cancer. Pediatrics 2008;121(5) e1461-9.

[69] Lee PA, Houk CP, Ahmed SF, Hughes IA, Achermann J, Ahmed F, et al. Consensus statement on management of intersex disorders. Pediatrics 2006;118(2):e488–500.

[70] Kudesia R, Chernyak E, McAvey B. Low fertility awareness in United States reproductive-aged women and medical trainees: creation and validation of the Fertility & Infertility Treatment Knowledge Score (FIT-KS). Fertil Steril 2017;108(4):711–17. Available from: https://doi.org/10.1016/j.fertnstert.2017.07.1158.

[71] Peterson B. A validated measure for fertility awareness: an essential step toward informed reproductive decision-making. Fertil Steril 2017;108(4):606–7. Available from: https://doi.org/10.1016/j.fertnstert.2017.08.027.

[72] Peterson BD, Pirritano M, Tucker L, Lampic C. Fertility awareness and parenting attitudes among American male and female undergraduate university students. Hum Reprod 2012;27(5):1375–82.

[73] Place JM, Peterson BD, Horton B, Sanchez M. Fertility awareness and parenting intentions among Mexican undergraduate and graduate university students. Hum Fertil (Camb) 2020;0(0):1–10. Available from: https://doi.org/10.1080/14647273.2020.1817577.

[74] Place JMS, Bireley MK. Exploring infertility from the cultural context of Latino college students: results from a preliminary focus group. J Racial Ethn Heal Disparities 2017;4(5):803–11. Available from: http://doi.org/10.1007/s40615-016-0282-4.

[75] Köhler TS, Kondapalli LA, Shah A, Chan S, Woodruff TK, Brannigan RE. Results from the survey for preservation of adolescent reproduction (SPARE) study: gender disparity in delivery of fertility preservation message to adolescents with cancer. J Assist Reprod Genet 2011;28(3):269–77.

[76] Loren AW, Brazauskas R, Chow EJ, Gilleece M, Halter J, Jacobsohn DA, et al. Physician perceptions and practice patterns regarding fertility preservation in hematopoietic cell transplant recipients. Bone Marrow Transplant 2013;48(8):1091–7.

[77] Vindrola-Padros C, Dyer KE, Cyrus J, Lubker IM. Healthcare professionals' views on discussing fertility preservation with young cancer patients: a mixed method systematic review of the literature. Psychooncology 2017;26(1):4–14.

[78] Addis ME, Mahalik JR. Men, masculinity, and the contexts of help seeking. Am Psychol 2003;58(1):5–14.

[79] Marcell AV, Morgan AR, Sanders R, Lunardi N, Pilgrim NA, Jennings JM, et al. The socioecology of sexual and reproductive health care use among young urban minority males. J Adolesc Health 2017;60(4):402–10. Available from: https://doi.org/10.1016/j.jadohealth.2016.11.014.

[80] Maeda E, Boivin J, Toyokawa S, Murata K, Saito H. Two-year follow-up of a randomized controlled trial: knowledge and reproductive outcome after online fertility education. Hum Reprod 2018;33(11):2035–42.

[81] Daniluk JC, Koert E. Fertility awareness online: the efficacy of a fertility education website in increasing knowledge and changing fertility beliefs. Hum Reprod 2015;30(2):353–63.

[82] Wiklander M, Strandquist J, Obol CM, Eriksson LE, Winterling J, Rodriguez-Wallberg KA, et al. Feasibility of a self-help web-based intervention targeting young cancer patients with sexual problems and fertility distress. Support Care Cancer 2017;25(12):3675–82.

[83] Faculty of Sexual and Reproductive Healthcare. Fertility Education Initiative (FEI) launches video aimed at young people, 2019. Available from: https://www.fsrh.org/news/fertility-education-initiative-video-young-people, (cited January 30, 2021).

[84] Moravek MB, Appiah LC, Anazodo A, Burns KC, Gomez-Lobo V, Hoefgen HR, et al. Development of a Pediatric Fertility Preservation Program: a report from the Pediatric Initiative Network of the Oncofertility Consortium. J Adolesc Health 2019;64(5):563–73. Available from: https://doi.org/10.1016/j.jadohealth.2018.10.297.

[85] Carlson CA, Kolon TF, Mattei P, Hobbie W, Gracia CR, Ogle S, et al. Developing a hospital-wide fertility preservation service for pediatric and young adult patients. J Adolesc Health 2017;61(5):571–6. Available from: https://doi.org/10.1016/j.jadohealth.2017.07.008.

PART II

Sexual dysfunctions and infertility

CHAPTER

2

Emotional consequences of male infertility

Vassili Glazyrine[1], Dane Stephens[1], Emily Wentzell[2], Kimberly Wallace-Young[3] and Ajay K. Nangia[4]

[1]Department of Urology, University of Kansas Medical Center, Kansas City, KS, United States [2]Department of Anthropology, University of Iowa, Iowa City, IA, United States [3]Department of Psychiatry and Behavioral Sciences, University of Kansas Medical Center, Kansas City, KS, United States [4]University of Kansas Medical Center, Kansas City, KS, United States

Introduction

Conceptualizing male infertility

Globally, 15% of couples suffer from infertility, defined as the inability to conceive after 1 year of regular unprotected intercourse [1–3]. Infertility is a complexly relational problem. Achieving pregnancy requires healthy reproductive physiology between partners; a person's desires regarding the timeline and experience of childbearing reflect their relationships to partners, families, and societal norms, including ideals of life course and gender [4–9]. Yet reproduction is often cast as only a women's issue [8,9]. This exclusion of men reflects cultural histories of women bearing the brunt of parenting and domestic life, and the related focus of reproductive medicine on women's bodies [10,11]. Yet focusing on women in infertility treatment is medically inaccurate, since male-factor infertility accounts for about half of infertile couples, with one-fifth of infertility cases solely dependent on the male [12]. It also problematically reproduces gendered social inequalities, while obscuring men's needs, difficulties, and lived experiences [13–15]. Social scientists have identified and critiqued the omission of men from studies of reproduction and infertility amid rising interest in studying the relational and embodied nature of masculinities more broadly [5,11,13–21]. This includes study of the intersecting roles played by factors like culture, law, economics, and religion.

Men's experiences of infertility can be challenging and traumatic [22]. These experiences often include shared suffering, with partners, family members, and groups beyond the family [23–26]. Yet, ideologies of masculinity also create specific forms of suffering related to infertility. Reproduction and fathering are important to a variety of masculinities, from "traditional" forms focused on procreation and virility to those which center emotional connection; infertility can thus hamper the performance of one's desired form of masculinity [27,28]. Further, men are often encouraged to conceal strong emotion. While some men find support through loved ones or in contexts like online support groups, others' sadness is amplified by the perceived necessity to appear strong or virile [29–32]. Related stress and sadness can even cause or worsen physical issues which further hamper fertility [33].

Fortunately, enhanced education on these issues has led healthcare providers to begin assessing men's as well as women's health as it contributes to a couple's infertility [27,29,34]. This focus on all members of a couple seeking to conceive can produce a more medically accurate picture of their reproductive difficulties, and help to avoid blame or guilt on the part of one partner. Men are also increasingly willing to engage in this medical process, reflecting their increasing participation in parenting and domestic labor more broadly [24,35].

There is a pressing need for clinicians to be able to support couples, including men, through the process of infertility treatment. Yet providers might lack the skills, knowledge, or confidence to provide social support. For instance, "siloing" among academic disciplines means that clinicians are unlikely to encounter the extensive social scientific research on men's experiences of infertility [31,36]. As a result, they might not recognize common social or emotional aspects of patients' experiences, or might not feel confident in raising or supporting patients through these social aspects of treatment. This lack might compound the awkwardness providers might already feel about addressing nonclinical aspects of care, especially the emotional consequences of issues they see as intimate, private, or taboo. Yet addressing these issues is necessary not only for providing high-quality care for patients as whole persons but also for identifying behavioral or psychosocial issues that might contribute to infertility itself (like stress affecting a male partner's sexual function).

Here, we provide information providers can use to address these "elephant in the room issues" and support their patients through infertility treatment. We overview key findings from the nonclinical literature on the relationships between cultural ideologies of manliness and male patients' experiences of infertility, so that providers can better understand how to recognize and address these social aspects of treatment. We then describe the biological aspects of several conditions that can reduce men's fertility and provide suggestions for addressing the particular social issues related to each. Our goal is to help clinicians move beyond basic physiological evaluation to diagnose contributing social factors to infertility more accurately, and to provide better care, support, and options counseling for couples experiencing infertility [13,20].

Patient and partner perceptions of reproductive health and conception

Clinicians must first understand that patients might have little or incorrect knowledge about the biology of reproduction and ways to enhance chances of conception (see Chapter 1: *The Acquisition of Sexual and Reproductive Health Knowledge*). School-based sexual education might be unavailable or poor quality, and people often learn about these issues in informal interactions like school-yard conversations between peers, from family, social media, support groups, and educational self-teaching tools [29,30,37]. There are gender-based differences in who learns what information about reproductive biology, and how they do so. For example, women with healthcare access are likely to see gynecological specialists or receive "women's health" exams that include information about reproduction, while men do not receive equivalent healthcare. Even so, women's access to, desire for, and comfort with that care, as well as its quality, vary widely [38,39]. So, many couples might not understand how to time intercourse, identify physical signs of ovulation, or how to correctly use tools like ovulation predictor kits [40,41]. They are also unlikely to know that while lubricants are advisable for pleasurable sex, certain types of lubricants can acts as spermicides and must be avoided for those trying to conceive [42].

Providers need to identify the misconceptions (pun intended) patients might have about their reproductive health and provide accurate information in a clear, nonjudgmental way [43,44]. Further, clinicians must identify whether social factors make it difficult for patients to put this knowledge into practice. For instance, clinicians can inform patients that the science of timing intercourse for natural conception starts 6 days or so before midcycle with intercourse every other day and is well outlined by the American Society for Reproductive Medicine (ASRM). Yet, social factors might make that difficult. These range from busy lives in which intercourse is not as frequent as "it used to be," work-related travel, for example, military deployment, or couples' difficulties due to other issues such as finances and work pressure. The common experience of couples trying to conceive that intercourse can feel like a goal-oriented "chore" rather than "making love" compounds these issues. This can lead to added stress and distress for both partners, which can hamper aspects of sexual function like penile erection or vaginal lubrication [45]. All aspects of the act of intercourse and trying to conceive often require extensive discussions and education at consultation. Providers should provide education about what is needed to optimize conception (using the most definitive source of information, the ASRM Practice Committee statement on optimizing reproduction) in the context of discussing patients' lived experiences of their current sexual relationship [41].

One aspect that can seem awkward for men is the discussion of masturbation to collect a semen sample. It is generally a private thought and activity. Of course, a semen analysis is an essential part of determining fertility potential and infertility. In a certain age group, usually teenage/puberty, discussion of getting a semen analysis in the past was taboo, but now, with some discussion with parents for minors, getting a semen analysis/cryopreservation for teenagers with cancer, adolescent varicoceles, etc. is often recommended. Sometimes this is the first time that a teenager has had to masturbate and as such is a sensitive and embarrassing conversation that must be taken into consideration when talking to a minor. Even later in a male's life, masturbation is a very private topic, and collecting a specimen in a collection room at an andrology or in vitro fertilization (IVF) clinic is difficult [46]. Patients may request to collect at home and data have shown that semen volume may be higher with home collection [47]. The issue of early sexual health education can try to "normalize" the conversation as masturbation is a normal part of sexual behavior [48,49]. However, often providers themselves find it difficult to bring up the topic due their own biases [48]. As long as the topic is discussed with no sense of embarrassment and part of normal bodily functions, it can reduce the anxiety of the conversation with patients [43].

Perception of duration of trying/infertility

One important but often overlooked social aspect of infertility is the potential difference in the ways male and female partners might experience suffering related to time and duration of conception attempts [22,25,44,50–52]. As time passes without conception, mutual insecurities might develop and clinicians can support couples in their increased need to comfort each other through the stress of perceived delay [46]. One in four couples achieve a pregnancy in the first 6 months of trying, and after that the success rate decreases, although 85% of couples achieve a pregnancy in the first 12 months and then another 7.5% achieve a pregnancy in the second 12 months of trying. So, even couples who are still likely to conceive without medical assistance might feel frustration or fear that they have not yet conceived. This is most likely an issue for women, whose social worlds more likely include discussions of other's conception experiences and timings than men [53]. Trying to explain the reality of conception over time is thus an important aspect of educating couples, often in the first consultation, to potentially ease anxieties. Unlike men, women are also likely to have engaged in long-standing peer and media conversations about how advanced female age and issues of ovulatory reserve can impact achieving a pregnancy [11]. This means that women might experience anxiety or frustration earlier in the process of attempting conception than men.

Men, however, are also likely to experience time-related distress as time-to-conception increases [31]. As noted in the introduction, they might begin to see the lack of conception as a failure of masculinity or virility [54]. Many men who hope to have children will experience the same sadness and anxiety as women undergoing fertility treatment [55]. Further, both because of cultural norms framing men as more stoic emotional supporters of female partners, and because of the desire to comfort their partners, men might also feel the need to comfort partners at the expense of seeking such comfort themselves [54,56]. Both partners might benefit from a clinician's acknowledgment that significant dates—like Mother's or Father's day, or the anniversary of a miscarriage—should be recognized as potentially painful and perhaps marked with some kind of ritual that acknowledges that fact [57]. Overall, this often unrecognized or silent issue has in fact shown that compared with infertile men, infertile women suffer from: lower self-esteem; higher depression; less life satisfaction; find childless living less acceptable; are more likely to blame themselves for the infertility; avoid triggers of the fertile world more, for example, pregnant women and children; and initiate infertility evaluation sooner than the male partner [31].

Further, time can become a sore spot in couples' interactions with family and friends as more and more time passes without a successful pregnancy [5,24]. One of the aspects that can require inquiry is the pressures placed on a couple from family and cultural expectations. For instance, patients from some cultural backgrounds might experience the desire—or pressure from relatives to produce—a male child, adding stress to their efforts to conceive [58]. Clinicians might discuss the common experiences of such couples making excuses to their families about why they have not had children yet, like "we are not ready," to "trying to establish a career at the moment"; to "we wanted a few years and time to ourselves." Some couples experience similar time-related stress due to their desire for "family balancing," that can result in some moral and ethical dilemmas. This does not take into consideration religious overtones to the situation. These pressures can result in suffering for couples even before the defined 1 year mark that instigates the medical label of "infertility."

The financial burden

Cost of out of pocket care for fertility treatment overall is a significant stressor for couples. This is often an extremely heavy financial burden for couples who do not have access to their needed or desired fertility interventions through state healthcare systems or private insurance. The fact that private insurance companies often consider such treatment a "desire" and not a "need," adds insult to the economic burden couples face as a result [59]. This is especially the case when assisted reproductive technology (ART) is needed [60]. While some country's national healthcare systems and some states in the United States have mandated infertility coverage, people in many places do not have infertility support for ART. This is a social, ethical, moral, and even constitutional health policy issue that is beyond the scope of this discussion [38]. Most relevant for clinicians is the need to frankly discuss the fact that couples might be left with a difficult decision to sacrifice the ability to have biological children over financial burden/ruin [61]. Openness about the financial aspects of proposed treatments and the social, emotional as well as economic burden is necessary to include in options counseling. Also, the time lost from work pursuing fertility care can be another significant stressor, with associated loss in pay [62].

Overall, all these issues cause increased stress for a couple, which each partner may express differently [54]. As such, it is important to recognize the experience of BOTH the male and female partners and not avoid these topics, to best help counsel the couple and support them through the journey. For many, infertility can have mental health consequences, equal to if not greater than the physical consequences. The pathophysiologic causes of male infertility vary a great deal and carry emotional responses based on the reversibility, treatment, and heritability of each unique disease process. This chapter next discusses some specific presentations of male infertility and the particular psychological burdens which they might pose.

Specific conditions

Diseases of male infertility are broadly divided into hormonal, anatomic, genetic, medical, and idiopathic. About 50%—80% of male infertility cases are ultimately idiopathic, that is, with no clear etiology defined as yet, while the most common diagnosable cause is anatomic in origin, most commonly a result of a varicocele [63,64]. Varicoceles account for about a quarter of all cases of infertility [36]. Vasectomy and other obstructive processes from scrotal surgery, trauma, and infection are other anatomic causes. Genetic causes only account for about 1% of all cause infertility, most commonly presenting as Klinefelter syndrome (KS) [39]. If patients appear phenotypically normal, Y chromosome deletion must be considered in the setting of azoospermia/severe oligospermia. Congenital bilateral absence of the vas deferens (CBAVD) can be considered both an anatomic defect and a known genetic cause. Hormonal causes of infertility can be classified into primary, related to the testicle, central, related to the hypothalamic—pituitary—adrenal (HPA) axis, or iatrogenic and related to medication or anabolic steroid use. In this section we will explore conditions in detail that highlight emotional and psychological challenges.

Hormonal

Iatrogenic testosterone replacement

Iatrogenic testosterone replacement is the current treatment of choice for males with documented testosterone deficiency. Testosterone deficiency is defined in the most recent American Urological Association (AUA) Guidelines as a serum testosterone of <300 ng/dL with signs and/or symptoms of testosterone deficiency [65]. The symptoms of testosterone deficiency can be divided into sexual and nonsexual categories. Sexual symptoms include but are not limited to: diminished libido and erectile dysfunction (ED). Nonsexual symptoms include fatigue, irritability, depressed mood, loss of muscle mass, and impaired cognition (short-term memory loss and reduced ability to focus). Measurable signs of testosterone deficiency include gynecomastia, anemia, and reduced bone density [65]. The diagnosis of testosterone deficiency must also take into account the patient's medical history, physical exam, and additional blood tests as indicated to rule out other potential causes.

The prevalence of testosterone deficiency is difficult to measure as definitions vary within the literature. The use of testosterone replacement increased dramatically during the last several years from an estimated 0.5% in 2002 to 1.7% in 2016 [66,67]. Testosterone prescriptions have increased for men of reproductive age (18—39 years) [68]. There are multiple reasons for this increase, ranging from increased research, medical awareness, advertising of men's health clinics, and direct-to-consumer advertising leading to initiation of therapy without thorough evaluation [44]. The mechanism by which testosterone replacement impairs fertility is through modulation of the hypothalamic—pituitary—gonadal (HPG) axis. During normal physiologic function, the hypothalamus secretes gonadotropin releasing hormone, which works on the pituitary to stimulate release of luteinizing hormone (LH) and follicle stimulating hormone (FSH). FSH will go on to function in the maturation of spermatozoa while LH works on Leydig cells of the testes to produce testosterone, and to a smaller extent, estrogen. Testosterone and estrogen make their way into the bloodstream where they exhibit an inhibitory function on both the level of the hypothalamus and pituitary on production of their respective products. Thus creating a negative feedback loop allowing for homeostasis and a balance of hormone production as needed. However, if exogenous testosterone is introduced to treat a diagnosed deficiency, the balance is shifted. Although the testosterone deficiency is now corrected, it will still impart its negative feedback on the HPG axis and result in decreased LH and more importantly, FSH from the pituitary. Without the cosecretion of FSH with LH, sperm maturation does not occur appropriately and may lead to infertility.

Use of medical testosterone has been abused to compensate for the fear of loss of virility and muscle mass. For example, a fear of so-called weakness can occur in professions that place a value on strength, like firefighting, police work, or athletes hoping to gain a sporting edge [69]. Testosterone replacement is not indicated for the decline in testosterone levels with age or metabolic syndrome, and requires a known specific etiology, for example, anorchia, along with both symptoms and signs to be utilized as a treatment. It is not to be used as a "fountain of youth" [69].

Unfortunately, the fertility status of men is not always considered in the prescription of testosterone. Kollettis et al. demonstrated that 9% of men presenting with infertility were inappropriately placed on testosterone at two academic hospitals in the United States, whereas 1% in Canada were placed on testosterone during their reproductive years [50,51]. It is unclear how much direct to patient advertising plays a role in this disparity. Ko et al. also showed that 25% of urologists inappropriately consider using testosterone to help men with infertility [52]. Lack of education or knowledge about the negative effects of testosterone on fertility can lead to patient anger and disappointment, especially if the couple have been trying to conceive for some time. Unfortunately, situations like this can become tragic for a couple: female age may advance to the point of affecting ovulatory reserve, and men may struggle to end what can become an addiction to testosterone treatment. In such situations, consultation can be difficult, and men can be placed on an alternative treatment, such as clomiphene citrate or human choriogonadotropin (HCG) with or without FSH [70]. Cessation of the testosterone supplementation can be an option. Return to baseline sperm numbers can take 4–9 months to occur, further delaying the timeline to natural conception, intrauterine insemination (IUI), or IVF [28].

There are some data to support the combined use of testosterone and HCG in men with symptomatic hypogonadism in their reproductive years, a combination that can result in maintained sperm production. This has been suggested in men who are not trying to achieve a pregnancy for at least 6 months [71]. While still controversial, this is sometimes a compromise that involves shared decision making with the patient. One concerning factor is how adamant patients are about not coming off testosterone or achieving only the minimum sperm count to result in conception via IVF or IUI.

Implementation of HCG ± FSH comes with "real-world" issues. The cost of HCG/FSH drug replacement can be significant. It may not be covered by insurance or could require significant petitioning, since FSH is considered a fertility drug and often not covered. From an individual patient perspective/preference, treatment can feel draining/taxing, especially to those with needle phobia since both HCG and FSH require an injection three times a week.

In the pediatric population, the issue of delayed puberty and testosterone replacement is a dilemma. Should testosterone be given to correct for bone age, growth, and development of secondary male characteristics without consideration of fertility versus use of HCG? With HCG, how long prior to any future fertility is considered should the medication be started, since plans to have children have not been determined yet for the adolescent? This leads to an extensive discussion with parents, pediatric endocrinologists, and the adolescent male patient as well. When the patient is not yet at an age to consider offspring, parents will often navigate the decision making. This process can be anxiety provoking for parents whose concerns about growth, secondary male issues, and the development of their sons often takes precedence over fertility at this stage. However, the reversibility of testosterone use at a later date, when fertility becomes the question, is often a large part of the consultation.

Overall, the use of exogenous testosterone for hypogonadism for medical reasons and inappropriate reasons, such as nonspecific symptoms and age, has led to a paradigm shift to iatrogenic causes of male infertility over the last 20 years. The relationship between provider and patient in this situation requires honest and careful discussion. In most cases, this issue is reversible to allow for conception.

Anabolic steroids

The mechanism by which illicit anabolic steroid use impairs fertility is nearly identical to the mechanism described for iatrogenic testosterone replacement. However, the glaring difference between the two is that the administration of anabolic steroids is not to treat a documented deficiency of testosterone, but rather to increase the normal physiologic levels in search of increased athletic performance. A 2014 study reports roughly 3,000,000 anabolic steroid users in the United States with an increasing prevalence [72]. To date, there are numerous synthetic derivatives to testosterone available without much in the form of regulation to govern their sale or use. With this in mind, many anabolic abusers are very sophisticated in their knowledge of how to acquire the medication, and know how to cycle anabolic steroids to recover testicular size and even potential fertility. However, many users may be unaware of the negative impact their use has on their reproductive potential or do not care about the effect on their fertility, especially when at early-stage adulthood with a different focus on life and image.

Many times, younger men ignore risky lifestyle behavior. In this situation the issues are: addiction, mental health issues with long-standing body image and sporting prowess insecurities, refusal to stop anabolic steroids, poor recovery of reproductive potential, and illegal drug behavior [73]. High school athletes, college athletes, bodybuilders, and professional athletes, may feel under increased pressure to excel to the point they turn to illegal, and sometimes poor quality anabolic, steroids on the black market. This behavior can lead to addiction and evasive techniques to avoid or cheat drug testing. Often, these men do not come off the drugs when they first meet their partners. Later, their fear of decreased strength or looks, despite the associated risks from such medication (e.g., cardiac and hematological), outweigh their concerns for personal health and fertility [74]. Sometimes convincing such men to stop anabolics is met with resistance or even distrust.

We see the same psychological patterns with men who abuse anabolic steroids and patients with eating disorders [75,76]. Both result in rigid thought processes. Examples of these thought processes include "tunnel vision" about needing a body to look a certain way despite evident medical consequences, a truncated ability to problem solve or consider long-term consequences, and a deep need for control in one area of life because other areas feel so out of control. Ironically, infertility could amplify the perceived "need" for anabolic steroid use, making it more psychologically threatening to stop use in an attempt to conceive.

The issue of converting to medications such as clomiphene citrate to HCG can seem like feeding into patient addiction and or legitimizing their behavior. Cessation of anabolic steroids without any "recovery medication" is a real option feasible for some patients. Some men are only willing to come off anabolic use just long enough to result in early recovery of sperm in the semen for IVF rather than enough for either IUI or natural conception. Many times anabolic drug abusers are not aware of the long-term consequences of their abuse [74]. Some men who abused anabolic steroids in the past do not recover sperm production or adequate intrinsic testosterone production, resulting in a condition called anabolic-induced hypogonadism [77,78]. This can result in issues of sexual dysfunction with persistent decreased libido and associated ED [79]. Overall, this can lead to significant regret on the part of the male partner, and can sometimes require marital counseling about "blame" [80].

Medications

Our collective understanding of pharmacology continues to advance [81]. However, as practitioners, we would be doing our patients a disservice by only presenting the benefits of such medications without also discussing the potential risks. The effect of medications on male fertility is too broad to review here, but some general issues are universal: need for the medication; chronicity of use of the medication; compliance with taking the medication; and limited knowledge regarding fertility when certain drugs are used long term [81]. Psychological issues that stem from taking medication need to be considered during consultation. Patients taking medication may experience feelings of denial or depression, or feel that because they are taking medication they are "getting old" and facing mortality. All of this can lead to issues of compliance [82]. The side effects of long-term use of ongoing medications for medical care are not often known or considered by providers. As shown with iatrogenic testosterone use, ignorance is not an excuse. However, lack of scientific evidence/knowledge in many cases is evident.

Modern antibiotics such as nitrofurantoin and tetracyclines affect testosterone production, while drugs of abuse, including opioids, can negatively impact testosterone and infertility as well [83]. The dose-dependent effect seen with opioids is thought to be due in part by increases in serum prolactin levels as well as decreased semen quality [72]. Short duration of use may have limited negative effects on fertility. With an increase of mental health issues in reproductive years, longer term/chronic need for medication, for example, psychotropic medications, may be a concern [84]. However, limited studies have failed to provide sufficient evidence that selective serotonin release inhibitors (SSRIs) reduce fertility to significant levels [85,86]. However, many psychotropic medications do affect sexual function, especially libido and erectile function. SSRIs used for significant clinical depression and anxiety can result in delayed ejaculation. In many severe psychiatric cases, withdrawal from medication is a concern, and requires close consultation with psychiatry. For fertility, anejaculation (AE) can require intervention with electroejaculation (EEJ) for IUI, IVF, or testicular biopsy with IVF.

Another medication that may be used by men in their reproductive years is low-dose finasteride, used for preventing hair loss. Again, issues of body image may affect fertility [87–90]. Finasteride is a 5-alpha reductase inhibitor that blocks the conversion of testosterone to dihydrotestosterone. Finasteride has been shown to reduce semen volume and sperm parameters. More concerning is a black box warning that irreversible sexual dysfunction may occur in 1%–2% of men [91]. The mechanism is not known, and is referred to as postfinasteride syndrome. In this situation, again there are issues of convincing a small group of men to stop this medication, thus resulting in hair loss and associated feelings of unattractiveness/issues of body image. In many cases, these men are already in a stable relationship trying to conceive and willing to stop the medication.

Chemotherapy is well known to affect male fertility, often permanently. Up to 46% of males who survive childhood cancer are infertile [92]. Alkylating agents in particular seem to be the most potent in causing azoospermia [93]. Discussion of fertility preservation before most chemotherapy is needed [94,95]. In the past, providers omitted the topic in the initial evaluation, resulting in significant bitterness and regret among long-term survivors [96]. This topic will be discussed in more detail in Chapter 7, *Reproductive and Sexual Health Concerns for Cancer Survivors*.

With fertility, many times couples are looking for a "magic pill" that can boost sperm counts or otherwise improve fertility, for example, clomiphene citrate. These hopes are difficult to rectify when 50% or more of male infertility is idiopathic [82]. Consequently continued research regarding mechanisms of male infertility to targeted drug development is needed. Over the counter nutraceutical supplements that are mainly vitamins and antioxidants have been promoted as possible methods to help with fertility/infertility. There is limited data on the benefits of these on sperm quality [97,98]. As such, many patients hope these supplements will provide some improvement. Appropriate counseling on their limited role is important. A major concern is the prevalence of inaccurate information available to patients, especially online [99].

Genetic

Klinefelter syndrome

KS is the most frequent chromosomal abnormality in males, present in about 1 in every 660 male births [100]. Genetically, the syndrome is based on the presence of an extra X chromosome, making the karyotype 47,XXY. Phenotypically, these men are characterized by infertility, small testes, gynecomastia, hypergonadotropic hypogonadism, and learning disability [100]. Because the phenotype varies greatly, there is a high degree of underdiagnosis, but virtually all men with KS are infertile [100]. The characteristic testicular germ cell loss is thought to start very early in life as spermatogonia carrying the extra X chromosome undergo apoptosis, whereas Leydig cell exhaustion is variable and can occur during puberty or adulthood [101]. As a result, KS patients suffer from hypergonadotropic hypogonadism which further attenuates fertility. Often during evaluation for infertility, previously undiagnosed men are identified with KS. Roughly 10%–15% of males with nonobstructive azoospermia are diagnosed with KS [102]. Microtesticular sperm extraction (microTESE), followed by intracytoplasmic sperm injection (ICSI) has successfully been used in men with KS allowing them to become biological fathers of healthy children [103].

The emotional consequences of a KS diagnosis are significant and thought to be a symptom of the syndrome. Patients with KS can have potential issues with learning when younger, including attention deficit, issues of cognition/retaining information, low self-esteem, depression, and anxiety [100,104,105]. This may be due to the genetic issue with the extra X chromosome with question of some receptor issues, but mostly thought to be low testosterone and a question of brain development during puberty and imprinting. This issue is poorly understood [100,104]. However, these factors are far from consistent with many males going unrecognized until they try to conceive naturally with their partners and present with infertility. At that time, the following can become the issue: shock of a genetic diagnosis of nonobstructive azoospermia; stress of options for ART and how sperm needs to be found (or not) through extensive surgical testicular dissection (microTESE); concern about possible transmission to a child (son); stress of health consequences; stress of alternative options; and finally, issues of correcting for testosterone deficiency and delayed puberty.

Most times men are diagnosed with KS when they present with infertility with azoospermia and in a relationship. However, sometimes the diagnosis is made due to preimplantation genetic screening (PGS), to in utero diagnosis with chorion villus biopsy or amniocentesis. This may lead to an emotional burden on parents several years before potential clinical consequences on the male offspring's endocrinology or puberty, to possible learning issues, fertility, and health issues in later life [106]. This begs the questions: when should a parent tell their child about their diagnosis and the potential effect on fertility/medical health? What effect will this have on relationships when the child grows up? How can that now-adult prepare to explain genetic issues and fertility status with his partner? Many times, the patient doesn't know what "he has been missing" in terms of testosterone deficiency. This can be enlightening to a patient when treated. The additional issue is testosterone replacement while still in the reproductive years, with exogenous testosterone treatment to be avoided during that time. This is controversial however and adds another level of dilemma especially in cases of delayed puberty or later due to issues with libido, etc. [107,108].

At what point in a relationship does a man tell his partner that he may be infertile? Testing can be done ahead of time with a semen analysis, but if low sperm counts to no sperm confirmed, the patient may fear or lose his confidence in maintaining a long-term relationship, especially if having a family becomes part of the discussion and the direct need for IVF-ICSI. This constitutes an added stress on a loving relationship, and how the desire of having future biological children plays into the equation, that is, when is the desire for biological children a "deal breaker or not" in the early part of a relationship if the male partner knows his diagnosis beforehand? Early relationships are a difficult time, at best, to introduce adoption or extensive and costly processes associated with IVF.

Y chromosome

Y chromosome deletions and microdeletions are a rare cause of infertility, with an estimated prevalence of around 1 in every 2000–3000 births [109]. Unlike men diagnosed with KS, men with Y chromosome infertility are usually phenotypically normal, with the exception of small testes as seen in 70% of patients [110]. Patients will have azoospermia or severe oligozoospermia on their semen analysis depending on size and location of the genetic insult [110]. A hemizygous deletion of the long arm of the Y chromosome, involving the azoospermic factor region which is responsible for spermatogenesis may be seen in 5%–10% of males with azoospermia [111]. Most of these mutations are *de novo* given the inheritance pattern of the Y chromosome. ART such as ICSI using either TESE or spermatozoa retrieved from ejaculate can otherwise be used in men with Y chromosome deletion to conceive biological offspring [112].

Like any time a patient is first diagnosed with azoospermia, there is typically shock and disbelief, followed by feeling numb and a sense of guilt related to what the male partner perceives the cause and his "fault" for infertility for the couple and possibly the loss of perceived manhood. The issue of past lifestyle often plays a role in that feeling of guilt. After that, the question of a "blockage"/obstruction over issues of nonobstructive azoospermia should be discussed with a specialist. With blood testing, a genetic cause related to the Y chromosome may become diagnosed [113]. At issue here is that the Y chromosome deletion will be transmitted to a male offspring if sperm are found and functional with IVF-ICSI [114,115]. That knowledge about transmission to a male offspring of passing on male infertility may be too abstract for a couple and a genetic counseling referral may be in order. Sex selection of the embryo for a female offspring, in this case for medical reasons, may be indicated. PGS with day 5 embryos will be recommended. This can limit the number of embryos available for transfer and also lead to social/cultural anxieties.

The potential of finding a few sperm through microTESE is like "finding a needle in a haystack" but can be achieved in 40%–70% of cases for use with IVF-ICSI. This can generate hope in a situation where a couple are told there are no sperm in the semen [116]. Care must be taken to not overexaggerate the likelihood of success. Creating realistic expectations is critical and we often indicate to the couple that the process is a "roller coaster ride" both clinically and emotionally. Finding sperm is only the starting point. Enough sperm must be found to fertilize the number of eggs retrieved. The potential anxiety is obvious. What if there are no sperm or not enough found? The role of donor sperm as a backup, normally a difficult topic, needs to be addressed at the consultation. Alternative treatment options such as donor sperm with IUI, to adoption and even foster care and child-free living are potential difficult topics for this consultation. Men often discuss that they "won't be able to love a baby that is not biologically related to them." The lack of control they feel around their own fertility then seems to be expanded, that is, "I can't conceive with my partner, so what other shortcomings will I have as a father." Each is specific and difficult in its own right.

Donor sperm use can create fears or perceptions requiring careful discussion and correction [117]. Men fear that the child will "not be theirs," fear their female partner is at risk for STIs from donor insemination, and have concerns about disclosure and how that may impact bonding with a child or be interpreted by family and friends if it is disclosed? [117] Options exist for directed donor sperm from a male family member, donation by an unknown donor from a sperm bank, identity release arrangements where the donor agrees to contact when the child turns 18 years of age are all possible [118,119]. True anonymity appears to be impossible given DNA testing services such as 23andMe and Ancestry.com which make it possible to find a donor and through donor-conceived sibling registries. Counseling men about what constitutes "parenting" versus fertilization is essential. Nonheteronormative family building is discussed in other chapters in this text.

For some azoospermic men and their partners using donated embryos or creating their families through adoption are additional solutions to family creation. The child is not genetically connected to either parent and as such this solution can seem more equitable. Unfortunately, the cost of adoption can be as high as IVF, with many social and legal matters to pursue.

Cystic fibrosis transmembrane conductance regulator/congenital bilateral absence of the vas deferens

CBAVD occurs in 1%–2% of males with infertility [120]. This is an anatomic malformation that has two genetic causes: one that results from mutations in the cystic fibrosis transmembrane conductance regulator (CFTR) gene, and another that results from alterations in other genes involved in mesonephric ductal development, which are not yet known [121]. Patients with CBAVD are azoospermic, have a normal HPA axis, and as the name implies an absent or beaded/obstructed vas deferens on physical exam. Although a small subset of men with infertility have CBAVD, 95% of patients with cystic fibrosis (CF) will have CBAVD [122]. Fortunately, most men with CBAVD are asymptomatic or subsequently diagnosed with milder/atypical CF, involving mild pulmonary disease, gastrointestinal issues, and even pancreatitis [123]. Spermatogenesis is typically normal in these patients so ART can be used to help father biological children via ICSI following surgical sperm extraction [124]. Since the carrier frequency of the CF gene mutation is 1:20 in the general Northern European population, it is important to screen the female partner and provide genetic counseling to the couple prior to undergoing any fertility treatments [121].

From an emotional/psychological perspective, there are several aspects of the clinical picture that need to be recognized and discussed as part of counseling: shock of diagnosis and association with CBAVD; role of CF work up and for patient and female partner; risk of passing disease or carrier status to offspring; and role of preimplantation genetic diagnosis (PGD) of the embryo if the female partner is a carrier for the CFTR.

Unless the patient has known CF and is sent for fertility consultation, because of the known association with CBAVD and obstructive azoospermia, most patients are seen primarily for azoospermia and diagnosed with CBAVD by an outside provider, usually a urologist. It is often the male infertility specialist that makes the diagnosis of CBAVD, then has to explain the association with CF/CFTR mutations. On one level it is reassuring to know that the problem is a "blockage," but often a shock that it is associated with CF, which in the past was a life-threatening condition. Patients and partners can be more concerned that the man's disease will advance, and could possibly explain past symptoms. For example, one patient presented with a history of pancreatitis and was labeled a juvenile delinquent and alcoholic, when in fact his later presentation for azoospermia was a form of CF. Distressed and relieved at the same time, the patient cried and felt he had been validated after several years. The diagnosis of "genetic" can often lead to anxiety. Added to this, CBAVD has a 10% association with having a congenitally missing kidney, creating another level of anxiety at the initial consultation stage [125]. Again, genetic testing of both partners is needed to determine risk of passing the disease to offspring. Referral for genetic counseling, the need for ART with IVF-ICSI, PGD, and associated costs, as noted previously, are all part of an overwhelming situation for many men.

Anatomic

Vasectomy and vasectomy reversal

Vasectomy is the most common procedure performed by a urologist, involving the surgical removal of a small piece of the vas deferens to prevent sperm from reaching the ejaculatory duct, functionally leading to obstructive azoospermia [126]. This elective form of sterilization for men is performed over half a million times per year in the United States and is relied on as the primary form of contraception for 10% of couples in the United States [127]. The failure rate following the procedure is less than 0.5% [128,129]. Up to 19.6% of men who previously underwent a vasectomy consider consultation for postvasectomy procreative management [127]. If a man is under 30 years of age when he has had his vasectomy, he is 12.5 times more likely to consider reversal compared with men over 30 years of age. Reasons for reversal are multifactorial, ranging from the number of existing children to change in partner status more likely under the age of 30 [130]. When does a man discuss with a new partner that he has had a vasectomy and how does that play into the relationship? This is an interesting question for mental health professionals to tackle. Similarly, if the partners are in the same relationship as prior to the vasectomy, why have they changed their minds as a couple? Reasons can include "we thought we were done, but then realized we are not" or the prospect of an empty nest removing something from their lives. Or the decision for the vasectomy may have been unilateral by the male partner. Marital or relationship issues are an obvious outcome of this. Counseling addressing secrets, power in the relationship, and other issues is recommended. Postvasectomy procreative management in a preexisting relationship may be the result of trauma in the relationship that led to male partner or couple to pursue vasectomy. These can include a difficult pregnancy, financial stress, or the death of a child [131]. Often decisions at this stage can seem reactive with later regret. In new relationships, the female partner may not have had children before, or if both partners have children with previous partners, then they may desire to have biological children together. In all cases, consensus from both partners about procreation seems essential for relationship stability.

A vasectomy reversal bypasses the previously created obstruction in the vas deferens with the goal of regaining fertility. Urologists typically perform a vasovasostomy or vasoepididymostomy and are able to achieve anastomotic patency 99.5% and 80% of the time, respectively [126]. These results translate to a 30%—75% pregnancy rate at greater than 15 years to less than 3 years from vasectomy, respectively [126,132]. Vasectomized patients also have a second option using newer ART via ICSI following surgical sperm extraction.

Vasectomy reversal is more cost effective, and advantageously has the potential of achieving further pregnancies [133]. However, the decision to proceed with reversal versus IVF is multifactorial and important to tailor for the couple, after discussing the relevant issues. If both partners have previous children and have experienced parenthood, the desire to have further children must be considered in the context of family dynamics and discussed honestly with the couple. Sometimes it is important to play "devil's advocate." The option to do nothing and enjoy the current status quo and children sometimes needs to be highlighted, as well as the health and social status of current children. It is important to understand the family dynamics. That does not mean that the provider is telling the couple what to do, but to facilitate the couple's wishes and understanding of success rates, timeline to success or not and cost of such a decision emotionally or financially. Along with these issues the need to consider age of the female partner with physiological issues and ovulatory reserve; effect of older male or female partner age and social consequences of raising a child and even posthumously, especially if there is a vast difference between male and female age; genetic risks to the child with older female and male partner age; and finally, timeline, with fear of failure, that is, failure of sperm return or pregnancy. All these factors should be discussed to counsel the couple effectively.

An important aspect to highlight specifically is the timeline to pregnancy. With advanced female age, the rate limiting issue is egg quality and success rates with pregnancy at 8% or less at female age of 40 for both reversal and IVF [134,135]. The role for PGS of the embryo is possible if the couple decide to proceed with IVF with sperm extraction and implantation of a euploid embryo, then pregnancy rates increase to up to 27% [136]. Genetic risk of a fetus cannot be assessed as early if pregnancy occurs naturally through a vas reversal, with only later chorion villus biopsy or amniocentesis possible. Finally, time to pregnancy, if it happens, is often shorter with IVF cases than a vasectomy reversal even though reversal allows for more months of trying naturally.

Alternative options, such as doing nothing, adoption, foster care, and use of donor sperm with ART with IUI versus IVF have to be discussed in a complete consultation. The role of the consultation asks a medical provider to be a clinician, surgeon, advocate, psychologist, financial advisor, and social worker all at once. Access to a team of professionals with competence in the wide range of reproductive healthcare issues is essential. Overall the decision for postvasectomy procreative management requires extensive counseling to weigh the risks and benefits of each option for postvasectomy procreative management and tailored to the couple to result in the healthiest and quickest outcome. The financial burden of each option often plays heavily on the medical and psychosocial decision.

Varicocele

Testicular varicocele is a dilation of the veins of the pampiniform plexus draining the testicle, resulting in an increase in the intratesticular temperature. This can lead to deleterious effects on semen parameters, and a subsequent decrease in fertility [137]. Testicular varicocele is the most common diagnosable cause of male infertility, with a presence in 15% of all men and 19%—41% of men with primary infertility [138]. A treatment paradigm exists in which not all men with varicoceles are infertile, and in fact most men are asymptomatic from their varicocele, though 20%—40% of men with a varicocele will suffer from fertility problems [139]. Due to the anatomic arrangement of venous drainage of the gonads, varicoceles are more common on the left-hand side. If an isolated right-sided varicocele is encountered, high suspicion must be maintained for retroperitoneal pathology like tumors/mass effect, and then subsequently investigated. Varicoceles are graded on an evidence-based clinical grading scale; Grade I is palpable only with valsalva; Grade II is palpable on exam, but not visible to the naked eye; and Grade III is visible through the scrotum [121]. Varicoceles that are evident clinically should be referred for either interventional radiology embolization or for surgical ligation.

There are significant biases amongst providers on the significance of varicoceles on fertility [140]. Gynecologists have often been taught that the rate of pregnancies with varicoceles are no different than natural conception [141]. Also, the teaching has been that a varicocele does not affect the outcome of ART [141,142]. Both issues are not supported by the literature. There is now growing data to show that correcting the varicocele can reduce the type of ART needed [143,144]. This is why multispecialty coordination of care and team meetings to discuss these issues are necessary. One of the reasons is that many times there is a delay in diagnosis of a varicocele and other treatments have been tried before a male is evaluated. This can lead to bitterness and disappointment for couples, which can be exaggerated especially with advanced female age. There is no guarantee that correction of the varicocele will lead to a pregnancy, but the goal is to maximize male and female reproductive health to result in pregnancy as soon as possible with the least cost. Overall, the best scenario for a couple is early evaluation of both partners with the aim to maximize each partner's health in the most efficient, timely, and least costly fashion. Varicocele management falls into this category.

Testicular cancer and retroperitoneal lymph node dissection

Testicular cancer is the most common solid tumor in men aged 15–35 years old. The incidence was estimated at 6.4 per 100,000 in 2014 [145]. The initial management of most testicular cancer cases is a radical orchiectomy. Preoperatively, sperm banking should be discussed as standard prior to the orchiectomy and especially before the first dose of chemotherapeutic agents such as etoposide- platinum based chemotherapy that carry a risk of gonadotoxicity [95,146]. Removing a testicle in a young man can result in issues of body image, especially a single male or one not in a committed relationship [147,148]. Patients often have concerns with confidence during foreplay with a testicle missing. In cases of bilateral testicular cancer, metachronous or rarely synchronous, the feeling of being emasculated is a real concern [149]. In all cases the placement of a testicular prosthesis can be performed providing some psychological and cosmetic benefit.

Retroperitoneal lymph node dissection (RPLND) is an important adjunct to treatment in certain testicular cancer patients with metastasis. RPLND is an operative procedure that involves the surgical removal of lymph nodes in a predetermined template of the retroperitoneum where most lymph node metastasis occurs. The hypogastric nerve plexus, containing sympathetic fibers required for ejaculation, also overlie this region and may be damaged during the procedure. Without a careful nerve sparing approach, AE is a risk postoperatively [121]. About 25% of couples divorcing after testicular cancer cite the cancer, sexual dysfunction, and its effect on fertility as a contributing factor [150].

Occasionally, other cancers of the genitourinary (GU) system may affect reproduction and sexual function. These include prostate cancer with prostatectomies and/or radiation; cystectomies for bladder cancer, and partial or complete penectomies for penile cancer (or trauma) [151–153]. Reproductive and sexual desires of patients should be addressed in conjunction with treatment of the cancer.

Some specific medical conditions

Diabetes mellitus

Diabetes mellitus (DM) is a complex metabolic disorder with the central feature being hyperglycemia leading to end organ dysfunction [154]. Type 1 DM is characterized by a destruction of pancreatic beta-islet cells, usually in childhood, while Type 2 DM is characterized by insulin resistance due to lifestyle and genetic risk factors that usually develops in middle age [155]. With both the rise in prevalence of this disease and its earlier onset, DM now affects an increased number of men of reproductive age [156]. Fertility is affected in those with DM due to macro and microvascular changes leading to ED, and lack of emission. ED is noted in more than half of men with this disease [157]. Furthermore, it has been noted that men with DM have lower levels of testosterone as well as impaired spermatogenesis and increased sperm DNA damage [158,159]. The associated use of medications, for example, antihypertensives can also affect ejaculation, erections, and sperm parameters.

Diabetic men can develop retrograde ejaculation (RE) and AE. RE is a relatively uncommon cause of infertility occurring in about 2% of men with infertility [160]. In a small case-control study, the prevalence of RE was estimated to be approximately 34% in men with diabetes aged between 35 and 55 years, though other studies of young male diabetics have estimated RE and AE to be present in only 6% of patients [161].

RE is a failure of the bladder neck to close during ejaculation causing a reflux of a semen into the bladder. Ejaculation is a complex process mediated by sympathetic nerve fibers working in concert to cause first the emission and then ultimately the expulsion of semen. Breakdown in this process can be caused by spinal cord injury (SCI), neuropathy from DM or MS (multiple sclerosis), prior retroperitoneal surgery, anatomic abnormality due to prior bladder neck surgery, congenital abnormalities, or pharmacological treatments (e.g., psychotropic medications and alpha-adrenergic blockers) or idiopathic [162]. Clinically, RE is diagnosed by five or more spermatozoa/high power field or greater than 5% of the anterograde amount present in the urine sediment immediately after masturbation [163]. Urinary sperm retrieval can be performed to extract sufficient viable sperm for ART [164]. Ejaculation has also been achieved with EEJ using a rectal probe with both the antegrade and retrograde ejaculate then used for ART also [165]. Ultimately, if sufficient viable sperm is not retrieved in the retrograde and antegrade ejaculate then testicular or epididymal sperm extraction can be used for sperm retrieval for ICSI.

AE also occurs in diabetic male patients and is often related to poor diabetic control. AE is defined by the complete absence of either antegrade or retrograde seminal emission from testicle to prostate but orgasm does occur [166]. One must also take care to distinguish AE with anorgasmisa [121]. Like RE, conditions that cause AE are primarily neurologic with SCI being the most common [167]. Diabetic neuropathy that damages the sympathetic nerves and sacral peripheral nerves can be a common cause also. In this situation, either vibratory stimulation without anesthesia or EEJ under anesthesia may be attempted to produce sperm for IUI or IVF [168]. Poor sperm quality may occur, but pregnancy using EEJ with ART can be successful [168]. If EEJ does not yield adequate sperm for ART then surgical extraction is indicated. The issue with EEJ is that many times insurance companies do not cover this treatment. Medicare in the United States and chronic illness status does cover EEJ in most cases, but not the ART that must accompany it.

Diabetic males can suffer from ED, which can affect their fertility. This will be covered in Chapter 4, *The Impact of Erectile Dysfunction on Infertility and its Treatment*. ED can affect issues of sexual intercourse and the delivery of sperm in the vagina/at the cervix and impacts overall fertility. ED often can cause psychological issues of confidence and manliness. ED also affects the timing of intercourse, and can be improved with medications such as phosphodiesterase inhibitors or penile injections. This can be difficult when couples are trying to coordinate intercourse mid female cycle, every other day prior to ovulation and just after. Referral to a sex therapist, especially one with reproductive health knowledge, is advisable.

Male reproductive and sexual health specialists frequently encounter poorly controlled diabetics and those who have developed pathology from the disease as indicated before. Many younger patients can be noncompliant about their diabetic care, resulting in reproductive consequences that must be addressed when they wish to have children. It is not unusual for these patients to have regret about their failure to monitor their disease better when they were younger.

Spinal cord injury

SCIs disproportionately affect young men of reproductive age, with a prevalence of 17,700 new cases in the United States each year [169]. Depending on the level of the injury virtually every part of the male reproductive mechanism can be affected leading to ED, ejaculatory dysfunction, and abnormal semen parameters [170]. Men with complete injury above T11 are unable to achieve psychogenic erections, whereas those with injuries below that level are typically unable to achieve reflexogenic erections. As previously described, emission and ejaculation are complex processes requiring coordination of sympathetic, parasympathetic, and somatic spinal centers. Again, antegrade ejaculation depends on the level and severity of the SCI. In patients with complete lower motor neuronal injury only 18% retain the ability to ejaculate whereas if the injury is incomplete, 70% will have preserved antegrade ejaculation. With upper motor neuron injury, only 11% preserve antegrade ejaculation versus 32% in incomplete SCI [169]. Semen parameters, specifically sperm motility and viability, are thought to be affected due to elevated proinflammatory cytokines and stasis of semen [171].

SCIs are often suffered by young men in their reproductive years, and often due to accidents from dangerous or risky behavior [172,173]. The physical and mental trauma of a SCI initially results in spinal shock as well as mental disbelief, followed by many stages of grief [174]. Once acceptance has been reached and the patient regains hope, often hope for potential fertility returns [175]. This leads to these men and their partners seeking consultation. Sperm can be obtained in some cases from vibratory stimulation for ejaculation to EEJ. Anesthesia is rarely needed in these cases. Surgical sperm extraction with IVF-ICSI is possible as well, as mentioned with DM.

The emotional, psychological, and reproductive issues should be discussed taking into account parenting with the physical challenges attached to a particular disability and assessing the degree of independence and caregiving needs [176]. Occasionally some men have continued medical issues ranging from urinary tract infections to decubiti. The chronicity of these issues can play a significant role in family building plans and a multiprofessional care team will help provide insights into more than the retrieval of sperm, fertilization, and pregnancy.

Cancer

The topic is complicated by concerns about mortality at the time of diagnosis, the overwhelming nature of ongoing medical care, hope for survival and, in many cases, fertility [95]. Many male cancer survivors in the reproductive years do consider future fertility [96]. As such the American Society of Clinical Oncology recommends that oncologists discuss fertility preservation with their patients [94]. However, many oncologists are not trained to discuss this issue especially the potential need for ART with the frozen sperm (see Chapter 7: *Reproductive and Sexual Health Concerns for Cancer Survivors*) [92]. Consultation with specially trained providers is recommended [177]. Management of fertility preservation for male adolescents that are not really considering fertility can put pressure on parents to assist the young man to make such decisions [92,178]. Sometimes young men have not learned how to masturbate, or have not seriously thought about having children. This can be an awkward, traumatic, and difficult time to discuss the issue [179].

The issues of potential posthumous sperm use, living wills, and the future use of cryopreserved sperm especially if there is no named partner are important for both patients and caregivers to consider [180]. There can be conflict within families that request sperm freezing for adults without partners. This issue is also a concern when minors with parents or guardians who wish to take control of cryopreserved specimens for potential grandchildren with an unknown/nonexistent and unnamed future partner. Grief and emotions cloud decision making and ethics of the issue [180]. The need to be compassionate and sensitive at the time of consultation is essential to navigate a potential desperate, emotional, and sometimes angry situation when a patient and family are unsure of life expectancy or when the patient is dying or has died. If there is no named partner and the patient dies, most situations indicate that the frozen sperm be discarded. Hallak et al. demonstrated that most of 342 patients with cancer discarded their specimens due to recovery of fertility or semen quality improving after cancer treatment. Twenty one specimens were discarded due to death [108]. Ultimately, local law must be considered and referral to an attorney well versed in reproductive law is advised.

Pediatric conditions and transitional care

Spina bifida

Spina bifida is a congenital neural tube defect where the spinal cord and surrounding tissues fail to develop in utero. Manifestations differ depending on the size and location of the defect along the spinal cord but may present with muscle weakness or paralysis and difficulties with gastrointestinal and GU system control. According to the Centers for Disease Control and Prevention, spina bifida affects 1500 newborns a year. In a 2013 study of spina bifida patients from 1983 to 2013, 85% of patients survived to at least 20 years of age [181]. Given this fact, it is important to understand the implications of spina bifida on potential fertility with patients surviving into adulthood. Barriers to fertility amongst men with spina bifida include ED, AE, and poor sperm quality [182]. ED and AE appear to be governed by the level of neurologic impairment. For instance, 86% of men with spina bifida lesion below T10 reported ED while only 36% of men with lesion above T10 reported ED [183]. Poor sperm quality relates to the higher than average rate of cryptorchidism found in patients born with spina bifida. The incidence of cryptorchidism at birth amongst males diagnosed with spina bifida was roughly 15%, from an average of 2%–5% amongst neurotypical male births [184].

As care for children with spina bifida has improved, more are reaching adulthood and seek relationships. Adult males with spina bifida mostly have normal sexual desire with 75% able to achieve an erection, although maintaining an erection may be difficult. Often, sexual education and access to intimacy are delayed compared to the general population. As such, it is important for providers to be cognizant of this topic and engage the individual in discussion [182]. The issue of fertility as male children grow into adulthood relates to the level of the defect very much like a traumatic SCI. The methods of treatment are similar to SCI.

Undescended testicles

Cryptorchidism is defined as the failure of one or both testes to descend into the scrotum prenatally. In full-term newborns, the prevalence is roughly between 2% and 5% [185]. However, most will descend by 6 months of age and only about 1% of males will have a persistent cryptorchidism after 6 months with limited impact on fertility if repaired before 1 year of age [186]. Cryptorchidism can be unilateral or bilateral with associated increasing negative effects on fertility. Those with untreated bilateral cryptorchidism have an 89% incidence of azoospermia and an associated 13% incidence in untreated unilateral cases [187]. The pathophysiology of decreased fertility relates to decreased numbers of Leydig cells and failure of maturation of germ cells [188]. It is important to note that cryptorchidism also confers a four to eight times increased risk of testicular cancer [189].

The main issue at consultation is management of infertility. Often parents and male patients who reach adulthood are surprised when either missed undescended testicles are diagnosed or correction takes place late, that is, after the age of 1 year. Patients with bilateral undescended testicles have often been warned about potential issues with fertility. As a result, many times, undiagnosed or untreated men entering their reproductive years must cope with potential infertility as they meet partners with whom they wish to have children. When does a man tell his partner that he may be infertile? Testing can be done ahead of time with a semen analysis, but if low to no sperm are confirmed, the patient may fear or lose confidence in maintaining a long-term relationship. This is similar to the situation faced by boys with Klinefelter and any other known issue with fertility. When and how to provide this information to a partner?

Transgender fertility issues

Gender dysphoria as defined by the DSM-5 as a marked incongruence between one's experienced/expressed and assigned gender for 6 months or more. The diagnosis is subject to meeting additional criteria and according to recent studies, including one long-term study from the Netherlands, has a prevalence of 1:3800 for men and 1:5200 for women in 2015 [190]. In this study, of the people who identified as trans and were subsequently diagnosed with gender dysphoria, between 65% and 90% initiated hormone therapy. Of those that began hormone therapy, 74.7% of transwomen and 83.8% of transmen went on to undergo gender affirmation surgery within 5 years [190].

About 50%–58% of transgender people desire children and 37%–76% consider fertility preservation [191,192]. In a multicenter German study only 9.6% of transwomen actually underwent fertility preservation [191]. It is imperative to counsel on goals for fertility before hormone therapy is initiated and best if done early by providers [193].

A thorough and detailed discussion of this topic is provided in Chapter 10, *Parenting in Transgender and Non-Binary Individuals*.

Lifestyle issues

Behaviors like the use of tobacco, illicit drugs, alcohol, and unhealthy diets causing obesity have known effects on sperm and male fertility [194]. They can also reflect patients' particular gender-role experiences, a fact clinicians must account for when discussing fertility enhancement through reduction or cessation of any of these habits. Globally, men are more likely than women to use tobacco, illicit drugs and alcohol, and to do so in greater amounts [195–197]. Researchers have attributed this gender imbalance in risk behavior in part to specific masculinity ideologies, which encourage some men to both engage in such health-demoting lifestyle activities and seek less medical care than women [198–200]. Tobacco use has long been associated with deleterious effects on female fertility [194]. Tobacco use in males also has been linked to infertility though less well understood and studied [201]. Tobacco use, specifically in men who chronically smoked >20 cigarettes per day, was linked to a 19% reduction in sperm concentrations compared to nonsmokers after controlling for age and overall health [202]. Importantly, a study using oral nicotine administered to male rats demonstrated similar decreases in sperm counts and sperm motility, suggesting that the adverse effects of tobacco are not exclusively due to smoking [203]. More research needs to be done to further elucidate the mechanism by which these deleterious effects occur.

Alcohol abuse has a long history of well-documented negative health effects, but its effect on male fertility may not be as widely known. It is estimated that roughly 9 million men in the United States suffer from alcohol-use disorder according to recent 2019 survey data from The National Institute on Alcohol Abuse and Alcoholism (SAMHSA) [204]. Globally, estimates are comparable for men. The effect of heavy alcohol use on male fertility cannot be overlooked. Greater than five drinks per day was associated with a decrease in sperm quality and concentration, especially after passing a threshold of 40 drinks or greater in a week yielding a 33% reduction in sperm concentration among Danish men [205].

Stigmatization by medical providers, on topics ranging from illicit drug use to body mass index (BMI), has been shown to harm patient health. Providers should be careful to discuss the evidence basis for behaviors that affect fertility [206,207]. As a men's health issue, maintaining good health results in lowered risk of chronic disease and use of medications. One aspect of this is diet [208]. However, worldwide structural barriers to healthy eating exist and are related to global and local inequalities [209,210]. While BMI does not specifically define an unhealthy lifestyle or eating habits, according to the WHO, in 2016 roughly 1.9 billion adults 18 years old or older were overweight (BMI ≥ 25) and over 650 million of these adults would classify as obese (BMI ≥ 30). The ratio of obesity is slightly higher in females but the impacts of obesity are felt by both sexes [211]. It has been well established that obesity reduces quality of life and life expectancy [212,213]. In addition, those living with obesity are at an increased risk of developing type II diabetes, coronary heart disease, stroke, asthma, and even certain forms of cancer [214–216]. There may be associated issues of body image, and other psychological factors. Obesity has been shown to affect male fertility with an effect on hormones and sperm [217]. The effects of obesity on the sexual health of men are less well documented than in women [218]. In a recent study conducted with couples from the United States, it was estimated that the odds of male infertility increased by 10% for every 9 kg a man is overweight [219]. This is likely multifactorial, including increased peripheral aromatization of androgens to estrogen by the excess adipose tissue leading to increased levels of estrogens to disrupt the HPG axis with effects similar to those discussed in the hypogonadism section [220]. In a recent meta-analysis of 28 cohort studies, it was shown that bariatric surgery leads to significant increases in testosterone levels as well as improvements in erectile function based on International Index of Erectile Function scores [218]. The results on semen parameters for men who undergo bariatric surgery is mixed [221]. One prospective study found an improvement in sperm concentration in men with azoospermia and oligospermia who underwent bariatric surgery while another found worsened sperm concentration after surgery [222,223]. At this time it is unclear what effects bariatric surgery has in reproductive function in men and whether pregnancy rates improve [221,224].

While some ideals of manliness encourage health-demoting habits, researchers also note that other masculinity ideologies—such as ideals of responsibility, strength, and "taking action"—can support men's adoption of healthier behaviors [225,226]. Clinicians know from experience that suggesting lifestyle change is often ineffective. For instance, men often fail to make healthy lifestyle changes in response to events like a disease diagnosis, for complex reasons, including masculinity ideologies and structural barriers like lack of access to necessary resources [227]. However, the experience of becoming a father—or perhaps even trying to via fertility treatment—presents a moment in which men's conceptions of themselves as men might be changing [35,228,229]. Linking the effects of men's lifestyle behaviors to their children's wellbeing is a strategy for persuading fathers to quit smoking, for example, and men presented with information about the possible effects of lifestyle behaviors on sperm health voiced desires to make healthy changes [11,230]. In their counseling regarding lifestyle change, clinicians might frame such changes as enabling paternal forms of responsibility, care, and strength. Providing examples of other men engaging in those behaviors might also help male patients to revise their normative ideas of manly health behavior [231]. As such, with the coresponsibility in a relationship, more of the "hunter-gatherer" mentality may develop, but the ignorance of being indestructible or not caring about the future may persist. Despite denial about infertility initially, especially male infertility, lifestyle habits may not change, despite a partner trying to encourage it. However, partners may also be complicit and enable each other's lifestyle issues, for example, both partners smoke. Communicating with the male partner, sometimes requires a different approach, sometimes talking in extreme consequences that could happen due to a particular behavior, for example, cancer and surgical excision. Sometimes the "guilt" of responsibility is a vehicle to the core of the patient. This involves indicating that if the male partner loves his significant other, he may not want to be so "selfish" and change his habits by being mindful and care about his partner and their future together, and hopefully the future child(ren). Also, the issue of wanting to live long enough, without personal long-term chronic illness or death, to enjoy the children and their future needs to be reiterated.

Conclusion

The goals of this chapter were to interlink medical, scientific knowledge with real-life understanding of human behavior and reproduction. The understanding of the fundamental drive in some men and women to desire biological children is stooped in science, psychology, social anthropology/behavior, and philosophy. It is a complex relationship between true knowledge, perceptions, with biases from cultural, social, or religious cues. All topics discussed are examples of the dilemmas that couples and providers have to navigate. For many couples, infertility can be devastating psychologically, resulting in a sense of grief. Physicians are usually trained in the medical side of care, but rarely formally in the science and art of psychology, social work, or financial advisor. Mental health professionals get extensive training in human behavior, motivation, and emotion but not as much in the medical science of human reproduction. For both categories of professional, empathy, compassion, and nonjudgmental sincerity are essential when working in this arena. This way providers can seek out the fundamentals of a sensitive problem to care for the patient/couple. It is important to provide a sense of "absolution" and eliminate the feeling of guilt or blame for both the male AND the female partner. Infertility is a couple's problem and not an individual issue despite past history or even indiscretions. Once blame is removed coping and healing can begin. A multidisciplinary approach as well as cross training is necessary for optimal care. Unfortunately this is rarely achieved in clinical training or in a single consult, and requires staged visits with several different specialists, from urologists, gynecologists, psychologists, social workers, genetic counselors, and financial counselors to achieve the most complete evaluation and most thorough treatment plan. Insuring that male patients seek comprehensive care can be difficult due to denial, masculine resistance, and issues too sensitive to discuss in public. The love and support between partners is needed to get them through this. With the guidance of professionals in this difficult journey, couples can be helped to cope and hopefully succeed in their family building goals.

References

[1] Thonneau P, Marchand S, Tallec A, Ferial ML, Ducot B, Lansac J, et al. Incidence and main causes of infertility in a resident population (1,850,000) of three French regions (1988–1989). Hum Reprod 1991;6(6):811–16.

[2] Zegers-Hochschild F, Adamson GD, de Mouzon J, Ishihara O, Mansour R, Nygren K, et al. International Committee for Monitoring Assisted Reproductive Technology (ICMART) and the World Health Organization (WHO) revised glossary of ART terminology, 2009. Fertil Steril 2009;92(5):1520–4.

[3] Sun H, Gong T-T, Jiang Y-T, Zhang S, Zhao Y-H, Wu Q-J. Global, regional, and national prevalence and disability-adjusted life-years for infertility in 195 countries and territories, 1990–2017: results from a global burden of disease study, 2017. Aging 2019;11(23):10952–91.

[4] Inhorn MC, editor. Reproductive disruptions: gender, technology, and biopolitics in the new millennium, vol. 11. New York: Berghahn Books; 2007.

[5] Hanna E, Gough B. Male infertility as relational: an analysis of men's reported encounters with family members and friends in the context of delayed conception. Fam Relatsh Soc 2021;10(1):51–65.

[6] Hampshire KR, Blell MT, Simpson B. 'Everybody is moving on': infertility, relationality and the aesthetics of family among British-Pakistani Muslims. Soc Sci Med 2012;74(7):1045–52.

[7] Millbank J. Exploring the ineffable in women's experiences of relationality with their stored IVF embryos. Body Soc 2017;23(4):95–120.

[8] Law C. Men on the margins? Reflections on recruiting and engaging men in reproduction research. Methodol Innov 2019;12(1) 2059799119829425.

[9] Locock L, Alexander J. Just a bystander'? Men's place in the process of fetal screening and diagnosis. Soc Sci Med 2006;62(6):1349–59.

[10] Daniels CR. Exposing men: the science and politics of male reproduction. Oxford: Oxford University Press; 2008.

[11] Almeling R. GUYnecology: the missing science of men's reproductive health. Oakland, CA: University of California Press; 2020.

[12] Anderson JE, Farr SL, Jamieson DJ, Warner L, Macaluso M. Infertility services reported by men in the United States: national survey data. Fertil Steril 2009;91(6):2466–70.

[13] Halcomb L. Men and infertility: insights from the sociology of gender. Sociol Compass 2018;12(10):12624.

[14] Mohr S, Almeling R. Men, masculinities, and reproduction—conceptual reflections and empirical explorations. NORMA 2020;163–71.

[15] Almeling R, Waggoner MR. More and less than equal: how men factor in the reproductive equation. Gend Soc 2013;27(6):821–42.

[16] Culley L, Hudson N, Lohan M. Where are all the men? The marginalization of men in social scientific research on infertility. Reprod Biomed Online 2013;27(3):225–35.

[17] Dudgeon MR, Inhorn MC. Gender, masculinity, and reproduction: anthropological perspectives. Int J Mens Health 2003;2(1):31–56.

[18] Lohan M, Marsiglio W, Lohan M, Culley L. Advancing research on men and reproduction. Int J Mens Health 2015;14(3):214.

[19] Dudgeon MR, Inhorn MC. Men's influences on women's reproductive health: medical anthropological perspectives. Soc Sci Med 2004;59(7):1379–95.

[20] Hanna E, Gough B. Experiencing male infertility: a review of the qualitative research literature. Sage Open 2015;5(4) 2158244015610319.

[21] Greene ME, Biddlecom AE. Absent and problematic men: demographic accounts of male reproductive roles. Popul Dev Rev 2000;26(1):81–115.

[22] Joja OD, Dinu D, Paun D. Psychological aspects of male infertility. An overview. Procedia Soc Behav Sci 2015;187:359–63.

[23] Daniluk JC. "If we had it to do over again…": couples' reflections on their experiences of infertility treatments. Fam J 2001;9(2):122–33.

[24] Inhorn MC. The new Arab man: emergent masculinities, technologies, and Islam in the Middle East. Princeton, NJ: Princeton University Press; 2012.

[25] Parrott FR. At the hospital I learnt the truth': diagnosing male infertility in rural Malawi. Anthropol Med 2014;21(2):174–88.

[26] Inhorn MC, Birenbaum-Carmeli D. Male infertility, chronicity, and the plight of Palestinian men in Israel and Lebanon. Chronic conditions, fluid states: chronicity and the anthropology from illness. New Brunswick, NJ: Rutgers University Press; 2010. p. 77–95.

References

[27] Wentzell E, Inhorn M. The male reproductive body. In: Mascia-Lees EFE, editor. A companion to the anthropology of the body and embodiment. New York: Wiley-Blackwell Publishers; 2011. p. 307—19.

[28] Gu Y, Liang X, Wu W, Liu M, Song S, Cheng L, et al. Multicenter contraceptive efficacy trial of injectable testosterone undecanoate in Chinese men. J Clin Endocrinol Metab 2009;94(6):1910—15.

[29] Malik SH, Coulson N. The male experience of infertility: a thematic analysis of an online infertility support group bulletin board. J Reprod Infant Psychol 2008;26(1):18—30.

[30] Hanna E, Gough B, Hudson N. Fit to father? Online accounts of lifestyle changes and help-seeking on a male infertility board. Sociol Health Illn 2018;40(6):937—53.

[31] Greil AL. Infertility and psychological distress: a critical review of the literature. Soc Sci Med 1997;45(11):1679—704.

[32] Mason MC. Male infertility—men talking. Philadelphia, PA: Psychology Press; 1993.

[33] Lenzi A, Lombardo F, Salacone P, Gandini L, Jannini EA. Stress, sexual dysfunctions, and male infertility. J Endocrinol Invest 2003;26(3 Suppl):72—6.

[34] Laitinen E, Vaaralahti K, Tommiska J, Eklund E, Tervaniemi M, Valanne L, et al. Incidence, phenotypic features and molecular genetics of Kallmann syndrome in Finland. Orphanet J Rare Dis 2011;6(1):41.

[35] Inhorn MC, Chavkin W, Navarro JA, editors. Globalized fatherhood, vol. 27. Oxford, NY: Berghahn Books; 2014.

[36] Wentzell E, Labuski C. Role of medical anthropology in understanding cultural differences. In: Rowland EDL, Jannini EA, editors. Cultural differences and the practice of sexual medicine: a guide for health practitioners. Cham: Springer Nature Switzerland AG; 2020. p. 23—35.

[37] Goldfarb ES, Lieberman LD. Three decades of research: the case for comprehensive sex education. J Adolesc Health 2021;68(1):13—27.

[38] Mehta A, Nangia AK, Dupree JM, Smith JF. Limitations and barriers in access to care for male factor infertility. Fertil Steril 2016;105(5):1128—37.

[39] Cussins C. Ontological choreography: agency through objectification in infertility clinics. Soc Stud Sci 1996;26(3):575—610.

[40] Pedro J, Brandão T, Schmidt L, Costa ME, Martins MV. What do people know about fertility? A systematic review on fertility awareness and its associated factors. Ups J Med Sci 2018;123(2):71—81.

[41] Bunting L, Tsibulsky I, Boivin J. Fertility knowledge and beliefs about fertility treatment: findings from the International Fertility Decision-making Study. Hum Reprod 2013;28(2):385—97.

[42] Weschler T. Taking charge of your fertility: the definitive guide to natural birth control, pregnancy achievement, and reproductive health. Random House; 2003.

[43] Barrett DG. Mum's the word: are we becoming silent on masturbation? Psychoanal Study Child 2012;66(1):173—96.

[44] Layton J, Kim Y, Alexander G, Emery S. Association between direct-to-consumer advertising and testosterone testing and initiation in the United States, 2009—2013. JAMA. 2017;317(11):1159.

[45] Tao P, Coates R, Maycock B. The impact of infertility on sexuality: a literature review. Australas Med J 2011;4(11):620—7.

[46] Kentenich H, Schmiady H, Radke E, Stief G, Blankau A. The male IVF patient—psychosomatic considerations. Hum Reprod 1992;7 (Suppl 1):13—18.

[47] Licht RS, Handel L, Sigman M. Site of semen collection and its effect on semen analysis parameters. Fertil Steril 2008;89(2):395—7.

[48] Shen JT. Adolescent sexual counseling. Postgrad Med 1982;71(5):91—3 96—7, 100.

[49] Smith AM, Rosenthal DA, Reichler H. High schoolers masturbatory practices: their relationship to sexual intercourse and personal characteristics. Psychol Rep 1996;79(2):499—509.

[50] Kolettis PN, Purcell ML, Parker W, Poston T, Nangia AK. Medical testosterone: an iatrogenic cause of male infertility and a growing problem. Urology 2015;85(5):1068—73.

[51] Samplaski MK, Loai Y, Wong K, Lo KC, Grober ED, Jarvi KA. Testosterone use in the male infertility population: prescribing patterns and effects on semen and hormonal parameters. Fertil Steril 2013;101(1):64—9.

[52] Ko EY, Siddiqi K, Brannigan RE, Sabanegh ES. Empirical medical therapy for idiopathic male infertility: a survey of the American Urological Association. J Urol 2012;187(3):973—8.

[53] Bute JJ. "Nobody thinks twice about asking": women with a fertility problem and requests for information. Health Commun 2009;24(8):752—63.

[54] Hanna E, Gough B. The social construction of male infertility: a qualitative questionnaire study of men with a male factor infertility diagnosis. Sociol Health Illn 2020;42(3):465—80.

[55] Wischmann T, Thorn P. (Male) infertility: what does it mean to men? New evidence from quantitative and qualitative studies. Reprod Biomed Online 2013;27(3):236—43.

[56] Naab F, Kwashie AA. 'I don't experience any insults, but my wife does': the concerns of men with infertility in Ghana. South Afr J Obstet Gynaecol 2018;24(2):45—8.

[57] Cui W. Mother or nothing: the agony of infertility. Bull World Health Organ 2010;88(12):881—2.

[58] Inhorn MC. Infertility and patriarchy: the cultural politics of gender and family life in Egypt. Philadelphia, PA: University of Pennsylvania Press; 1996.

[59] Strasser MO, Dupree JM. Care delivery for male infertility: the present and future. Urol Clin N Am 2020;47(2):193—204.

[60] Katz P, Showstack J, Smith JF, Nachtigall RD, Millstein SG, Wing H, et al. Costs of infertility treatment: results from an 18-month prospective cohort study. Fertil Steril 2011;95(3):915—21.

[61] Wu AK, Odisho AY, Washington SL, Katz PP, Smith JF. Out-of-pocket fertility patient expense: data from a multicenter prospective infertility cohort. J Urol 2014;191(2):427—32.

[62] Wu AK, Elliott P, Katz PP, Smith JF. Time costs of fertility care: the hidden hardship of building a family. Fertil Steril 2013;99(7):2025—30.

[63] Punab M, Poolamets O, Paju P, Vihljajev V, Pomm K, Ladva R, et al. Causes of male infertility: a 9-year prospective monocentre study on 1737 patients with reduced total sperm counts. Hum Reprod 2017;32(1):18—31.

[64] Niederberger C. WHO manual for the standardized investigation, diagnosis and management of the infertile male. Urology 2001;57(1):208.
[65] Mulhall JP, Trost LW, Brannigan RE, Kurtz EG, Redmon JB, Chiles KA, et al. Evaluation and management of testosterone deficiency: AUA guideline. J Urol 2018;200(2):423–32.
[66] Handelsman DJ. Global trends in testosterone prescribing, 2000–2011: expanding the spectrum of prescription drug misuse. Med J Aust 2013;199(8):548–51.
[67] Baillargeon J. Screening and monitoring in men prescribed testosterone therapy in the United States, 2001–2010. Public Health Rep 2015;130(2):143–52.
[68] Layton JB, Li D, Meier CR, Sharpless JL, Stürmer T, Jick SS, et al. Testosterone lab testing and initiation in the United Kingdom and the United States, 2000 to 2011. J Clin Endocrinol Metab 2014;99(3):835–42.
[69] Irwig MS, Fleseriu M, Jonklaas J, Tritos NA, Yuen KCJ, Correa R, et al. Off-label use and misuse of testosterone, growth hormone, thyroid hormone, and adrenal supplements: risks and costs of a growing problem. Endocr Pract 2020;26(3):340–53.
[70] Kim ED, Crosnoe L, Bar-Chama N, Khera M, Lipshultz LI. The treatment of hypogonadism in men of reproductive age. Fertil Steril 2013;99(3):718–24.
[71] Tatem AJ, Beilan J, Kovac JR, Lipshultz LI. Management of anabolic steroid-induced infertility: novel strategies for fertility maintenance and recovery. World J Mens Health 2020;38(2):141–50.
[72] Pope H, Wood R, Rogol A, Nyberg F, Bowers L, Bhasin S. Adverse health consequences of performance-enhancing drugs: an endocrine society scientific statement. Endocr Rev 2013;35(3):341–75.
[73] Mędraś M, Brona A, Jóźków P. The central effects of androgenic-anabolic steroid use. J Addict Med 2018;12(3):184–92.
[74] Quaglio G, Fornasiero A, Mezzelani P, Moreschini S, Lugoboni F, Lechi A. Anabolic steroids: dependence and complications of chronic use. Intern Emerg Med 2009;4(4):289–96.
[75] Foster AC, Shorter GW, Griffiths MD. Muscle dysmorphia: could it be classified as an addiction to body image? J Behav Addict 2015;4(1):1–5.
[76] Wroblewska AM. Androgenic–anabolic steroids and body dysmorphia in young men. J Psychosom Res 1997;42(3):225–34.
[77] Coward RM, Rajanahally S, Kovac JR, Smith RP, Pastuszak AW, Lipshultz LI. Anabolic steroid induced hypogonadism in young men. J Urol 2013;190(6):2200–5.
[78] Rahnema CD, Lipshultz LI, Crosnoe LE, Kovac JR, Kim ED. Anabolic steroid-induced hypogonadism: diagnosis and treatment. Fertil Steril 2014;101(5):1271–9.
[79] Armstrong JM, Avant RA, Charchenko CM, Westerman ME, Ziegelmann MJ, Miest TS, et al. Impact of anabolic androgenic steroids on sexual function. Transl Androl Urol 2018;7(3):483–9.
[80] Kovac JR, Scovell J, Ramasamy R, Rajanahally S, Coward RM, Smith RP, et al. Men regret anabolic steroid use due to a lack of comprehension regarding the consequences on future fertility. Andrologia 2015;47(8):872–8.
[81] Drobnis EZ, Nangia AK. Introduction to medication effects on male reproduction. Adv Exp Med Biol 2017;1034:1–4.
[82] Brown MT, Bussell J, Dutta S, Davis K, Strong S, Mathew S. Medication adherence: truth and consequences. Am J Med Sci 2016;351(4):387–99.
[83] Wieder JA. Pocket guide to urology. 5th ed. Oakland, CA: Medical; 2014.
[84] Sultan RS, Correll CU, Schoenbaum M, King M, Walkup JT, Olfson M. National patterns of commonly prescribed psychotropic medications to young people. J Child Adolesc Psychopharmacol 2018;28(3):158–65.
[85] Sylvester C, Menke M, Gopalan P. Selective serotonin reuptake inhibitors and fertility. Harv Rev Psychiatry 2019;27(2):108–18.
[86] Samplaski MK, Nangia AK. Adverse effects of common medications on male fertility. Nat Rev Urol 2015 Jul;12(7):401–13.
[87] Drobnis EZ, Nangia AK. 5α-Reductase inhibitors (5ARIs) and male reproduction. Adv Exp Med Biol 2017;1034:59–61.
[88] Samplaski MK, Lo K, Grober E, Jarvi K. Finasteride use in the male infertility population: effects on semen and hormone parameters. Fertil Steril 2013;100(6):1542–6.
[89] Amory JK, Wang C, Swerdloff RS, Anawalt BD, Matsumoto AM, Bremner WJ, et al. The effect of 5alpha-reductase inhibition with dutasteride and finasteride on semen parameters and serum hormones in healthy men. J Clin Endocrinol Metab 2007;92(5):1659–65.
[90] Tu HYV, Zini A. Finasteride-induced secondary infertility associated with sperm DNA damage. Fertil Steril 2011;95(6):2125.e13–14.
[91] Traish AM. Post-finasteride syndrome: a surmountable challenge for clinicians. Fertil Steril 2020;113(1):21–50.
[92] Klosky JL, Flynn JS, Lehmann V, Russell KM, Wang F, Hardin RN, et al. Parental influences on sperm banking attempts among adolescent males newly diagnosed with cancer. Fertil Steril 2017;108(6):1043–9.
[93] Green DM, Liu W, Kutteh WH, Ke RW, Shelton KC, Sklar CA, et al. Cumulative alkylating agent exposure and semen parameters in adult survivors of childhood cancer: a report from the St Jude Lifetime Cohort Study. Lancet Oncol 2014;15(11):1215–23.
[94] Lee SJ, Schover LR, Partridge AH, Patrizio P, Wallace WH, Hagerty K, et al. American Society of Clinical Oncology recommendations on fertility preservation in cancer patients. J Clin Oncol 2006;24(18):2917–31.
[95] Nangia AK, Krieg SA, Kim SS. Clinical guidelines for sperm cryopreservation in cancer patients. Fertil Steril 2013;100(5):1203–9.
[96] Schover LR, Brey K, Lichtin A, Lipshultz LI, Jeha S. Oncologists' attitudes and practices regarding banking sperm before cancer treatment. J Clin Oncol 2002;20(7):1890–7.
[97] Buhling K, Schumacher A, Eulenburg CZ, Laakmann E. Influence of oral vitamin and mineral supplementation on male infertility: a meta-analysis and systematic review. Reprod Biomed Online 2019;39(2):269–79.
[98] Yao DF, Mills JN. Male infertility: lifestyle factors and holistic, complementary, and alternative therapies. Asian J Androl 2016;18(3):410–18.
[99] Samplaski MK, Clemesha CG. Discrepancies between the internet and academic literature regarding vitamin use for male infertility. Transl Androl Urol 2018;7(Suppl 2):S193–197.
[100] Groth KA, Skakkebæk A, Høst C, Gravholt CH, Bojesen A. Clinical review: Klinefelter syndrome—a clinical update. J Clin Endocrinol Metab 2013;98(1):20–30.
[101] Zitzmann M, Rohayem J. Gonadal dysfunction and beyond: clinical challenges in children, adolescents, and adults with 47,XXY Klinefelter syndrome. Am J Med Genet C Semin Med Genet 2020;184(2):302–12.

References

[102] Tournaye H, Krausz C, Oates RD. Novel concepts in the aetiology of male reproductive impairment. Lancet Diabetes Endocrinol 2017;5(7):544–53.

[103] Schiff JD, Palermo GD, Veeck LL, Goldstein M, Rosenwaks Z, Schlegel PN. Success of testicular sperm injection and intracytoplasmic sperm injection in men with Klinefelter syndrome. J Clin Endocrinol Metab 2005;90(1):6263–7. Available from: https://doi.org/10.1210/jc.2004-2322.

[104] Gravholt CH, Chang S, Wallentin M, Fedder J, Moore P, Skakkebæk A. Klinefelter syndrome: integrating genetics, neuropsychology, and endocrinology. Endocr Rev 2018;39(4):389–423.

[105] Skakkebæk A, Wallentin M, Gravholt CH. Neuropsychology and socioeconomic aspects of Klinefelter syndrome: new developments. Curr Opin Endocrinol Diabetes Obes 2015;22(3):209–16.

[106] Davis SM, Rogol AD, Ross JL. Testis development and fertility potential in boys with Klinefelter syndrome. Endocrinol Metab Clin N Am 2015;44(4):843–65.

[107] Paduch DA, Bolyakov A, Cohen P, Travis A. Reproduction in men with Klinefelter syndrome: the past, the present, and the future. Semin Reprod Med 2009;27(2):137–48.

[108] Mehta A, Paduch DA. Klinefelter syndrome: an argument for early aggressive hormonal and fertility management. Fertil Steril 2012;98(2):274–83.

[109] de Vries JW, Repping S, van Daalen SK, Korver CM, Leschot NJ, van der Veen F. Clinical relevance of partial AZFc deletions. Fertil Steril 2002;78(6):1209–14.

[110] Fan Y, Silber SJY. Chromosome infertility In: Adam MP, Ardinger HH, Pagon RA, Wallace SE, Bean LJ, Stephens K, et al., editors. GeneReviews®. Seattle, WA: University of Washington, Seattle; 1993Available from:. Available from: http://www.ncbi.nlm.nih.gov/books/NBK1339.

[111] Colaco S, Modi D. Genetics of the human Y chromosome and its association with male infertility. Reprod Biol Endocrinol 2018;16(1):14.

[112] Faddy MJ, Silber SJ, Gosden RG. Intra-cytoplasmic sperm injection and infertility. Nat Genet 2001;29(2):131.

[113] Choi JM, Chung P, Veeck L, Mielnik A, Palermo GD, Schlegel PN. AZF microdeletions of the Y chromosome and in vitro fertilization outcome. Fertil Steril 2004;81(2):337–41.

[114] Mau Kai C, Juul A, McElreavey K, Ottesen AM, Garn ID, Main KM, et al. Sons conceived by assisted reproduction techniques inherit deletions in the azoospermia factor (AZF) region of the Y chromosome and the DAZ gene copy number. Hum Reprod 2008;23(7):1669–78.

[115] Page DC, Silber S, Brown LG. Men with infertility caused by AZFc deletion can produce sons by intracytoplasmic sperm injection, but are likely to transmit the deletion and infertility. Hum Reprod 1999;14(7):1722–6.

[116] Corona G, Pizzocaro A, Lanfranco F, Garolla A, Pelliccione F, Vignozzi L, et al. Sperm recovery and ICSI outcomes in Klinefelter syndrome: a systematic review and meta-analysis. Hum Reprod Update 2017;23(3):265–75.

[117] Eisenberg ML, Smith JF, Millstein SG, Walsh TJ, Breyer BN, Katz PP. Perceived negative consequences of donor gametes from male and female members of infertile couples. Fertil Steril 2010;94(3):921–6.

[118] Lampic C, Skoog Svanberg A, Sydsjö G. Attitudes towards disclosure and relationship to donor offspring among a national cohort of identity-release oocyte and sperm donors. Hum Reprod 2014;29(9):1978–86.

[119] Blyth E, Crawshaw M, Frith L, Jones C. Donor-conceived people's views and experiences of their genetic origins: a critical analysis of the research evidence. J Law Med 2012;19(4):769–89.

[120] de Souza D a S, Faucz FR, Pereira-Ferrari L, Sotomaior VS, Raskin S. Congenital bilateral absence of the vas deferens as an atypical form of cystic fibrosis: reproductive implications and genetic counseling. Andrology 2018;6(1):127–35.

[121] Wein AJ, Kavoussi LR, Campbell MF. Campbell-Walsh urology. 10th ed. Philadelphia, PA: Elsevier Saunders; 2012.

[122] Chillón M, Casals T, Mercier B, Bassas L, Lissens W, Silber S, et al. Mutations in the cystic fibrosis gene in patients with congenital absence of the vas deferens. N Engl J Med 1995;332(22):1475–80.

[123] Noone PG, Knowles MR. CFTR-opathies': disease phenotypes associated with cystic fibrosis transmembrane regulator gene mutations. Respir Res 2001;2(6):328–32.

[124] Kamal A, Fahmy I, Mansour R. Does the outcome of ICSI in cases of obstructive azoospermia depend on the origin of the retrieved spermatozoa or the cause of obstruction? A comparative analysis. Fertil Steril 2010;94(6):2135–40.

[125] McCallum T, Milunsky J, Munarriz R, Carson R, Sadeghi-Nejad H, Oates R. Unilateral renal agenesis associated with congenital bilateral absence of the vas deferens: phenotypic findings and genetic considerations. Hum Reprod 2001;16(2):282–8.

[126] Bernie AM, Osterberg EC, Stahl PJ, Ramasamy R, Goldstein M. Vasectomy reversal in humans. Spermatogenesis 2012;2(4):273–8.

[127] Barone MA, Hutchinson PL, Johnson CH, Hsia J, Wheeler J. Vasectomy in the United States, 2002. J Urol 2006;176(1):232–6.

[128] Jamieson DJ, Costello C, Trussell J, Hillis SD, Marchbanks PA, Peterson HBUnited States Collaborative Review of Sterilization Working Group. The risk of pregnancy after vasectomy. Obstet Gynecol 2004;103(5 Pt 1):848–50.

[129] Sharlip ID, Belker AM, Honig S, Labrecque M, Marmar JL, Ross LS, et al. Vasectomy: AUA guideline. J Urol 2012;188(6 Suppl):2482–91.

[130] Potts JM, Pasqualotto FF, Nelson D, Thomas AJ, Agarwal A. Patient characteristics associated with vasectomy reversal. J Urol 1999;161(6):1835–9.

[131] Howard G. Who asks for vasectomy reversal and why? Br Med J (Clin Res Ed) 1982;285(6340):490–2.

[132] Belker AM, Thomas AJ, Fuchs EF, Konnak JW, Sharlip ID. Results of 1,469 microsurgical vasectomy reversals by the Vasovasostomy Study Group. J Urol 1991;145(3):505–11.

[133] Pavlovich CP, Schlegel PN. Fertility options after vasectomy: a cost-effectiveness analysis. Fertil Steril 1997;67(1):133–41.

[134] Kolettis PN, Sabanegh ES, Nalesnik JG, D'Amico AM, Box LC, Burns JR. Pregnancy outcomes after vasectomy reversal for female partners 35 years old or older. J Urol 2003;169(6):2250–2.

[135] Hourvitz A, Machtinger R, Maman E, Baum M, Dor J, Levron J. Assisted reproduction in women over 40 years of age: how old is too old? Reprod Biomed Online 2009;19(4):599–603.

[136] Munné S, Fischer J, Warner A, Chen S, Zouves C, Cohen J, et al. Preimplantation genetic diagnosis significantly reduces pregnancy loss in infertile couples: a multicenter study. Fertil Steril 2006;85(2):326–32.

[137] Pastuszak AW, Wang R. Varicocele and testicular function. Asian J Androl 2015;17(4):659−67.
[138] Agarwal A, Deepinder F, Cocuzza M, Agarwal R, Short RA, Sabanegh E, et al. Efficacy of varicocelectomy in improving semen parameters: new *meta*-analytical approach. Urology. 2007;70(3):532−8.
[139] Chiba K, Ramasamy R, Lamb DJ, Lipshultz LI. The varicocele: diagnostic dilemmas, therapeutic challenges and future perspectives. Asian J Androl 2016;18(2):276−81.
[140] Maheshwari A, Muneer A, Lucky M, Mathur R, McEleny K. British Association of Urological Surgeons and the British Fertility Society. A review of varicocele treatment and fertility outcomes. Hum Fertil (Camb) 2020;7:1−8.
[141] Nieschlag E, Hertle L, Fischedick A, Abshagen K, Behre HM. Update on treatment of varicocele: counselling as effective as occlusion of the vena spermatica. Hum Reprod 1998;13(8):2147−50.
[142] Evers JL, Collins JA. Surgery or embolisation for varicocele in subfertile men. Cochrane Database Syst Rev 2004;3(3):CD000479.
[143] Samplaski MK, Lo KC, Grober ED, Zini A, Jarvi KA. Varicocelectomy to "upgrade" semen quality to allow couples to use less invasive forms of assisted reproductive technology. Fertil Steril 2017;108(4):609−12.
[144] Kirby EW, Wiener LE, Rajanahally S, Crowell K, Coward RM. Undergoing varicocele repair before assisted reproduction improves pregnancy rate and live birth rate in azoospermic and oligospermic men with a varicocele: a systematic review and *meta*-analysis. Fertil Steril 2016;106(6):1338−43.
[145] Howlader N, Noone AM, Krapcho M, Miller D, Brest A, Yu M, et al., editors. SEER Cancer Statistics Review, 1975−2017. Bethesda, MD: National Cancer Institute; 1975Available from:. Available from: https://seer.cancer.gov/csr/1975_2017/.
[146] Ishikawa T, Kamidono S, Fujisawa M. Fertility after high-dose chemotherapy for testicular cancer. Urology 2004;63(1):137−40.
[147] Incrocci L, Bosch JL, Slob AK. Testicular prostheses: body image and sexual functioning. BJU Int 1999;84(9):1043−5.
[148] Srivatsav A, Balasubramanian A, Butaney M, Thirumavalavan N, McBride JA, Gondokusumo J, et al. Patient attitudes toward testicular prosthesis placement after orchiectomy. Am J Mens Health 2019;13(4) 1557988319861019.
[149] Chapple A, McPherson A. The decision to have a prosthesis: a qualitative study of men with testicular cancer. Psychooncology 2004;13(9):654−64.
[150] Schover LR, von Eschenbach AC. Sexual and marital relationships after treatment for nonseminomatous testicular cancer. Urology 1985;25(3):251−5.
[151] Chambers SK, Occhipinti S, Schover L, Nielsen L, Zajdlewicz L, Clutton S, et al. A randomised controlled trial of a couples-based sexuality intervention for men with localised prostate cancer and their female partners. Psychooncology 2015;24(7):748−56.
[152] Schover LR, von Eschenbach AC, Smith DB, Gonzalez J. Sexual rehabilitation of urologic cancer patients: a practical approach. CA Cancer J Clin 1984;34(2):66−74.
[153] Schover LR, Evans R, von Eschenbach AC. Sexual rehabilitation and male radical cystectomy. J Urol 1986;136(5):1015−17.
[154] Zaccardi F, Webb DR, Yates T, Davies MJ. Pathophysiology of type 1 and type 2 diabetes mellitus: a 90-year perspective. Postgrad Med J 2016;92(1084):63−9.
[155] Haffner SM. Epidemiology of type 2 diabetes: risk factors. Diabetes Care 1998;21(Suppl 3):C3−6.
[156] La Vignera S, Condorelli RA, Di Mauro M, Lo Presti D, Mongioì LM, Russo G, et al. Reproductive function in male patients with type 1 diabetes mellitus. Andrology 2015;3(6):1082−7.
[157] Kouidrat Y, Pizzol D, Cosco T, Thompson T, Carnaghi M, Bertoldo A, et al. High prevalence of erectile dysfunction in diabetes: a systematic review and meta-analysis of 145 studies. Diabet Med 2017;34(9):1185−92.
[158] Kasturi SS, Tannir J, Brannigan RE. The metabolic syndrome and male infertility. J Androl 2008;29(3):251−9.
[159] Ding G-L, Liu Y, Liu M-E, Pan J-X, Guo M-X, Sheng J-Z, et al. The effects of diabetes on male fertility and epigenetic regulation during spermatogenesis. Asian J Androl 2015;17(6):948−53.
[160] Vernon M, Wilson E, Muse K, Estes S, Curry T. Successful pregnancies from men with retrograde ejaculation with the use of washed sperm and gamete intrafallopian tube transfer (GIFT). Fertil Steril 1988;50(5):822−4.
[161] Kam J, Tsang VH, Chalasani V. Retrograde ejaculation: a rare presenting symptom of type 1 diabetes mellitus. Urol Case Rep 2016;10:9−10.
[162] Jefferys A, Siassakos D, Wardle P. The management of retrograde ejaculation: a systematic review and update. Fertil Steril 2012;97(2):306−312.e6.
[163] Otani T. Clinical review of ejaculatory dysfunction. Reprod Med Biol 2019;18(4):331−43.
[164] Philippon M, Karsenty G, Bernuz B, Courbiere B, Brue T, Saïas-Magnan J, et al. Successful pregnancies and healthy live births using frozen-thawed sperm retrieved by a new modified Hotchkiss procedure in males with retrograde ejaculation: first case series Basic Clin Androl 2015;25:5Available from:. Available from: https://www.ncbi.nlm.nih.gov/pmc/articles/PMC4450833/.
[165] Rosenlund B, Sjöblom P, Törnblom M, Hultling C, Hillensjö T. In-vitro fertilization and intracytoplasmic sperm injection in the treatment of infertility after testicular cancer. Hum Reprod 1998;13(2):414−18.
[166] Colpi G, Weidner W, Jungwirth A, Pomerol J, Papp G, Hargreave T, et al. EAU guidelines on ejaculatory dysfunction. Eur Urol 2004;46(5):555−8.
[167] Gray M, Zillioux J, Khourdaji I, Smith RP. Contemporary management of ejaculatory dysfunction. Transl Androl Urol 2018;7(4):686−702.
[168] Heruti RJ, Katz H, Menashe Y, Weissenberg R, Raviv G, Madjar I, et al. Treatment of male infertility due to spinal cord injury using rectal probe electroejaculation: the Israeli experience. Spinal Cord 2001;39(3):168−75.
[169] Anderson R, Moses R, Lenherr S, Hotaling JM, Myers J. Spinal cord injury and male infertility—a review of current literature, knowledge gaps, and future research. Transl Androl Urol 2018;7(Suppl 3):S373−382.
[170] Ibrahim E, Lynne CM, Brackett NL. Male fertility following spinal cord injury: an update. Andrology 2016;4(1):13−26.
[171] Kumar N, Singh AK. Trends of male factor infertility, an important cause of infertility: a review of literature. J Hum Reprod Sci 2015;8(4):191−6.
[172] Sekhon LH, Fehlings MG. Epidemiology, demographics, and pathophysiology of acute spinal cord injury. Spine 2001;26(24 Suppl):S2−12.
[173] Hagen EM, Rekand T, Gilhus NE, Grønning M. Traumatic spinal cord injuries—incidence, mechanisms and course. Tidsskr Den Laegeforen 2012;132(7):831−7.

[174] Klyce DW, Bombardier CH, Davis TJ, Hartoonian N, Hoffman JM, Fann JR, et al. Distinguishing grief from depression during acute recovery from spinal cord injury. Arch Phys Med Rehabil 2015;96(8):1419–25.

[175] Simpson LA, Eng JJ, Hsieh JTC, Wolfe DLSpinal Cord Injury Rehabilitation Evidence Scire Research Team. The health and life priorities of individuals with spinal cord injury: a systematic review. J Neurotrauma 2012;29(8):1548–55.

[176] Stiens SA, Kirshblum SC, Groah SL, McKinley WO, Gittler MS. Spinal cord injury medicine. 4. Optimal participation in life after spinal cord injury: physical, psychosocial, and economic reintegration into the environment. Arch Phys Med Rehabil 2002;83(3 Suppl 1): S72–81 S90–98.

[177] Canada AL, Schover LR. Research promoting better patient education on reproductive health after cancer. J Natl Cancer Inst Monogr 2005;2005(34):98–100.

[178] Klosky JL, Wang F, Russell KM, Zhang H, Flynn JS, Huang L, et al. Prevalence and predictors of sperm banking in adolescents newly diagnosed with cancer: examination of adolescent, parent, and provider factors influencing fertility preservation outcomes. J Clin Oncol 2017;35(34):3830–6.

[179] Klosky JL, Lehmann V, Flynn JS, Su Y, Zhang H, Russell K, et al. Patient factors associated with sperm cryopreservation among at-risk adolescents newly diagnosed with cancer. Cancer 2018;124(17):3567–75.

[180] Ethics Committee of the American Society for Reproductive Medicine. Posthumous retrieval and use of gametes or embryos: an Ethics Committee opinion. Fertil Steril 2018;110(1):45–9.

[181] Shin M, Kucik JE, Siffel C, Lu C, Shaw GM, Canfield MA, et al. Improved survival among children with spina bifida in the United States. J Pediatr 2012;161(6):1132–7.

[182] Bong GW, Rovner ES. Sexual health in adult men with spina bifida. ScientificWorldJournal 2007;7:1466–9.

[183] Gamé X, Moscovici J, Gamé L, Sarramon J-P, Rischmann P, Malavaud B. Evaluation of sexual function in young men with spina bifida and myelomeningocele using the International Index of Erectile Function. Urology 2006;67(3):566–70.

[184] Ferrara P, Rossodivita A, Ruggiero A, Pulitanò S, Tortorolo L, Salvaggio E. Cryptorchidism associated with meningomyelocele. J Paediatr Child Health 1998;34(1):44–6.

[185] Toppari J, Kaleva M. Maldescendus testis. Horm Res 1999;51(6):261–9.

[186] Docimo SG, Silver RI, Cromie W. The undescended testicle: diagnosis and management. Am Fam Physician 2000;62(9):2037–44 2047–8.

[187] Kobayashi H, Nagao K, Nakajima K. Therapeutic advances in the field of male infertility: stem cell research. Adv Stud Med Sci 2013;1(1–4):39–54.

[188] Huff DS, Hadziselimovic F, Snyder HM, Blythe B, Ducket JW. Histologic maldevelopment of unilaterally cryptorchid testes and their descended partners. Eur J Pediatr 1993;152(Suppl 2):S11–14.

[189] Thorup J, McLachlan R, Cortes D, Nation TR, Balic A, Southwell BR, et al. What is new in cryptorchidism and hypospadias—a critical review on the testicular dysgenesis hypothesis. J Pediatr Surg 2010;45(10):2074–86.

[190] Wiepjes CM, Nota NM, de Blok CJM, Klaver M, de Vries ALC, Wensing-Kruger SA, et al. The Amsterdam cohort of gender dysphoria study (1972–2015): trends in prevalence, treatment, and regrets. J Sex Med 2018;15(4):582–90.

[191] Auer MK, Fuss J, Nieder TO, Briken P, Biedermann SV, Stalla GK, et al. Desire to have children among transgender people in Germany: a cross-sectional multi-center study. J Sex Med 2018;15(5):757–67.

[192] Wierckx K, Van Caenegem E, Pennings G, Elaut E, Dedecker D, Van de Peer F, et al. Reproductive wish in transsexual men. Hum Reprod 2012;27(2):483–7.

[193] Neblett MF, Hipp HS. Fertility considerations in transgender persons. Endocrinol Metab Clin N Am 2019;48(2):391–402.

[194] Sansone A, Di Dato C, de Angelis C, Menafra D, Pozza C, Pivonello R, et al. Smoke, alcohol and drug addiction and male fertility Reprod Biol Endocrinol 2018;16(1):3Available from:. Available from: https://www.ncbi.nlm.nih.gov/pmc/articles/PMC5769315/.

[195] Holmila M, Raitasalo K. Gender differences in drinking: why do they still exist? Addiction 2005;100(12):1763–9.

[196] Kodriati N, Pursell L, Hayati EN. A scoping review of men, masculinities, and smoking behavior: the importance of settings. Glob Health Action 2018;11(Suppl 3):1589763.

[197] Korcha RA, Cherpitel CJ, Witbrodt J, Borges G, Hejazi-Bazargan S, Bond JC, et al. Violence-related injury and gender: the role of alcohol and alcohol combined with illicit drugs. Drug Alcohol Rev 2014;33(1):43–50.

[198] Courtenay WH. Constructions of masculinity and their influence on men's well-being: a theory of gender and health. Soc Sci Med 2000;50(10):1385–401.

[199] Galdas PM, Cheater F, Marshall P. Men and health help-seeking behaviour: literature review. J Adv Nurs 2005;49(6):616–23.

[200] O'Brien R, Hunt K, Hart G. "It's caveman stuff, but that is to a certain extent how guys still operate": men's accounts of masculinity and help seeking. Soc Sci Med 2005;61(3):503–16.

[201] Kovac JR, Khanna A, Lipshultz LI. The effects of cigarette smoking on male fertility. Postgrad Med 2015;127(3):338–41.

[202] Ramlau-Hansen CH, Thulstrup AM, Aggerholm AS, Jensen MS, Toft G, Bonde JP. Is smoking a risk factor for decreased semen quality? A cross-sectional analysis. Hum Reprod 2007;22(1):188–96.

[203] Oyeyipo IP, Raji Y, Emikpe BO, Bolarinwa AF. Effects of nicotine on sperm characteristics and fertility profile in adult male rats: a possible role of cessation. J Reprod Infertil 2011;12(3):201–7.

[204] SAMHSA. Section 2 PE Tables—Results from the 2019 National Survey on Drug Use and Health: Detailed Tables, SAMHSA, CBHSQ. Available from: <https://www.samhsa.gov/data/sites/default/files/reports/rpt29394/NSDUHDetailedTabs2019/NSDUHDetTabsSect2pe2019.htm> [cited February 24, 2021].

[205] Jensen TK, Gottschau M, Madsen JOB, Andersson A-M, Lassen TH, Skakkebæk NE, et al. Habitual alcohol consumption associated with reduced semen quality and changes in reproductive hormones; a cross-sectional study among 1221 young Danish men. BMJ Open 2014;4(9):e005462.

[206] Ginn SK, Clark E. The medical profession and stigma against people who use drugs. Br J Psychiatry 2017;211(6):400.

[207] Tomiyama AJ, Carr D, Granberg E, Major B, Robinson E, Sutin A, et al. How and why weight stigma drives the obesity 'epidemic' and harms health. BMC Med 2018;16:123.

[208] Salas-Huetos A, Bulló M, Salas-Salvadó J. Dietary patterns, foods and nutrients in male fertility parameters and fecundability: a systematic review of observational studies. Hum Reprod Update 2017;23(4):371−89.
[209] Gewertz DB, Errington FK. Cheap meat: flap food nations in the Pacific Islands. Oakland, CA: University of California Press; 2010.
[210] Gough B, Conner MT. Barriers to healthy eating amongst men: a qualitative analysis. Soc Sci Med 2006;62(2):387−95.
[211] WHO. Obesity and overweight. Available from: <https://www.who.int/news-room/fact-sheets/detail/obesity-and-overweight>, [cited February 24, 2021].
[212] Grover SA, Kaouache M, Rempel P, Joseph L, Dawes M, Lau DCW, et al. Years of life lost and healthy life-years lost from diabetes and cardiovascular disease in overweight and obese people: a modelling study. Lancet Diabetes Endocrinol 2015;3(2):114−22.
[213] Taylor VH, Forhan M, Vigod SN, McIntyre RS, Morrison KM. The impact of obesity on quality of life. Best Pract Res Clin Endocrinol Metab 2013;27(2):139−46.
[214] Poirier P, Giles TD, Bray GA, Hong Y, Stern JS, Pi-Sunyer FX, et al. Obesity and cardiovascular disease: pathophysiology, evaluation, and effect of weight loss: an update of the 1997 American Heart Association Scientific Statement on Obesity and Heart Disease from the Obesity Committee of the Council on Nutrition, Physical Activity, and Metabolism. Circulation 2006;113(6):898−918.
[215] Guh DP, Zhang W, Bansback N, Amarsi Z, Birmingham CL, Anis AH. The incidence of co-morbidities related to obesity and overweight: a systematic review and meta-analysis. BMC Public Health 2009;9:88.
[216] Lauby-Secretan B, Scoccianti C, Loomis D, Grosse Y, Bianchini F, Straif K. Body fatness and cancer—viewpoint of the IARC Working Group. N Engl J Med 2016;375(8):794−8.
[217] Du Plessis SS, Cabler S, McAlister DA, Sabanegh E, Agarwal A. The effect of obesity on sperm disorders and male infertility. Nat Rev Urol 2010;7(3):153−61.
[218] Lee Y, Dang JT, Switzer N, Yu J, Tian C, Birch DW, et al. Impact of bariatric surgery on male sex hormones and sperm quality: a systematic review and meta-analysis. Obes Surg 2019;29(1):334−46.
[219] Sallmén M, Sandler DP, Hoppin JA, Blair A, Baird DD. Reduced fertility among overweight and obese men. Epidemiology (Cambridge, Mass) 2006;17(5):520−3.
[220] Fui MNT, Dupuis P, Grossmann M. Lowered testosterone in male obesity: mechanisms, morbidity and management. Asian J Androl 2014;16(2):223−31.
[221] Di Vincenzo A, Busetto L, Vettor R, Rossato M. Obesity, male reproductive function and bariatric surgery Front Endocrinol (Lausanne) 2018;9:769Available from:. Available from: https://www.ncbi.nlm.nih.gov/pmc/articles/PMC6305362/.
[222] Wood GJA, Tiseo BC, Paluello DV, de Martin H, Santo MA, Nahas W, et al. Bariatric surgery impact on reproductive hormones, semen analysis, and sperm DNA fragmentation in men with severe obesity: prospective study. Obes Surg 2020;30(12):4840−51.
[223] El Bardisi H, Majzoub A, Arafa M, AlMalki A, Al Said S, Khalafalla K, et al. Effect of bariatric surgery on semen parameters and sex hormone concentrations: a prospective study. Reprod Biomed Online 2016;33(5):606−11.
[224] Moxthe LC, Sauls R, Ruiz M, Stern M, Gonzalvo J, Gray HL. Effects of bariatric surgeries on male and female fertility: a systematic review. J Reprod Infertil 2020;21(2):71−86.
[225] Farrimond H. Beyond the caveman: rethinking masculinity in relation to men's help-seeking. Health (London) 2012;16(2):208−25.
[226] Sloan C, Gough B, Conner M. Healthy masculinities? How ostensibly healthy men talk about lifestyle, health and gender. Psychol Health 2010;25(7):783−803.
[227] Mróz LW, Chapman GE, Oliffe JL, Bottorff JL. Men, food, and prostate cancer: gender influences on men's diets. Am J Mens Health 2011;5(2):177−87.
[228] Coltrane S. Making men into fathers: men, masculinities, and the social politics of fatherhood by Barbara Hobson (reviewed work). Contemp Sociol 2003;32(6):739−40.
[229] Crespi I, Ruspini E. Transition to fatherhood: new perspectives in the global context of changing men's identities. Int Rev Sociol 2015;25(3):1−6.
[230] Kwon J-Y, Oliffe JL, Bottorff JL, Kelly MT. Masculinity and fatherhood: new fathers' perceptions of their female partners' efforts to assist them to reduce or quit smoking. Am J Mens Health 2015;9(4):332−9.
[231] Courtenay W. Making health manly: social marketing and men's health. J Mens Health Gend 2004;1(2−3):275−6.

CHAPTER 3

Female sexual function and fertility

Elizabeth A. Grill[1], Alison J. Meyers[2] and Alice D. Domar[2]

[1]Center for Reproductive Medicine, Weill Cornell Medical College, New York, NY, United States [2]Domar Centers for Mind/Body Health, Waltham, MA, United States

Highlights

Purpose of chapter:
   The objective of this chapter was to provide a general framework for understanding the complex struggles that women face along the family building journey and to understand the affect this stress has on female sexual function. This chapter will provide direction to providers about how to assess and treat these complicated issues.

Importance:
   The psychological and sexual implications of infertility and its treatment on women can have long-term effects even after withdrawal or completion of fertility treatment. Diagnosing, understanding, and addressing these issues early may ease the distress women experience during fertility treatment and eliminate long-term consequences.

Main ideas:
   While often overlooked or concealed, the sexual effects of infertility can have serious implications on a woman's psychological health and clinical outcomes. Sexual challenges can impact interpersonal relationships, sexual desire and satisfaction, self-esteem, and can often negatively affect fertility treatment outcomes. There are numerous sexual, psychosocial, and clinical interventions which may be efficacious in decreasing the impact of infertility on sexuality and reducing distress.

Summary:
   Healthcare professionals can prevent, assess, and treat female sexual dysfunction that further complicates the family building experience and interferes with wellbeing. Given the reported levels of distress experienced by women diagnosed with infertility, medical treatment should be in conjunction with counseling, emphasizing the importance of emotional health and well-being in couples struggling to build their families.

Case

Mark (42) and Marcie (38) have been married for 5 years and have tried unsuccessfully to start a family for the past 2 years. Marcie wanted to start trying to conceive as soon as they got married because she had a history of endometriosis and was worried it could impact her fertility. Mark wished to wait until he was promoted at work. They tried to conceive on their own for 1 year before seeking help from a reproductive endocrinology and infertility (REI) specialist. After receiving a combined factor diagnosis, they attempted three cycles of intrauterine insemination (IUI) and two cycles of in vitro fertilization (IVF). They became pregnant during the last IVF cycle but miscarried at 8 weeks. They plan to do another cycle but their REI advised them to start thinking about alternative family building options. Prior to starting a third IVF cycle, they decided to talk with a mental health professional who specializes in couple's issues related to reproductive medicine.

The constant barrage of shots, blood tests, and surgical procedures left Marcie feeling physically and emotionally exhausted. Mark found it difficult to connect with Marcie as she became more withdrawn, depressed, anxious, lethargic, and uninterested in the things they both used to enjoy doing together. Mark complained that he no longer recognized Marcie and feared that he would never get the woman he married and fell in love with back. Over time, this couple began to feel that the very foundation of their relationship was shaken as they were challenged to cope with stress and vulnerability, the loss of a dream, a sense of powerlessness, and feelings of guilt as well as blame.

While their marital and sexual relationships were strong at the beginning of treatment, the cumulative stresses of the infertility experience started to take a toll on their marital and sexual satisfaction. In prior relationships, Marcie struggled with vaginismus but worked with a pelvic floor physical therapist and sex therapist who were able to help her have sexual intercourse without pain. Throughout the course of infertility treatment, this couple reported sexual problems ranging from lack of desire, pleasure, and spontaneity to erectile dysfunction and repeat problems of vaginismus. Common feelings of infertility such as loss, anger, guilt, despair, depression, shame, and anxiety, began to overshadow intimate feelings of warmth, affection, and emotional connection so that sex became methodical, predictable, and unexciting. This added additional pressure for Mark and Marcie who felt the responsibility of performing on demand (e.g., during ovulation, producing semen samples, etc.).

Their differing emotional reactions, communication styles, and coping strategies left each of them feeling alone in the struggle, and the stresses resulting from multiple treatment failures put a strain on their personal and emotional wellbeing as well as their sexual/intimate connection. Both felt a sense of profound loss and hopelessness from the unsuccessful IUI and IVF cycles and the miscarriage. Both Mark and Marcie reported feeling isolated, emotionally unsupported, depressed, and rejected by the other.

The aforementioned case illustrates the typical stressors and psychosocial complications of a couple struggling to conceive. This chapter will address an overview of the psychosocial interplay between infertility and relationship health, specifically focusing on the female and will provide a framework to providers about how to address these complex issues.

Introduction

Infertility is defined as the "failure to establish a clinical pregnancy after 12 months of regular and unprotected sexual intercourse" [1]. The diagnosis affects approximately 12%—18% of women aged 15—44 [1,2]. The reasons for infertility can include both female and male factors. In females, reproduction can be impaired by altered function of the reproductive organs, illnesses, or by psychological factors. Women over the age of 35 are advised to only initiate medical evaluation after 6 months of trying to conceive, despite a lower likelihood of becoming pregnant each month compared to younger patients [3]. In patients who have preexisting factors that predispose them to an infertility diagnosis such as history of endometriosis, irregular periods, and factors that may result in tubal occlusion, including pelvic inflammatory disease, or a suspected male factors such as undescended testicles, or prior chemotherapy treatment, a medical evaluation is recommended after only 3 months of attempting to conceive [3]. Women with a suspected infertility diagnosis will likely undergo an examination by their obstetrician/gynecologist (OB/GYN), reproductive endocrinologist, or a physician trained in female reproductive tract abnormalities [3].

The misconception that a couple will get pregnant after having sex once, or that pregnancy will happen within the first month of trying in spite of the increasing age of the female partner is a widely accepted belief [3]. With this belief, initial attempts to conceive often begin as spontaneous with the intention of just seeing what happens when contraception is stopped. The frequency, erotic pleasure, and spontaneity of sex may increase during this time. Nevertheless, the stress, frustration, and anxiety of failed pregnancy attempts escalate each month after each unwanted menstrual period signifying such failure. Sex becomes methodical and scheduled around the female partner's "fertile window" and ovulation. This type of regimented sex can put an emotional and psychological burden on both partners that further impacts sexual function and creates sexual challenges [3].

Psychological effects of infertility in women

There is a known link between the physical, financial, and emotional challenges associated with a diagnosis of infertility and increased rates of distress, including anxiety and depression [4,5]. The inability to conceive naturally often results in feelings of low self-esteem, distress, guilt, and shame. Motherhood is seen by many women as a primary role in life and as an integral part of their femininity, gender identity, and sexuality. Women tend to assume that they are the cause of the infertility and begin (often fruitlessly) to search for a cause. They reproach themselves for past "misdeeds" and may even offer to leave their partners so as to free them to have children with another partner. Those who have difficulty getting pregnant or carrying a pregnancy may also feel like a failure as a human being. It is common for some infertile women to describe themselves as "defective" or "damaged goods." Clearly this self-perception can lead to depression, anxiety, and a loss of self-confidence and competence.

Despite the high incidence of infertility, the majority of infertile patients do not share their story with friends and family, thereby isolating themselves and increasing their vulnerability to psychological distress.

Individuals that undergo assisted reproductive technology (ART) treatment are at extreme risk of experiencing psychological symptoms of distress. Studies have shown higher rates of depression and anxiety in infertile women than fertile women [6]. Researchers from one study reported that approximately 40.8% of infertile women suffer from clinical depression, in addition to 86.8% women reporting an experience of anxiety [7]. Additional research has shown that the psychological effects of infertility affect 25%—53% of women before commencing and 40%—75% during reproductive medical treatment [8,9]. In one study consisting of 352 women seeking infertility treatment, 56.5% of the participants scored in the clinically depressed range and 75.9% of the women scored in the clinical range for anxiety. Further, only 21% of the women reported receiving mental health services [8]. A large study in Denmark consisting of 42,000 women who underwent ART treatment evaluated women for depression, reporting 35% of positive cases [10]. In a recent study, 60 married women, 30 with infertility and 30 controls, were evaluated for depression, anxiety, and stress. The results of the study indicate significantly higher rates of depression (10.83 + 8.37 vs 4.17 + 3.21; $P < .000$), anxiety (11.60 + 8.48 vs 5.50 + 4.24; $P < .001$), and stress (19.67 + 8.40 vs 12.10 + 6.76; $P < .000$) in infertile women compared to fertile controls [11]. Finally, as the number of failed conceptions increase, the rates of distress follow the same pattern. One study found that 15% of women reported severe depression after 1 year of unsuccessful infertility treatment [12]. Unfortunately, the main factor predicting the success of fertility treatments is age, thus, as age increases, fertility treatments fail, and the likelihood that the treatments will someday be successful lessen, the psychological impacts of infertility only worsen affecting all realms of life [3].

A diagnosis of infertility and its accompanied stress has been compared to devastating illnesses, including cancer and AIDS. Domar et al. [13] evaluated 149 women with infertility, 136 with chronic pain, 22 in the process of cardiac rehabilitation, 93 with cancer, 77 with hypertension, and 11 with human immunodeficiency virus (HIV). This study showed that women with infertility had scores regarding psychological wellbeing comparable to cancer, cardiac rehabilitation, and hypertension patients, and had lower scores than the HIV-positive and chronic patient participants; the anxiety and depression scores of women with infertility were not significantly different from all other groups excluding the chronic pain patients. Women frequently classify their infertility diagnosis as their most stressful life experience, and this study validated that the stress associated with infertility is comparable to other devastating medical manifestations [13]. Further, a recent study by Vaughan et al. [14] reported that infertility-related stress was still dominant even during the global COVID-19 pandemic affecting everyone across the world. About 2202 nonpregnant women with infertility completed a questionnaire assessing the top three stressors of women with infertility over three separate time courses between January 1, 2019 and April 1, 2020. While Coronavirus was reportedly the third most common stressor in early March, at all time-points, infertility was reportedly the most common top stressor [14].

Women with infertility experience severe stress daily, and as fertility treatments fail, this stress only intensifies. While trying to conceive, patients no longer feel in control of their bodies or their life plan. Lives are put on hold, attempts to conceive become all consuming, and couples are beholden to treatment [15]. Trying to juggle medical appointments and medicine regimes with job responsibilities can increase pressure and put stress on careers. Not surprisingly, the most common reason why insured patients drop out of treatment is psychological burden resulting from infertility, including treatment [16].

Women with infertility often experience greater levels of psychological distress than their male partners related to guilt, grief, denial, depression, anxiety, cognitive disturbance, and hostility [3]. Reproduction and sexuality may be more entangled for women than men, so challenges in one area may resonate in others. Typically, women initiate medical intervention for infertility and are more invested in having a child than their partner. Further, women are frequently more willing to consider extreme or alternative measures to achieve parenthood. Many factors contribute to driving women's distress levels higher than their male spouses. Firstly, the social obligation of pregnancy is mainly attributed to the female. Women tend to feel more failure and guilt regarding sexual and reproductive functions that are further reinforced by medical language such as premature ovarian "failure" and "incompetent" cervix. Additionally, women view motherhood as an imperative part of their gender identity, femininity, and sexuality; therefore anything that threatens this role may create social pressure and internal conflict [3]. Secondly, treatments for infertility are often more invasive, time consuming, and painful for the female partner. Thus infertility-related distress may be associated with both the diagnosis and the treatment interventions which are physically, psychologically, or pharmacologically intrusive. A diagnosis can lead to a loss of spontaneity and erotic value in a sexual relationship, as the goal becomes conceiving and sexual intercourse becomes scheduled to the "fertility window." The distortion of a couple's sexual relationship can be long lasting even after treatment [3]. Thirdly, coping strategies between men and women differ. Men tend to deny the diagnosis and remain active. Opposingly, women cannot image a life without children and often develop depressive reactions. Researchers have found that active coping strategies and positive reinterpretation has a positive impact on sexual functioning, while self-restraint coping and excess planning negatively affected sexual functioning [3].

Further, the medicalization of an infertility diagnosis and the stigmatization of infertility-related stress only increases the need for effective and accessible psychological treatments. A lack of mental health treatments is problematic for infertility-treatment success and continuation, in addition to one's psychological wellbeing [8,17].

Psychological distress and female sexual function

Sexual dysfunction (SD) is common in females with 40%–45% of adult women reporting one or more manifestation of SD [18]. In females, excessive stress can have negative effects on menstruation, resulting in more irregular cycles, changes in cycle duration, and intensification of menstrual symptoms such as pain. Excessive stress may also worsen premenstrual symptoms. Additionally, extreme stress can result in a decline in sexual desire and a decrease in the ability to conceive naturally due to these sexual challenges. Excess stress greatly increases the likelihood of developing psychological disruptions, such as anxiety and depression. In fact, depression caused by excess stress is one of the leading complications in pregnancy and postpartum adjustment [19]. The researchers from one study sought to investigate the effects of chronic stress on female sexual arousal. The results revealed that women in the high stress groups had lower levels of genital arousal and higher levels of cortisol, a hormone produced with excess stress. Interestingly, psychological arousal was not decreased between the group with high stress and the control [20]. In a 2004 study examining the effects of prolonged stress on female rat sexual function, results showed that the high-stress experimental group experienced reduced receptivity to male mates. Additionally, the high-stress group reported alterations in sex hormones, endocrine factors, and neurotransmitters, demonstrating how chronic stress may modify sexual behavior [21]. Evidently, excessive stress can have negative effects on psychological wellbeing and sexual function in females. Sexual challenges may also facilitate the development of psychological distress symptoms. In one study, over 50% of women who met the diagnostic and statistical manual of mental disorders (DSM) criteria for female orgasm disorder (FOD), a form of SD, also met the criteria for depression. Additionally, over 27% of women with FOD are also suffering from anxiety [22,23]. Furthermore, stress exacerbated by an infertility diagnosis can intensify psychological and sexual effects, and sexual challenges secondary to infertility can also lead to psychological symptoms.

Infertility leading to female sexual dysfunction

SD may play an etiological role in infertility, but it may also be a consequence of the infertility diagnosis secondary to psychological stress of one or both partners. Regardless of the cause of infertility, studies have shown that women experience greater psychological and emotional distress to infertility and its treatment than men, often due to more feelings of personal responsibility and having to deal with the bulk of the medical treatment procedures [24]. Furthermore, sexual challenges are high in all women with infertility. Research statistics estimate a range from 10% to 60% of couples have sexual problems related to infertility [25,26]. Moreover, sexual challenges are highest in secondary infertility patients, or individuals who have already conceived successfully once, and now cannot have another child [3,27]. Tanha et al., evaluated 191 primary and 129 secondary infertility female patients compared with 87 fertile controls. The results showed that sexual function was deprived in all infertile women, and importantly, secondary infertility was linked to worse results [27]. Similarly, Pakpour et al., examined 410 women with primary infertility and 194 women with secondary infertility in comparison to healthy controls based on sexual satisfaction. Results showed that infertile women reported significantly lower sexual satisfaction than fertile controls, and women with secondary infertility reported the worst scores [28]. As previously discussed, as infertility drags on, feelings of depression, anxiety, and sexual inadequacy can emerge as a result of the close association between sexuality and fertility [29]. The psychological implications of infertility, the physical and financial burdens of treatment, in addition to the social "defectiveness" individuals who are unable to conceive experience, all contribute to the manifestation of sexual challenges.

This section will address the prevalence of infertility-related sexual challenges in the female partner compared to nonfertile women. Notably, sexual challenges can range from clinical SD to sexual issues not related to a medical cause. The studies mentioned subsequently utilize various terminology for sexual challenges women with infertility may face.

Bakhtiari et al. examined 236 infertile women for SD. The results revealed that 55.5% of the infertile women reported some form of impaired sexual function [30]. Additionally, Czyżkowska et al. found that the incidence of SD between 50 infertile women and 50 fertile women was determined. About 90% of infertile women suffered from some form of SD, while 26% of fertile women did [31]. Carter et al. assessed the emotional and sexual state of 50 women with infertility and reported that 33% of the participants were clinically depressed, 59% with high distress, and a mean Female Sexual Function Index (FSFI) score indicating SD [32]. In one research study, 88 women and 45 couples receiving fertility treatments completed measures of sexual functioning. The researchers reported that the frequency of SD varied from 14.8% pain-related and 58% desire-driven in women [33]. In a recent study (2019), Ozturk et al. evaluated 269 females with infertility aged 24–45 and investigated the effects of infertility-related distress on sexual function during assisted reproductive treatment (ART). SD, sexual distress, dyspareunia, and frequency of intercourse per month was examined, in addition to infertility-related distress. The results of this study showed that women with higher reported infertility-related distress were more likely to report SD (95% CI, 1.01–1.03, odds ratio = 1.02 per point of score, $P = .001$) [34]. Finally, 96 infertile and 96 fertile women were evaluated on the Beck Depression Inventory and FSFI. The rate of SD (87.5% vs 69.8%) and FSFI total score (31.8 ± 7.8 vs 35.7 ± 6.3) was significantly higher in women with infertility compared to fertile controls. Sexual satisfaction and discomfort during sexual intercourse scales on FSFI was significantly lower for infertile women ($P < .001$). There was no significant difference in Beck Depression Inventory total score between the groups (infertile: 11.5 ± 9.7 vs fertile: 9.9 ± 9.0), but it was found that sexual functions decreased when depressive symptoms increased for both infertile and fertile women [35]. These studies not only indicate the higher incidence of sexual challenges in women with infertility compared to fertile controls but also highlight the role of psychological distress on sexual functioning.

Female sexual function disorders leading to infertility

Statistically, preexisting clinical SDs have only a minor etiological role in infertility, impacting approximately 5% of infertility cases. In these cases, male erectile dysfunction and anejaculation, in addition to female vaginismus, are the only clinical SDs inhibiting natural conception [36]. In females, disruption in desire, arousal, orgasm, or resolution, the four phases of sexual response, may contribute to infertility, in addition to pain disorders [3]. Research has shown that the most common causes of female SD are vaginismus and dyspareunia (now combined as *genitopelvic pain/penetration disorder in the DSM-V*) [3,37]. This section will address the clinical manifestations that may impact sexual function and in turn, impact fertility.

Vaginismus is the only clinical manifestation in women that can directly inhibit pregnancy. Nevertheless, the SD in women and couples tends to be a product of infertility rather than a direct cause [36]. Vaginismus affects approximately 1% of the population and is a condition in which vaginal spasms occur and prevent penetration during intercourse. Vaginismus may influence a woman's ability to conceive and impact her sexual identity and femininity. Interestingly, the disease often signifies a somatic manifestation of an underlying psychological problem, but most commonly, it is the result of gynecological disorders, including endometriosis, pelvic pain, or vestibulitis. In one study examining pregnant women with vaginismus, 100% of the participants described feelings of anxiety and anger immediately before sexual intercourse [38].

Hypoactive sexual desire disorder (HSDD), now known as *female sexual interest/arousal disorder* in the DSM-V, involving the loss of sexual desire or libido may also be relevant. HSDD may be episodic or situational, long standing, or a result of a problem that is not primarily sexual in nature [3]. Furthermore, an interference in desire, arousal, orgasm, or resolution may be related to HSDD and can significantly impact the ability to biologically conceive due to frequency of sex and sexual satisfaction for both partners. Women with HSDD may avoid sex except when ovulating, or may limit or avoid foreplay to facilitate a more rapid ejaculation from their male partner. This often leads to marital tension, a reduction in nonsexual affection, and feelings of disconnection within a relationship [3,39,40]. Studies have found that sexual function is dyadic; therefore it is important to note that a disruption in female sexual function may result in sexual challenges for the other partner affecting the couple's ability to sexually respond and successfully conceive [3,36].

Additional psychological or psychiatric problems may also factor into the cause of SDs and must be considered [3,41]. For instance, selective serotonin reuptake inhibitors (SSRIs) are used for a wide range of psychological disorders, including major depressive disorder, general anxiety, posttraumatic stress disorder, eating disorders, panic disorder, and more. SSRIs have sexual side effects that can impact desire and performance. Therefore psychological issues leading to antidepressant use can suppress or disrupt sexual function. Additionally, these side effects often lead to changes in the patient's compliance with the antidepressant medication and ultimately result in complete cessation of the treatment facilitating negative psychological consequences [42].

Furthermore, a loss of libido or other sexual challenges in women could be a consequence of infertility, or the result of a specific treatment procedure for infertility. Conversely, sexual challenges may play an etiological role in infertility diagnoses. Finally, the stresses and demands of infertility on financial resources, work-life, marital or social relationships, or general self-perception may also impact female sexual function [3]. Regardless, sexual challenges and psychological disruptions associated with infertility should not be overlooked and must be addressed with appropriate treatments and therapies.

Treatment outcomes

If female sexual challenges associated with infertility and infertility-related stress are neglected, the likelihood for successful conception may be affected. For instance, a decrease in sexual activity due to psychological distress or sexual difficulties may lead to a decrease in the probability of successfully conceiving. Research has also demonstrated that infertility-related stress and associated symptoms may negatively impact the success of fertility treatments.

As mentioned previously, sexual impairment in infertile couples is often due to the performance pressure experienced in response to planned sex, pressure to perform on demand, extensive and painful tests, intense feelings of anxiety, and the highly personal matter of sexuality being turned over to the external control of a physician and the psychological feeling of the medical team in the bedroom [29,43]. As infertility drags on, feelings of sexual inadequacy and depression can occur due to the close association between sexuality and fertility. If these tensions are not addressed they could lead to a reduction in nonsexual affection, resulting in feelings of disconnection and exacerbating relationship problems [44].

A commonly debated area in reproductive medicine is the prospective influence of psychological factors such as stress, depression, anxiety, and so on, on pregnancy rates. Dozens of studies have assessed the relationship between pregnancy rates and psychological symptoms prior to and during ART cycles. Some have shown no connection; however, many have revealed that higher rates of distress before and during treatment correlate with lower pregnancy rates [45]. One study found that the more distressed a female patient is prior to starting IVF treatment, the less likely it is that she will conceive. This study showed that stress levels were correlated to number of retrieved oocytes, number fertilized, pregnancy success rates, live birth rates, and birth weight [45,46]. While there are no conclusive studies confirming the positive linear relationship between psychological amelioration and pregnancy rates, only contradictory investigations, one can conjecture that improved psychological function and associated sexual function is undoubtedly a constructive result of clinical and psychological intervention [47].

Neglecting sexual disruption and psychological challenges may negatively impact a woman's ability to conceive and sustain a pregnancy. Furthermore, appropriate treatment interventions should be offered to help mitigate these effects associated with infertility.

Referral, consultation, and treatment

Couples often have a reluctance to discuss the psychological and sexual aspects of their relationship normally, but this reluctance intensifies even more so when they fear it may lead to interruption of medical treatment [48]. Sexual problems of infertility are often disregarded with the hope that they will dissipate on their own or not result in long-term consequences. Research has shown that some sexual problems may lessen following infertility treatment; however, some sexual challenges may persist or become more problematic after treatment ends or even when parenthood is achieved, ceaselessly affecting the individual's marital, psychological, and social relationships [49,50]. Even couples who never encounter major or disrupting sexual problems often experience episodic or situational diminished sexual desire and satisfaction in response to the emotional distress or physical strains of infertility or a specific treatment. Episodic loss of libido in one or both partners can usually be addressed with minimal education and reassurance. However, consistent and extensive diminished sexual desire in infertile men and women is more problematic and usually multifactorial. Females experiencing psychological distress and sexual challenges associated with infertility should be properly evaluated, referred to the appropriate facility, and offered treatment intervention to alleviate these effects.

Appropriate assessment should evaluate whether the sexual impact is: "(1) preexisting or secondary to infertility; (2) generalized or situation specific (e.g., problems more likely to occur when collecting a sperm sample, when the woman is ovulating); and (3) related to medical conditions or medications associated with infertility (e.g., endometriosis, prostatitis, medications, such as clomiphene or gonadotropins; Daniluk et al., 2014)" [56]. Depending on the rapport, relationship, comfort level, preference, and resource availability, a physician or infertility specialist may choose to personally treat a female's psychological and sexual symptoms, or refer them to a sex therapist, infertility counselor, or psychological counselor [36,39].

Sex therapy

One option to address female sexual function related to infertility is sex therapy. Sex therapists should strive to provide patient education and emphasize the importance of female sexual health and psychological wellbeing, even if the individual continues to proceed with medical infertility treatments [3].

SD involves an interruption in an individual's or couple's enjoyment or performance of sexual activity. SD is defined as any impairment or disturbance in one or more of the four phases of the sexual response cycle. A primary (lifelong) dysfunction has always been present, while a secondary (acquired) dysfunction is one that occurs after a period of normal, healthy sexual functioning. Dysfunctions are further specified as generalized when they occur in all situations and with all partners or situations when their sexual problem is limited to certain situations or partners.

The most important cause of SD is lack of adequate friction and/or erotic fantasy, or insufficient stimulation. Sex is fantasy and friction, mediated by frequency [51]. To function sexually, people need sexy thoughts, not only adequate friction. Negative thinking/antifantasy thoughts, whether a reflection of the infertility and treatment or partner anger, is often a significant contributor to SD. Depression may present as another obstacle. As previously reviewed, there are statistically significant increases in the incidence of depression in individuals with SD and infertility.

The sexual status examination is the single most important diagnostic tool available to the sex therapist and is a focused sex status that assists in understanding and identifying the immediate cause of the SD (i.e., the actual behavior and/or cognition causing or contributing to the sexual disorder). The sex status examination involves obtaining a description of a recent experience that incorporates the sexual symptoms reported. One question that will help pin down many of the immediate and remote causes is, "Tell me about your last sexual experience" and "Tell me about one of your best sexual experiences before you started trying to conceive." Common immediate causes of SD are quickly evoked by the patient's response. Unlike the fertility specialist, the sex therapist follows up with focused, open-ended questions to obtain a mental "video picture." Inquiries are made about desire, fantasy, frequency of sex, and effects of drugs and alcohol prior to and during infertility treatment. Answers to these questions provide awareness of the patient's sexual script and expectations before and after infertility, leading to more precise and improved recommendations and management of patient expectations [51].

Prevention of SD may involve targeting either issues related to the medical treatment or the couple's relationship. Sometimes, the most effective means of preventing SD is simply addressing with the couple the importance of their sexual relationship and specifically asking each partner about common sexual problems both related and unrelated to the infertility experience. It is important to carefully assess with a couple (and medical caregivers) the pros and cons of a treatment procedure in terms of its potential for contributing to or exacerbating sexual difficulties. By the same token, every effort should be made to accommodate medical treatment plans related to infertility as it may be the primary goal for the couple.

Couples usually respond with relief at being given permission to discuss sexual problems. For these couples, preventing problems may involve basic education; offering helpful tips; or encouraging them to discuss the problems with their physician, infertility counselor, and/or a sex therapist. This can also normalize sexual problems for the infertile couple, minimizing guilt and stigma, while helping them understand the nature of common sexual problems in infertility. In this manner, the importance of their sexual relationship is validated, and they are encouraged not to "sacrifice" sexual rewards for the sake of a pregnancy, parenthood, or infertility treatment [24]. For less serious problems, prevention may simply involve encouraging couples to keep their sexual relationship rewarding, interesting, and enlivened. Couples may wish to explore nonintercourse sexual expression, such as massage or sensate-focus exercises that emphasize physical closeness and nongenital pleasuring.

Although prevention of sexual distress should be a goal for all infertility caregivers and patients, it often is not. Infertile couples that are typically focused on having a baby believe that achieving pregnancy will solve all their problems and their sexual relationship will return to its "preinfertility" level of satisfaction. Of course, this is one of the myths that the infertility counselor must address, helping couples understand that achieving a pregnancy may further impair individual, couple, or family functioning.

Infertility counseling

Oftentimes, sexual disruption is related to the psychological effects of infertility. Therefore addressing the psychological symptoms may help alleviate some of the sexual issues women with infertility face. Psychological interventions emphasizing stress management and coping-skills have been associated with decreasing some of the most deleterious emotional effects accompanying infertility [52]. Frederikson et al. reviewed 39 studies assessing the effects of psychological intervention not only psychological effects of infertility (depression, anxiety, stress, and marital function) but also pregnancy outcomes. The results showed that there were statistically significant effects of alleviating a variety of psychological symptoms (Hedges $g = 0.59$; CI 0.38–0.80; $P = .001$) and correspondingly increasing pregnancy rates (risk ratio = 2.01; CI 1.48–2.73; $P < .001$) from the psychosocial interventions [53]. Boivin performed a review of some of the psychosocial interventions for infertility, examining the results of 380 studies. The results showed three main themes: psychosocial interventions were most successful in diminishing negative affect than changing interpersonal functioning such as marital and social functioning; pregnancy rates were largely unaffected by psychosocial interventions; and group programs highlighting education and skills training were considerably more effective than counseling interventions emphasizing emotional expression, thoughts, and feeling related to infertility [54]. Domar et al. [55] conducted a study of 143 women less than 40 years of age who were about to begin their first IVF cycle. Women were randomly assigned to complete a ten-session mind/body program (MB) comprised of psychological intervention and education on appropriate coping skills for infertility, or assigned to a control group without intervention. The women were followed for two IVF cycles. The researchers found that at cycle 1, pregnancy rates for all subjects was 43%. Notably, the majority of the patients in the intervention group had not attended the MB prior to undergoing their cycle. At cycle 2, pregnancy rates for the MB group was 52% and only 20% for the controls [55]. Therefore a psychosocial intervention treating the psychological effects of infertility was correlated to higher pregnancy rates in infertile patients, underscoring the necessity to address nonclinical implications of infertility.

Studies have also explicitly shown that decreasing psychological consequences of infertility has positive implications on sexual function. One study with 70 women with infertility revealed that those who received two psychoeducational sexual counseling sessions had higher sexual function and satisfaction 4 months later in comparison to the control group [26,56]. Similarly, Sahraeian et al. examined 52 women with infertility who were randomly divided into intervention and control groups. The intervention group underwent a group-based six-session sexual counseling using a cognitive behavioral therapy approach. Sexual function was evaluated using FSFI at three points in time. The results of this study showed no significant difference at baseline between groups. One month after intervention, a significant difference was found in the FSFI mean scores of the intervention group (29.35 ± 2.71) versus the control group (25.84 ± 2.52, $P < .001$, effect size 0.32). These significant differences were found in all sexual-function domains: sexual desire, arousal, lubrication, orgasm, satisfaction, and pain [57].

The field of fertility counseling comprises an eclectic use of a variety of treatment modalities, including but not limited to psychoeducational counseling, therapeutic counseling (e.g., cognitive behavioral), supportive counseling, grief counseling, and counseling that assists couples in decision making about treatment and next steps. The key is to match the right intervention at the right time to serve the emotional needs of the individual and couple. Table 3.1 provides a list of some of the goals and techniques of therapeutic intervention.

The form of counseling provided will be determined by the needs of the couple, the timing of treatment (e.g., initiation, treatment, and resolution), the couples' level of distress, and individual personality and coping factors. The timing of interventions and assessments might be particularly important to their effectiveness since the issues facing the couple at each phase of treatment can differ and require different therapeutic approaches.

TABLE 3.1 Therapeutic interventions and techniques.

Therapeutic interventions	Examples of techniques
Psychoeducational counseling	Provide information about treatment to empower patients and to manage expectations.
Supportive counseling	Improve patients' emotional health and wellbeing through empathy, validation of feelings, and normalizing distress.
Improve communication with doctor/staff/bosses/friends/family members	Role play typical interactions, assertiveness training, boundary setting.
Reduce the stress and demands of fertility treatment	Relaxation techniques, mindfulness, cognitive behavioral strategies.
Help make informed decisions about family building options or ending treatment	Enhance problem-solving skills.
Improve couple communication	Acknowledge different coping styles, learn to fight fairly, teach empathic listening skills.
Improve intimacy and sexual relationship	Psychosexual education, dispute male/female myths about desire and performance, nonprocreative sex, date night without fertility discussion, devote time to activities and interests that they enjoy together.
Promote healthy coping strategies	Replace bad habits with positive coping strategies like exercise, healthy-eating habits, relaxation techniques.
Grief counseling	Introduce rituals that validate loss and help with acceptance and resolution.
Encourage patients to make meaning of the infertility experience	Journaling, resilience training.
Improve wellbeing	Self-care strategies, positive coping, restoring hope.
Help set boundaries with friends and family members	Role-play conversations, develop self-protective strategies.
Understand social, cultural, and religious factors that contextualize infertility and treatment.	Ask questions to become culturally competent and respectful, consult with clergy, healers, family members, etc. (with permission).

Psychoeducational counseling most commonly occurs before treatment begins but can also take place throughout the fertility journey as couples navigate treatment options at different stages. Psychoeducational counseling is aimed at reducing feelings of helplessness and the stress of treatment though preparation. Psychoeducation enhances patient control, addresses decision making and treatment options, and manages expectations.

Less distressed couples may benefit from written psychosocial information provided at key times in treatment or brief counseling that emphasizes education. For example, counselors have developed interventions tailored to specific challenges, such as coping with the 2-week waiting period before the pregnancy test and preparing couples for treatment [11,12].

For those whose coping resources are inadequate and/or depleted, such interventions might not be sufficient and ongoing supportive or therapeutic counseling can be used to decrease psychological distress and improve relationship satisfaction for couples experiencing more moderate to severe levels of distress.

Longer-term therapeutic and grief counseling can be used when psychological stressors are more severe or after an unsuccessful fertility treatment cycle when stress is greatest. Grief counseling can occur at any point throughout the fertility journey. Couples can process frustration about starting later than desired, sadness about the number of eggs/embryos yielded or unsuccessful ART attempts. Couples may need to mourn miscarriages, selective reduction or termination. If couples decide to pursue third-party reproduction or adoption, they will need to grieve the loss associated with giving up a genetic connection. Ultimately, if couples end treatment and decide to remain childless, they will need to process despair and make meaning of their fertility struggle.

Pharmacological and medical treatment

Clinical intervention for psychological distress and sexual challenges is also an option to mediate these effects in infertile women. Antidepressants may be prescribed to mitigate the psychological effects of infertility; nevertheless, it is important to keep in mind the potential effects on sexual function secondary to these medications

[58]. Pharmacological treatments may be appropriate for addressing the clinical manifestations leading to sexual challenges in women with infertility. For example, vaginismus may be treated with local anesthetics (e.g., lidocaine), muscles relaxants (e.g., nitroglycerin ointment or botulinum toxin), and anxiolytic medications [59]. Other treatments for vaginismus may involve an eclectic approach of education, Kegel's exercises, gradual insertion of fingers or dilators, and psychological intervention [60]. It is also necessary to address any underlying medical conditions contributing to the sexual, psychological, and clinical effects of infertility, including preexisting diagnoses, medications, and discontinuing the use of alcohol, tobacco, and recreational drugs that may interfere [61].

Whether sexual challenges play an etiological role in infertility or are a symptom of infertility and related stresses, an integrated approach of clinical and psychological intervention addressing all aspects of the diagnosis will be most efficacious. Medical and fertility treatments should be in combination with psychotherapy and/or sex therapy, emphasizing the importance of sexual health and wellbeing in women and couples experiencing infertility [3].

Conclusion

The purposes of this chapter is to provide a general framework for understanding the complex struggles that women face along the family building journey and to provide direction to providers about how to assess and treat these complicated issues. Mental health professionals trained in the field of reproductive medicine can intervene on several different therapeutic levels by providing patient education, supportive and grief counseling, and helping patients with treatment decisions. Sex therapists can prevent, assess, and treat SD that further complicates the family building experience and interferes with wellbeing. Given the reported levels of distress experienced by women experiencing infertility, medical treatment should be in conjunction with counseling, emphasizing the importance of emotional health and wellbeing in couples struggling to build their families.

While often overlooked or concealed, the sexual effects of infertility can have serious implications on a woman's psychological health and clinical outcomes. Furthermore, accurately diagnosing the etiology of sexual challenges, whether they are causative or a result of infertility, and offering appropriate treatment is crucial for the patient's emotional and sexual wellbeing, in addition to increasing the likelihood of successful fertility treatment products.

Extensive research highlights the psychological effects of infertility affecting women. Further, research has found links between psychological function and sexual health. Similarly, sexual disruption has been found to increase the rates of psychological challenges. Consequently psychological treatments and sex therapy are viable options for addressing these effects commonly associated with infertility. Additionally, clinical manifestations that result in both infertility and SD should be treated in an integrated approach with pharmaceuticals and psychological intervention.

Furthermore, the sexual challenges women with infertility may experience should never be neglected, and appropriate treatment interventions should be emphasized to the patient by all medical professionals addressing the patient's infertility diagnosis.

References

[1] Vander Borght M, Wyns C. Fertility and infertility: definition and epidemiology. Clin Biochem 2018;62:2–10. Available from: https://doi.org/10.1016/j.clinbiochem.2018.03.012.
[2] Lotti F, Maggi M. Ultrasound of the male genital tract in relation to male reproductive health. Hum Reprod Update 2015;21(1):56–83. Available from: https://doi.org/10.1093/humupd/dmu042.
[3] Grill E, Schattman GL. Female sexual dysfunction and infertility. In: Lipshultz LI, Pastuszak AW, Goldstein AT, Giraldi A, Perelman MA, editors. Management of sexual dysfunction in men and women. New York: Springer; 2016. p. 337–42. 10.1007/978-1-4939-3100-2_29.
[4] Whiteford LM, Gonzalez L. Stigma: the hidden burden of infertility. Soc Sci Med 1995;40(1):27–36. Available from: https://doi.org/10.1016/0277-9536(94)00124-C.
[5] Andrews FM, Abbey A, Jill Halman L. Is fertility-problem stress different? The dynamics of stress in fertile and infertile couples. Fertil Steril 1992;57(6):1247–53. Available from: https://doi.org/10.1016/S0015-0282(16)55082-1.
[6] Rooney KL, Domar AD. The impact of stress on fertility treatment. Curr Opin Obstet Gynecol 2016;28(3):198–201. Available from: https://doi.org/10.1097/GCO.0000000000000261.
[7] Ramezanzadeh F, Aghssa MM, Abedinia N, et al. A survey of relationship between anxiety, depression and duration of infertility. BMC Womens Health 2004;4(1):9. Available from: https://doi.org/10.1186/1472-6874-4-9.

References

[8] Pasch LA, Holley SR, Bleil ME, Shehab D, Katz PP, Adler NE. Addressing the needs of fertility treatment patients and their partners: are they informed of and do they receive mental health services? Fertil Steril 2016;106(1):209–215.e2. Available from: https://doi.org/10.1016/j.fertnstert.2016.03.006.

[9] Clifton J, Parent J, Seehuus M, Worrall G, Forehand R, Domar A. An internet-based mind/body intervention to mitigate distress in women experiencing infertility: a randomized pilot trial. PLoS One 2020;15(3):e0229379. Available from: https://doi.org/10.1371/journal.pone.0229379.

[10] Sejbaek CS, Hageman I, Pinborg A, Hougaard CO, Schmidt L. Incidence of depression and influence of depression on the number of treatment cycles and births in a national cohort of 42 880 women treated with ART. Hum Reprod 2013;28(4):1100–9. Available from: https://doi.org/10.1093/humrep/des442.

[11] Khan AR, Iqbal N, Afzal A. Impact of infertility on mental health of women. Int J Indian Psychol 2019;7(1):804–9. Available from: https://doi.org/10.25215/0701.089.

[12] Lund R, Sejbaek CS, Christensen U, Schmidt L. The impact of social relations on the incidence of severe depressive symptoms among infertile women and men. Hum Reprod 2009;24(11):2810–20. Available from: https://doi.org/10.1093/humrep/dep257.

[13] Domar AD, Zuttermeister PC, Friedman R. The psychological impact of infertility: a comparison with patients with other medical conditions. J Psychosom Obstet Gynaecol 1993;14(Suppl.):45–52.

[14] Vaughan DA, Shah JS, Penzias AS, Domar AD, Toth TL. Infertility remains a top stressor despite the COVID-19 pandemic. Reprod Biomed Online 2020;41(3):425–7. Available from: https://doi.org/10.1016/j.rbmo.2020.05.015.

[15] Benyamini Y, Gozlan MKE. Variability in the difficulties experienced by women undergoing infertility treatments. Fertil Steril 2005;83:275–83.

[16] Gameiro S, Boivin J, Peronace L, Verhaak CM. Why do patients discontinue fertility treatment? A systematic review of reasons and predictors of discontinuation in fertility treatment. Hum Reprod Update 2012;18(6):652–69. Available from: https://doi.org/10.1093/humupd/dms031.

[17] Shreffler K, Gallus K, Peterson B, Greil AL. Couples and infertility. 1st ed. The handbook of systemic family therapy, vol. 3. New York: John Wiley & Sons Ltd; 2020. p. 385–405.

[18] McCabe MP, Sharlip ID, Lewis R, et al. Incidence and prevalence of sexual dysfunction in women and men: a consensus statement from the fourth international consultation on sexual medicine 2015. J Sex Med 2016;13(2):144–52. Available from: https://doi.org/10.1016/j.jsxm.2015.12.034.

[19] Stress effects on the body. American Psychological Association. Published online 2020. https://www.apa.org/helpcenter/stress/effects-male-reproductive.

[20] Hamilton LD, Meston CM. Chronic stress and sexual function in women. J Sex Med 2013;10(10):2443–54. Available from: https://doi.org/10.1111/jsm.12249.

[21] Yoon H, Chung WS, Park YY, Cho IH. Effects of stress on female rat sexual function. Int J Impot Res 2005;17(1):33–8. Available from: https://doi.org/10.1038/sj.ijir.3901223.

[22] Laan E, Rellini AH, Barnes T. Standard operating procedures for female orgasmic disorder: consensus of the International Society for Sexual Medicine. J Sex Med 2013;10(1):74–82. Available from: https://doi.org/10.1111/j.1743-6109.2012.02880.x.

[23] Mintz LB, Guitelman J. Orgasm problems in women. In: Hall KSK, Binik YM, editors. Principles and practice of sex therapy. 6th ed. New York and London: The Guilford Press; 2020.

[24] Burns L. Sexual counseling and infertility. Infertility counseling: a comprehensive handbook for clinicians. New York: Parthenon Publishing; 2006. p. 212–35.

[25] Wischmann TH. Sexual disorders in infertile couples. J Sex Med 2010;7(5):1868–76. Available from: https://doi.org/10.1111/j.1743-6109.2010.01717.x.

[26] Sexuality in the transition to parenthood. In: Hall KSK, Binik YM, Rosen NO, Byers S, editors. Principles and practice of sex therapy. 6th ed. New York and London: The Guilford Press; 2020.

[27] Tanha FD, Mohseni M, Ghajarzadeh M. Sexual function in women with primary and secondary infertility in comparison with controls. Int J Impot Res 2014;26(4):132–4. Available from: https://doi.org/10.1038/ijir.2013.51.

[28] Pakpour AH, Yekaninejad MS, Zeidi IM, Burri A. Prevalence and risk factors of the female sexual dysfunction in a sample of infertile Iranian women. Arch Gynecol Obstet 2012;286(6):1589–96. Available from: https://doi.org/10.1007/s00404-012-2489-x.

[29] Daniluk JC. Women's sexuality across the life span: challenging myths, creating meanings. New York: Guilford Press; 2003.

[30] Bakhtiari A, Basirat Z, Aghajani Mir M-R. Sexual dysfunction in men seeking infertility treatment: the prevalence and associations. Casp J Reprod Med 2015;1(3):2–6.

[31] Czyżkowska A, Awruk K, Janowski K. Sexual satisfaction and sexual reactivity in infertile women: the contribution of the dyadic functioning and clinical variables. Int J Fertil Steril 2016;9(4):465–76. Available from: https://doi.org/10.22074/ijfs.2015.4604.

[32] Carter J, Applegarth L, Josephs L, Grill E, Baser R, Rosenwaks Z. A cross-sectional cohort study of infertile women awaiting oocyte donation: the emotional, sexual, and quality-of-life impact. Fertil Steril 2011;95(2):711–16. Available from: https://doi.org/10.1016/j.fertnstert.2010.10.004.

[33] Purcell-Lévesque C, Brassard A, Carranza-Mamane B, Péloquin K. Attachment and sexual functioning in women and men seeking fertility treatment. J Psychosom Obstet Gynecol 2019;40(3):202–10. Available from: https://doi.org/10.1080/0167482X.2018.1471462.

[34] Facchin F, Somigliana E, Busnelli A, Catavorello A, Barbara G, Vercellini P. Infertility-related distress and female sexual function during assisted reproduction. Hum Reprod 2019;34(6):1065–73. Available from: https://doi.org/10.1093/humrep/dez046.

[35] Ozturk S, Sut HK, Kucuk L. Examination of sexual functions and depressive symptoms among infertile and fertile women. Pak J Med Sci 2019;35(5):1355–60. Available from: https://doi.org/10.12669/pjms.35.5.615.

[36] Grill E, Khavari R, Zurawin J, Flores Gonzales JR, Pastuszak AW. Infertility and sexual dysfunction (SD) in the couple. In: Lipshultz LI, Pastuszak AW, Goldstein A, Giraldi A, Perelman MA, editors. Management of sexual dysfunction in men and women: an interdisciplinary approach. New York: Springer; 2016.

[37] Meana M, Binik YM, Khalifé S, Bergeron S, Pagidas K, Berkley KJ. Dyspareunia: more than bad sex. Pain 1997;71(3):211–12.

[38] Achour R, Koch M, Zgueb Y, Ouali U, Rim BH. Vaginismus and pregnancy: epidemiological profile and management difficulties. Psychol Res Behav Manag 2019;12:137−43. Available from: https://doi.org/10.2147/PRBM.S186950.

[39] Perelman MA. Sex coaching for physicians: combination treatment for patient and partner. Int J Impot Res 2003;15(S5):S67−74. Available from: https://doi.org/10.1038/sj.ijir.3901075.

[40] Keye W. The impact of infertility on psychosexual function. Fertil Steril 1980;34:308−9.

[41] Kucur Suna K, Ilay G, Aysenur A, et al. Effects of infertility etiology and depression on female sexual function. J Sex Marital Ther 2016;42(1):27−35. Available from: https://doi.org/10.1080/0092623X.2015.1010673.

[42] Atmaca M. Selective serotonin reuptake inhibitor-induced sexual dysfunction: current management perspectives. Neuropsychiatr Dis Treat 2020;16:1043−50.

[43] Applegarth L, Grill EA. Psychological issues in reproductive disorders. In: Chan P, Goldstein M, Rosenwaks Z, editors. Reproductive medicine secrets. Philadelphia: Hanley & Belfus; 2004.

[44] Perelman M. The impact of relationship variables on the etiology, diagnosis and treatment of erectile dysfunction. Adv Primary Care Med: Clin Updat 2007;3:3−6.

[45] Rooney KL, Domar AD. The relationship between stress and infertility. Dialogues Clin Neurosci 2018;20(1):41−7.

[46] Rooney Domar KAD. Emotional and social aspects of infertility treatment. In: Dubey AK, editor. Infertility: Management and Treatment. New Delhi, India: Jaypee Brothers Medical Publishers; 2012.

[47] Klonoff-Cohen H, Chu E, Natarajan L, Sieber W. A prospective study of stress among women undergoing in vitro fertilization or gamete intrafallopian transfer. Fertil Steril 2001;76(4):675−87. Available from: https://doi.org/10.1016/S0015-0282(01)02008-8.

[48] Bachmann GA, Leiblum SR, Grill J. Brief sexual inquiry in gynecologic practice. Obstet Gynecol 1989;73(3 Pt 1):425−7.

[49] Wright J, Duchesne C, Sabourin S, Bissonnette F, Benoit J, Girard Y. Psychosocial distress and infertility: men and women respond differently. Fertil Steril 1991;55(1):100−8.

[50] Benazon N, Wright J, Sabourin S. Stress, sexual satisfaction, and marital adjustment in infertile couples. J Sex Marital Ther 1992;18(4):273−84. Available from: https://doi.org/10.1080/00926239208412852.

[51] Perelman M. Integrated sex therapy: a psychosocial−cultural perspective integrating behavioral, cognitive and medical approaches. In: Carson C, Kirby R, Goldstein I, Wyllie M, editors. Textbook of erectile dysfunction. 2nd ed. CRC Press; 2008. p. 298−305. 10.3109/9780203091807-41.

[52] Cousineau TM, Domar AD. Psychological impact of infertility. Best Pract Res Clin Obstet Gynaecol 2007;21(2):293−308. Available from: https://doi.org/10.1016/j.bpobgyn.2006.12.003.

[53] Frederiksen Y, Farver-Vestergaard I, Skovgard NG, Ingerslev HJ, Zachariae R. Efficacy of psychosocial interventions for psychological and pregnancy outcomes in infertile women and men: a systematic review and *meta*-analysis. BMJ Open 2015;5(1):e006592. Available from: https://doi.org/10.1136/bmjopen-2014-006592.

[54] Boivin J. A review of psychosocial interventions in infertility. Soc Sci Med 2003;57(12):2325−41. Available from: https://doi.org/10.1016/S0277-9536(03)00138-2.

[55] Domar AD, Rooney KL, Wiegand B, et al. Impact of a group mind/body intervention on pregnancy rates in IVF patients. Fertil Steril 2011;95(7):2269−73. Available from: https://doi.org/10.1016/j.fertnstert.2011.03.046.

[56] Karakas S, Aslan E. Sexual counseling in women with primary infertility and sexual dysfunction: use of the BETTER model. J Sex Marital Ther 2019;45(1):21−30. Available from: https://doi.org/10.1080/0092623X.2018.1474407.

[57] Sahraeian M, Lotfi R, Qorbani M, Faramarzi M, Dinpajooh F, Ramezani, et al. The effect of cognitive behavioral therapy on sexual function in infertile women: a randomized controlled clinical trial. J Sex Marital Ther 2019;45(7):574−84. Available from: https://doi.org/10.1080/0092623X.2019.1594476.

[58] Evans-Hoeker EA, Eisenberg E, Diamond MP, et al. Major depression, antidepressant use, and male and female fertility. Fertil Steril 2018;109(5):879−87. Available from: https://doi.org/10.1016/j.fertnstert.2018.01.029.

[59] Lahaie M-A, Boyer S, Amsel R, Khalife S, Binik YM. Vaginismus: a review of the literature on the classification/diagnosis, etiology and treatment. Womens Health 2010;6(5):705−19.

[60] Harish T, Muliyala K, Murthy P. Successful management of vaginismus: an eclectic approach. Indian J Psychiatry 2011;53(2):154. Available from: https://doi.org/10.4103/0019-5545.82548.

[61] Grill EA, Perelman MA. The role of sex therapy for male infertility. In: Goldstein M, Schlegel PN, editors. Surgical and medical management of male infertility. New York: Cambridge University Press; 2013. p. 204−19.

CHAPTER

4

The impact of erectile dysfunction on infertility and its treatment

Amir Ishaq Khan[1], Jennifer Lindelof[2] and Stanton Honig[1]

[1]Department of Urology, Yale School of Medicine, Yale University, New Haven, CT, United States [2]Division of Urology, UConn Health, Farmington, CT, United States

Historical and anatomical overview of erectile dysfunction

Introduction

The interface between sexuality and male reproduction has been a complicated relationship since the beginning of time. Sexuality, virility, and fertility share a common link of "manliness" that can result in significant effects on reproduction. This chapter reviews the history of this relationship, causes of male sexual dysfunction, and treatment options available to optimize reproduction in the infertile couple.

History, prevalence, and incidence

Erectile dysfunction (ED) is a type of sexual dysfunction defined as the consistent inability to achieve or keep an erection for satisfactory sexual intercourse [1]. ED has a high prevalence, estimated to affect up to 10%–20% of adult men globally and up to 12 million American men each year, with 20%–40% of men in their sixties and 50%–70% of men in their seventies to eighties experiencing ED [2–5]. In an analysis of the 2001–02 National Health and Nutrition Examination Survey, researchers found an estimated 18.4% incidence of ED, while the international MALES study found an overall global prevalence of 16% [4,6,7].

ED has been noted in history as far back as the ancient Egyptian civilization in 2000 BCE [8]. Philosophers such as Hippocrates noted a link between horseback riding and ED, and Aristotle postulated a theory that there were three nerves to the penis and a contribution of inhaled air to the development of an erection [8,9]. Leonardo da Vinci connected the role of blood flow through the penis in achieving an erection [8,9]. Studies in the 1970s and 1980s confirmed this impact of vascular blood flow using duplex Doppler ultrasound to evaluate penile hemodynamics [10–12]. These studies acknowledged the role of increased inflow of blood, smooth muscle function, and corporal venoocclusive function in maintaining an erection, with the additional, on a more cellular level, regulatory roles of nitric oxide (NO) in erections (or tumescence) and the enzymatic effect of phosphodiesterases in detumescence [10–12].

While ED is further impacted by numerous comorbidities and lifestyle factors such as obesity, cardiovascular disease, diabetes mellitus, hypertension, hyperlipidemia, metabolic syndrome, tobacco use, and depression, age is a significant factor in the incidence of ED. The Massachusetts Male Aging Study (MMAS) showed that an estimated 40% of men aged 40 years old had some level of ED, with ED incidence increasing with increased age [4]. The National Health and Social Life Survey measured an estimated 31% of men ages 18–59 had sexual dysfunction, including ED [5]. Alfred Kinsey estimated that 25% of men have ED by 65, although there is a role for the confounding comorbidities and their increasing incidence with age to explain this complex relationship [13]. Nevertheless, age-related decrease in androgens and endothelial function contributes to the decline of sexual function in healthy aging men, which can include increased latency to erection, decreased ejaculate and decreased force of ejaculation, prolonged refractory periods, decreased penile sensitivity, as well as decreased nocturnal penile tumescence [14–16]. Age-related vascular change includes increased smooth muscle tone and dysfunction, and increased endothelial dysfunction, which both impact the ability for penile vascular smooth muscle to relax [15,16]. The prevalence of ED has been reported in up to 10% of men under the age of 40 and can exist due to a variety of organic and psychosocial factors explained further [17]. This overall prevalence of ED can be important in the context of couples dealing with infertility.

Anatomy

The penis consists of three cylinders, with the two paired vascular corpora cavernosa dorsally, and a ventral vascular corpus spongiosum, which envelops the urethra, all covered by subcutaneous tissue and skin (Fig. 4.1). The corpora contain spongy vascular sinusoids that are interconnected and can serve as a reservoir for significant volumes of blood. The corporal sinusoids are enveloped by trabeculated smooth muscle and the tunica albuginea, which consists of fibrous sheaths, elastic fibers, and collagen, all of which contribute to penile expansion during tumescence. There can be a wide variability in penile length, girth, and curvature [18–20].

Superficial penile arterial supply derives from the external pudendal arteries from the femoral artery, while deep penile arterial blood blow derives from the internal pudendal arteries, which arise from the internal iliac arteries. They then become the common penile arteries, as well as the cavernous, dorsal, and bulbourethral arteries (Fig. 4.1) [21–23]. The cavernous arteries have helicine arterial branches, which provide blood flow to erectile tissue within the corpora. The dorsal penile artery provides blood flow to the glans and distal penis, while the

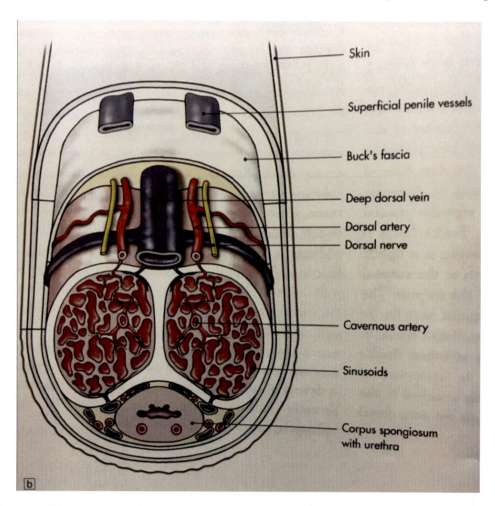

FIGURE 4.1 Anatomy of the penis. *Obtained and published with permission from the American Urological Association AUA Update Series, volume 13, lesson 2; 1994.6.*

bulbourethral artery supplies the penile bulb and corpus spongiosum. In an estimated one-third of men, there can also be accessory arterial blood flow supplying the penis, deriving from various origins such as the external iliac, obturator, vesical, and femoral arteries [22,23].

Sexual arousal and sensory stimulation can precipitate the initiation of an erection (or tumescence), which is a complex and delicate process, involving the release of neurotransmitters, relaxation of penile smooth muscle, dilation of penile arterioles and arteries with expansion of sinusoids due to rapid entry of arterial blood flow, and compressive venous occlusion of outflow via penile venous plexuses, culminating in the erect penis [12,19–21]. Flaccid penile blood is similar to venous blood flow with an overall slow rate of blood flow, but tumescence involves rapid entry of arterial blood, with consequent arterial blood gas levels within the penis and compression of subtunical venules [18,20]. Detumescence involves the vasoconstriction of arterial flow, with compression of the penile sinusoid cavities and a subsequent decrease in pressure with the opening of venous outflow.

Both tumescence and detumescence are mediated and reliant on this vascular contribution to the penis, in the context of somatic and autonomic neural input, as well as some degree of hormonal modulation. Somatic afferent sensory nerves for the penis are abundant from the free nerve endings and sensory receptors of the glans, penile skin, and urethra and travel in the dorsal nerve of the penis, joining the pudendal nerve, which transmits to levels S2–S4 [24]. These somatic afferent sensory inputs travel to spinal erection centers, where they both ascend the spinal cord for sensory perception in the central nervous system (CNS) and activate autonomic nuclei for tumescence [25,26]. Tumescence is primarily mediated in parasympathetic nerve centers from S2–S4 spinal levels. Detumescence is primarily mediated by sympathetic nerves originating from the sympathetic trunk at T11-L2 spinal levels. Both sympathetic and parasympathetic nerve fibers join in the pelvic plexus, which then contributes to the cavernous nerves to the penis [24,25].

The neural signaling pathways for erections classify them into psychogenic or reflexogenic erections. Psychogenic erections arise from audiovisual sensory stimulation and are preserved in men with spinal cord injuries below T9 [27,28]. Reflexogenic erections are a result of tactile stimulation of the genitalia and are maintained in patients with upper spinal cord injury [29,30].

At a biochemical level, nitric oxide (NO) is the primary neurotransmitter of erectile function, released from neurons and the endothelium and contributing to tumescence. NO activates guanylate cyclase, which can then produce cyclic guanylate monophosphate (cGMP) for relaxation of the penile smooth muscle [12,31,32]. The degradation of cGMP by phosphodiesterase enzymes allows for contraction of penile smooth muscle necessary for detumescence. There is also a central nervous component to erectile function, with proerectile contribution of the dopaminergic neuropathways and antierectile component of some adrenergic and serotonergic neuropathways [12,33,34]. Norepinephrine is the primary neurotransmitter of detumescence. When situational anxiety occurs in the male of an infertile couple, sympathomimetic overdrive (release of norepinephrine) may result in lack of initiation or maintenance of erections for intimacy. This situation may "mimic" a true blood flow issue [33,34].

Infertility and its relationship with erectile dysfunction

Infertility is defined by the World Health Organization (WHO) as the inability of a couple to attain pregnancy with unprotected intercourse for greater than 12 months, which can affect more than 72 million couples worldwide and 6 million American couples [35–37]. Infertility is estimated to affect approximately 15% of couples, with 7% of all men likely to experience fertility problems over a lifetime [35,38–40]. In couples with infertility, an estimated 20% can be attributed to male factor, with combined infertility in 27%, female infertility in 27%, and unknown cause in 15% [35,38]. Another study suggests that in 40% of cases, there is a male factor, 40% female factor, and in 20%, there is a combined issue [41].

With such global prevalence and complex causality, infertility has significant socioeconomic, clinical, and psychological implications. Infertility has been associated with increased sexual dysfunction in both men and women [42,43]. Multiple studies have demonstrated an increased level of ED in men within infertile couples. An Italian consecutive series of 244 men by Lotti et al. found that 17.8% of men, or an estimated one in six infertile patients, experienced ED, at a level that is double that seen in the general population [35]. A Chinese study by Gao et al. studied over 2000 men and found that ED, depression, and anxiety were significantly higher in infertile men [44]. Sexual dysfunction also extended to women in infertile couples, with female partners of infertile couples having increased depression and sexual dysfunction, with a direct correlation to male partner sexual function [42,45–48]. Male partners dealing with couple infertility also report less sexual satisfaction than female partners, with likely contribution of psychological stress and pressure [37,49,50].

There is a significant association between male sexual dysfunction, psychological distress, and infertility [44]. Infertile men have been noted to be more prone to psychological feelings of guilt, depression, inadequacy, and anxiety, which can impact the occurrence of ED, although causality is likely bidirectional and often difficult to determine [35,51]. Men in infertile couples carry a significant psychological burden, with higher levels of anxiety and depression than men in the general population [44,52]. There is a likely synergistic effect of both infertility and sexual dysfunction in this psychological context that can impact the fertility process [42]. Song et al. found that 46.2% of men in infertile couples had higher stress and more sexual dysfunction during timed intercourse during women's fertile period [53]. Moreover, Gao et al. found that 62% of infertile men do not perceive the link between psychological distress and sexual dysfunction [44]. In the setting of the numerous other medical contributions to ED, this can present a complicated barrier in not only fertility counseling and treatment but also for addressing general physical and emotional wellbeing and sexual satisfaction among men [5,42].

Causes of erectile dysfunction

A variety of medical comorbidities, medications, psychological factors, and lifestyle habits can contribute to ED. The many interconnected causes of ED will be categorized as follows: vascular, neurogenic, medication-induced, hormonal, psychological, and lifestyle.

Vascular

The erectile process depends on the increase in vascular blood flow with the coordination of the relaxation of the smooth muscle of the corpus cavernosum. Atherosclerosis can reduce arterial perfusion and penile blood flow, subsequently impacting penile rigidity and increasing the time to erection [54–57]. In fact, ED and abnormalities of penile arterial blood flow on Doppler ultrasonography are significant as early indicators of systemic vascular disease and cardiac risk stratification in terms of adverse major cardiac events [58–60]. Atherosclerosis and arterial insufficiency can be increased with risk factors such as age, hypertension, diabetes mellitus, hyperlipidemia, smoking, pelvic trauma, obesity, metabolic syndrome, and kidney disease [61].

Increased age is not only associated with increased comorbidities but also contributes age-dependent changes in vasculature, such as increased smooth muscle tone and increased endothelial dysfunction, which can contribute to ED through impaired penile vascular smooth muscle relaxation [15,54,62]. Hypertension has been noted to be an independent risk factor for the development of ED, as it is associated with long-term changes in vascular contractility and tone [63,64]. Patients with diabetes mellitus are three times more likely to have ED, with neurogenic, hormonal, and vascular contributions, including disrupting penile arterial blood flow, impairing the venoocclusive function for tumescence, increased oxidative stress, and endothelial dysfunction [4,33,65,66]. Uncommonly, pelvic and perineal trauma can contribute to stenosis of penile vasculature or can also manifest as fibroelastic alterations or impairment in tunica albuginea that impacts venoocclusion and relaxation of smooth muscle for tumescence [67]. Metabolic syndrome, defined as factors that increase risk for diabetes mellitus, coronary artery disease, and early mortality, is said to result from the interaction between genetic risk and lifestyle habits (such as smoking, stress, and caloric excess) and is also associated with endothelial dysfunction, oxidative stress, insulin resistance, and atherosclerosis [57,61]. All of the aforementioned factors can contribute to ED, which is common in metabolic syndrome [68]. Chronic renal failure is another condition significantly linked to ED, with uremia being associated with chronic disruptions in the hypothalamic-pituitary-gonadal axis (HPG axis) and atherosclerotic damage to vessels [69,70]. As delays in family building occur and male reproductive age increases, it is more likely that a vascular component may contribute to ED in the infertile male.

Neurologic

Loss of cavernosal innervation is a core component to neurogenic ED, limiting the ability for smooth muscle relaxation to allow for increased blood flow to the penis. Diabetes mellitus, particularly if uncontrolled, can lead to demyelination and neuropathy that can damage both the neuropathways and vasculature of the penis [33,71]. Multiple sclerosis, tumors, and spinal lesions such as spina bifida, syringomyelia, and herniated disk can be associated with neurogenic ED, with disruption of somatic and autonomic spinal erection pathways [72,73]. Injury to the CNS, as in cerebrovascular accident, Parkinson's disease, epilepsy, malignancy, dementia, and traumatic brain injury, can also impair cerebral regions involved in the erectile process, such as the medial preoptic area, hypothalamus, thalamus, and hippocampus, all of which can play a role in the interaction of libido and sensory stimuli with erectile function [26,72−74]. Traumatic or iatrogenic nerve injury can also lead to ED. Pelvic fracture has been associated with ED secondary to injury to the cavernous nerves [75]. Iatrogenic cavernosal nerve injury was historically common after pelvic surgery such as radical prostatectomy, radical cystectomy, or abdominoperineal resection [76−80]. Advances in understanding of pelvic neuroanatomy and surgical technique led to the development of nerve-sparing approaches, which have allowed for reduction in cavernosal and pelvic nerve injury and lowered secondary effects on erectile function [76−84]. Age also plays a neurogenic role in ED, with decline of sensory tactile sensitivity with age, partly contributing to age-related increase in ED [85]. While this may be a small portion of patients with ED in the infertile couple, understanding the etiology may direct therapy.

Medication-induced

Multiple medications have been linked to ED, with various mechanisms in disrupting the pathway of tumescence. Certain antihypertensives have commonly been linked to ED. Diuretics such as thiazide diuretics are notably linked to ED, with effects on decreased blood flow to the penis and decreased testosterone and libido [86]. Beta blockers, especially nonselective beta blockers such as propranolol, have also been associated with ED, by disrupting smooth muscle relaxation and impacting CNS sensory processing pathways [12,87]. Of the common antihypertensives, angiotensin-converting enzyme inhibitors, angiotensin receptor blockers, and calcium channel blockers have been associated with minimal disruption of sexual and erectile function [87,88]. However, some calcium channel blockers are thought to affect fertility through effects on mannose receptors [87,89]. In general, however, in hypertensive patients, it is the disease process more than the medication that is likely responsible for the ED.

Certain psychiatric and pain medications are also significantly associated with ED. Antipsychotics can block the effects of dopamine, and result in impairment of libido and/or elevation of prolactin, thus contributing to ED. Studies have shown that antipsychotics have been associated with sexual dysfunction in 40%−70% of users, likely due to a mixture of antidopaminergic, anticholinergic, and hyperprolactinemic effects [90]. Prolactin, which is associated with milk production and lactation in pregnancy, can have a direct effect on smooth muscle relaxation in the corpora, and elevated prolactin levels can also disrupt androgen receptors and the HPG axis, all of which can lead to increased incidence of ED with antipsychotic use [91−93]. Selective serotonin reuptake inhibitors (SSRIs) have also been associated with ED, anorgasmia, and impaired ejaculation, as increased serotonin is generally associated with inhibited libido and erectile function [94,95]. SSRIs can stimulate serotonergic receptors (particularly 5-HT_2 and 5-HT_3 receptors) to inhibit proerectile spinal neuropathways, as well as disrupt metabolism of NO and impair dopaminergic effects in the CNS [94−97]. Up to 50% of users of SSRIs have been reported to experience some sexual dysfunction [98]. Tricyclic antidepressants can affect erectile function and orgasm due to their significant anticholinergic effects [99]. Monoamine oxidase inhibitors can also affect orgasm and libido due to disruption in autonomic pathways [99]. Additionally, antiepileptic medications, including carbamazepine and valproate, have been associated with sexual dysfunction, ED, and loss of libido [100,101].

Pain and anxiolytic medications have also played a role in ED. Opioids can impair the HPG axis and decrease testosterone synthesis, leading to hypogonadotropic hypogonadism and potentially associated ED [102,103]. This has become an increasingly common cause, as opiate addiction has increased over the last 10−15 years [103]. Benzodiazepines and their GABAergic influence can impair CNS dopaminergic activity and affect libido and erectile function to a lesser degree [104,105].

Hormonal antiandrogens, such as 5-alpha reductase blockers used for benign prostatic hyperplasia and antiandrogens for therapy in prostate cancer, have also been associated with ED via the blockade of androgenic action via receptors [106,107]. The short-term and long-term effects on sexual function have not been clearly established. However, these causes of ED are not common in the infertile male patient.

Hormonal

There are numerous hormones that both modulate and affect erectile function and have interplay with male reproduction and spermatogenesis. The HPG axis is the primary hormonal network involved in testosterone and sperm production [108]. The hypothalamus controls episodic release of gonadotropin-releasing hormone (GnRH), which is involved in stimulating episodic release of both follicle-stimulating hormone (FSH) and luteinizing hormone (LH) from the anterior pituitary gland. FSH and LH modulate specific testicular function [109]. FSH binds to Sertoli cells to initiate and maintain spermatogenesis. LH affects steroidogenesis and testosterone production in Leydig cells in the testis.

Age-related impact on this hormonal axis can play a role in the increased incidence of ED with age. Testosterone and sperm production are noted to decline with age [109]. Age is also associated with decrease in seminiferous tubule volume and length, decreased sperm production and germ cell proliferation, and decreased Leydig cells, which can disrupt erectile function [109]. Low testosterone can sometimes be noted in cases of ED, and its effects are more pronounced with age [110–112]. Although ED symptoms have been noted in studies across a range of testosterone from 200 to 400 ng/dL, one study found testosterone <225 ng/dL as significantly associated with increased frequency of ED [113]. In addition to age, diabetes mellitus, hyperlipidemia, anemia, and obesity have all been associated with low testosterone, although causality is difficult to determine [114]. Certain conditions may result in hypogonadotropic hypogonadism such as anabolic steroid use, opioid usage, etc. Direct specific causes of this may result from pituitary adenomas, Allman's syndrome, brain lesions, etc.

Dysfunction of thyroid hormone has uncommonly been associated with low libido and ED, with increased estrogen noted in hyperthyroidism and low testosterone and increased prolactin noted in hypothyroidism [115,116]. All of these conditions may be seen in men of reproductive age (Fig. 4.2).

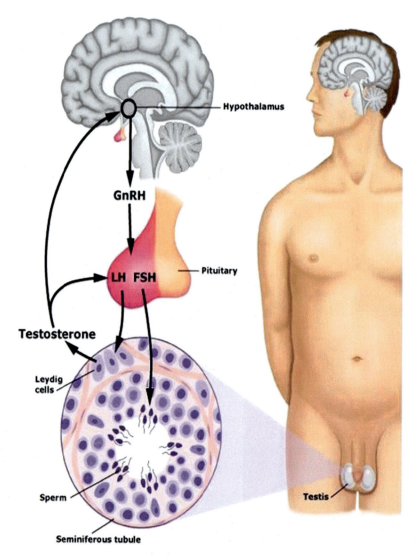

FIGURE 4.2 Hypothalamic-pituitary-gonadal axis. *Obtained and published with permission from UpToDate.*

Psychological or situational anxiety–related

There is a significant association between psychological distress and ED [35,42,44,53]. This is likely the most common cause of ED in the infertile male, and we like to describe it as "situational anxiety–related ED." As discussed in the context of infertile couples, the psychological burden of the diagnosis can lead to heightened stress, depression, anxiety, and a greater prevalence of ED, which can affect the frequency of intercourse and infertility treatment [35,41,43,52]. Stress can also have some modulatory effects on semen quality. Sociocultural norms regarding gender and masculinity can often impact the way psychology and sexual function interact. Some men tend to associate fertility and erectile function with masculinity [117]. In addition, studies have shown that men seek social support less than women, which can deepen the psychological impact and complex management of ED, as well as infertility [118]. ED can often be of clinical psychogenic origin and can be classified further as generalized, situational, performance related, or distress/adjustment related. Psychogenic or situational ED is thought to involve an excessive CNS response that inhibits the spinal erection center and leads to increased smooth muscle contraction, thereby contributing to ED [119,120]. This is typically the result of increased adrenergic tone from excess sympathetic output prior to or during intimacy. Generalized psychogenic ED can include a lack of sexual arousability, an age-related decline in libido, or general sexual inhibition. Situational ED can be partner related within a relationship, due to sexual preferences, or within the context of conflict. Performance-related ED is very common in the infertility population and can be associated with other forms of sexual dysfunction such as premature ejaculation, delayed ejaculation, or inability to ejaculate inside of partner due to anxiety or a fear of failure [35,42,44,53]. Adjustment-related ED can be linked to an overall mood state in response to life stressors such as depression, loss of job, or recent death of a partner. Overall, the prevalence of ED in mental illness can be as high as 80%, and there is a close association between psychological distress and ED [121]. Counseling can be extremely valuable in these settings to ameliorate these issues.

Lifestyle

There is a significant contribution of lifestyle components and habits to the incidence of ED. Overall, globally, men have a shorter life expectancy than women and are more vulnerable to major chronic diseases and comorbidities. Men also have four times as high tobacco consumption as women, are less compliant with medications and screenings, and do not visit primary care physicians as often as women. These may all increase the risk of various comorbidities that can contribute to ED [122–124]. Tobacco use itself has a significant impact on erectile and sexual function, impairing semen quality, increasing oxidative stress, and impairing NO activity in erectile function [125]. Alcohol use, when consumed in small amounts in moderation, may improve erectile quality due to vascular blood flow and anxiolytic effects [126]. However, chronic heavy alcohol use is associated with decreased testosterone, decreased libido, diminished sperm quality, increased estrogen, and neuropathy, all of which can commonly lead to ED [127]. A few studies have also shown that cannabis can be associated with low testosterone [128,129]. Chronic bicycling can also play a role in ED, with potential neurogenic and vascular dysfunction related to chronic cycling-associated perineal compression [67]. Caloric excess and associated obesity is also associated with metabolic syndrome, diabetes mellitus, and low testosterone, often in a synergistic and bidirectional manner [130,131]. However, in addition to the various treatment options for ED, improved dietary habits, exercise, weight loss, moderation of alcohol intake, and tobacco cessation have all demonstrated significant containment of ED, suggesting the importance of counseling on lifestyle changes [130,131].

Treatment of erectile dysfunction: effects on infertility

Sperm needs to reach the cervix during coitus for the pregnancy process to begin. ED can result in coital factor infertility. This is a treatable and reversible cause of male infertility. There are a number of Food and Drug Administration (FDA)-approved oral and nonoral treatments available for ED. ED impacts millions of Americans every year, including many where infertility is also an issue. In looking to evaluate men for ED, it is important to understand the underlying mechanism for the patient's ED. Depending on the mechanism, monotherapy with oral treatments may prove to be effective, while in other more refractory cases, a multimodal approach to ED is merited. Phosphodiesterase 5 inhibitors (PDE5is) are the first-line therapy of choice given their ease of use; however, they are not fully effective in all men and a number of second-line therapies are available. Second-line therapies available at this time include intracavernosal injections, vacuum erection devices (VEDs), intraurethral application of vasodilatory drugs, and placement of penile prostheses. Therapy will also include counseling and hormone therapy based on specific issues. Much of infertility-associated ED involves situational anxiety. First-line options, including counseling and medical therapy, are the mainstay of reversing ED. If natural intercourse is not possible, methods to obtain sperm in combination with assisted reproductive technologies (ART) may be necessary.

Treatment options

Phosphodiesterase 5 inhibitors

PDE5is are considered the gold standard initial therapy for ED. Part of the appeal of these drugs as first-line treatment for ED is that PDE5is have demonstrated efficacy regardless of the cause of ED, including situational or psychogenic etiologies [132]. Currently four major PDE5is are commercially available, including sildenafil, vardenafil, tadalafil, and avanafil. Sildenafil was first approved by the FDA in 1998, with vardenafil (2003), tadalafil (2003), and avanafil (2013) thereafter (Fig. 4.3).

These drugs differ slightly in onset and duration of action; however, their mechanism of action and effectiveness is very similar [133]. Penile erections are the result of smooth muscle relaxation [134]. Sexual stimulation triggers the release of nitric oxide in smooth muscle cells, which through a number of intracellular reactions results in cGMP. Phosphodiesterase 5 inhibitors work to treat ED in the context of sexual arousal by inhibiting the enzyme that breaks down cGMP, the main moderator of smooth muscle relaxation in the penis. By increasing the concentration of cGMP in the penile tissues an erection is possible [134]. These drugs are usually taken on a "on-demand" basis; however, tadalafil is FDA-approved for daily dose use as well. Some men find that daily-dose medication works better for them as a steady state develops of drug levels after about 2 weeks and there is no need for "timing things" for medication use in addition to timed intercourse for fertility purposes.

While all four drugs have been shown to be effective, patients may prefer one over another for a variety of reasons. These include patient preference for efficacy, side-effect profile, and duration of action. A number of reviews indicate that PDE5i are safe, well tolerated, and effective drugs [132,133,135,136]. Given the effectiveness of PDE5i in treating ED, many patients prefer to try another PDE5i if one fails or results in significant side effects before proceeding with other therapies [135,136].

With regards to their effect on fertility, any of the PDE5is available may prove to be helpful in patients whose primary obstacle is the inability to achieve and maintain erection, but have otherwise normal sperm transport and function [137]. PDE5is are prescribed to assist in achieving an erection, as well as to increase ejaculatory latency [138]. To date, PDE5is have not been shown to have a negative effect on spermatogenesis [132,133,139–141].

While highly effective, it is important to review the side effects and contraindications to use of PDE5i. The most common side effects reported include flushing, dyspepsia, headache, dizziness, and visual changes, including color changes and palpitations [132]. Some patients find the side effects bothersome enough to discontinue use, though the drugs are generally very well tolerated. Tadalafil has the added side effect of musculoskeletal pain in legs and back, although this rarely limits use. The main contraindications are for patients who are taking nitrates and those with angina, as PDE5i can potentiate the hypotensive effects of nitrates. Alpha blockers can also be associated with orthostatic hypotension when used with PDE5i, but this synergistic effect is uncommon [132,134].

These drugs work extremely well in situational anxiety–related ED that is very commonly seen in the infertile couple [138]. Many times, with time, confidence returns, anxiety departs, and the need for long-term PDE5i use

Drug Name	Usual Dosage	Tmax	Half Life
Sildenafil (Viagra®)	25-100 mg/day	0.5 - 2 hours	4 hours
Vardenafil (Levitra®)	5-20 mg/day	0.5 - 2.5 hour	4-6 hours
Tadalafil (Cialis®)	5-20 mg/day (PRN) 2.5-5mg/day (QD)	0.5 – 6 hours	17.5 hours
Avanafil (Stendra™)	50-200mg/day	0.5-0.75 hours	5 hours

FIGURE 4.3 Comparison of the phosphodiesterase 5 inhibitors currently on the market in the United States. *Obtained and published with permission from Smith WB, McCaslin IR, Gokce A, Mandava SH, Trost L, Hellstrom WJ. PDE5 inhibitors: considerations for preference and long-term adherence. Int J Clin Pract. 2013;67(8):768–80.*

is uncommon. Combining a PDE5i with psychological interventions has been thought to improve erectile response, as counseling can help to contextualize the problem allowing men to understand the effects of their negative thoughts, anxiety, and feelings of hopelessness that often interfere with erectile function [142].

Counseling

Historically, psychogenic or better described as "situational anxiety"-related issues were thought to be the root cause of most cases of ED and while there remains a high correlation with ED in men with mental health conditions most agree that ED is predominantly a functional or physical disorder. Review of current evidence suggests couples with an unfilled desire for children do not display psychological disorders with more frequency than couples without fertility disorders, regardless of the cause of infertility [143,144]. However, situational anxiety relating to low sperm quality, demand for "timed intercourse," and anxiety of the partner can contribute to a high rate of situational-anxiety-related ED in the couple struggling with infertility [138].

Male factor infertility is estimated to occur at similar rates to female factor infertility, yet counseling resources and psychological support are vastly skewed toward female infertility [145]. Additionally, the most effective resources appear to be underutilized and inaccessible for most men. In one study by Furman et al., it was found that men responded more positively to group counseling than individual counseling sessions and that counseling was an effective tool for mitigating the emotional impact of infertility [146].

Another area of infertility research that is gaining attention in recent years is counseling in the setting of advanced paternal age. Unlike females, where age is the most significant factor in fertility treatments, fertility in men does not have as clear of a timeline with spermatogenesis and androgen production occurring throughout life [147]. While paternity is still possible until a late age, there is evidence that semen parameters decrease after age 35 making conception more difficult. This may create some level of situational-anxiety-related ED that can contribute to fertility issues.

Hormonal replacement

Low serum testosterone is commonly identified in men with ED. For men with hypogonadism, the most common treatment is with exogenous testosterone. Supplementation of this low serum testosterone may improve symptoms of ED; however, use of exogenous testosterone alone will result in suppression of the HPG axis and have a negative effect on spermatogenesis. Exogenous testosterone therefore leads to decreased production of LH and FSH, which impairs sperm production and may induce testicular atrophy [148]. This happens by suppression of Leydig cell production of intratesticular testosterone, which is important for spermatogenesis. The number of individuals especially in the reproductive age undergoing testosterone replacement therapy has increased over the last decade. It is estimated that 7% of men with infertility have been undergoing testosterone replacement therapy and is likely the etiology of infertility in the majority of these patients [149]. *Therefore exogenous testosterone alone is contraindicated in males of reproductive age considering fertility.* Unfortunately, this is a common finding in patients who present for a fertility evaluation with low testosterone.

AUA guidelines on the management and evaluation of testosterone deficiency state that men with testosterone deficiency who are interested in fertility should have a reproductive health evaluation performed prior to treatment [150]. In addition to a detailed history and physical, FSH levels are recommended to assess for impaired spermatogenesis. Guidelines also recommend a discussion of the long-term impact of exogenous testosterone on spermatogenesis, as there is a variable time course for return of sperm in the ejaculate [150]. Recovery of sperm is highly variable, and, while it usually takes about 3–4 months to return, it may take a year or more to return to pretreatment levels. Additionally, sudden withdrawal of testosterone supplementation can result in symptomatic hypogonadism until production of endogenous testosterone returns to normal levels [151].

In patients with hypogonadotropic hypogonadism who are interested in initiating or maintaining fertility, treatment regimens with human gonadotrophins, recombinant FSH, and human chorionic gonadotropin are used to stimulate spermatogenesis [152]. Stimulation of hypothalamic-pituitary-thyroid axis can take several months; however, onset of spermatogenesis can sometimes take 12–24 months of therapy [153]. AUA guidelines, conditionally recommend use of aromatase inhibitors, human chorionic gonadotropin, selective estrogen receptor modulators, or a combination thereof in men with testosterone deficiency desiring to maintain fertility [150].

Clomiphene citrate is a selective estrogen receptor modulator that is used to treat hypogonadal men interested in preserving fertility [148]. Clomiphene citrate works by inhibiting negative feedback of estrogen at the hypothalamic pituitary axis, resulting in increased LH and FSH secretion which acts to stimulate Leydig cells. While there is evidence that use of clomiphene citrate improves symptoms of hypogonadism, preserves fertility, and improves bone density over time, little is known about its effects on ED [154]. Human chorionic gonadotropin can be used independently or supplemented with clomiphene citrate, tamoxifen, anastrozole, or a combination can be used to restore spermatogenesis [151].

Penile injection therapy

If oral PDE5is fail to provide patients with a satisfactory erection, minimally invasive methods such as penile injection therapy can be tried. Three different types of intracavernosal medications are commonly used. They are prostaglandin E1 (alprostadil), a combination of phentolamine and papaverine (Bimix), or a combination of all three drugs prostaglandin E1, phentolamine, and papaverine (Trimix). By combining papaverine, phentolamine, and PGE1, the amount of each drug needed to provide an effect is less than if the components were used individually, increasing the safety profile of the therapy [155]. Efficacy for intracavernosal injections is high, with a natural appearing erection in most cases, especially those from situational anxiety—induced ED that are refractory to oral therapy.

While highly successful, one of the issues with intracavernosal injections is a high rate of attrition, as many patients have difficulty with the concept of penile injections [155]. With reasonable counseling, risks of treatment are low, but include hematoma and fibrosis in tissue, and in rare cases, prolonged painful erections or priapism. Fig. 4.4 illustrates the recommended procedure for intracavernosal therapy [156]. In men with spinal cord injury, it should be noted that denervated tissue seems to be more sensitive, require lower doses of medication and have

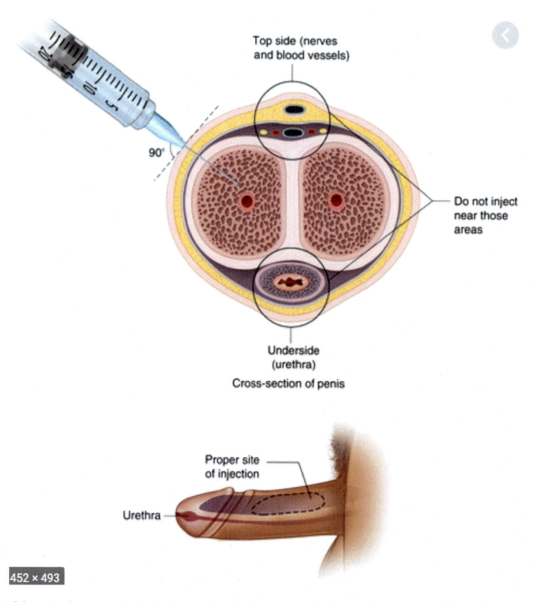

FIGURE 4.4 Schematic of recommended injection procedure for intracavernosal therapy. *Obtained and published with permission from Narus JB. Intracavernosal injection training. In: Atlas of office based andrology procedures. Cham: Springer International Publishing; 2017, p. 117–27.*

a higher success rate, along with an elevated risk of priapism [157]. In some cases of situational anxiety—induced ED, patients may be candidates for temporary use of penile injection therapy to allow for normal intercourse. This may allow for normal semen deposition in the vagina and pregnancy through natural intercourse.

Vacuum erection device

VEDs, also known as vacuum constriction devices are among the oldest nonsurgical treatments available for men with ED. With VEDs, the penis is inserted into a rigid cylinder and negative pressure is applied causing blood flow into the penis, resulting in an erection. A constriction band is then placed around the base of the penis, allowing for penetrative sex. VEDs are often thought of as second-line therapy behind oral PDE5is; however, in some patient populations such as those with neurogenic, psychiatric, or arteriogenic causes of ED they may prove to be more effective [158,159]. While use as a standalone device is seen, the VED has also shown promising results when used in combinations with other therapies for ED [160]. Unfortunately, use of this device is somewhat limited in the infertile male since it will typically block the ejaculate from forward propulsion out of the urethra. The following is a summary of its value; however, it is somewhat limited in this population.

The VED is increasingly being touted as a key factor in penile rehabilitation postprostatectomy, as a means to help recover natural erections [161]. Radical prostatectomy (robotic or open) is one of the standards of treatment for intermediate-grade prostate cancer. With improved screening and early diagnosis for prostate cancer, there is an increasing population of younger, more sexually active patients, who are receiving treatment where infertility may be an issue [159]. In general, erectile function prior to prostatectomy dictates what degree of ED will be present after surgery, with younger, healthier men having better outcomes [162]. With a VED, the proposed mechanism of rehabilitation is that blood flows retrograde thru the venous system into the tissues maintaining the integrity of smooth muscle and preventing fibrotic changes within the corpora during the period of neuropraxia that occurs even after nerve-sparing radical prostatectomy [155]. With the mechanism of action of retrograde venous flow, the corpus cavernosum does not see as high oxygenated flow as with PDE5is or penile injection therapy.

Despite being a cost-effective treatment regimen, dropout rates with VEDs are high due to lack of spontaneity and difficulty with device placement. One of the drawbacks of the tool is a nonphysiologic erection, where the erection is only present distal to the constriction band leading to a "hinged" effect where an awkward angle may be present during intercourse [163]. Additionally, patients describe a bluish or cyanotic look to the penis, as well as a cool to the touch erection due to the constriction of blood flow [159]. Patients also need to be aware of how long the device has been in use, as leaving the constriction band in place for longer than 30—60 minutes can rarely result in damage to the skin. This is particularly important in patients who are insensate in the genital area, such as after spinal cord injury, as they may be unable to detect the pain associated with tissue damage [158]. As stated earlier with regards to fertility, one of the reported adverse effects of treatment with a VED is discomfort with ejaculation or in many cases obstructed ejaculation, thus limiting its use with this population [157].

MUSE (intraurethral therapy)

Alprostadil is a synthetic vasodilator that is chemically identical to the natural vasodilator prostaglandin E1. Alprostadil was first developed for use as an intracavernosal injection, but has been adapted to other delivery mechanisms, including the medicated urethral system for erections or MUSE [164]. With this system, a pellet containing alprostadil suspended in polyethylene glycol is administered using an applicator directly in the urethra. MUSE is intended to bypass some of the complications seen with intracavernosal injections, including fibrosis, priapism, pain, and hematoma, while still providing a vasodilatory effect and erection [165].

MUSE therapy works indirectly by diffusion of PGE1 from corpus spongiosum to corpus cavernosum, is associated with vasodilation of the corpora cavernosa and an increase in cavernosal artery blood flow. Alprostadil also stimulates the production of cAMP in smooth muscle cells leading to calcium sequestration and eventual relaxation, allowing for an erection to occur. Given its localized mechanism of action, MUSE is not dependent on nitric oxide or an intact nervous system and can be utilized in men who are unable to take or do not respond to oral PDE5is [136,137,164]. As a result, patients who are more likely to be refractory to PDE5 inhibitors such as those with peripheral nerve injury after radical prostatectomy, severe vascular disease, diabetic neuropathy, or vascular disease can benefit from MUSE, similar to penile injections [164].

The overall success rate of MUSE therapy is reported to be between 15% and 56%, making it another choice as a second-line therapy or in combination with other therapies [155,160,166,167]. Most common side effects are burning and pain in the urethra and periphery leg pain. Although MUSE application of alprostadil is less effective than intracavernosal injection therapy, MUSE may be a treatment option for men due to its comparative ease of use and minimal discomfort [136,164,166,168]. It can be used effectively regardless of the origin of a patient's ED and is in general preferred by patients over intracavernosal injections for those who are needle phobic [164]. Efficiency is not nearly as good as penile injection therapy and can be very expensive since it is a proprietary drug delivery system. In addition, there is no data evaluating the effect of MUSE on semen given that is present within the sperm transport system, that is, the urethra. Therefore its role in the infertile male is unclear.

Penile implant

The most involved treatment for men with ED is the placement of a penile implant. Penile prostheses come in three different models, a three-piece pump, a two-piece pump, and malleable devices. Penile prosthesis is an effective treatment for ED, as it allows patients to engage in penetrative sex without interfering with urination, ejaculation, sensation, or orgasm and no limitation of spontaneity. It is frequently used as a treatment for ED in cases refractory to other noninvasive approaches or as a matter of patient preference [169]. Penile prosthesis implantation is one of the few treatments available that works for almost all men, provided they have the manual dexterity to manipulate the device. In patients with poor manual dexterity to work an inflatable device, a malleable penile implant can be utilized. Patient and partner satisfaction is also extremely high compared to other treatments [169,170].

Infection remains one of the most significant long-term complications with inflatable penile prosthesis [171]. Several patient populations are known to exhibit higher rates of infection. These include patients with prior radiation therapy, prior scarring such as priapism or prior implant infection and spinal cord injury patients. Infection rates for penile prosthesis are variable from 1% to 10% [171–174]. For patients with spinal cord injury, the rate of infection is reported to be 7% versus 2% in the general population. Erosion rates are also higher, with a rate of 11% versus 1% [175]. To combat infections, several steps have been implemented from antibiotic dips prior to implantation, to standardized operating room teams, to modified surgical technique such as the no touch technique [169,176]. Other risks include device malfunction, migration of reservoir, and organ injury.

Treatment of infertility when erectile dysfunction is an issue

ED is just one of many causes of male factor infertility, as without an adequate erection, sperm are unable to be deposited into the vagina for conception to possibly occur during coitus. For some patients, correcting ED with therapies previously discussed, is enough to overcome fertility challenges leading to conception. But for other men who also suffer from ejaculatory dysfunction and/or poor semen parameters, additional interventions may be required to achieve a viable pregnancy.

Reproductive function in males is dependent on many factors, including the neurologic integrity of both the pelvic floor and spinal cord [157]. Erectile function and ejaculatory function are separate events that require the involvement of different neural pathways, as such it is possible for one to occur in the absence of the other. Conditions such as diabetes, multiple sclerosis, injuries to the sympathetic nerves, and spinal cord injuries are associated with diminished ejaculatory function [157]. In the case of men with spinal cord injury, anejaculation is noted in upward of 90% of patients [177]. In addition, psychogenic ejaculatory dysfunction does occur and may limit deposition of semen into the vagina via natural intercourse.

The health, age, and concurrent medical problems facing the female partner is another important component to selecting the right treatment modality for an infertile couple. A thoughtful approach, considering the goals and limitations of both partners is necessary for successful conception. For example, in a couple where the male partner suffers from obstructive azoospermia, surgical correction could be the best approach to fix the problem. However, taking that same male patient with a female partner of advanced age and the treatment decision becomes more complicated. Considering the risks, benefits, and both partners, in couples with a female partner with advanced age, sperm retrieval and in vitro fertilization (IVF) may make more sense than fixing the underlying problem.

Treat the underlying problem

ED is not uncommon, with prevalence increasing in men over 50 as described previously. This is especially true in patients with multiple comorbidities, including obesity, diabetes mellitus, hypertension, hyperlipidemia, coronary artery disease, smoking, or depression. Additionally, social behaviors such as alcohol consumption, smoking, and drug use all negatively impact erectile function [136]. While many options exist to treat ED, given the often multifactorial nature of the disorder, conservative management with lifestyle modifications should always be considered as part of the treatment algorithm. Improving underlying health can improve erectile function and subsequently fertility.

Multiple drugs are known to impact erectile function, through modifications of the hypothalamic pituitary axis hormones or by nonhormonal mechanisms. A wide variety of drugs interfere with sexual function and may cause ED, impairment of spermatogenesis, or alteration of epididymal maturation [178]. A drug-induced dopamine or androgen deficiency can cause loss of sexual desire, as well as erectile disorders [152,153]. With GnRH analogs and antiandrogens, the mechanism of action appears to be related to the natural physiology of an erection, whereas with alpha blockers there is an association with ejaculatory dysfunction, specifically with tamsulosin. The mechanism of action of other drug classes such as antihypertensives, diuretics, antiretrovirals, antidepressants, and antipsychotics is more difficult to ascertain as the effects of the medical condition on sexuality are hard to separate from treatment modalities [178]. The key factor is treatment of ED, regardless of etiology to allow for deposition of semen in the vagina to allow for pregnancy via natural intercourse.

Move the sperm closer to the eggs via assisted reproductive techniques

Natural cycle intrauterine insemination with ejaculated sperm

Natural cycle intrauterine insemination (IUI) or intravaginal insemination is an option for couples who struggle with male factor infertility that are either refractory to ED treatments discussed previously or have an additional component of ejaculatory dysfunction. Some men will have issues with ejaculation inside of his partner, while able to ejaculate via masturbation. If semen quality is good, this may be amenable to natural cycle insemination. If there is a female factor, it may be combined with ovarian stimulation. With IUI, sperm must be present at high enough concentrations, with adequate morphology and motility to achieve a successful outcome. In couples with subfertility only one accepted male semen analysis parameter has been shown to be predictive of IUI outcomes, total motile sperm count [179]. This usually is 5 million motile sperm after sperm processing. Natural cycle inseminations rely on normal female anatomy and are performed timed with the female's ovulatory cycle, with or without hormonal stimulation (controlled ovarian stimulation) of the female partner [180]. IUI is minimally invasive and associated with less risk to the female partner and has been shown to be more cost-effective than IVF/ICSI when enough sperm is present [181]. However, reasons contributing to infertility are often multifactorial and as such some couples would benefit from bypassing IUI and going straight to IVF or ICSI. Advanced female age and duration of subfertility are amongst the most significant negative predictive factors for the success of IUI [182]. Total motile sperm count, less than 5 million motile sperm as described above [179,183] has also been associated with a lower chance of pregnancy after IUI compared to IVF, and has been suggested as a potential marker to distinguish which couples should jump straight to IVF/ICSI [182,184].

Sperm retrieval/ICSI (more for ejaculatory dysfunction)

While most men with ED have normal ejaculatory function, some patient populations require assisted ejaculation techniques or surgical removal of sperm. For example, patients with obstructive azoospermia who elect to proceed with IVF or intracytoplasmic sperm injection (ICSI) rather than undergo corrective surgery. Additionally, patients who present with nonobstructive azoospermia from either congenital or inheritable causes will need to undergo one of several retrieval techniques [185]. The probability of retrieving sperm is almost 100% in men with obstructive azoospermia; however, the odds are about 50% for nonobstructive azoospermia [186].

There are several surgical options for sperm retrieval for men with obstructive azoospermia. Testicular sperm extraction, testicular sperm aspiration, percutaneous epididymal sperm aspiration, or microsurgical epididymal sperm aspiration, where a microscope is utilized in the operating room to help retrieve sperm from the epididymis can be utilized. ICSI provides fertilization rates of 45%–75% per injected oocyte when epididymal or testicular spermatozoa from men with obstructions are used, with reasonably high pregnancy rates [187].

When ED is accompanied by ejaculatory dysfunction, the aforementioned methods of sperm retrieval may be necessary. Sometimes ejaculates can also be collected via electroejaculation (EEJ). With EEJ, a rectal probe is positioned to apply current to the seminal vesicles and prostate until ejaculation occurs (Fig. 4.5). This requires a general anesthetic and semen quality tends to be quite variable. EEJ is successful in obtaining semen in upward of 90% of men with spinal cord injury [177]. Ohl et al. showed that for 653 cycles of EEJ only 57 pregnancies or 8.7% resulted [183]. The median number of cycles to achieve pregnancy in those that were ultimately successful was three. Overall reported rates of success for pregnancy through IUI range from 5% to 20% per cycle [179]. In most cases at the present time, EEJ is combined with IVF and ICSI to optimize success rates. One study reported a fertilization rate of 75% per injected oocyte and clinical pregnancy rate of 55% per fresh semen retrieval attempt when ICSI was coupled to EEJ [188].

EEJ has also been shown to be helpful in retrieving sperm of men with psychogenic anejaculation. EEJ in combination with ART for psychogenic anejaculation has been shown to have variable success rates. One Danish study performed with patients with strong religious beliefs observed an overall fertilization rate of 65%, and a pregnancy rate of 19.2% [189]. Treatment of psychogenic ejaculatory dysfunction was first reported in the Orthodox Jewish population in 1996 [190]. EEJ may provide spermatozoa with good motility, one of the key factors to success with IUI [190]. If semen quality is excellent, this may be combined with IUI [179]. If not, IVF/ICSI is required (Fig. 4.6).

Testis sperm retrieval techniques as described before should be close to 100% if patients have been shown to have sperm in the ejaculate but cannot reliably collect a sample on demand; that is, psychogenic ejaculatory dysfunction. These can be performed under local anesthesia in office in most cases as any technique of testis sperm aspiration or extraction may be performed as described before for obstructive azoospermia. However, sperm

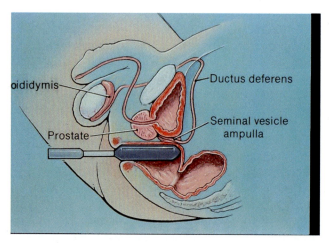

FIGURE 4.5 Electroejaculation. *Obtained and published with permission from Krane, et al. Clinical urology. Philadelphia, PA: J.B. Lippincott Company; 1994.*

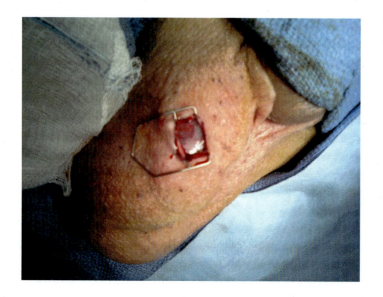

FIGURE 4.6 Open testis sperm extraction. *Obtained and published with permission from Honig S, MD.*

source should be testis not epididymis, unless concomitant obstruction is present. With sperm retrieval techniques listed before, motility of sperm is usually significantly reduced. Pregnancy rates continue to be high in these cases as sperm quality is good and if the female partner appears with normal quality oocytes, it is usually a straightforward clinical endeavor.

While the advancement of technology has allowed men with inability to ejaculate sperm to father children, one of the limitations of ICSI/IVF is the cost to execute each cycle of treatment. Costs associated with surgical sperm retrieval, storage of semen, hyperstimulation of female partner, as well as the procedural cost associated with IVF and embryo transfer are significant and have proven to be a barrier to access. Low-cost IVF has been gaining traction globally as a reproductive justice mission, driven by helping those in resource poor settings [191]. Low-cost ART is based on the use of affordable protocols, clinical judgment, and streamlining use of products to optimize well-established protocols for laboratory analysis [191,192].

Conclusions

In the infertile couple, sexual dysfunction may result in barriers to pregnancy. Treating the underlying problem and allowing for sexual intercourse and pregnancy through natural intercourse is the best first-line step. Excellent therapies are available and should be utilized early in the course of treatment in these couples. Treatment of ED should restore couples to achieve a pregnancy via natural intercourse if semen quality is good. In couples where a combined ED and ejaculatory dysfunction are present, sperm retrieval techniques, including EEJ and standard testis sperm retrieval techniques are available in conjunction with assisted reproductive techniques to achieve a pregnancy in these situations.

References

[1] Montorsi F, Adaikan G, Becher E, Giuliano F, Khoury S, Lue TF, et al. Summary of the recommendations on sexual dysfunctions in men. J Sex Med 2010;7(11):3572–88.
[2] Lewis RW, Fugl-Meyer KS, Corona G, Hayes RD, Laumann EO, Moreira Jr. ED, et al. Definitions/epidemiology/risk factors for sexual dysfunction. J Sex Med 2010;7(4 Pt 2):1598–607.
[3] Derogatis LR, Burnett AL. The epidemiology of sexual dysfunctions. J Sex Med 2008;5(2):289–300.
[4] Feldman HA, Goldstein I, Hatzichristou DG, Krane RJ, McKinlay JB. Impotence and its medical and psychosocial correlates: results of the Massachusetts Male Aging Study. J Urol 1994;151(1):54–61.
[5] Laumann EO, Paik A, Rosen RC. Sexual dysfunction in the United States: prevalence and predictors. JAMA 1999;281(6):537–44.
[6] Rosen RC, Fisher WA, Eardley I, Niederberger C, Nadel A, Sand M, et al. The multinational Men's Attitudes to Life Events and Sexuality (MALES) study: I. Prevalence of erectile dysfunction and related health concerns in the general population. Curr Med Res Opin 2004;20(5):607–17.
[7] Selvin E, Burnett AL, Platz EA. Prevalence and risk factors for erectile dysfunction in the United States. Am J Med 2007;120(2):151–7.
[8] Shah J. Erectile dysfunction through the ages. BJU Int 2002;90(4):433–41.
[9] van Driel MF. Physiology of penile erection—a brief history of the scientific understanding up till the eighties of the 20th century. Sex Med 2015;3(4):349–57.
[10] Shirai M, Ishii N, Mitsukawa S, Matsuda S, Nakamura M. Hemodynamic mechanism of erection in the human penis. Arch Androl 1978;1(4):345–9.
[11] Lue TF, Hricak H, Marich KW, Tanagho EA. Vasculogenic impotence evaluated by high-resolution ultrasonography and pulsed Doppler spectrum analysis. Radiology 1985;155(3):777–81.
[12] Andersson KE, Wagner G. Physiology of penile erection. Physiol Rev 1995;75(1):191–236.
[13] Gades NM, Jacobson DJ, McGree ME, St Sauver JL, Lieber MM, Nehra A, et al. Longitudinal evaluation of sexual function in a male cohort: the Olmsted county study of urinary symptoms and health status among men. J Sex Med 2009;6(9):2455–66.
[14] Masters WH, Johnson VE. The sexual response of the human male. I. Gross anatomic considerations. West J Surg Obstet Gynecol 1963;71:85–95.
[15] Toda N. Age-related changes in endothelial function and blood flow regulation. Pharmacol Ther 2012;133(2):159–76.
[16] Christ GJ, Maayani S, Valcic M, Melman A. Pharmacological studies of human erectile tissue: characteristics of spontaneous contractions and alterations in alpha-adrenoceptor responsiveness with age and disease in isolated tissues. Br J Pharmacol 1990;101(2):375–81.
[17] Rastrelli G, Maggi M. Erectile dysfunction in fit and healthy young men: psychological or pathological? Transl Androl Urol 2017;6(1):79–90.
[18] Sattar AA, Wespes E, Schulman CC. Computerized measurement of penile elastic fibres in potent and impotent men. Eur Urol 1994;25(2):142–4.
[19] Lue TF, Tanagho EA. Physiology of erection and pharmacological management of impotence. J Urol 1987;137(5):829–36.
[20] Dean RC, Lue TF. Physiology of penile erection and pathophysiology of erectile dysfunction. Urol Clin North Am 2005;32(4):379–95.
[21] Nelson RP, Lue TF. Physiology, hemodynamics and pharmacology of penile erection. Arch Ital Urol Nefrol Androl 1988;60(1):63–6.

[22] Breza J, Aboseif SR, Orvis BR, Lue TF, Tanagho EA. Detailed anatomy of penile neurovascular structures: surgical significance. J Urol 1989;141(2):437–43.
[23] Bare RL, DeFranzo A, Jarow JP. Intraoperative arteriography facilitates penile revascularization. J Urol 1994;151(4):1019–21.
[24] Halata Z, Munger BL. The neuroanatomical basis for the protopathic sensibility of the human glans penis. Brain Res 1986;371(2):205–30.
[25] Giuliano F. Neurophysiology of erection and ejaculation. J Sex Med 2011;8(Suppl 4):310–15.
[26] McKenna KE. Central control of penile erection. Int J Impot Res 1998;10(Suppl 1):S25–34.
[27] Courtois FJ, Macdougall JC, Sachs BD. Erectile mechanism in paraplegia. Physiol Behav 1993;53(4):721–6.
[28] Chapelle PA, Durand J, Lacert P. Penile erection following complete spinal cord injury in man. Br J Urol 1980;52(3):216–19.
[29] Hess MJ, Hough S. Impact of spinal cord injury on sexuality: broad-based clinical practice intervention and practical application. J Spinal Cord Med 2012;35(4):211–18.
[30] Biering-Sorensen F, Sonksen J. Sexual function in spinal cord lesioned men. Spinal Cord 2001;39(9):455–70.
[31] Hurt KJ, Musicki B, Palese MA, Crone JK, Becker RE, Moriarity JL, et al. Akt-dependent phosphorylation of endothelial nitric-oxide synthase mediates penile erection. Proc Natl Acad Sci U S A 2002;99(6):4061–6.
[32] Ignarro LJ, Bush PA, Buga GM, Wood KS, Fukuto JM, Rajfer J. Nitric oxide and cyclic GMP formation upon electrical field stimulation cause relaxation of corpus cavernosum smooth muscle. Biochem Biophys Res Commun 1990;170(2):843–50.
[33] Saenz de Tejada I, Goldstein I, Azadzoi K, Krane RJ, Cohen RA. Impaired neurogenic and endothelium-mediated relaxation of penile smooth muscle from diabetic men with impotence. N Engl J Med 1989;320(16):1025–30.
[34] Prieto D. Physiological regulation of penile arteries and veins. Int J Impot Res 2008;20(1):17–29.
[35] Lotti F, Corona G, Rastrelli G, Forti G, Jannini EA, Maggi M. Clinical correlates of erectile dysfunction and premature ejaculation in men with couple infertility. J Sex Med 2012;9(10):2698–707.
[36] Brugh 3rd VM, Lipshultz LI. Male factor infertility: evaluation and management. Med Clin North Am 2004;88(2):367–85.
[37] Boivin J, Bunting L, Collins JA, Nygren KG. International estimates of infertility prevalence and treatment-seeking: potential need and demand for infertility medical care. Hum Reprod 2007;22(6):1506–12.
[38] Krausz C. Male infertility: pathogenesis and clinical diagnosis. Best Pract Res Clin Endocrinol Metab 2011;25(2):271–85.
[39] Anderson JE, Farr SL, Jamieson DJ, Warner L, Macaluso M. Infertility services reported by men in the United States: national survey data. Fertil Steril 2009;91(6):2466–70.
[40] Eisenberg ML, Betts P, Herder D, Lamb DJ, Lipshultz LI. Increased risk of cancer among azoospermic men. Fertil Steril 2013;100(3):681–5.
[41] Kumar N, Singh AK. Trends of male factor infertility, an important cause of infertility: a review of literature. J Hum Reprod Sci 2015;8(4):191–6.
[42] Nelson CJ, Shindel AW, Naughton CK, Ohebshalom M, Mulhall JP. Prevalence and predictors of sexual problems, relationship stress, and depression in female partners of infertile couples. J Sex Med 2008;5(8):1907–14.
[43] Wischmann TH. Sexual disorders in infertile couples. J Sex Med 2010;7(5):1868–76.
[44] Gao J, Zhang X, Su P, Liu J, Shi K, Hao Z, et al. Relationship between sexual dysfunction and psychological burden in men with infertility: a large observational study in China. J Sex Med 2013;10(8):1935–42.
[45] Sand M, Fisher WA. Women's endorsement of models of female sexual response: the nurses' sexuality study. J Sex Med 2007;4(3):708–19.
[46] Fisher WA, Rosen RC, Eardley I, Sand M, Goldstein I. Sexual experience of female partners of men with erectile dysfunction: the female experience of men's attitudes to life events and sexuality (FEMALES) study. J Sex Med 2005;2(5):675–84.
[47] Ichikawa T, Takao A, Manabe D, Saegusa M, Tanimoto R, Aramaki K, et al. The female partner's satisfaction with sildenafil citrate treatment of erectile dysfunction. Int J Urol 2004;11(9):755–62.
[48] Montorsi F, Althof SE. Partner responses to sildenafil citrate (Viagra) treatment of erectile dysfunction. Urology 2004;63(4):762–7.
[49] Monga M, Alexandrescu B, Katz SE, Stein M, Ganiats T. Impact of infertility on quality of life, marital adjustment, and sexual function. Urology 2004;63(1):126–30.
[50] O'Brien JH, Lazarou S, Deane L, Jarvi K, Zini A. Erectile dysfunction and andropause symptoms in infertile men. J Urol 2005;174(5):1932–4 discussion 4.
[51] Seidman SN, Roose SP. The relationship between depression and erectile dysfunction. Curr Psychiatry Rep 2000;2(3):201–5.
[52] Drosdzol A, Skrzypulec V. Depression and anxiety among Polish infertile couples—an evaluative prevalence study. J Psychosom Obstet Gynaecol 2009;30(1):11–20.
[53] Song SH, Kim DS, Yoon TK, Hong JY, Shim SH. Sexual function and stress level of male partners of infertile couples during the fertile period. BJU Int 2016;117(1):173–6.
[54] Bacon CG, Mittleman MA, Kawachi I, Giovannucci E, Glasser DB, Rimm EB. Sexual function in men older than 50 years of age: results from the health professionals follow-up study. Ann Intern Med 2003;139(3):161–8.
[55] Martin-Morales A, Sanchez-Cruz JJ, Saenz de Tejada I, Rodriguez-Vela L, Jimenez-Cruz JF, Burgos-Rodriguez R. Prevalence and independent risk factors for erectile dysfunction in Spain: results of the Epidemiologia de la Disfuncion Erectil Masculina Study. J Urol 2001;166(2):569–74 discussion 74–5.
[56] Shabsigh R, Fishman IJ, Schum C, Dunn JK. Cigarette smoking and other vascular risk factors in vasculogenic impotence. Urology. 1991;38(3):227–31.
[57] Schulster ML, Liang SE, Najari BB. Metabolic syndrome and sexual dysfunction. Curr Opin Urol 2017;27(5):435–40.
[58] Corona G, Monami M, Boddi V, Cameron-Smith M, Lotti F, de Vita G, et al. Male sexuality and cardiovascular risk. A cohort study in patients with erectile dysfunction. J Sex Med 2010;7(5):1918–27.
[59] Gandaglia G, Briganti A, Montorsi P, Mottrie A, Salonia A, Montorsi F. Diagnostic and therapeutic implications of erectile dysfunction in patients with cardiovascular disease. Eur Urol 2016;70(2):219–22.
[60] Vlachopoulos CV, Terentes-Printzios DG, Ioakeimidis NK, Aznaouridis KA, Stefanadis CI. Prediction of cardiovascular events and all-cause mortality with erectile dysfunction: a systematic review and meta-analysis of cohort studies. Circ Cardiovasc Qual Outcomes 2013;6(1):99–109.

[61] Gandaglia G, Briganti A, Jackson G, Kloner RA, Montorsi F, Montorsi P, et al. A systematic review of the association between erectile dysfunction and cardiovascular disease. Eur Urol 2014;65(5):968–78.

[62] Seidman SN. The aging male: androgens, erectile dysfunction, and depression. J Clin Psychiatry 2003;64(Suppl 10):31–7.

[63] Shimizu S, Tsounapi P, Honda M, Dimitriadis F, Taniuchi K, Shimizu T, et al. Effect of an angiotensin II receptor blocker and a calcium channel blocker on hypertension associated penile dysfunction in a rat model. Biomed Res 2014;35(3):215–21.

[64] Johannes CB, Araujo AB, Feldman HA, Derby CA, Kleinman KP, McKinlay JB. Incidence of erectile dysfunction in men 40 to 69 years old: longitudinal results from the Massachusetts male aging study. J Urol 2000;163(2):460–3.

[65] Belba A, Cortelazzo A, Andrea G, Durante J, Nigi L, Dotta F, et al. Erectile dysfunction and diabetes: association with the impairment of lipid metabolism and oxidative stress. Clin Biochem 2016;49(1–2):70–8.

[66] Condorelli RA, Calogero AE, Favilla V, Morgia G, Johnson EO, Castiglione R, et al. Arterial erectile dysfunction: different severities of endothelial apoptosis between diabetic patients "responders" and "non responders" to sildenafil. Eur J Intern Med 2013;24(3):234–40.

[67] Sommer F, Goldstein I, Korda JB. Bicycle riding and erectile dysfunction: a review. J Sex Med 2010;7(7):2346–58.

[68] Chitaley K, Kupelian V, Subak L, Wessells H. Diabetes, obesity and erectile dysfunction: field overview and research priorities. J Urol 2009;182(6 Suppl):S45–50.

[69] Lew-Starowicz M, Gellert R. The sexuality and quality of life of hemodialyzed patients—ASED multicenter study. J Sex Med 2009;6(4):1062–71.

[70] Lai CF, Wang YT, Hung KY, Peng YS, Lien YR, Wu MS, et al. Sexual dysfunction in peritoneal dialysis patients. Am J Nephrol 2007;27(6):615–21.

[71] Ziegler D. Diagnosis and treatment of diabetic autonomic neuropathy. Curr Diab Rep 2001;1(3):216–27.

[72] Chaudhuri KR, Schapira AH. Non-motor symptoms of Parkinson's disease: dopaminergic pathophysiology and treatment. Lancet Neurol 2009;8(5):464–74.

[73] Jung JH, Kam SC, Choi SM, Jae SU, Lee SH, Hyun JS. Sexual dysfunction in male stroke patients: correlation between brain lesions and sexual function. Urology. 2008;71(1):99–103.

[74] Jeon SW, Yoo KH, Kim TH, Kim JI, Lee CH. Correlation of the erectile dysfunction with lesions of cerebrovascular accidents. J Sex Med 2009;6(1):251–6.

[75] Mouraviev VB, Coburn M, Santucci RA. The treatment of posterior urethral disruption associated with pelvic fractures: comparative experience of early realignment vs delayed urethroplasty. J Urol 2005;173(3):873–6.

[76] Aboseif S, Shinohara K, Breza J, Benard F, Narayan P. Role of penile vascular injury in erectile dysfunction after radical prostatectomy. Br J Urol 1994;73(1):75–82.

[77] Catalona WJ, Bigg SW. Nerve-sparing radical prostatectomy: evaluation of results after 250 patients. J Urol 1990;143(3):538–43 discussion 44.

[78] Hekal IA, El-Bahnasawy MS, Mosbah A, El-Assmy A, Shaaban A. Recoverability of erectile function in post-radical cystectomy patients: subjective and objective evaluations. Eur Urol 2009;55(2):275–83.

[79] Liang JT, Lai HS, Lee PH, Chang KJ. Laparoscopic pelvic autonomic nerve-preserving surgery for sigmoid colon cancer. Ann Surg Oncol 2008;15(6):1609–16.

[80] Walsh PC, Brendler CB, Chang T, Marshall FF, Mostwin JL, Stutzman R, et al. Preservation of sexual function in men during radical pelvic surgery. Md Med J 1990;39(4):389–93.

[81] Kendirci M, Hellstrom WJ. Current concepts in the management of erectile dysfunction in men with prostate cancer. Clin Prostate Cancer 2004;3(2):87–92.

[82] Khorrami MH, Moosaie MR, Javid A. Erectile function after radical cystectomy: comparing surgical stapler with LigaSure in division of vascular pedicles. Int J Urol 2019;26(12):1157–8.

[83] Tal R, Valenzuela R, Aviv N, Parker M, Waters WB, Flanigan RC, et al. Persistent erectile dysfunction following radical prostatectomy: the association between nerve-sparing status and the prevalence and chronology of venous leak. J Sex Med 2009;6(10):2813–19.

[84] Vale J. Erectile dysfunction following radical therapy for prostate cancer. Radiother Oncol 2000;57(3):301–5.

[85] Rowland DL, Greenleaf WJ, Dorfman LJ, Davidson JM. Aging and sexual function in men. Arch Sex Behav 1993;22(6):545–57.

[86] Grimm Jr. RH, Grandits GA, Prineas RJ, McDonald RH, Lewis CE, Flack JM, et al. Long-term effects on sexual function of five antihypertensive drugs and nutritional hygienic treatment in hypertensive men and women. Treatment of Mild Hypertension Study (TOMHS). Hypertension 1997;29(1 Pt 1):8–14.

[87] Suzuki H, Tominaga T, Kumagai H, Saruta T. Effects of first-line antihypertensive agents on sexual function and sex hormones. J Hypertens Suppl 1988;6(4):S649–51.

[88] Toblli JE, Cao G, Casas G, Mazza ON. In vivo and in vitro effects of nebivolol on penile structures in hypertensive rats. Am J Hypertens 2006;19(12):1226–32.

[89] Fovaeus M, Andersson KE, Hedlund H. Effects of some calcium channel blockers on isolated human penile erectile tissues. J Urol 1987;138(5):1267–72.

[90] Wirshing DA, Pierre JM, Marder SR, Saunders CS, Wirshing WC. Sexual side effects of novel antipsychotic medications. Schizophr Res 2002;56(1–2):25–30.

[91] Milano W, Colletti C, Capasso A. Hyperprolactinemia induced by antipsychotics: from diagnosis to treatment approach. Endocr Metab Immune Disord Drug Targets 2017;17(1):38–55.

[92] Rehman J, Christ G, Alyskewycz M, Kerr E, Melman A. Experimental hyperprolactinemia in a rat model: alteration in centrally mediated neuroerectile mechanisms. Int J Impot Res 2000;12(1):23–32.

[93] Paick JS, Yang JH, Kim SW, Ku JH. The role of prolactin levels in the sexual activity of married men with erectile dysfunction. BJU Int 2006;98(6):1269–73.

[94] Foreman MM, Hall JL, Love RL. The role of the 5-HT2 receptor in the regulation of sexual performance of male rats. Life Sci 1989;45(14):1263–70.

[95] Foreman MM, Wernicke JF. Approaches for the development of oral drug therapies for erectile dysfunction. Semin Urol 1990;8(2):107–12.

[96] Angulo J, Peiro C, Sanchez-Ferrer CF, Gabancho S, Cuevas P, Gupta S, et al. Differential effects of serotonin reuptake inhibitors on erectile responses, NO-production, and neuronal NO synthase expression in rat corpus cavernosum tissue. Br J Pharmacol 2001;134(6):1190–4.

[97] Tang Y, Rampin O, Calas A, Facchinetti P, Giuliano F. Oxytocinergic and serotonergic innervation of identified lumbosacral nuclei controlling penile erection in the male rat. Neuroscience 1998;82(1):241–54.

[98] Keltner NL, McAfee KM, Taylor CL. Mechanisms and treatments of SSRI-induced sexual dysfunction. Perspect Psychiatr Care 2002;38(3):111–16.

[99] Harrison WM, Rabkin JG, Ehrhardt AA, Stewart JW, McGrath PJ, Ross D, et al. Effects of antidepressant medication on sexual function: a controlled study. J Clin Psychopharmacol 1986;6(3):144–9.

[100] Kuba R, Pohanka M, Zakopcan J, Novotna I, Rektor I. Sexual dysfunctions and blood hormonal profile in men with focal epilepsy. Epilepsia 2006;47(12):2135–40.

[101] Herzog AG, Drislane FW, Schomer DL, Pennell PB, Bromfield EB, Kelly KM, et al. Differential effects of antiepileptic drugs on sexual function and reproductive hormones in men with epilepsy: interim analysis of a comparison between lamotrigine and enzyme-inducing antiepileptic drugs. Epilepsia 2004;45(7):764–8.

[102] Melis MR, Succu S, Spano MS, Argiolas A. Morphine injected into the paraventricular nucleus of the hypothalamus prevents noncontact penile erections and impairs copulation: involvement of nitric oxide. Eur J Neurosci 1999;11(6):1857–64.

[103] Zhao S, Deng T, Luo L, Wang J, Li E, Liu L, et al. Association between opioid use and risk of erectile dysfunction: a systematic review and meta-analysis. J Sex Med 2017;14(10):1209–19.

[104] Zarrindast MR, Shokravi S, Samini M. Opposite influences of dopaminergic receptor subtypes on penile erection. Gen Pharmacol 1992;23(4):671–5.

[105] Zarrindast MR, Farahvash H. Effects of GABA-ergic drugs on penile erection induced by apomorphine in rats. Psychopharmacology (Berlin) 1994;115(1–2):249–53.

[106] Tosti A, Piraccini BM, Soli M. Evaluation of sexual function in subjects taking finasteride for the treatment of androgenetic alopecia. J Eur Acad Dermatol Venereol 2001;15(5):418–21.

[107] Helsen C, Van den Broeck T, Voet A, Prekovic S, Van Poppel H, Joniau S, et al. Androgen receptor antagonists for prostate cancer therapy. Endocr Relat Cancer 2014;21(4):T105–18.

[108] Tapanainen JS, Aittomaki K, Min J, Vaskivuo T, Huhtaniemi IT. Men homozygous for an inactivating mutation of the follicle-stimulating hormone (FSH) receptor gene present variable suppression of spermatogenesis and fertility. Nat Genet 1997;15(2):205–6.

[109] Vermeulen A, Kaufman JM. Ageing of the hypothalamo-pituitary-testicular axis in men. Horm Res 1995;43(1–3):25–8.

[110] Granata AR, Rochira V, Lerchl A, Marrama P, Carani C. Relationship between sleep-related erections and testosterone levels in men. J Androl 1997;18(5):522–7.

[111] Bhasin S, Cunningham GR, Hayes FJ, Matsumoto AM, Snyder PJ, Swerdloff RS, et al. Testosterone therapy in men with androgen deficiency syndromes: an Endocrine Society clinical practice guideline. J Clin Endocrinol Metab 2010;95(6):2536–59.

[112] Wu FC, Tajar A, Beynon JM, Pye SR, Silman AJ, Finn JD, et al. Identification of late-onset hypogonadism in middle-aged and elderly men. N Engl J Med 2010;363(2):123–35.

[113] Marberger M, Roehrborn CG, Marks LS, Wilson T, Rittmaster RS. Relationship among serum testosterone, sexual function, and response to treatment in men receiving dutasteride for benign prostatic hyperplasia. J Clin Endocrinol Metab 2006;91(4):1323–8.

[114] Hall SA, Esche GR, Araujo AB, Travison TG, Clark RV, Williams RE, et al. Correlates of low testosterone and symptomatic androgen deficiency in a population-based sample. J Clin Endocrinol Metab 2008;93(10):3870–7.

[115] Maggi M, Buvat J, Corona G, Guay A, Torres LO. Hormonal causes of male sexual dysfunctions and their management (hyperprolactinemia, thyroid disorders, GH disorders, and DHEA). J Sex Med 2013;10(3):661–77.

[116] Freeman ME, Kanyicska B, Lerant A, Nagy G. Prolactin: structure, function, and regulation of secretion. Physiol Rev 2000;80(4):1523–631.

[117] Fisher JR, Baker GH, Hammarberg K. Long-term health, well-being, life satisfaction, and attitudes toward parenthood in men diagnosed as infertile: challenges to gender stereotypes and implications for practice. Fertil Steril 2010;94(2):574–80.

[118] Peterson BD, Newton CR, Rosen KH, Skaggs GE. Gender differences in how men and women who are referred for IVF cope with infertility stress. Hum Reprod 2006;21(9):2443–9.

[119] Kim SC, Oh MM. Norepinephrine involvement in response to intracorporeal injection of papaverine in psychogenic impotence. J Urol 1992;147(6):1530–2.

[120] Steers WD. Neural pathways and central sites involved in penile erection: neuroanatomy and clinical implications. Neurosci Biobehav Rev 2000;24(5):507–16.

[121] Mosaku KS, Ukpong DI. Erectile dysfunction in a sample of patients attending a psychiatric outpatient department. Int J Impot Res 2009;21(4):235–9.

[122] Berg KM, Demas PA, Howard AA, Schoenbaum EE, Gourevitch MN, Arnsten JH. Gender differences in factors associated with adherence to antiretroviral therapy. J Gen Intern Med 2004;19(11):1111–17.

[123] Monane M, Bohn RL, Gurwitz JH, Glynn RJ, Levin R, Avorn J. Compliance with antihypertensive therapy among elderly Medicaid enrollees: the roles of age, gender, and race. Am J Public Health 1996;86(12):1805–8.

[124] Galdas PM, Cheater F, Marshall P. Men and health help-seeking behaviour: literature review. J Adv Nurs 2005;49(6):616–23.

[125] Imamura M, Waseda Y, Marinova GV, Ishibashi T, Obayashi S, Sasaki A, et al. Alterations of NOS, arginase, and DDAH protein expression in rabbit cavernous tissue after administration of cigarette smoke extract. Am J Physiol Regul Integr Comp Physiol 2007;293(5):R2081–9.

[126] Chew KK. Alcohol consumption and male erectile dysfunction: an unfounded reputation for risk? J Sex Med 2009;6(8):2340.

[127] Miller NS, Gold MS. The human sexual response and alcohol and drugs. J Subst Abuse Treat 1988;5(3):171–7.

[128] Gundersen TD, Jorgensen N, Andersson AM, Bang AK, Nordkap L, Skakkebaek NE, et al. Association between use of marijuana and male reproductive hormones and semen quality: a study among 1,215 healthy young men. Am J Epidemiol 2015;182(6):473–81.

[129] Gorzalka BB, Hill MN, Chang SC. Male-female differences in the effects of cannabinoids on sexual behavior and gonadal hormone function. Horm Behav 2010;58(1):91–9.
[130] Gupta BP, Murad MH, Clifton MM, Prokop L, Nehra A, Kopecky SL. The effect of lifestyle modification and cardiovascular risk factor reduction on erectile dysfunction: a systematic review and meta-analysis. Arch Intern Med 2011;171(20):1797–803.
[131] DeLay KJ, Haney N, Hellstrom WJ. Modifying risk factors in the management of erectile dysfunction: a review. World J Mens Health 2016;34(2):89–100.
[132] Giuliano F, Jackson G, Montorsi F, Martin-Morales A, Raillard P. Safety of sildenafil citrate: review of 67 double-blind placebo-controlled trials and the postmarketing safety database. Int J Clin Pract 2010;64(2):240–55.
[133] Yuan J, Zhang R, Yang Z, et al. Comparative effectiveness and safety of oral phosphodiesterase type 5 inhibitors for erectile dysfunction: a systematic review and network meta-analysis. Eur Urol 2013;63(5):902–12.
[134] Corbin JD. Mechanisms of action of PDE5 inhibition in erectile dysfunction. Int J Impot Res 2004;16(Suppl 1):S4–7.
[135] Smith WB, McCaslin IR, Gokce A, Mandava SH, Trost L, Hellstrom WJ. PDE5 inhibitors: considerations for preference and long-term adherence. Int J Clin Pract 2013;67(8):768–80.
[136] Lee M, Sharifi R. Non-invasive management options for erectile dysfunction when a phosphodiesterase type 5 inhibitor fails. Drugs Aging 2018;35(3):175–87.
[137] Nehra A. Oral and non-oral combination therapy for erectile dysfunction. Rev Urol 2007;9(3):99–105.
[138] Lotti F, Maggi M. Sexual dysfunction and male infertility. Nat Rev Urol 2018;15(5):287–307.
[139] Hellstrom WJ, Overstreet JW, Yu A, et al. Tadalafil has no detrimental effect on human spermatogenesis or reproductive hormones. J Urol 2003;170(3):887–91.
[140] Glenn DR, McVicar CM, McClure N, Lewis SE. Sildenafil citrate improves sperm motility but causes a premature acrosome reaction in vitro. Fertil Steril 2007;87(5):1064–70.
[141] Rago R, Salacone P, Caponecchia L, Marcucci I, Fiori C, Sebastianelli A. Effect of vardenafil on semen parameters in infertile men: a pilot study evaluating short-term treatment. J Endocrinol Invest 2012;35(10):897–900.
[142] Khan S, Amjad A, Rowland D. Potential for long-term benefit of cognitive behavioral therapy as an adjunct treatment for men with erectile dysfunction. J Sex Med 2019;16(2):300–6.
[143] Wischmann TH. Psychogenic infertility—myths and facts. J Assist Reprod Genet 2003;20(12):485–94.
[144] Wischmann T, Scherg H, Strowitzki T, Verres R. Psychosocial characteristics of women and men attending infertility counselling. Hum Reprod 2009;24(2):378–85.
[145] Petok WD. Infertility counseling (or the lack thereof) of the forgotten male partner. Fertil Steril 2015;104(2):260–6.
[146] Furman I, Parra L, Fuentes A, Devoto L. Men's participation in psychologic counseling services offered during in vitro fertilization treatments. Fertil Steril 2010;94(4):1460–4.
[147] Jennings MO, Owen RC, Keefe D, Kim ED. Management and counseling of the male with advanced paternal age. Fertil Steril 2017;107(2):324–8.
[148] Wheeler KM, Sharma D, Kavoussi PK, Smith RP, Costabile R. Clomiphene citrate for the treatment of hypogonadism. Sex Med Rev 2019;7(2):272–6. https://doi.org/10.1016/j.sxmr.2018.10.001.
[149] Scovell JM, Khera M. Testosterone replacement therapy vs clomiphene citrate in the young hypogonadal male. Eur Urol Focus 2018;4(3):321–3.
[150] Mulhall JP, Trost LW, Brannigan RE, et al. Evaluation and management of testosterone deficiency: AUA guideline. J Urol 2018;200(2):423–32.
[151] Wenker EP, Dupree JM, Langille GM, et al. The use of HCG-based combination therapy for recovery of spermatogenesis after testosterone use. J Sex Med 2015;12(6):1334–7.
[152] Haidl G. Management strategies for male factor infertility. Drugs. 2002;62(12):1741–53.
[153] Pitteloud N, Dwyer A. Hormonal control of spermatogenesis in men: therapeutic aspects in hypogonadotropic hypogonadism. Ann Endocrinol (Paris) 2014;75(2):98–100.
[154] Moskovic DJ, Katz DJ, Akhavan A, Park K, Mulhall JP. Clomiphene citrate is safe and effective for long-term management of hypogonadism. BJU Int 2012;110(10):1524–8.
[155] Raina R, Pahlajani G, Agarwal A, Zippe CD. Treatment of erectile dysfunction: update. Am J Mens Health 2007;1(2):126–38.
[156] Narus JB. Intracavernosal injection training. Atlas of office based andrology procedures. Cham: Springer International Publishing; 2017,. p. 117–27.
[157] Fode M, Krogh-Jespersen S, Brackett NL, Ohl DA, Lynne CM, Sønksen J. Male sexual dysfunction and infertility associated with neurological disorders. Asian J Androl 2012;14(1):61–8.
[158] Brackett NL. Infertility in men with spinal cord injury: research and treatment. Scientifica (Cairo) 2012;2012:578257.
[159] Zippe CD, Pahlajani G. Vacuum erection devices to treat erectile dysfunction and early penile rehabilitation following radical prostatectomy. Curr Urol Rep 2008;9(6):506–13.
[160] Dhir RR, Lin HC, Canfield SE, Wang R. Combination therapy for erectile dysfunction: an update review. Asian J Androl 2011;13(3):382–90.
[161] Raina R, Pahlajani G, Agarwal A, Jones S, Zippe C. Long-term potency after early use of a vacuum erection device following radical prostatectomy. BJU Int 2010;106(11):1719–22.
[162] Gandaglia G, Suardi N, Cucchiara V, et al. Penile rehabilitation after radical prostatectomy: does it work? Transl Androl Urol 2015;4(2):110–23.
[163] Wassersug R, Wibowo E. Non-pharmacological and non-surgical strategies to promote sexual recovery for men with erectile dysfunction. Transl Androl Urol 2017;6(Suppl 5):S776–94.
[164] Costa P, Potempa AJ. Intraurethral alprostadil for erectile dysfunction: a review of the literature. Drugs 2012;72(17):2243–54.
[165] Guay AT, Perez JB, Velásquez E, Newton RA, Jacobson JP. Clinical experience with intraurethral alprostadil (MUSE) in the treatment of men with erectile dysfunction. A retrospective study. Medicated urethral system for erection. Eur Urol 2000;38(6):671–6.

[166] Padma-Nathan H, Yeager JL. An integrated analysis of alprostadil topical cream for the treatment of erectile dysfunction in 1732 patients. Urology 2006;68(2):386–91.
[167] Padma-Nathan H, Hellstrom WJ, Kaiser FE, et al. Treatment of men with erectile dysfunction with transurethral alprostadil. Medicated urethral system for erection (MUSE) study group. N Engl J Med 1997;336(1):1–7.
[168] Shokeir AA, Alserafi MA, Mutabagani H. Intracavernosal vs intraurethral alprostadil: a prospective randomized study. BJU Int 1999;83(7):812–15.
[169] Levine LA, Becher EF, Bella AJ, et al. Penile prosthesis surgery: current recommendations from the international consultation on sexual medicine. J Sex Med 2016;13(4):489–518.
[170] Levine LA, Benson J, Hoover C. Inflatable penile prosthesis placement in men with Peyronie's disease and drug-resistant erectile dysfunction: a single-center study. J Sex Med 2010;7(11):3775–83.
[171] Hebert KJ, Kohler TS. Penile prosthesis infection: myths and realities. World J Mens Health 2019;37(3):276–87.
[172] Lipsky MJ, Onyeji I, Golan R, et al. Diabetes is a risk factor for inflatable penile prosthesis infection: analysis of a large statewide database. Sex Med 2019;7(1):35–40.
[173] Mahon J, Dornbier R, Wegrzyn G, et al. Infectious adverse events following the placement of a penile prosthesis: a systematic review. Sex Med Rev 2020;8(2):348–54.
[174] Herati AS, Lo EM. Penile prosthesis biofilm formation and emerging therapies against them. Transl Androl Urol 2018;7(6):960–7.
[175] Yarkony GM. Enhancement of sexual function and fertility in spinal cord-injured males. Am J Phys Med Rehabil 1990;69(2):81–7.
[176] Lokeshwar SD, Bitran J, Madhusoodanan V, Kava B, Ramasamy R. A surgeon's guide to the various antibiotic dips available during penile prosthesis implantation. Curr Urol Rep 2019;20(2):11.
[177] Brackett NL, Ibrahim E, Iremashvili V, Aballa TC, Lynne CM. Treatment for ejaculatory dysfunction in men with spinal cord injury: an 18-year single center experience. J Urol 2010;183(6):2304–8.
[178] Semet M, Paci M, Saïas-Magnan J, et al. The impact of drugs on male fertility: a review. Andrology 2017;5(4):640–63.
[179] Luco SM, Agbo C, Behr B, Dahan MH. The evaluation of pre and post processing semen analysis parameters at the time of intrauterine insemination in couples diagnosed with male factor infertility and pregnancy rates based on stimulation agent. A retrospective cohort study. Eur J Obstet Gynecol Reprod Biol 2014;179:159–62.
[180] Ye F, Cao W, Lin J, et al. The pregnancy outcomes of intrauterine insemination with husband's sperm in natural cycles vs ovulation stimulated cycles: a retrospective study. BioSci Trends 2018;12(5):463–9.
[181] Bahadur G, Homburg R, Bosmans JE, et al. Observational retrospective study of UK national success, risks and costs for 319,105 IVF/ICSI and 30,669 IUI treatment cycles. BMJ Open 2020;10(3):e034566.
[182] Tjon-Kon-Fat RI, Tajik P, Custers IM, et al. Can we identify subfertile couples that benefit from immediate in vitro fertilisation over intrauterine insemination? Eur J Obstet Gynecol Reprod Biol 2016;202:36–40.
[183] Ohl DA, Wolf LJ, Menge AC, et al. Electroejaculation and assisted reproductive technologies in the treatment of anejaculatory infertility. Fertil Steril 2001;76(6):1249–55.
[184] Ombelet W, Dhont N, Thijssen A, Bosmans E, Kruger T. Semen quality and prediction of IUI success in male subfertility: a systematic review. Reprod Biomed Online 2014;28(3):300–9.
[185] Corona G, Minhas S, Giwercman A, et al. Sperm recovery and ICSI outcomes in men with non-obstructive azoospermia: a systematic review and meta-analysis. Hum Reprod Update 2019;25(6):733–57.
[186] Ghanem M, Bakr NI, Elgayaar MA, El Mongy S, Fathy H, Ibrahim AH. Comparison of the outcome of intracytoplasmic sperm injection in obstructive and non-obstructive azoospermia in the first cycle: a report of case series and meta-analysis. Int J Androl 2005;28(1):16–21.
[187] Esteves SC, Miyaoka R, Agarwal A. Sperm retrieval techniques for assisted reproduction. Int Braz J Urol 2011;37(5):570–83.
[188] Chung PH, Palermo G, Schlegel PN, Veeck LL, Eid JF, Rosenwaks Z. The use of intracytoplasmic sperm injection with electroejaculates from anejaculatory men. Hum Reprod 1998;13(7):1854–8.
[189] Soeterik TF, Veenboer PW, Lock TM. Electroejaculation in psychogenic anejaculation. Fertil Steril 2014;101(6):1604–8.
[190] Hovav Y, Kafka I, Horenstein E, Yaffe H. Prostatic massage as a method for obtaining spermatozoa in men with psychogenic anejaculation. Fertil Steril 2000;74(1):184–5.
[191] Inhorn MC, Patrizio P. Infertility around the globe: new thinking on gender, reproductive technologies and global movements in the 21st century. Hum Reprod Update 2015;21(4):411–26.
[192] Bahamondes L, Makuch MY. Infertility care and the introduction of new reproductive technologies in poor resource settings. Reprod Biol Endocrinol 2014;12:87.

CHAPTER 5

Ejaculatory dysfunction and infertility

Daniel N. Watter[1] and Kathryn S.K. Hall[2]

[1]Morris Psychological Group, P.A., Parsippany, NJ, United States [2]Private Practice, Princeton, NJ, United States

Introduction

Problems with ejaculation are among the greatest sexual vexations for men and their partners. Whether we are considering premature or rapid ejaculation, or delayed or absent ejaculation, the experience of having no control over the timing of their ejaculation has been a source of frustration and befuddlement for men through the ages. While the literature on the link between ejaculatory disorders and infertility is scant, it is obvious that problems with male ejaculation will frustrate attempts to conceive via sexual intercourse, and such problems frequently are the precipitant for a couple's visit to a fertility clinic [1].

Treatment of male ejaculatory problems has met with mixed results, but most clinicians and researchers agree that the successful management of infertility and sexual dysfunction should involve appropriate psychological and medical therapies [2]. Attending to both the presenting sexual dysfunction as well as the psychosocial needs of the couple is required to efficaciously bring about a positive resolution for the couple.

According to Kondoh [3], ejaculatory dysfunction is the most common male sexual disorder, and can be divided into four categories: premature ejaculation (PE), delayed ejaculation, retrograde ejaculation, and anejaculation. Premature and delayed ejaculation are significant sources of sexual dissatisfaction among men and their partners, but patients with these conditions may retain normal fertility. However, those patients with retrograde ejaculation or anejaculation are unable to deliver sperm into the female genital tract and are therefore considered subfertile [4]. Premature and delayed ejaculation will be examined in detail. Retrograde ejaculation (ejaculation into the bladder) and anejaculation (the complete absence of ejaculation) will be given less consideration since they are not typically seen as being within the purview of sex therapy and are therefore beyond the scope of this chapter.

Retrograde ejaculation and anejaculation

According to Barazani et al. [4], retrograde ejaculation is marked by the propulsion of seminal fluid into the bladder. The diagnosis of retrograde ejaculation is confirmed by a postejaculatory urine that reveals spermatozoa, seminal fluid, or fructose [5]. Retrograde ejaculation has multiple causes, but more than 80% of the cases are caused by either diabetes, retroperitoneal surgery, bladder neck surgery, or transurethral resection of the prostate [6]. Psychotropic medications and alpha-adrenergic blockers are also frequent causes of retrograde ejaculations.

Anejaculation, or the complete absence of ejaculation, can have the same etiologies as retrograde ejaculation. Any disease, surgical procedure, or trauma that interferes with the afferent or efferent innervation of the seminal vesicles, vas deferens, bladder neck, or posterior urethra can potentially result in anejaculation [4]. The most common causes of anejaculation are retroperitoneal lymph node dissection and spinal cord injury. However, diabetes, multiple sclerosis, and psychotropic medications can also result in this condition [4].

Kondoh [3] asserts that oral pharmacotherapy is the simplest, least invasive, and if successful, offers the most desirable possibility to conceiving via sexual intercourse. For those men who do not respond to pharmacological intervention, or for whom such intervention is otherwise contraindicated, assisted ejaculation procedures to harvest sperm are often utilized. Some patients will respond well to penile vibratory stimulation (PVS). PVS is an office-based procedure that involves placing a vibrator against the penis for several minutes and mechanical stimulation is delivered to induce antegrade ejaculation [7,8].

Electroejaculation (EEJ) is an alternative approach to PVS. EEJ utilizes a specifically designed electric probe that is inserted into the rectum. General anesthesia is required, with the exception of some cases of complete spinal cord injuries in which painful sensation from the action of the probe is not an issue [4].

Those patients who are not successful with the assisted stimulation methods may be candidates for surgical sperm retrieval (SSR). While sperm retrieval can occasionally be achieved by nonsurgical means (i.e., prostate massage, bladder catheterization, or sperm obtained from nocturnal emissions in men with psychogenic anejaculation), SSR appears to be the more efficacious strategy [4].

Premature or rapid ejaculation

While premature, or rapid, ejaculation is the most frequent sexual complaint among men, it is nevertheless, a poorly understood condition [9]. Although not implicated in fertility problems at nearly the rate of delayed ejaculation, the inability to deposit semen into the vagina can result in significant distress for both the man and his partner [10].

Our ability to more fully understand this condition is confounded by a lack of agreement on the precise definition of the dysfunction. The definition of premature, or rapid, ejaculation is complicated due to the highly subjective nature of the terms *premature* and *rapid*. In considering premature or rapid ejaculation, how fast is too fast? How long is one *supposed* to be able to engage in sexual intercourse before ejaculating?

There have been many attempts to try to standardize the definition of premature or rapid ejaculation. One of the first was Masters and Johnson's [11] assertion that ejaculation is premature if the man is unable to delay his ejaculation long enough for his partner to reach orgasm on 50% of intercourse attempts. Unfortunately, this definition has several substantive limitations. As pointed out by Parnham and Serefoglu [9], much of the burden for diagnosis lay with the female partner, whose ability to climax during sexual intercourse becomes the primary determinant of dysfunction. According to Mintz and Guitelman [12], there is a large "orgasm gap" between men and women in terms of frequency of orgasm during intercourse. They point out that research and clinical experience has clearly demonstrated that men are significantly more likely to experience orgasm during sexual intercourse than are women. Therefore the notion of diagnosing a male's sexual dysfunction based on his *partner's* responsiveness is not only unfair, but clinically unsound. For example, if we were to use Masters and Johnson's definition of PE, a man could engage in sexual intercourse with a female partner for 30 minutes and if he ejaculates before she reached orgasm, he would qualify for the diagnosis of PE. Of course, it is highly doubtful that Masters and Johnson would aver that a man in such circumstances was, indeed, a premature ejaculator, but it highlights a weakness and imperfection in their proposed definition.

Since the time of Masters and Johnson, there have been several attempts to refine the definition of premature or rapid ejaculation. Unfortunately, all have had their shortcomings. The latest issue of the Diagnostic and Statistical Manual of Mental Disorders, DSM-V [13] has offered the following definition of what they refer to as premature (early) ejaculation:

A. *A persistent or recurrent pattern of ejaculation occurring during partnered sexual activity within approximately 1 minute following vaginal penetration and before the individual wishes it. [Note: Although the diagnosis of premature (early) ejaculation may be applied to individuals engaged in nonvaginal sexual activities, specific duration criteria have not been established for these activities.]*
B. *The symptom in Criterion A must have been present for at least 6 months and must be experienced on almost all or all (approximately 75%–100%) occasions of sexual activity (identified situational contexts or, if generalized, in all contexts).*
C. *The symptom in Criterion A causes clinically significant distress in the individual.*
D. *The sexual dysfunction is not better explained by a nonsexual mental disorder or as a consequence of severe relationship distress or other significant stressors and is not attributable to the effects of a substance/medication or another medical condition.*

Specify whether:
Lifelong: The disturbance has been present since the individual became sexually active.
Acquired: The disturbance began after a period of relatively normal sexual dysfunction.

Specify whether:
Generalized: Not limited to certain types of stimulation, situations, or partners.
Situational: Only occurs with certain types of stimulation, situations, or partners.
Specify current severity:
Mild: Ejaculation occurring within approximately 30 seconds to 1 minute of vaginal penetration.
Moderate: Ejaculation occurring within approximately 15–30 seconds of vaginal penetration.
Severe: Ejaculation occurring prior to sexual activity, at the start of sexual activity, or within approximately 15 seconds of vaginal penetration (pp. 579–580).

While this definition is clearly an improvement over that put forth by Masters and Johnson, it is not without its own serious flaws and limitations. On the most basic level, the criterion of less than 1 minute is still highly subjective and arbitrary. Why not 30 seconds? 2 minutes? 4 minutes? The choice to identify a time frame reflects the desire of diagnosticians to provide an answer to the question we posed before: *How long is one supposed to be able to engage in sexual intercourse before ejaculating?* So, the attribution of time has come to be seen as necessary to create a more standardized assessment of ejaculatory duration. Althof et al. and Althof [14,15] has described the concept of intravaginal ejaculatory latency time (IELT) as the standard of measurement for ejaculatory disorders. According to Althof [15] and Waldinger [16], IELT refers to the time between the start of vaginal penetration and the start of intravaginal ejaculation. Clearly many men feel distressed about the timing of ejaculation with IELTs of longer than 1 minute. So, while statistically sensible, the criterion of 1 minute for a diagnosis of PE may nonetheless be clinically arbitrary and capricious.

With regard to what is likely to be seen in an infertility clinic, Burns [17] reports that while lifelong PE is the most common male sexual dysfunction in the general population, it is actually acquired PE that is most likely seen in the infertility clinic. In addition, it is also the severe level of severity that is likely most commonly seen in couples presenting with fertility concerns because while early ejaculations may certainly be distressing and disappointing for couples in terms of sexual satisfaction, it is the severe level that is going to impede the depositing of semen intravaginally. In addition, Burns [17] points out that if PE was a problem before infertility, it will likely be exacerbated by an infertility diagnosis and treatment. Therefore if we look at aforementioned Criteria D, would problems related to infertility that would exacerbate an already rapid ejaculation pattern be considered a relationship or other stressor and therefore negate the diagnosis of PE?

In 2014 the International Society for Sexual Medicine (ISSM) [18] attempted to further refine the definition of premature or rapid ejaculation with different time frames differentiating lifelong and acquired forms of the dysfunction. They have suggested that a diagnosis of PE may be made when:

1. *Ejaculation always or nearly always occurs prior to or within about 1 minute of vaginal penetration from the first sexual experience (lifelong PE) or a clinically significant and bothersome reduction in latency time, often to about 3 minutes or less (acquired).*
2. *The inability to delay ejaculation on all or nearly all vaginal penetrations.*
3. *Negative personal consequences, such as distress, bother, frustration, and/or the avoidance of sexual intimacy.*

Here, too, we see an improvement of specificity over the Masters and Johnson definition, but ISSM has also been unable to avoid the subjectivity of timing.

The World Health Organization has recently ratified the 11th revision of the International Classification of Diseases and Related Health Problems (ICD-11) [19]. Adding to the growing and somewhat confusing nomenclature for this condition, the ICD-11 has replaced the term *premature ejaculation* with the diagnostic label *early ejaculation*. Importantly, the ICD-11 does not reference IELTs but defines early ejaculation as "ejaculation that occurs prior to or within a very short duration of the initiation of vaginal penetration or other relevant sexual stimulation, with no or little perceived control over ejaculation" [19]. Althof [20] bemoans the lack of objectivity noting that according to these diagnostic criteria a man who ejaculates within a statistically normal amount of time can still be diagnosed as suffering from PE. Indeed, the ICD-11 has added a third type of PE, which is roughly equivalent to what Waldinger and Schweitzer [21] and Janssen and Waldinger [22] have labeled subjective PE in which men worry that they have no control over the timing of their ejaculation despite being able to last as long as 5 minutes of penile-vaginal intercourse. And so, the debate continues as to what exactly defines PE. Is it a time frame or a lack of control over timing? Whatever the definition that is used, PE is a highly distressing condition for men and their partners.

Premature ejaculation and infertility

To highlight Burns [17], noted earlier, if PE was a problem before infertility, it will likely be exacerbated by an infertility diagnosis and treatment.

Thus when assessing premature or rapid ejaculation as a cause for infertility, we can use a much more functional definition: if the man is unable to hold back his ejaculation to enable intravaginal penetration and thus expels semen prior to penile insertion into the vagina, we can proceed under the verifiable certainty that ejaculation is, indeed, premature, rapid, or early. What the preceding discussion of diagnostic nosology does highlight however is that PE is best understood as an umbrella term for a variety of clinical presentations, all of which cause relationship and individual distress. There is often anxiety about sexual competence (*Am I too quick?*), a concern about the pleasure one is missing or denying a partner, the negative self-perception that one does not have control over the timing of ejaculation, and the resulting avoidance of sex and other forms of intimacy. When PE interferes with fertility, the blame and shame is magnified. Not only is one's ejaculatory incompetence interfering with pleasure, it is denying one's partner the opportunity to conceive. Understanding the importance of these issues will help the clinician sensitively and more effectively initiate treatment protocols for PE.

In all cases, the relational context in which the sexual dysfunction occurs is important. The stress of infertility is most disruptive in those couples who already have a difficult relationship. Another important factor involves the sociocultural expectations and pressures that are often magnified when fertility is at issue. The following case vignette highlights the clinical presentation of a couple in distress with sociocultural factors highlighted.

Javaan and Ahmed were a couple in their early twenties when they were referred for sex therapy. The couple had been trying to conceive since their marriage 1 year prior and were highly anxious given the pressure they felt from their extended family in Pakistan to begin their family. However, while Ahmed had no sexual difficulties prior to his marriage, he had begun to experience severe PE almost immediately after the wedding, ejaculating prior to intercourse. Javaan was highly critical of Ahmed and accused him of selfishly enjoying his own pleasure and questioned his commitment to her and to starting a family. Almost as soon as Ahmed had an erection Javaan would exhort him to insert his penis into her vagina "Just put it in! What is wrong with you? Just do it!" Their sex life soon deteriorated to the point where Ahmed masturbated alone to get an erection and then would approach his waiting wife and try to insert his penis into her vagina before he ejaculated. Worried that he would lose his erection, and distracted by his anxiety and his dread of his wife's unhappiness, Ahmed invariably ejaculated before penetration. Soon, Ahmed was avoiding sexual interactions with his wife and resisted her suggestion that they use a turkey baster or other means to achieve conception. It was important to him and to his sense of his masculinity that they conceive "the natural way" wondering "How will I ever feel like a real father?" They arrived at therapy a couple in much distress.

Treatment for premature or rapid ejaculation

Historically, premature or rapid ejaculation has been treated as a psychological disorder [23]. To be more precise, while this condition has been treated mostly by mental health professionals, it has often been viewed more as a skill deficit that needed to be improved. This is particularly so in the case of lifelong PE. Elliot and Fluker [10] suggest that although premature or rapid ejaculation may have medical causes, it is usually considered a conditioned reflex that requires behavioral techniques, or retraining, and/or pharmacological assistance.

The etiology of lifelong PE or rapid ejaculation is not well understood. According to Zilbergeld [24], ejaculation is a reflex, and some men have better control over their ejaculatory trigger than others. Perhaps some men have a greater sensitivity level than others. Others may have conditioned a quick ejaculatory response through a hurried and furtive masturbation pattern as an adolescent. Still others may have some genetic or neurological predisposition to ejaculate quickly [25]. Clinical reports and global survey data indicate that there is a higher prevalence of PE in traditional cultures and Asian and Middle Eastern countries. But whether these differences reflect a genetic predisposition, differential learning or sexual opportunities, or expectations is not clear [26,27]. None of these possible etiologies have received widespread acceptance or empirical support. Nevertheless, many sex therapists have proclaimed that this is a fairly easy and straightforward condition to treat successfully [20,24,28], regardless of the specific etiology.

Waldinger [23] asserts that our approach to treating premature or rapid ejaculation has not evolved much over the last several decades. In 1956 urologist James Semans reported on using a behavioral intervention known as the stop/start technique. This technique involves the man, or the man's partner, to arouse him to the point of "ejaculatory inevitability," or just prior to the point of ejaculation. The man would then (or signal his partner to) cease stimulation to allow the ejaculatory urge to pass. Once the urge passes, stimulation would then resume and again cease as the man again approaches ejaculatory inevitability. He or his partner would then again cease stimulation prior to ejaculation, and this pattern would be repeated for a specified amount of time. In 1970 Masters and Johnson made a slight modification to the stop/start technique that became known as the squeeze technique, in which the man, or his partner would squeeze the penis by placing the thumb on the frenulum just beneath the glans penis, and the first and second fingers on the coronal ridge, as the man approaches ejaculatory inevitability. Both variations have become the standard protocol for the behavioral retraining of the ejaculatory reflex. Zilbergeld [24] has devised a series of self-help exercises based on the stop/start technique that can be done by the man via masturbation retraining. Zilbergeld asserts that 80%–90% of men who follow his protocol will achieve improved ejaculatory control in approximately 8–20 weeks, provided they are willing to devote the necessary time and energy to the program. Waldinger [23] cautions, however, that there have been few studies on the effectiveness of our behavioral treatments of PE, and those studies that have been conducted note that the gains in control had been lost 3 years after the cessation of treatment.

Recent years have seen the utilization of medications, particularly the selective serotonin reuptake inhibitors (SSRIs) in the treatment of premature or rapid ejaculation. Althof [20] reports that since 1995, clinicians began to experiment with off-label uses of SSRIs to improve ejaculatory latency. It had long been reported that one of the frequent side effects of SSRI use experienced by men and women was difficulty reaching the point of climax. As a result, small doses of an SSRI were thought to be an effective resolution to premature, or rapid ejaculation. Althof [20] cautions, however, that even though we have had success with medications and behavioral retraining exercises, the treatment of premature or rapid ejaculation may be more complicated than it may seem. While improving ejaculatory control has become fairly straightforward, restoring the man's sexual confidence, and reversing the harmful effects on the relationship, may be substantially more challenging.

Consider the following case vignette[1]:

Sheryl and George consulted with me (DW) due to their inability to conceive a child. Specifically, George's difficulty controlling his ejaculation made intercourse impossible, and before embarking on a complex and expensive course of treatment at a fertility clinic, they were advised to pursue sex therapy.

By way of history, Sheryl and George were both in their late twenties. They married right out of college and had been hoping to conceive for the past 4 years. However, the couple was never able to successfully have intercourse as George would ejaculate prior to vaginal penetration. Masturbation for George was frequent, but also completed very quickly. While not timed, George estimated that his masturbatory time from erection to orgasm was less than 1 minute. Sheryl was not George's first sex partner, and he was unable to control his ejaculation with all of the women he had been with, and thus has never had successful sexual intercourse. This was highly frustrating for George, but it rarely produced great distress in his relationships since he was a generous lover, providing both manual and oral stimulation for his partners. Sheryl was similarly accepting of George's ejaculatory difficulties, since he was a good sexual and life partner in many other ways. Following consultation with a local urologist and given a clean bill of urologic health, George was referred for sex therapy. Given this history, George would be considered to have a generalized lifelong case of PE.

George and Sheryl were presented with the treatment protocol for utilizing the squeeze technique in a modified Masters and Johnson format. George would first learn better ejaculatory control via masturbation retraining, and then he and Sheryl would transition to couples' exercises, first without intercourse and then with intercourse. They were also told about the use of an SSRI as an alternative mode of treatment. Since their primary goal was conception, George and Sheryl opted to try an SSRI as a first line of treatment since the effects would be felt more quickly, easily, and cheaply. If this was not effective, they would move to ejaculatory retraining treatment. George and Sheryl were also made aware that should they desire to try medication until conception, they could later return for sex therapy when they were less focused on the goal of conception.

George was prescribed 50 mg of sertraline to be taken once daily. Within 2 weeks, George found that he was able to delay ejaculation long enough to have a brief sexual intercourse experience with Sheryl, and conception followed 2 months later. George and Sheryl have yet to pursue sex therapy and ejaculation retraining exercises, as they expressed being satisfied with the effects of the sertraline.

The case of Sheryl and George was straightforward and uncomplicated. While many clinicians may not be pleased with their desire to continue the reliance on medication as opposed to pursuing a more behavioral treatment, Sheryl and George were quite pleased, especially since neither desired a long intercourse, and their

---

[1] Please note that patients described in all case vignettes have had their identities and identifying details altered to preserve their confidentiality.

primary goal of conception had been satisfied. Regardless of the treatment regimen chosen, most cases of generalized lifelong PE are fairly easily resolved to permit the depositing of sperm via sexual intercourse.

Some cases of acquired PE are also amenable to psychopharmacological interventions but the addition of behavioral techniques is often desirable given the wish to restore a previously enjoyable level of sexual function.

Revisiting the case of Javaan and Ahmed, Ahmed was prescribed paroxetine 40 mg and the couple were instructed in the use of stop-start techniques. Javaan's frustration and hopelessness dissipated with therapy which allowed her to see a path forward to pregnancy. She stopped berating Ahmed and began to participate more in their sexual interactions, first as necessary for stop-start and then for her own pleasure. Within 6 weeks, Javaan was successful in ejaculating intravaginally. The couple remained in therapy with the goal to improve their relationship, especially their communication and their ability to handle stress prior to becoming parents.

Many cases of acquired PE or rapid ejaculation situations are not so easily resolved. As Waldinger [23] has pointed out, those men experiencing acquired PE or rapid ejaculation follow a different pattern. These are men who have not had problems with ejaculatory control in the past, but for some reason have now developed an uncontrolled ejaculatory response. This may occur with gradual or sudden onset. In our clinical experience, those acquired PE or rapid ejaculation cases related to fertility complaints most often present with a rather sudden arrival. Such cases may, indeed, have a medical or physiological basis (i.e., illnesses such as prostatitis or epididymitis, or some form of penile injury or trauma), but most of what is seen in fertility clinics are those cases in which there is some underlying psychological conflict or relationship difficulty. These cases require a much more complex and nuanced treatment approach as their origins are usually multidetermined and not generally amenable to a simple treatment algorithm. Given the multiplicity of personal and relational dynamics involved in human sexual expression, most cases of acquired premature or rapid ejaculation must be carefully assessed as underlying psychological issues are often creating the problem. As a result, it is difficult to apply treatments on the basis of symptom manifestation alone [29]. Perelman [30], Althof [20,31], and Watter [28] have all suggested that in cases of acquired PE or rapid ejaculation an approach that combines psychotherapeutic and pharmacological interventions will likely be the treatment of choice.

Often men with acquired PE or rapid ejaculation are expressing through their penis the message that they are either displeased with something in their relationship or experiencing some ambivalence about engaging in sexual intercourse. Van der Kolk [32] and Mate [33] have noted that often the body "speaks" for us when we are otherwise unable to express our underlying fears, unacknowledged traumas, or negative emotions. For example, in cases in which the PE or rapid ejaculation begins when the couple decides to begin the process of conception, it is not unusual for the man to experience a high degree of ambivalence about the commitment to parenthood. If he is fearful or otherwise uncomfortable acknowledging this ambivalence to his partner, his body may unconsciously react by disrupting the completion of sexual intercourse by triggering an ejaculation prior to vaginal penetration. Similarly, if the man feels "objectified" or that he is only being desired as a sperm producer instead of an object of love and affection, he may unconsciously express this displeasure through an interrupted sexual interaction. Consider the following case vignette.

The case of Joan and Maxwell

Joan and Maxwell were both in their early thirties. They had dated for approximately 3 years and married 2 years ago. Maxwell had doubts about marrying but loved and enjoyed Joan so much that he decided to bend to her desire to marry. Soon after marriage, both reported that sexual frequency began to diminish, but dismissed this as the result of increased familiarity and the passage of time. Approximately 18 months into marriage, Joan expressed her desire to seriously begin a family. Maxwell was ambivalent at best and expressed his hesitations to Joan. Joan, however, felt that Maxwell always reacted negatively to change and believed that if she persisted, he would eventually come around and join her in her enthusiasm for a family. Maxwell was highly conflicted. On the one hand, he did not want to disappoint Joan and knew that her decisions most often turned out to be for the best. However, he was very concerned about giving up another piece of his perceived freedom and autonomy. He said little after their initial conversations and behaved as if he was in agreement with Joan. Interestingly, sexual intercourse almost immediately became problematic as Joan felt as if she was "chasing" Maxwell to have sex, and when they did engage in sex (especially during what she believed were the most fertile times in her cycle) Maxwell would ejaculate prior to vaginal entry. This had never been an issue for Maxwell before, and he was perplexed as to what was creating this disruption in his sexual functioning. Joan thought they should consult a therapist, but Maxwell resisted. They began to fight with an increasing frequency as they both became ever more frustrated. Eventually, Maxwell had to concede that this had become a problem he could not resolve on his own and consulted his primary care physician who then referred him to a local urologist. After a complete urologic examination, Maxwell's urologist recommended consultation with a sex therapist.

By way of history, Maxwell was raised in a highly dysfunctional and traumatic family environment. His father left Maxwell, his mother, and two younger siblings when Maxwell was 9 years old. His mother's drinking increased dramatically after that, and Maxwell was soon left to care for himself, his two younger siblings, and his actively alcoholic mother. This situation became increasingly burdensome to Maxwell, and he felt trapped, confined, and suffocated by his family responsibilities. He essentially had no childhood to speak of and recalls feeling an extreme level of anger and resentment toward his entire family. Family life was experienced as a confining, smothering, and enmeshing ruse, and he swore to himself that once his siblings were old enough to fend for themselves, he would be gone. Unfortunately, this was easier said than done for Maxwell. He sacrificed his time with friends, participation in school activities, residential college, and visions for an exciting career as he felt responsible for the care and wellbeing of his family. It was not until he met Joan that he was able to pull himself away from the ensnarement of his family and begin to consider the development of his own life. Joan made him feel alive, vibrant, vital, and pulsating with excitement. He saw Joan as a vivacious, animated, and effervescent soul and he longed to have as much of her as possible. She also made him feel free for the first time he could recall. She placed few demands on him, encouraged him to explore opportunities in life, and applauded his strides toward autonomy and independence. Of course, Maxwell also experienced substantial guilt for leaving his family, but they seemed to be doing well, and his siblings who recognized all he had sacrificed for them, lovingly urged him to move on.

Maxwell reveled in his newfound independence and was truly joyful until Joan suggested marriage. Maxwell's initial response was one of panic, as the trauma of family entrapment was triggered within him. He feared his long-awaited free-spirited life was about to be snatched away from him, but calmed himself by reminding himself how his relationship with Joan was so markedly different from his relationship with his family of origin, how much he loved and cherished Joan, and how much better his life had become since they found each other. He agreed to marriage, and despite his anxieties, settled into a gratifying and agreeable married life. However, when Joan expressed a desire to have children, Maxwell's internal alarms went off in a violent, blustery, and uncontrollable outburst. His internal experience of angst felt like a foreboding signal of impending doom. He felt as if his greatest fears were about to be realized and he considered his urgent sense of internal panic as an omen that portended a calamitous outcome. Not being able to acknowledge what was going on inside him to either Joan or to himself, Maxwell tried to press on as if nothing was wrong. However, his protective unconscious used his body to manifest his terror, and it began to disrupt the sexual encounter so that Maxwell could be "saved" from a return to a life of captivity and restriction.

Sex therapy for Joan and Maxwell began with a thorough history of the presenting symptom, their life together, and their experiences with their families of origin. Following the initial psychological assessment, it was determined that Maxwell would benefit from individual psychotherapy to deal with his unacknowledged and unexpressed expressions of trauma from his childhood. This approach was agreeable to both Maxwell and Joan, and it elucidated for them what was likely causing the ambivalence on Maxwell's part. Maxwell's individual psychotherapy sessions were supplemented with occasional couples' therapy sessions to work on residual relationship tensions incurred during the course of their stressful pretreatment months. Within about 4 months, Maxwell was able to function well enough during sexual encounters, but he elected to remain in therapy to continue to work on the sequelae of his early childhood trauma, and to remain aware of unconscious triggers going forward. Maxwell has been seen in a therapy that has now passed the 5-year mark, and he and Joan are the parents of two boys. Maxwell reports reveling in family life, and he has been an engaged, adoring father while still being able to preserve an essential sense of autonomy within the context of mutually rewarding interpersonal familial relationships.

The case of Maxwell and Joan is clearly more nuanced and complex than the case of Sheryl and George or Javaan and Ahmed. This is also a much more common case presentation that is likely to be seen in fertility clinics [17]. Maxwell and Joan's situation was resolvable, but Maxwell's sexual difficulties went well beyond the need to simply retrain his ejaculatory trigger and increase his intravaginal ejaculatory latency. Althof [20] reminds us that often it is not enough to simply offer a drug or behavioral intervention to help delay ejaculation or increase ejaculatory control. The causes, as well as the impacts, of sustained, unexplained sexual dysfunction are profound and painful for both the man and his partner. Often, a course of deep psychotherapy is required to fully understand the meaning behind the presenting symptom and to allow an individual or a couple to return to satisfying relational functionality.

Delayed ejaculation

While premature or rapid ejaculation is occasionally seen as being implicated in fertility problems, delayed ejaculation is seen with substantially greater frequency. Indeed, many couples in which the man experiences delayed ejaculation will only present for sexual medicine or sex therapy treatment when the couple would like to conceive via sexual intercourse and are unable to do so [1].

Defining delayed ejaculation is subject to many of the same constraints and concerns as with PE or rapid ejaculation. In many instances, the diagnosis of delayed ejaculation is arbitrary and subjective. The capriciousness of the diagnosis may be best reflected in our inability to find a suitable diagnostic label for the condition that the sex therapy community can agree upon. While delayed ejaculation is the currently accepted diagnostic label, the condition has also been referred to as ejaculatory incompetence [11], retarded ejaculation [34], inhibited ejaculation [1,10], male orgasmic disorder [25], and inhibited orgasm [35]. None of these labels has been able to accurately capture the clinical picture that best describes the phenomenon since what is termed delayed ejaculation can refer to those who take a long time to ejaculate, those who are unable to ejaculate during intercourse, those who are unable to ejaculate during masturbation, and those who are able to ejaculate via solo masturbation but not in the presence of a partner. It would seem, then, that a diagnosis of delayed ejaculation provides little specificity of the actual condition being experienced by the man and his partner.

Masters and Johnson [11] defined the condition in rather vague terms suggesting that ejaculatory incompetence should be assessed clinically as the reverse of, or counterpart to, PE. Masters and Johnson relied on an imprecise and highly subjective measure of assessment that provides little diagnostic guidance or specificity.

In an effort to be more precise, the World Health Organization 2nd Consultation on Sexual Dysfunction [36] defined delayed ejaculation as the persistent or recurrent difficulty, delay in, or absence of attaining orgasm after sufficient sexual stimulation, which causes personal distress. This definition, too, suffers from a lack of specificity, but importantly adds the dimension of "personal distress." Still, however, adding personal distress as a criterion leaves the clinician with a diagnostic label of limited utility. How much distress does one need to experience to be diagnoseable? Can it be mild disappointment, or does the level of distress need to have some demonstrated level of impairment? In addition, whose distress are we referring to? The man's? His partner's? Either? Both?

The most recent edition of the DSM-V [13] offers the following diagnostic criteria:

A. *Either of the following symptoms must be experienced on almost all or all occasions (approximately 75%–100%) of all partnered sexual activity (in identified situational contexts, or if generalized, in all contexts), and without the individual desiring delay:*
  1. *Marked delay in ejaculation.*
  2. *Marked infrequency or absence of ejaculation.*
B. *The symptoms in Criterion A have persisted for a minimum duration of approximately 6 months.*
C. *The symptoms in Criterion A cause clinically significant distress in the individual.*
D. *The sexual dysfunction is not better explained by a nonsexual mental disorder or as a consequence of severe relationship distress or other significant stressors and is not attributable to the effects of a substance/medication or another medical condition.*

Specify whether:
Lifelong: The disturbance has been present since the individual became sexually active.
Acquired: The disturbance began after a period of relatively normal sexual dysfunction.
Specify whether:
Generalized: Not limited to certain types of stimulation, situations, or partners.
Situational: Only occurs with certain types of stimulation, situations, or partners.
Specify current severity:
Mild: Evidence of mild distress over the symptoms in Criterion A.
Moderate: Evidence of moderate distress over the symptoms in Criterion A.
Severe: Evidence of severe or extreme distress over the symptoms in Criterion A.

At first glance, the DSM-V diagnostic guidelines would appear to be more comprehensive and useful than its counterparts. In truth, however, many of the same limitations apply here. How "marked" does an ejaculation need to be to be considered a marked delay? How does one objectively distinguish between mild and severe distress? Most all clinicians have seen patients who minimize or catastrophize their experience of the symptoms.

The ICD-11 has likewise published criteria that are also notably vague: *Male delayed ejaculation is characterized by an inability to achieve ejaculation or an excessive or increased latency of ejaculation, despite adequate sexual stimulation and the desire to ejaculate. The pattern of delayed ejaculation has occurred episodically or persistently over a period at least several months and is associated with clinically significant distress* [17]. In essence, none of our efforts to develop a precise and broadly useful definition of delayed ejaculation have proved to be satisfactory. Abdel-Hamid and Ali

[37] have lamented that the ability of an agreed upon internationally accepted definition, combined with the absence of consensus about normative data for defining the duration of "normal" ejaculatory latency has severely limited our ability to understand the scope of ejaculatory disorders, or their true prevalence. There are currently efforts underway to standardize and apply objective measures to the diagnosis of delayed ejaculation, but this is still preliminary [38]. As a result, delayed ejaculation is generally considered a poorly understood disorder, with inconsistent practice patterns seen among practicing sexual medicine and sex therapy clinicians [39,40].

Fortunately, for the purposes of the infertility clinician, these diagnostic vagaries are of no greater importance than was the case for PE or rapid ejaculation. When assessing the impact of delayed ejaculation on fertility, we are again able to use a much more functional definition. That is, if the man is unable to ejaculate and deposit sperm into the woman's vagina, we can proceed under the verifiable and objective certainly that a diagnosis of delayed or inhibited ejaculation is indicated. The clinician can then initiate the appropriate treatment protocols for delayed ejaculation.

Etiological factors in delayed ejaculation

While defining delayed ejaculation has been oftentimes vexing, there are several factors that have been implicated in the etiology of the disorder. For example, we know that as men age their ejaculatory latency will increase. Jenkins [35] and Watter [41] have pointed out that ejaculatory latency and ejaculatory inconsistency will increase for men between the ages of 50 and 80 +. Of course, this is a natural and expected result of the aging process, and thus would not be technically considered a disorder. Nevertheless, men who are unaware of the typical and ordinary effects aging may have on their sexual function, or those who are unwilling to accept the reality of the aging process, may still experience significant distress over their ejaculatory changes. Similarly, men who take an SSRI for depression or some other psychiatric condition may also notice that ejaculation will become more difficult to achieve or may be completely absent. Watter [29], Perelman and Watter [40], Jenkins [35], Abdel-Hamid and Ali [37], and Zilbergeld [24] have all noted that SSRI use is often associated with delayed ejaculation. However, while the level of distress may be equivalent, the fact that these ejaculatory difficulties are the result of an identifiable process (i.e., aging or medication side effects), and thus would constitute a secondary effect, they would exclude them from an actual diagnosis of delayed ejaculation. Again, in cases of infertility, this distinction would be moot since the fertility clinician would base the diagnosis and resulting treatment protocol on a more functional and less academic diagnostic assessment.

Certain physiological or medical conditions have been associated with delayed ejaculation. In addition to medications, a loss of penile sensitivity often associated with diabetes or other illnesses may be a causative factor. Abdel-Hamid and Ali [37] have also identified factors such as congenital abnormalities that may compromise the functions of the vas deferens, ejaculatory duct, prostate, seminal vesicle, and urethra, surgical procedures that may affect the male reproductive system, infection/inflammation, and traumatic injuries to the spinal cord as potential causes of ejaculatory difficulties in men.

Perelman [42] and Perelman and Watter [40] have discussed three factors that disproportionally characterize men with delayed ejaculation. They often have: (1) a high-frequency masturbation pattern, (2) an idiosyncratic masturbation style, and (3) experience a high degree of disparity between reality of sex with a partner and their preferred masturbation fantasy. Perelman [43] coined the term "idiosyncratic masturbatory style" to describe the phenomenon in which a man masturbates in a way that is not easily duplicated by a partner's hand, mouth, vagina, or anus. Of the 250 men complaining of delayed ejaculation studied by Perelman [43], 70% described engaging in masturbatory patterns notable for one or more of the following characteristics: speed, pressure, duration, body posture/position, and specificity of focus on a particular spot of sensitivity to produce orgasm/ejaculation.

Other noted psychosocial factors cited in the etiology of delayed ejaculation have included underlying fears of loss of control and autonomy, fears of abandonment or rejection, and fears of intimacy, to name but a few [40,44]. In addition, paraphilic inclinations/interests may also result in ejaculatory difficulties for some men [40,45]. Apfelbaum [34] has proposed the intriguing concept of an "autosexual" orientation. He suggests that there are some men who are aroused more by the feel of their own hand than that of any stimulation provided by a partner. Apfelbaum suggests that some men with delayed or absent ejaculation that is situational (i.e., only in the presence of a partner) may, in fact, have a low desire for partnered sex and only experience a high enough level of desire to result in orgasm/ejaculation when engaged in self-stimulation. These men often present with what initially appears to be an essentially sexless marriage. In reality, however, they are often quite sexual on their own, preferring solo masturbation to partnered sexual activity.

Cultural issues are also relevant in the etiology of delayed ejaculation. The value accorded to semen varies greatly cross culturally with seminal fluid considered the basis of vitality and a life force for many men in Asia and the Middle East. As such, many men from these traditional cultures are motivated to conserve semen as semen loss is believed to lead to physical ailments and sexual dysfunction. Dhat syndrome (excessive preoccupation about physical weakness or other ailments as a result of semen loss) is very prevalent around the world being a more common complaint than erectile disorders in some parts of the world [46]. In practice, therefore, men from traditional cultures may not masturbate to ejaculation and may purposefully delay or defer ejaculation during sexual intercourse. A learned pattern of arousal without ejaculation combined with a concern about losing vitality can contribute to difficulty ejaculating when it suddenly becomes a desired outcome. Consider the case of Jung Kim, a recent immigrant to the United States from Korea who was referred for sex therapy after being unable to provide a semen sample at the infertility clinic. Jung was 52 years old and married to a 32-year-old woman who was eager to start a family. However, Jung prided himself on his ability to control his ejaculation and had, throughout his adulthood ejaculated only about once a month, despite having much more frequent (solo and partnered) sexual activity. Now he found that he was not able to masturbate to orgasm, nor could he ejaculate intravaginally according to a schedule based on his wife's ovulation.

While certain sociocultural beliefs may contribute to the etiology and maintenance of delayed ejaculation, other learning experiences may also be factors. Consider the following case:

Jared was a 27-year-old man who was unable to ejaculate in the presence of a woman. He had in the past faked orgasm, but now he and his girlfriend were discussing the option of marriage and children and Jared knew he had to address this problem. Jared described growing up in a close family, in a very small, two-bedroom house. Since he could remember until early adolescence, Jared slept in the same bed as his mother. His father worked the night shift, and his older sister required her own room. As Jared entered middle school, he felt uncomfortable about this arrangement and never had friends over to his house lest they ask to see his bedroom. Although he does not recall ever having a nocturnal emission when he was in his mother's bed, he does recall being anxious about that possibility and trying to "will" himself not to. When he was 14 and his sister went to college Jared finally had his own bedroom. Nevertheless, he recalled continuing anxiety about ejaculating when anyone was home, and this anxiety transferred to sexual activity with girlfriends through high school and now in his adulthood.

What likely will be of particular concern to the infertility clinician may be the often-noted correlation between delayed ejaculation and relationship distress, as well as the man's fears or ambivalence of pregnancy, commitment, and/or responsibility. These issues are likely to emerge when the couple is deliberately trying to conceive. Perelman and Watter [40], Perelman [42], and Abdel-Hamid and Ali [37] all note that these diverse elements of etiological factors need not be mutually exclusive. There is no reason to believe that a single pathogenetic pathway to delayed ejaculation exists, as there are likely to be several.

Treatment of delayed ejaculation

At the present time, there are no FDA-approved treatments for delayed ejaculation [37,42]. However, for the fertility specialist dealing with men who are unable to produce an ejaculation suitable for intravaginal insemination, the aforementioned assistive ejaculation methods may be considered. Procedures such as PVS [7,8], EEJ [3,4], and both surgical and non-SSR [4,10] have all been utilized successfully in cases of infertility due to the man's inability to voluntarily produce sperm.

The cases of delayed ejaculation that have a more psychological etiology are more varied in their presentation and require a more complicated and nuanced treatment. Most clinicians who have studied this clinical phenomenon agree that the key to effective treatment begins with a detailed, thorough sexual and psychosocial history [28,35,37,40,47]. Such a history would involve the clinician attempting to obtain as clear a timeline of the presenting symptom as possible. Often, the timing of the onset of the symptom is not coincidental and provides substantial insight into the understanding of, or meaning behind, the appearance of the delay in ejaculation. This is particularly so in the cases of acquired and situational ejaculatory disorders.

According to Perelman [48], Burns [17], and Perelman and Watter [40], the classic presentation of delayed ejaculation will consist of a man who has little or no difficulty achieving and maintaining penile erection but finds it difficult or impossible to achieve ejaculation despite an "adequate" amount of stimulation. Abdel-Hamid and Saleh [49] and Rowland et al. [50] have also suggested that these men report less coital activity, higher levels of relationship distress, higher levels of sexual dissatisfaction, lower levels of sexual arousal, higher levels of anxiety about sexual performance, and higher levels of general health-related issues as compared to sexually functional men. The most common clinical presentation of delayed ejaculation likely to present in an infertility clinic is of a man who has little difficulty reaching orgasm/ejaculation during solo masturbation but is unable to do so when in the presence of a partner. Diagnostically this would be considered acquired, situational delayed ejaculation.

There is no one preferred manner of treatment for these cases. Given that the underlying factors creating this dysfunction are varied and case specific, little data exist to support the endorsement of any evidence-based treatments. As a result, treatment will often have to be tailored to the individual man and the particulars of his intrapersonal and interpersonal situation [28,29]. This is not to say, however, that effective treatments are not available. Quite the contrary. The experienced sexual medicine and sex therapy clinician will recognize the etiology of these cases is multifactorial and multidetermined [51]. As such, mechanistic, reductionist, and perfunctory views of psychogenic sexual problems and their solutions need be set aside to assist the man and his partner in finding a successful resolution to his ejaculatory dilemma.

While Jung decided not to pursue therapy, preferring instead to continue to practice conserving his semen and believing that he would still be able to impregnate his wife. Jared was able to resolve his sexual issues through a combination of psychotherapy, sex therapy techniques to increase arousal and awareness, as well as relaxation training and systematic desensitization. Jared had a supportive girlfriend and was not under time pressure as he accessed therapy before fertility was a pressing issue.

Perelman [42] has suggested that men with delayed ejaculation curtail noncoital sexual activity for a period of time. He cautions that this alone is not likely to resolve the problem but will increase the probability for success. He further recommends that since the man with delayed ejaculation enjoys a masturbatory fantasy life that does not match the reality of sexual activity with his partner, the identification and use of fantasy and bodily movements during coitus that approximate the thoughts and sensations experienced in successful solo masturbation may be effective for achieving the desired level of sexual arousal required for orgasmic/ejaculatory release during coitus.

The behavioral techniques advocated by Masters and Johnson in 1970 remain the mainstay of most sex therapy protocols for the treatment of delayed ejaculation [44]. In the Masters and Johnson approach, the man will begin to masturbate with his partner present until he reaches a significant level of sexual arousal. His partner will then take over and continue to aggressively and forcefully stimulate the man's penis and then quickly switch to vaginal intromission as the man reaches ejaculatory inevitability. The idea is that once even a small amount of semen is placed into the vagina, the unconscious fear of intravaginal ejaculation will be erased and future coital experiences will become easier. While this technique may allow a small amount of semen to be deposited into the woman's vagina and therefore result in conception, the likelihood that this will then create a satisfying sexual experience or way of being is low. However, for the couple struggling with infertility, this may be enough to allow them to succeed in their primary goal of having a sexual experience that results in a pregnancy.

Apfelbaum [34] has been highly critical of this approach to treatment, however. He describes this as a "demand" strategy and "aggressive attack" on a symptom. Apfelbaum advocates for a more depth-oriented psychotherapy to fully understand and resolve the symptom of delayed ejaculation. If a man's ejaculatory inabilities are the result of some underlying psychological conflict, demand strategies are likely to be resisted, sabotaged, and become increasingly impervious to successful resolution.

Those cases of delayed ejaculation presenting in fertility clinics that have underlying psychological conflicts as significant etiological factors are likely to include some of the following psychological concerns. The sexual medicine or sex therapy clinician will need to evaluate for the presence of any relationship concerns or issues. If the relationship has been troubled, the man may be experiencing substantial ambivalence about wanting to deepen the relationship commitment by adding a child to the mix. This is especially true of those men who are unable to either acknowledge to themselves or to their partners their sizeable degree of ambivalence and conflict. Mate [33] and van der Kolk [32] have noted that oftentimes unacknowledged or unexpressed psychological stresses and traumas will take up residence in the body and be expressed in some somatic or functional manner. For the man who is attempting to deny or contain his ambivalence regarding conception, a sexual disruption would certainly be an effective tool for his protective unconscious to employ.

Other psychological complications that may be present for the man include concerns about the loss of freedom and autonomy, as well as fears of the increased responsibility and commitment associated with having children. Often these men have had early childhood trauma that has yet to be resolved and is currently manifesting in an intense ambivalence and existential panic regarding the event of conception and emergence of parenthood. Many of these conflicts and dilemmas will be illustrated in the cases further.

The case of Philip and Yolanda: lifelong, situational delayed ejaculation

Philip and Yolanda had been married for 10 years when they presented for sex therapy. Philip was 39 years old and Yolanda was 35. Both reported being in good health, took no medications, and had no difficulties with alcohol or other drugs. Philip and Yolanda met at a party hosted by a mutual friend, and both said that their attraction to each other was immediate and intense. They began dating and engaging in frequent sexual activity. While pleasurable for both of them, their sexual activity was limited by Philip's inability to ejaculate in Yolanda's presence. Whether via sexual intercourse, manual stimulation, or oral sex Philip reported enjoying sex with Yolanda but never being able to reach the point of orgasm or ejaculation. Masturbation, however, was no problem at all. Philip found masturbation to be highly enjoyable and satisfying. Yolanda was aware of this but was flummoxed as to why this was the case. Philip reported being similarly unaware of the causality for his sexual constraints. Approximately 4 years prior to our consultation, Yolanda began to express her strong desire for children. This was not a surprise to Philip as they had always planned to have a family, but Yolanda was becoming increasingly concerned about her age once she entered her thirties. As the years went by and Yolanda reached the age of 35, she found herself becoming increasingly anxious about Philip's ejaculatory difficulties and pushed for medical or psychological intervention. After Philip was evaluated by a urologist who found no organic explanation for his ejaculatory frustrations, he referred them for sex therapy.

In an individual meeting, Philip revealed that he actually had a very specific masturbatory fantasy that aroused him to the point of ejaculation/orgasm. He reported having a paraphilic interest in women who wore large framed glasses and bright red nail polish. During masturbation, he would concentrate on the woman's glasses and nails becoming quickly and decidedly aroused. Climax would be reached in a matter of minutes. Philip had never told Yolanda about his fantasy due to his fear that she would find it unpalatable and would reject him. At their next joint session, Philip told Yolanda about his masturbatory arousal and much to his surprise and relief she was accepting of it and offered to role play the fantasy with him. Philip was hesitant, but grateful that Yolanda was so understanding. They planned to try it that week.

When Philip and Yolanda returned for their next joint session, they had both expressed disappointment that even though Yolanda had purchased a pair of large framed glasses and had worn bright red nail polish, Philip was still unable to reach climax with her. Philip was also saddened and requested another individual session to explore the events further. Yolanda was agreeable inasmuch as she was eager for Philip to find a resolution to his ejaculatory vexation. An individual session for Philip was scheduled for the next day. At that session, Philip revealed that while he was appreciative of Yolanda's efforts, he had trouble seeing her in the role of his fantasy partner. He said that Yolanda, while looking the part, did not move or make sounds like his fantasy partner. He tried to tell her how to make adjustments, but the real movements and sounds of an actual partner had actually been a distraction for Philip, and his arousal levels would stagnate. It became increasingly apparent that Philip's ejaculatory difficulties would not remit to a simple and straightforward intervention. As a result, couples' therapy was suspended for the time being while Philip engaged in individual psychotherapy to explore his personal sexuality in greater depth.

Philip spent a good deal of time discussing his family of origin and resulting childhood trauma. According to Philip, his mother suffered from a debilitating depression. She was often nonfunctional and had attempted suicide three times. Philip recalled being so frightened that his mother would succeed in killing herself that he became hypervigilant and extraordinarily tuned in to the slightest indication that her mood was slipping. He took it upon himself to be his mother's protector and would rarely leave her side. He essentially relinquished his childhood in service of his mother's mental health. He rarely played with friends and refused to participate in activities that would take him away from home such as sports, clubs, and other school or community-sponsored activities. Philip reported a childhood filled with anxiety, tension, and dread. Given these circumstances, Philip was never able to allow himself to recognize or focus on his wants or desires when in his mother's presence.

Philip came to see through psychotherapy that his relationship with his mother positioned him to be unable to relax when he was in the presence of another person. He would become so focused on the needs of the other that he would lose sight of any sense of having needs of his own. This translated into Philip's sexual life as well. When he was with Yolanda, or any of his previous partners, he would be so focused on their level of arousal and whether they were enjoying the experience that he would be unable to focus attention on his own physical or mental sensations to allow his level of arousal to proceed and intensify. Solo masturbation was the only time Philip was able to relax enough to focus on his own sexual pleasure, and orgasm and ejaculation came easily under those conditions.

With this new insight and understanding of how his early childhood trauma was affecting his current sexual functioning, Philip was able to participate in some ejaculatory retraining exercises. He became better able to focus on his own sensations when with Yolanda sexually, and became less consumed with the need to focus on and interpret Yolanda's reactions. Eventually, Philip was able to use his fantasy to his advantage while engaged in sexual intercourse with Yolanda, and even though it was still a lengthy process, Philip was able to ejaculate intravaginally. Yolanda, while not being completely comfortable that Philip was thinking of someone else while having sex with her, was pleased that they were able to finally bring intercourse to completion, and she was pregnant within 4 months of Philip's ability to ejaculate during intercourse. Philip reported being relieved that they were able to conceive via sexual intercourse, but he still found solo masturbation to be considerably more satisfying (at least in terms of orgasmic release) than partnered sexual activity. At last follow up, that preference had not changed.

The case of Philip and Yolanda contained many of the elements common in cases of delayed ejaculation. Assessment required a thoughtful and exploratory approach as the specifics of Philip's etiology were nuanced and complex. Philip apparently possessed an autosexual orientation as described by Apfelbaum [34]. This was likely the result of Philip's unacknowledged and unexpressed childhood trauma from becoming the emotional caretaker of his ill mother. Until this aspect of his being was uncovered and explored, Philip was unable to find his way past the obstruction created by the emergence of his ejaculatory dysfunction. Once the trauma was uncovered and better understood, Philip was able to make progress on what had become a long-standing and perplexing conundrum, and he and Yolanda were able to reach their goal of conception.

Let's turn to another common presentation of delayed ejaculation that is likely encountered in the fertility clinic.

The case of Desmond and Mollie: acquired situational delayed ejaculation

Desmond and Mollie had been together for 14 years when they presented for consultation. They met in college, and while they both found their relationship extremely enjoyable and satisfying, marriage never was important to either of them until recently. Now in their late thirties, they decided they would like to begin a family, and given that Mollie's fertility clock was ticking, they were eager to solidify their commitment to each other move forward as quickly as possible. They married 3 years prior to this consultation, and both reported being in good health with neither taking any medications nor having any challenges with substance use.

In the early years of their relationship, sex had been frequent, relaxed, and mutually fulfilling. Both Desmond and Mollie reported being quite pleased with their relationship, both personally and sexually. However, approximately 3 years ago Desmond began to have difficulty ejaculating during intercourse with Mollie. Masturbation for Desmond remained unimpaired and nonproblematic, but to his and Mollie's surprise, sex between them became more difficult. Although not recognized by Desmond or Mollie at the time, it was likely not happenstance that Desmond's ejaculatory difficulties began shortly after marriage to Mollie. Desmond had never made this association prior to our meeting inasmuch as he authentically loved Mollie and was genuinely happy to be spending his life with her. It had never occurred to either of them that marriage would have triggered such a dramatic change in his sexual functioning.

By way of history, Desmond grew up in a chaotic and dysfunctional family. His mother was an undiagnosed, and therefore untreated, paranoid schizophrenic whose illness wreaked havoc on the family. She would continually fight with the neighbors, and the family would have to move frequently. Desmond was frightened of his mother, and particularly concerned about her violent and irrational outbursts of anger. Desmond could never understand why his father stayed with her and was willing to abdicate any parental responsibility for protecting Desmond and his siblings. His feelings toward his father vacillated between anger and pity. Anger for not being more protective of him, and pity for wasting his life with such an unruly wife. Desmond recalled as a child vowing to never be like his father, and swore to himself that he would never allow himself to be trapped in such a ghastly, unhappy marital situation. He believed his father had chosen a life of putrid nonexistence and vowed to not allow the same fate to befall him.

Desmond experienced severe childhood trauma, but interestingly did not see his situation as traumatic. He said he was never physically or sexually abused, never without food, clothing, or shelter, and never experienced a significant loss or death of someone close to him. Desmond was unaware of the fact that living a life of terror, unhappiness, and parental instability could create a significant level of emotional trauma that would carry over onto his adult relationships. For Desmond, the act of marriage-triggered unconscious fears of being trapped in another harsh and severely flawed family situation and he began to experience an existential panic signaling to him that his very existence was about to be threatened. Since this was largely an unconscious process, Desmond was unable to acknowledge or express his dysphoric state and his penis was utilized as the mechanism for communication of his angst and terror of impending doom. Psychotherapy for Desmond focused on awakening and bringing to consciousness the trauma of his childhood and helping him work through the residual effects of growing up in such a nonnurturing and frightening childhood home. Over time, Desmond was able to come to terms with the reality of his trauma and its impact on his current life and sexual functioning. He and Mollie were able to resume successful sexual intercourse and they were eventually able to conceive and begin a family. Desmond continued his psychotherapy to continue to increase his awareness and understanding of how his early childhood experiences have impacted many of the relationships throughout his life, and to more effectively cope with the sequelae of his childhood pain and suffering.

It is clear from the cases of Philip and Yolanda, as well as Desmond and Mollie, that the treatment for delayed ejaculation is often significantly more complicated and difficult than the treatment of PE or rapid ejaculation. Delayed ejaculation cases are often the result of underlying psychological conflict or trauma, and these cases rarely lend themselves to a rapid or simple amelioration. Psychotherapeutic treatment for cases of delayed ejaculation are usually much lengthier and more involved than that of PE or rapid ejaculation, and successful resolution of delayed ejaculation is much less assured than cases of PE or rapid ejaculation. In addition, since many of those couples presenting for concerns related to infertility may no longer have the patience to wait for the psychotherapeutic approach for the treatment of delayed ejaculation to be demonstrated, medical approaches, such as PVS, EEJ, or SSR may be elected to achieve the goal of conception, and sex therapy can be conducted either in concert or at a later time.

Conclusions

This chapter explored the impact of ejaculatory dysfunction on fertility. Problems such as premature or rapid ejaculation and delayed or absent ejaculation have often brought couples to fertility clinics due to an inability to successfully engage in sexual intercourse that would result in conception. While the literature on the relationship between ejaculatory dysfunction and fertility problems is scant, the connection is readily apparent, and the distress experienced by individuals and couples is palpable. Discussed in this chapter are both the medical and psychological etiological factors that often result in ejaculatory disorders, as well as treatment options from both sexual medicine and sex therapy. While there is a dearth of research critically examining the efficacy of treatment for ejaculatory problems, clinical acumen and patient outcomes attest to the fact that effective treatment can be reliably expected.

Notable in this chapter is the discrepancy between the hierarchy of goals that couples experiencing infertility present as opposed to those of the typical sex therapy patient. Couples struggling with infertility are primarily concerned with treatments that will result in conception. Sexual satisfaction or pleasure is, at best, a secondary goal or concern. Therefore most of the treatments for ejaculatory disorders within the context of problems with fertility place their primary emphasis, and gage their primary efficacy, on whether or not the man is able to impregnate his partner. Even after successful treatment, many men will still find greater sexual enjoyment and pleasure from their nonintercourse, or nonpartnered sexual activities. Some men, either individually or with their partner, may decide to continue sex therapy treatment to improve the sexual enjoyment in partnered sex play, but many will be satisfied with achieving their goal of pregnancy. This is especially true in the case of delayed ejaculation in which many men's masturbation style is highly pleasurable and satisfying.

It is important for sexual medicine and sex therapy clinicians to remain mindful of the fact that male ejaculatory disorders that impede fertility affect both the man and his partner. The concerns of both, as well as the anticipated relationship distress and disruption must all be attended to in order for treatment to be effective.

References

[1] Perelman MA, Rowland DL. Retarded ejaculation. World J Urol 2006;24(6):645—52.
[2] Berger MH, Messore M, Pastuszak AW, Ramasamy R. Association between infertility and sexual dysfunction in men and women. Sex Med Rev 2016;4(4):353—65.
[3] Kondoh N. Ejaculatory dysfunction as a cause of infertility. Reprod Med Biol 2012;11(1):59—64.
[4] Barazani Y, Stahl PJ, Nagler HM, Stember DS. Management of ejaculatory disorders in infertile men. Asian J Androl 2012;14(4):525—9.
[5] Rowland D, McMahon CG, Abdo C, Chen J, Jannini E, Waldinger MD, et al. Disorders of orgasm and ejaculation in men. J Sex Med 2010;7(4):1668—86.
[6] Kamischke A, Nieschlag E. Update on medical treatment of ejaculatory disorders. Int J Androl 2002;25(6):333—44.
[7] Ohl DA, Quallich SA, Sonksen J, Brackett NL, Lynne CM. Anejaculation: an electrifying approach. Semin Reprod Med 2009;27(2):179—85.
[8] Stewart DE, Ohl DA. Idiopathic anejaculation treated by electroejaculation. Int J Psychiatry Med 1989;19(3):263—8.
[9] Parnham A, Serefoglu EC. Classification and definition of premature ejaculation. Transl Androl Urol 2016;5(4):416—23.

References

[10] Elliott S, Fluker MR. Fertility options for men with ejaculatory disorders. J Obstet Gynaecol Can 2000;22(1):26−32.

[11] Masters WH, Johnson VE. Human sexual inadequacy. Boston, MA: Little Brown and Co; 1970.

[12] Mintz LB, Guitelman J. Orgasm problems in women. In: Hall KSK, Binik YM, editors. Principles and practice of sex therapy. 6th ed. New York: Guilford Press; 2020. p. 109−33.

[13] American Psychiatric Association. The diagnostic and statistical manual of mental disorders. 5th ed. Washington, DC: American Psychiatric Association; 2013.

[14] Althof SE, Levine SB, Corty EW, Risen CB, Stern EB, Kurit DM. A double-blind crossover trial of clomipramine for rapid ejaculation in 15 couples. J Clin Psychiatry 1995;56(9):402−7.

[15] Althof SE. Patient reported outcomes in the assessment of premature ejaculation. Transl Androl Urol 2016;5(4):470−4.

[16] Waldinger MD. The neurobiological approach to premature ejaculation. J Urol 2002;168(6):2359−67.

[17] Burns LH. Sexual problems during disrupted reproduction and pregnancy. In: Levine SB, Risen CB, Althof SE, editors. Handbook of clinical sexuality for mental health professionals. 3rd ed. New York: Routledge; 2016. p. 195−208.

[18] Serefoglu EC, McMahon CG, Waldinger MD, Althof SE, Shindel A, Adaikan G, et al. An evidence-based unified definition of lifelong and acquired premature ejaculation: report of the second International Society for Sexual Medicine Ad Hoc Committee for the Definition of Premature Ejaculation. J Sex Med 2014;11(6):1423−41.

[19] World Health Organization. International classification of diseases 11th revision. Geneva: World Health Organization;; 2018.

[20] Althof SE. Treatment of premature ejaculation: psychotherapy, pharmacotherapy, and combined therapy. In: Hall KSK, Binik YM, editors. Principles and practice of sex therapy. 6th ed. New York: Guilford Press; 2020. p. 134−55.

[21] Waldinger MD, Schweitzer DH. Method and design of drug treatment research of subjective premature ejaculation in men differs from that of lifelong premature ejaculation in males: proposal for a new objective measure (Part 1). Int J Impot Res 2019;31(5):328−33.

[22] Janssen PKC, Waldinger MD. Men with subjective premature ejaculation have a similar lognormal IELT distribution as men in the general male population and differ mathematically from males with lifelong premature ejaculation after an IELT of 1.5 minutes (Part 2). Int J Impot Res 2019;31(5):341−7.

[23] Waldinger MD. Premature ejaculation. In: Levine SB, Risen CB, Althof SE, editors. Handbook of clinical sexuality for mental health professionals. 3rd ed. New York: Routledge; 2016. p. 134−49.

[24] Zilbergeld B. The new male sexuality, revised edition. New York: Bantam Books; 1999.

[25] Strassberg DS, Perelman MA. Sexual dysfunction in males. In: Grossman L, Walfish S, editors. Translating psychological research into practice. New York: Springer; 2014. p. 435−40.

[26] McCabe MP, Sharlip ID, Lewis R, Atalla E, Balon R, Fisher AD, et al. Incidence and prevalence of sexual dysfunction in women and men: a consensus statement from the 4th international consultation on sexual medicine. J Sex Med 2015;12(2):144−52.

[27] Richardson D, Goldmeier D. Premature ejaculation—does country of origin tell us anything about etiology? J Sex Med 2005;2(4):508−12.

[28] Watter DN. Commentary: Clinical evaluation and treatment of disorders of ejaculation. In: Lipshultz LI, Pastuszak AW, Goldstein AT, Giraldi A, Perelman MA, editors. Management of sexual dysfunction in men and women. New York: Springer; 2016. p. 153−7.

[29] Watter DN. Sexual dysfunction in males: clinical application. In: Grossman L, Walfish S, editors. Translating psychological research into practice. New York: Springer; 2014. p. 440−2.

[30] Perelman MA. A new combination treatment for premature ejaculation: a sex therapist's perspective. J Sex Med 2006;3(6):1004−12.

[31] Althof SE. Treatment of premature ejaculation. In: Binik YM, Hall KSK, editors. Principles and practice of sex therapy. 5th ed. New York: Guilford Press; 2014. p. 112−37.

[32] van der Kolk B. The body keeps the score: brain, mind, and body in the healing of trauma. E. Rutherford, NJ: Penguin Books; 2015.

[33] Mate G. When the body says no: understanding the stress-disease connection. Hoboken, NJ: Wiley; 2011.

[34] Apfelbaum B. Retarded ejaculation: a much misunderstood syndrome. In: Leiblum SR, Rosen RC, editors. Principles and practice of sex therapy. 3rd ed. New York: Guilford Press; 2000. p. 205−41.

[35] Jenkins LC. Delayed orgasm and anorgasmia. Fertil Steril 2015;104(5):1082−8.

[36] McMahon CG, Althof SE, Waldinger MD, Porst H, Dean J, Sharlip ID, et al. An evidence-based definition of lifelong premature ejaculation: report of the International Society for Sexual Medicine (ISSM) Ad Hoc Committee for the Definition of Premature Ejaculation. J Sex Med 2008;5(7):1590−606.

[37] Abdel-Hamid IA, Ali OI. Delayed ejaculation: pathophysiology, diagnosis, and treatment. World J Mens Health 2018;36(1):22−40.

[38] Rowland DL, Cote-Ledger P. Moving toward empirically based standardization in the diagnosis of delayed ejaculation. J Sex Med 2020;17(10):1896−902.

[39] Butcher MJ, Welliver Jr RC, Sadowski D, Botchway A, Kohler TS. How is delayed ejaculation defined and treated in North America? Andrology 2015;3(3):626−31.

[40] Perelman MA, Watter DN. Delayed ejaculation. In: Levine SB, Risen CB, Althof SE, editors. Handbook of clinical sexuality for mental health professionals. 3rd ed. New York: Routledge; 2016. p. 150−63.

[41] Watter DN. Sexuality and aging: navigating the sexual challenges of aging bodies. In: Hall KSK, Binik YM, editors. Principles and practice of sex therapy. 6th ed. New York: Guilford Press; 2020. p. 357−70.

[42] Perelman MA. Delayed ejaculation. In: Hall KSK, Binik YM, editors. Principles and practice of sex therapy. 6th ed. New York: Guilford Press; 2020. p. 156−79.

[43] Perelman MA. The urologist and cognitive behavioral sex therapy. Contemp Urol 1994;6(3):27−31.

[44] Rowland DL, Cooper SE. Treating men's orgasmic difficulties. In: Peterson ZD, editor. The Wiley handbook of sex therapy. Malden, MA: John Wiley and Sons, Inc; 2017. p. 72−97.

[45] Perelman MA, Watter DN. Delayed ejaculation. In: Kirana PS, Tripodi MF, Reisman Y, Porst H, editors. The EFS and ESSM syllabus of clinical sexology. Amsterdam: Medix;; 2014. p. 660−72.

[46] Hall KS. Cultural differences in the treatment of sex problems. Curr Sex Health Rep 2019;11(1):29−34.

[47] Althof SE, Rosen RC, Perelman MA, Rubio-Aurioles E. Standard operating procedures for taking a sexual history. J Sex Med 2013;10(1):26−35.

[48] Perelman MA. Delayed ejaculation. In: Binik YM, Hall KSK, editors. Principles and practice of sex therapy. 5th ed. New York: Guilford Press; 2014. p. 138−55.

[49] Abdel-Hamid I, Saleh E. Primary lifelong delayed ejaculation: characteristics and response to bupropion. J Sex Med 2011;8(6):1772–9.
[50] Rowland DL, van Diest S, Incrocci I, Slob A. Psychosocial factors that differentiate men with inhibited ejaculation from men with no dysfunction or another sexual dysfunction. J Sex Med 2005;2(3):383–9.
[51] Kleinplatz PJ, editor. New directions in sex therapy: innovations and alternatives. 2nd ed. New York: Routledge; 2012.

CHAPTER

6

Early menopause: diagnosis and management

Tanya Glenn and Amanda Kallen

Division of Reproductive Endocrinology and Infertility, Department of Obstetrics, Gynecology and Reproductive Sciences, Yale School of Medicine, New Haven, CT, United States

Introduction

Ovarian aging is a critical determinant of overall healthspan and lifespan. With age, a drastic decline in the quantity of ovarian follicles and oocytes (the "ovarian reserve") occurs [1], leading to infertility. Aging oocytes and follicles also accumulate DNA damage, causing deterioration of gamete quality and increasing the risk of birth defects and miscarriage [2–4]. Menopause, the culmination of the ovarian aging process, represents a major hormonal, psychological, and physiological event and confers increased risk for comorbidities and overall mortality unrelated to fertility. In women with primary ovarian insufficiency (POI), this process is catastrophically accelerated, causing loss of fertility and early menopause (EM). Women who experience earlier onset of natural menopause (e.g., POI) or surgical menopause (e.g., following oophorectomy) live shorter lives [5], with a higher incidence of diabetes, ischemic heart disease, cardiovascular disease (CVD) mortality, bone fracture, and earlier cognitive decline than women who experience normal or late menopause [5–12]. Moreover, human chronological life span has extended dramatically over the last century [13], while the timing of menopause has remained relatively constant [14]. Thus women now spend a larger portion of their lives in the postmenopausal period [15,16]. It is clear, then, that reproductive aging plays a critical role in overall population health and longevity.

The effects of ovarian aging on overall health are largely due to the progressive, irreversible loss of follicles and oocytes that occurs with age, which results in declining feedback from the somatic cells of the aging ovary, changes in endocrine hormones, and ultimately, menopause. Natural menopause is diagnosed after 12 months of amenorrhea without any obvious pathological cause and occurs, on average, at age 51.4 [17]. At this time, ovarian function and menses cease entirely. EM is defined as the disruption of ovarian function and menstrual cycles between the ages of 40 and 44 [17,18]. EM occurs in approximately 5% of the population (1 in 20 women) [17,18]. By contrast, primary ovarian insufficiency (POI) is a disorder characterized by the depletion or dysfunction of ovarian follicles with cessation of menses before age 40 [19]. This condition has borne many monikers over the past several decades (including premature menopause or EM, premature ovarian failure, primary ovarian failure, ovarian hypofunction, hypergonadotropic hypogonadism, gonadal dysgenesis, and menopause praecox [19–22]), reflective of our evolving understanding of the disorder itself. However, these terms are now understood to be either incorrect or insufficient as they do not reflect the fact that women with POI may have fluctuations in ovarian function and even spontaneous ovulation [23]. Primary ovarian insufficiency is a relatively rare condition with a prevalence of 1 in 100 in women under the age of 40, dropping to 1 in 10,000 under the age of 20 [29]. The prevalence of POI appears to differ among ethnic backgrounds, with increased prevalence observed in African American and Hispanic women and a lower prevalence of POI seen in women who are Chinese, Japanese, or Caucasian [24].

Etiologies of primary ovarian insufficiency

Even as our diagnostic capabilities and understanding of POI continue to improve, the underlying etiology remains elusive in 50%–90% of cases [25]. Etiologies of spontaneous POI include genetic causes, exposure to gonadotoxins (e.g., chemotherapy or radiation, which can result in temporary or permanent follicle loss), metabolic causes, infectious causes, and autoimmune disorders. Underlying biological mechanisms which have been proposed to result in POI in these situations include follicle depletion (either due to oocyte/follicle destruction or a congenital absence of follicles), and follicle dysfunction [such as a follicle stimulating hormone (FSH) receptor mutation]. POI may also result from surgical removal of the ovaries (oophorectomy) or extensive ovarian surgery which compromises ovarian reserve. Importantly, due to these risks, the American College of Obstetricians and Gynecologists (ACOG) strongly recommends against the surgical removal of the ovaries at time of hysterectomy in premenopausal women who do not have an elevated risk for ovarian cancer [26]. If no etiology is found, POI is considered to be idiopathic.

Genetics causes play a large role in the etiology of POI; the younger the woman is when diagnosed with POI, the more likely a genetic cause will be found. Indeed, approximately 50% of adolescents with POI will have an abnormal karyotype, versus only 13% of younger adult women <30 years old [19]. The most common heritable genetic cause of POI is an expansion in the *FMR1* gene, known as an *FMR1* gene premutation, which can cause POI of variable severity. Overall, this condition is found in approximately 6% of women with POI [27]. However, in women with a positive family history of POI the prevalence is much higher, at 14%, while the prevalence of POI is only 2% in those without any family history [19,20]. POI is also caused by chromosomal defects, such as Turner syndrome (monosomy X); women with mosaic Turner syndrome in whom the ovaries are affected may also have POI [28,29]. Other aberrations in the X chromosome such as deletions, duplications, or structural defects can also result in POI. Individuals with XX gonadal dysgenesis, like Turner syndrome, exhibit an embryologic abnormality in the formation of the appropriate gonads and can often manifest streak ovaries that do not produce estrogen or contain oocytes. However, unlike Turner syndrome, where these events are due to a chromosomal aberration, the etiology of XX gonadal dysgenesis is often unexplained [30]. Although extremely heterogenous in phenotype, individuals with XY gonadal dysgenesis, or Swyer syndrome, may be born with nonfunctioning ovaries (bilateral streak gonads), and consequently exhibit primary amenorrhea [31]. Abnormalities in the FSH receptor have also been described [28]. Even when a specific genetic disorder cannot be determined, POI may still have a genetic etiology, and 10%–15% of women with POI have a first-degree relative suffering from the same disorder [25]. Researchers have described a multitude of single gene defects that are linked to POI, such as inhibin alpha subunit (INHA), NOBOX, FOX03, or POF1B [28]. However, these gene defects should not be specifically evaluated unless a syndrome is expected based on personal or family history.

Autoimmunity and endocrinopathies are among other conditions associated with POI, with studies showing a large range of autoantibodies in 34%–92% in POI patients [32]. Autoimmune disorders in general represent an abnormality in the immune system to appropriately recognize self; autoimmune disorders are often clustered together, and the ovary is a common target [33]. Indeed, it has been suggested that when a patient has POI and a concurrent autoimmune disorder, an underlying immune dysfunction can be considered to be the likely primary etiology of POI, even if the exact mechanism cannot be elucidated [33]. However, if no autoimmune disorder is associated with POI, then an immune relationship is unlikely. Women with POI have been found to have alterations in the populations of certain immune-regulated cells in the peripheral blood, such as natural killer cells, CD4 T cells, and CD8 T cells, which further support the important relationship between the immune and reproductive systems [32].

In keeping with these findings, POI symptoms may be the first indication of another underlying autoimmune syndrome [19]. The most common endocrinopathy in women with POI is hypothyroidism; 20% of women with POI will have hypothyroidism or be later diagnosed with hypothyroidism [23]. It is important to note that hypothyroidism is not considered a cause of POI, but rather likely reflects an underlying autoimmune dysfunction often seen in POI patients [32]. Because women with POI are at increased risk of developing autoimmune hypothyroidism, a reasonable option is to check thyroid levels and thyroid peroxidase antibodies at time of diagnosis, then perform thyroid screening every 1–2 years thereafter, or sooner if symptoms of hypothyroidism develop. Adrenal autoimmunity is also associated with POI, and adrenal dysfunction is seen in 15% of POI cases [20]. Approximately 4% of women with POI have adrenal or ovarian antibodies. Due to the severity of adrenal insufficiency, an annual corticotropin stimulation test should be considered in those with adrenal antibodies, as patients with primary ovarian insufficiency also have a 50% chance of developing adrenal insufficiency if they have adrenal autoimmunity [27]. However, the presence of adrenal or ovarian antibodies does not universally predict a future diagnosis of POI. Regardless, all POI individuals should be educated on the warning signs of adrenal insufficiency. Other autoimmune disorders known to be associated with POI include diabetes mellitus, rheumatoid arthritis, systemic lupus erythematosus, and myasthenia gravis, and testing should be based on symptomatology. However, as with hypothyroidism and adrenal insufficiency, many of these are not considered specific causes of POI; rather, their association with POI supports a link between immune dysregulation and POI.

Other potential POI etiologies include infectious causes (e.g., mumps oophoritis) infiltrative diseases, or metabolic or enzyme aberrations, such as galactosemia or 17-alpha hydroxylase deficiency. One area of increasing interest is the role of environmental exposures in ovarian function (and dysfunction). Current tobacco users have been shown to have a twofold risk of POI versus nonusers, which increases to 15-fold in those with over a 15-year history [34]. Additionally, a strong dose response was noted and current smokers who had a 11–15 pack-year history had over a fourfold increased risk of POI. Fortunately, those who have quit smoking for over 10 years have an equivalent risk of POI to those who have never smoked. Research has also identified exposures from endocrine disrupting chemicals (EDCs), which have been shown to impact ovarian function at a variety of levels in animal models. Some of these include the plastic, bisphenol A (BPA), the pesticides or pesticide byproduct, methoxychlor (MXC), and genestein, an isoflavone phytoestrogen found in plants. In mouse models, BPA was seen to alter growth of follicles, promote atresia, and impede normal steroidogenesis. In similar fashion, MXC inhibits normal follicular growth and steroidogenesis. Last, genistein exposures have been demonstrated to have a detrimental effect on follicular growth, from accelerating recruitment to inhibiting growth or increasing apoptosis. Although all these studies were conducted in animal models, this body of work highlights a potentially adverse effect of fertility from EDC exposures [35].

Diagnosis of primary ovarian insufficiency and early menopause

Overt POI can be diagnosed by oligomenorrhea or amenorrhea, symptoms of estrogen deficiency, and a menopausal-range FSH (secreted by the pituitary gland) before the age of 40 [23,24,36]. However, POI encompasses a spectrum of impaired ovarian function; women with spontaneous POI may intermittently produce estrogen, ovulate, menstruate, and even conceive. Thus while some women with POI may experience symptoms of menopause, such as hot flashes and vaginal dryness due to hypoestrogenism, others may remain more or less asymptomatic [37]. This is especially true in adolescents with POI who experience primary amenorrhea [20,36].

Guidelines defining a "menopausal FSH" include >40 IU/L twice (repeated 4–6 weeks apart, from the National Institute of Health and Care Excellence) or two values >25 IU/L at least 4 weeks apart (from the European Society of Human Reproduction and Embryology) [23,24]. These values reflect unsuppressed hypothalamic-pituitary-ovarian axis function due to a lack of negative feedback from ovarian-produced estradiol. Serum estradiol levels may be quite low in these women, but because of potentially intermittent ovulatory function, a specific cutoff for estradiol is not used. Antimullerian hormone (AMH), a glycoprotein produced by the granulosa cells of growing follicles which serves as a measure of ovarian reserve, is also typically low in women with POI, reflecting decreased follicle counts. However, no cut-off value of AMH for POI has been established. EM can be differentiated from POI by the age of the woman (between 40 and 44); additionally, some small studies suggest that women with EM are more likely to present with amenorrhea [17,18].

The first steps in the diagnostic workup of POI remains the same as for any patient who presents with abnormal uterine bleeding, and includes the consideration of different etiologies for abnormal uterine bleeding or amenorrhea, such as pregnancy, thyroid abnormalities, congenital adrenal hyperplasia, hyperprolactinemia, and polycystic ovarian syndrome [19,20]. These can be evaluated by a careful menstrual history, assessment for associated symptoms some as hair growth or loss, acne, changes in voice, visual changes, heat/cold intolerance, hot flashes, family history of menstrual abnormalities, hyperpigmentation, and mood swings. Laboratory assessment should include serum FSH (on menstrual cycle day 3 in women with menstrual cycles), prolactin and thyroid-stimulating hormone, and a pregnancy test [19]. If this testing is normal and the FSH is found to be >25–40 mIU/L, particularly with a low estrogen (<50 pg/mL) [19], then POI should be suspected. To confirm, a repeat FSH should be ordered in 1 month, and additional testing for possible etiologies of POI should be performed. This testing should include a karyotype, FMR1 premutation, and adrenal antibodies (21-hydroxylase or CYP21) [19,20,24]. While European Society for Human Reproduction and Embryology guidelines indicate that transvaginal ultrasound is not required for the diagnosis of POI, an ultrasound may reveal decreased numbers of small growing follicles, although some individuals will have larger follicles noted [24]. One study showed that an FSH in the lower range (i.e., less than 33–40 mIU/mL) suggests a higher likelihood of visible follicles [38]. This also differed by primary versus secondary amenorrhea. No follicles were seen in women with primary amenorrhea when FSH > 33 mIU/mL whereas a cut off of greater than 40 was required for secondary amenorrhea. It is important for both the patient and provider to realize that the presence of follicles in the presence of an elevated FSH does not rule out POI, as the elevated gonadotropins reflect insufficient estradiol production from the follicle.

As reviewed before, after determining a woman has POI based upon her history, age, and FSH level, the remainder of the diagnostic workup is designated toward determining the etiology and other health complications. For women with EM, due to the myriad causes of abnormal uterine bleeding or hot flashes, it is still prudent in this population to conduct a complete workup as for POI if there is not an obvious etiology, such as surgical removal of the ovaries.

Comorbidities associated with early menopause

Similar to our knowledge of the etiology of POI, our understanding of the numerous health related comorbidities associated with EM has grown considerably of late yet remains incomplete. The majority of health effects are likely due to the effects of low estrogen. The health problems women with POI face include infertility, decline in sexual/urogenital health, mental/neurocognitive affects, CVD, adverse bone health, and associated endocrinopathies. One study of women who experienced surgical menopause prior to the age of 45 showed a decreased life expectancy in women after surgical menopause (hazard ratio 1.67 [25]). This reduction in life expectancy by 2 years was also seen in POI patients in a large retrospective Dutch study; the differences were observed regardless of ethnicity, particularly in the areas of CVD and fracture risk [6]. This shorter life expectancy was more notable in women who did not receive estrogen up until the age of 45.

The elevated risk of CVD in women with POI is well detailed, with an 80% increase in mortality from ischemic heart disease and a hazard ratio of 1.69 for a diagnosis of, or death from, CVD [24]. As mentioned earlier, this is likely due to suboptimal levels of estrogen. Women who undergo natural menopause, and thus a decline in estrogen, have increased activity of the renin-angiotensin-aldosterone system, and modified lipid profiles that support atherogenesis [17]. These changes can lead to potential vascular damage or alterations through inflammatory, immune, and endothelial dysfunction. Studies have shown other systemic effects related to CVD, such as modifications in renal function and an increased risk of hypertension, stroke, and abdominal adiposity [25,36]. The potential link between low estrogen and CVD is supported by one study that showed an increased risk of stroke by 44% in women who underwent surgical menopause who did not receive hormone therapy (HT), as compared to a 13% increased risk in those treated with HT, although the sample size was small and the result was not statistically significant [39]. Additionally, one study of cancer survivors with gonadotoxin-induced POI who were treated with HT demonstrated decreased activation of the renin-angiotensin-aldosterone system, as well as improvements in blood pressure and renal function, all supporting the potential protective effect of estrogen on these systems [40].

An inverse relationship between androgen levels and carotid artery thickness (a marker for future atherosclerotic disease) has been noted with postmenopausal women, where higher levels of androgens were noted to have a beneficial impact [41]. Likewise, it can be postulated that the lower levels of androgens seen in women with POI may also contribute to adverse effects on the carotid artery wall and thus an increased risk of CVD [25,36,41]. Of note, this increased risk of CVD is observed despite the fact that the average woman with POI has a lower body mass index than the general population [42]. Because of these risks, it is imperative that POI patients continue regular visits with their primary care providers (including appropriate screening for CVD and blood pressure monitoring), and that a healthy lifestyle (including tobacco cessation, diet, and exercise) be encouraged. It is also important to note that women diagnosed with Turner syndrome should be referred to a cardiologist to have a complete workup for potential congenital cardiac disease and management, specifically aortic abnormalities [24].

It is commonly understood that the risk of decreased bone density greatly intensifies as a woman ages. The reduction in estrogen seen in women with POI likely contributes to this phenomenon, as lower estrogen levels increase both osteoclast and osteoblast activities, but bone formation lags behind its destruction [43]. Women with POI have much lower bone mineral density than women of similar age, with one cross-sectional studying noting a reduction of 2%−3% at all surveyed sites and a Z-score of ≤ -2.0; however, no data are available on how this relates to fracture risk. One small, randomized control trial demonstrated improvement in lumbar bone density with the use of transdermal 17β-estradiol and micronized progesterone over combined oral contraceptives (COCs) [44]. Due to the potential long-term ramifications of bisphosphonates (a well-known treatment for osteoporosis), specifically to the theoretical possibility of harm if pregnancy occurs while bisphosphonates are taken, these medications are not recommended in women <40 years old [45]. The knowledge deficit regarding optimal monitoring and management for low bone density is even more problematic in the adolescent age group, in whom bone density is still accruing and the consequences of a diagnosis of low bone density may be more drastic. Some sources recommended a baseline dual energy x-ray absorption (DEXA) scan at diagnosis of POI, but do not specify whether this depends on the age of diagnosis [20,24]. After this initial screen, recommendations range from annual/biannual screening to no further DEXA testing needed. For example, the European Society of Human Reproduction and Embryology recommends performing a DEXA at diagnosis, and repeating a DEXA only if the initial one is abnormal or if HT is not provided [24]. Other guidance for treatment or prevention of low bone density should focus on lifestyle modifications, such as diet, weight bearing exercise, reduction of alcohol, smoking cessation, and adequate intake of calcium (1000 mg/day) and vitamin D (800 IU/day) [24].

Recently, research has examined the potential negative impact POI and EM may have on neurocognition. Studies performed in rat models have shown that estrogen has a neurotropic effect on dendritic synapses, thus forming a protective response in aging [46]. Data extrapolated from premenopausal women after undergoing oophorectomy had a decrease in visual memory, verbal fluency, cognitive impairment, and an increased risk of Parkinson's disease, neuritic plaques, and dementia [47]. A systematic review and meta-analysis showed that bilateral oophorectomy ≤45 years old was associated with increased risk of dementia [relative risk 1.70, confidence interval (CI) 1.07–2.69] and a faster rate of decline/memory [47]. It is important to emphasize that these studies were not conducted in women with POI, and thus may be more applicable to woman experiencing EM. However, given the low prevalence, identifying a large cohort of POI patients for study can be difficult; therefore extrapolating information from surgical menopause can provide insight into potential POI complications. There has been some limited information of women with POI or Turner syndrome on HT versus a control population that showed no loss of cognitive function when HT was provided [48]. However, POI women diagnosed with Turner syndrome still had some cognitive decline, even with HT [48].

Treatment of early menopause

There are many critical issues to consider in the management of women with a diagnosis of primary ovarian insufficiency (POI), including symptoms related to estrogen deficiency, fertility and contraception, bone and cardiovascular health, and emotional health.

HT: a changing landscape

Estrogen has many roles within the human body, including maintenance of vaginal health. Estrogen deficiency, as a result of natural or surgical menopause, is often associated with altered sexual function. One study evaluated the presence of sexual dysfunction in the context of serum estradiol levels. When levels of estradiol were below 50 pg/mL, women reported greater levels of vaginal dryness, dyspareunia, pain from intercourse, and burning. When estradiol levels were brought to above 50 pg/mL, these symptoms abated [49]. The use of hormonal replacement therapy dates back to 1899, while the more familiar conjugated equine estrogen (CEE) was approved by the FDA in 1942 for the treatment of menopausal symptoms.

HT was deployed as a preventive strategy against common postmenopausal ailments, including skeletal fragility and CVD. However, evidence of its success was mixed. While the Nurses' Health Study reported a 50% decline in coronary heart disease (CHD) in never-users versus ever-users of estrogen [5,7,8], the Framingham Heart Study (1985), reported a twofold increase in CVD risk among ever-users of estrogen. Moreover, the Heart and Estrogen/Progestin Replacement Study (HERS), a randomized controlled trial of 2763 postmenopausal women (mean age 63), identified no difference in CVD events and CVD death among users of daily CEE plus medroxyprogesterone acetate (MPA) or placebo; a significant increase in CHD risk was also observed in HT users [10]. While the postmenopausal estrogen/progestins clinical trial did demonstrate an improvement in HDL with the use of CEE, daily MPA (a synthetic progestin added to protect the endometrium from estrogen-induced hyperplasia), reduced this effect [9].

Against this backdrop, the landmark Women's Health Initiative (WHI) hormone trial was designed to evaluate the risks and benefits of estrogen plus progesterone (E + P) on women with a uterus, and of estrogen alone (E alone) on women who had undergone a hysterectomy. The primary outcome in both trials was CHD; invasive breast cancer was the primary adverse outcome [11,12]. Significant outcomes from the WHI included an increase in stroke in women aged 60–69 years assigned to estrogen and progestin as compared to placebo (Hazard Ratio-HR 1.65). Despite benefits, including a decrease in colorectal cancer for women aged 70–79 years (HR 2.09), and a decrease in hip fracture in women aged 60–69 years (HR 0.33, 95% CI 0.13–0.83), the identified risks resulted in the premature cessation of the WHI E + P trial, followed by cessation of the WHI E alone trial. However, the majority (64%) of the women randomized in WHI were more than 10 years postmenopause, representing an older group of women in whom the processes of atherosclerosis had likely already begun. Moreover, many of the subjects had comorbid conditions, including hypertension, smoking, and obesity, all of which are risk factors for CHD, further increasing the likelihood of subclinical or undiagnosed atherosclerosis. Thus it became clear from the WHI that the timing of initiation of HT (specifically, the number of years after menopause that HT is initiated) may be very important in determining the outcome of therapy.

Moreover, it is important to emphasize that, although the results of the WHI demonstrated increased health risks related to use of HT, young women with POI and EM by contrast are in a pathologic state of estrogen deficiency compared to their peers with normal ovarian function. Thus the strikingly different situation in women with POI requires careful consideration of how best to provide long-term hormone replacement for that group. Without estrogen replacement, women with POI are at greater risk for CHD, overall mortality, cognitive decline, and dementia. Thus these women differ from those who have reached menopause "normally" menopausal women in critical ways, with respect to the risk-benefit ratio of estradiol therapy.

Choice of HT

Despite the controversies surrounding HT in the postmenopausal population, in women with POI, physiologic replacement of estrogen is essential for health, and the data from the WHI suggesting an increase in CVD and breast cancer with HT, do not apply to these women (WEBBER). The goal of hormone replacement in this population is to mimic normal ovarian function, thereby treating symptoms of estrogen deficiency, improving quality of life and sexual health, and mitigating the long-term health risk associated with POI (such as osteoporosis, CHD, stroke, overall mortality, cognitive decline, and dementia). However, data comparing various regimens in this population are limited compared to the general menopause literature. Estrogen replacement should be administered unless absolutely contraindicated (e.g., in women with breast cancer [19]) and may be achieved with several regimens (Table 6.1), with dosing guided by symptom. Serum estradiol testing is not recommended. Treatment should continue until the average age of menopause (approximately age 52) [19], and may be continued past that age with shared decision making for an individual who has clinical symptoms or indications. To further decrease the risk of venous thromboembolism related to estrogen use, consideration should be given to a transdermal or vaginal route of estrogen administration. This approach eliminates the "first pass" effect of estrogens on the liver, although as noted previously, the advantages of transdermal and vaginal estrogens related to vascular safety are more important in older, postmenopausal women. Examples of these approaches include transdermal estradiol (100 mcg daily), estradiol vaginal ring (100 mcg daily), or oral micronized estradiol (2 mg daily). These doses both mimic the average daily ovarian production rate of estradiol across the menstrual cycle in women with normal ovarian function (100 pg/mL) [50].

In women with a uterus, estrogen therapy should be combined with progestin therapy to prevent the sequelae of estrogen-induced endometrial hyperplasia and cancer. One exception to the use of estrogen-progestin combination therapy is in girls and young women with primary amenorrhea and POI in whom secondary sex characteristics have not yet developed; these individuals should initially receive very low doses of estrogen alone, with later addition of a progestin, to mimic gradual pubertal maturation. For women who need a progestin, options include micronized progesterone or oral MPA, or a levonorgestrel intrauterine device (IUD). As with estrogens, there is a paucity of data comparing different progestin options in women with EM, although data suggest that micronized progesterone may be preferable over MPA in postmenopausal women due to adverse effects of MPA on lipids and clotting factors. One randomized controlled trial of MPA in women with POI demonstrated that long-term transdermal estradiol replacement in combination with oral MPA restored normal femoral bone mineral density [51]. Notably, this trial also included a testosterone arm; the use of physiologic transdermal T did not provide additional benefit. With respect to progestin-containing IUDs, a randomized trial of 40 postmenopausal women receiving transdermal estradiol (50 mcg daily) and either a 52 mg levonorgestrel IUD (Mirena) or oral norethisterone showed that both treatments conferred endometrial protection, resulting in an atrophic endometrium developing from a proliferative one [52]. Other levonorgestrel IUDs (e.g., the 12 mcg/day IUD, Skyla) have not been studied for endometrial protection.

Standard postmenopausal HT, which has a much lower dose of estrogen than COCs with estrogen and progestin, does not provide effective contraception. There are a paucity of randomized trials compares COCs with HT in women with POI and EM. In an open randomized trial comparing the effect of HT versus COCs or no

TABLE 6.1 Hormone therapy (HT) options for POI.

Estrogen		
Oral 17β-estradiol	1–2 mg daily	
Transdermal 17β-estradiol	100 mcg daily	
Conjugated equine estrogen	0.625–1.25 mg daily	
Estradiol vaginal ring	100 mcg daily	
Progestin		
Oral micronized progesterone	*Sequential*	*Continuous*
	200 mg daily for 12 days per month	100 mg daily
Oral medroxyprogesterone acetate	5–10 mg daily for 12 days per month	2.5–5 mg daily
Levonorgestrel intrauterine device (IUD)	52 mg IUD (release rate approximately 20 mcg daily)	

treatment on bone density and turnover among 59 women with spontaneous POI, HR was found to be superior to COCs in increasing bone density at the lumbar spine (+0.050 g/cm; [1] 95% CI 0.007–0.092; $P = .025$). In the no treatment group, bone density dropped at all sites. While the study was limited by small sample size and a high drop-out rate, it is reasonable to conclude that either treatment (HT or COCs) is superior to no treatment [53]. If oral contraceptives are used, a continuous regimen is ideal because vasomotor symptoms may recur during the placebo week (Table 6.1).

Contraceptive needs

About 75% of women with karyotypically normal, spontaneous POI have potentially functional ovarian follicles, and these women have an approximately 4% chance of spontaneous ovulation per month [54,55]. Limited data extrapolated from perimenopausal women (who also have high serum gonadotropins and low fecundity) suggests that COCs prevent spontaneous ovulation and pregnancy more reliably than HT [56], a critical consideration for women who need contraception. Thus one approach to HT in women with EM and contraceptive needs is the use of COCs, which also provide ease of dosing and potentially less stigma than HT. However, contraceptive-dose options provide significantly more estrogen and progestin than HT. Moreover, due to the extremely elevated FSH at baseline, there is a potential that hormonal contraceptives will be unable to suppress FSH to a level to prevent escape ovulation, and case reports of pregnancies while on oral contraceptives have been documented [57]. For women who prefer HT but also desire highly effective contraception, a levonorgestrel IUD, or a contraceptive barrier method, may be utilized. Alternatively, if HT is prescribed, a cyclic regimen which induces regular monthly withdrawal bleeding, and the use of a menstrual calendar, allows for easier recognition of a spontaneous pregnancy. A missed withdrawal bleed should prompt an evaluation for pregnancy.

Fertility

The adverse impact a diagnosis of POI has on current or future fertility can be one of the most upsetting realizations for many patients. This requires extensive counseling, not only to discuss the difficulties with pregnancy but also the potential ramifications for future offspring if POI has resulted from a heritable genetic anomaly. Intermittent ovarian function (defined as serum estradiol >50 pg/mL) or ovulation has been demonstrated in up to 50% of patients with POI; however, only 16%–23.7% will exhibit ovulation [27,37,58], and the frequency and timing of these ovulations is unpredictable. This potential for ovulation, as well as an overall 5%–10% spontaneous conception rate, differentiates POI from natural menopause [27,37,58]. In one study of 100 women with POI, intermittent ovulation was more likely to occur in those with secondary amenorrhea versus primary amenorrhea [37,55,59]. Thus although some women with POI conceive without treatment, the low chance of ovulation renders this approach, as well as the use of ovulation induction, ineffective. Monitoring for spontaneous ovulation may be considered, however, to help provide closure for an individual with POI, and to ease the transition to other options. Likewise, while in vitro fertilization with autologous oocytes may be effective for women with POI with residual ovarian reserve for ovarian stimulation, most commonly, these women exhibit a poor ovarian response to ovarian stimulation and overall low success. Small case reports and observational studies have utilized various protocols utilizing estrogen, progesterone, and gonadotropins, and have not noted any significant change from baseline pregnancy rate of 5%—10% [29,59]. A systematic review in 1999, including seven controlled studies, six of which were randomized, demonstrated that no treatment can improve ovarian function or pregnancy rates greater than the baseline rates of 5%—10% [59—61]. Moreover, while women with POI may exhibit visible ovarian follicles on ultrasound, as yet there is no universally accepted method for collecting and maturing these oocytes in vitro. While a recent report described a case of successful in vitro maturation (IVM) after failure to produce oocytes from traditional gonadotropin stimulation, in which the patient eventually froze eight cleavage stage embryos and delivered twins at term [62], at present, such options remain experimental.

Therefore the best chance for conception remains in vitro fertilization utilizing donor oocytes or donor embryos. These approaches can have cumulative success rates in excess of 80%, with the chance of conception being dependent primarily on the age of the oocyte donor. Notably, women with POI due to Turner syndrome require a careful cardiovascular evaluation prior to attempting to conceive, as these women are at risk of aortic dissection during pregnancy [63]. In cases in which pregnancy is contraindicated, the use of a gestational carrier can be a viable option for family building.

Sexual health

POI/EM also impacts sexual wellbeing. One study which surveyed 81 POI patients and 68 women with regular menstrual cycles revealed that women with POI report distress concerning decreased arousal (45.3%), sexual satisfaction (20%—25%), negative emotions concerning their sexual life (18.7%), and increased pain that did not improve with HT (44%) [64]. Overall, some type of sexual dysfunction can be noted in 25%—62% of women who experience EM/POI [65]. This can be more pronounced in women who have undergone surgical menopause due to the sudden loss of hormones. One large cross-sectional survey performed in Europe observed that women undergoing oophorectomy had twice the rate of hypoactive sexual desire disorder as compared to women who underwent natural menopause [66]. Decreased estrogen can also result in a reduction in sexual satisfaction from a loss of lubrication. Moreover, a person's sexual drive and ability to be aroused may be affected, which has been thought to be due to a decrease in sex steroids [64]. One cross-sectional Danish study of over 500 women between the ages of 19 and 65 analyzed the relationship between sexual desire and androgen levels (free testosterone, androstenedione, total testosterone, DHEAS, and androstenedione). Lower serum levels of free testosterone and androstenedione were associated with a reduction in sexual desire [64].

Androgens have been utilized to help increase sexual desire, but their use should be managed carefully and for only a short duration due to uncertain long-term effects [67]. Some randomized control studies have shown improvement in sexual desire, arousal, and satisfaction when using various forms of testosterone [68]. However, it is important to realize that no single testosterone formulation has been specifically designed to treat women. In fact, the Endocrine Society recommends against making a diagnosis of "androgen deficiency" in healthy women, and that only women with hypoactive sexual desire disorder are prescribed any type of testosterone for a maximum of a 6-month trial [69]. The use of androgens for the purpose of treating sexual desire presents challenges due to a lack of a universally accepted definition for "low" testosterone or its precursors (especially age related cut offs), a limited ability to accurately measure testosterone [70], and the decision of which androgen to evaluate [71]. If utilized, testosterone levels should be measured at baseline and at 3—6 weeks after initiation to ensure that patients are not being overtreated. It is also important that providers understand that there is a paucity of information of testosterone formulation or dose in women, and patients should be informed that there is a complete lack of data beyond 24 months of testosterone use [69]. Unfortunately, the aforementioned studies regarding testosterone therapy were not conducted in women with POI; thus there is even more limited data concerning testosterone therapy in POI patients in general. One study noted that although women with POI overall have lower sexual satisfaction scores than control women, the one area that did not differ from a control population was sexual desire, which is the only true indication to use testosterone therapy in women [72].

In women whose primary complaint is discomfort during intercourse, rather than desire, some alternative strategies include lubrication, pelvic floor exercises, local estrogen (e.g., vaginal estrogen), or a combination of the two [24,73,74]. A Cochrane review concerning vaginal health in postmenopausal women concluded that, while there was no evidence of a difference in efficacy between the various intravaginal estrogenic preparations (e.g., rings, creams, and tablets) when compared with each other, low-quality evidence suggests that that vaginal estrogen preparations improve the symptoms of vaginal atrophy in postmenopausal women when compared to placebo [75]. In general, for women with menopausal vulvovaginal symptoms and no contraindications to local estrogen, the most effective therapy for these symptoms is local estrogen, in any formulation [76]. However, one small cross-sectional study comparing sexual symptoms in women with POI on either 1–2 mg estradiol or 0.625 mg conjugated estrogen with progesterone demonstrated a decrease in lubrication and increase in pain despite use of HT [77]. There is thus limited information concerning what is deemed adequate dosing to ameliorate vaginal symptoms in women with POI or postmenopausal women. Regardless of the choice of HT, in one study, over 40% of POI patients discontinue therapy within the first year of treatment [78]. Thus the patient's preferences for optimal route, drug, and type of hormonal therapy should be a foremost consideration in the choice of treatment.

Emotional health

It is important to remember that a diagnosis of POI is life-changing, resulting in increased morbidity and altered potential future family building plans. Therefore it is not a surprise that the psychological ramifications of POI can be monumental, with increased rates of depression, anxiety, self-esteem, and a decrease in quality of life. One long-term study of women who had undergone bilateral oophorectomy prior to menopause, with an average follow up of over 20 years, showed an increase in depression or anxiety diagnosed by a psychiatrist in these women (HR 1.72, 95% CI 1.00–2.96, $P = .05$ and HR 2.52, 95% CI 1.15–5.53, $P = .02$, respectively) [79]. Importantly, symptoms of anxiety did not improve with the use of HT. A diagnosis of POI is shocking, confusing, and devastating for patients, and is associated with intense feelings of grief and loss. When a diagnosis of POI is made, it is crucial that the patient be informed in a sensitive and caring manner, and that she receives accurate information and appropriate resources for emotional support. Clinicians should also address the potential development of depression and anxiety disorders. For women who experience significant anxiety or depression related to the diagnosis, referral to a mental health provider with expertise in POI and reproductive health should be made.

Moreover, a multidimensional approach to POI should be utilized to address the long-term impact on physical health, fertility, and of particular importance is the discussion of the impact on mental health and a referral to a mental health provider and/or support groups. Numerous resources are available for providers and patients alike to help with support and discussion on this difficult topic. Examples of these resources include the Daisy Network (https://www.daisynetwork.org/), Resolve (http://resolve.org/support), and Early Menopause (https://www.earlymenopause.com). Notably, terms such as "menopause" or "failure" can be exceedingly distressing to a young woman and should be avoided.

Looking toward the future of POI treatment

The consequence of POI and EM can range from psychological devastation relating to the diagnosis and loss of fertility, to the long-term health consequences of premature loss of ovarian function, including bone loss, cardiovascular and neurocognitive disorders. Until recently, therapeutic options have been limited to the use of HT to treat symptoms and minimize long-term risks of estrogen deprivation, as well as the use of donor eggs for biological parenting. However, recent advances in the reproductive field have begun to unravel the complex pathways involved in the pathophysiology of POI and EM, and development of promising future diagnostic and treatment modalities is already underway. Emerging diagnostic tests and tools may allow earlier diagnosis of POI in sporadic cases. For example, efforts to detect novel genes related to POI have included genotyping via genome-wide association studies as well as genome-wide sequencing through next-generation sequencing, which allow for the identification of genetic variations associated with POI. Timely interventions in women at risk for POI may offer the hope of preserving residual reproductive potential. Elective egg freezing offers a preemptive approach to fertility preservation in women at risk for POI, such as those with Turner syndrome, pediatric cancer survivors [80], FMR1 premutation carriers [81,82], or autoimmune conditions [32]. Ovarian tissue cryopreservation, which has been increasingly utilized to safeguard fertility in young girls and women undergoing cancer treatment, may also be a consideration in women with benign conditions which confer risk of POI. More than 130 live births have been reported after transplantation of cryopreserved ovarian tissue [83]. Other novel (and more controversial) areas of study include the administration of stem cell therapy to promote residual follicle rescue [84], the use of platelet-rich plasma to support follicular growth [85], and in vitro activation of follicles as a strategy for reactivating dormant primordial follicles.

Conclusion

The problem of ovarian aging has considerable impact on public health, and presently no viable preventative or treatment options are available. It is critical that research continue with the goal of improving our understanding of the mechanisms underpinning the ovarian aging process. This is an essential first step toward the development of novel therapies for treatment of conditions such as POI and EM.

References

[1] Kallen A, Polotsky AJ, Johnson J. Untapped reserves: controlling primordial follicle growth activation. Trends Mol Med 2018;24(3):319–31.
[2] Winship AL, Stringer JM, Liew SH, Hutt KJ. The importance of DNA repair for maintaining oocyte quality in response to anti-cancer treatments, environmental toxins and maternal ageing. Hum Reprod Update 2018;24(2):119–34.
[3] Mailhes JB, Marchetti F, Phillips GL, Barnhill DR. Preferential pericentric lesions and aneuploidy induced in mouse oocytes by the topoisomerase II inhibitor etoposide. Teratog Carcinog Mutagen 1994;14(1):39–51.
[4] Barekati Z, Gourabi H, valojerdi MR, Yazdi PE. Previous maternal chemotherapy by cyclophosphamide (Cp) causes numerical chromosome abnormalities in preimplantation mouse embryos. Reprod Toxicol 2008;26(3–4):278–81.
[5] Asllanaj E, Bano A, Glisic M, Jaspers L, Ikram MA, Laven JSE, et al. Age at natural menopause and life expectancy with and without type 2 diabetes. Menopause 2019;26(4):387–94.
[6] Ossewaarde ME, Bots ML, Verbeek ALM, Peeters PHM, Van Der Graaf Y, Grobbee DE, et al. Age at menopause, cause-specific mortality and total life expectancy. Epidemiology 2005;16(4):556–62.
[7] Muka T, Oliver-Williams C, Kunutsor S, Laven JSE, Fauser BCJM, Chowdhury R, et al. Association of age at onset of menopause and time since onset of menopause with cardiovascular outcomes, intermediate vascular traits, and all-cause mortality: a systematic review and meta-analysis. JAMA Cardiol 2016;1(7):767–76.
[8] Georgakis MK, Kalogirou EI, Diamantaras AA, Daskalopoulou SS, Munro CA, Lyketsos CG, et al. Age at menopause and duration of reproductive period in association with dementia and cognitive function: a systematic review and meta-analysis. Psychoneuroendocrinology 2016;73:224–43. Available from: https://doi.org/10.1016/j.psyneuen.2016.08.003.
[9] Poorthuis MHF, Algra AM, Algra A, Kappelle LJ, Klijn CJM. Female-and male-specific risk factors for stroke a systematic review and meta-analysis. JAMA Neurol 2017;74(1):75–81.
[10] Ley SH, Li Y, Tobias DK, Manson JAE, Rosner B, Hu FB, et al. Duration of reproductive life span, age at menarche, and age at menopause are associated with risk of cardiovascular disease in women. J Am Heart Assoc 2017;6(11):e006713.
[11] Sullivan SD, Lehman A, Thomas F, Johnson KC, Jackson R, Wactawski-Wende J, et al. Effects of self-reported age at nonsurgical menopause on time to first fracture and bone mineral density in the Women's Health Initiative Observational Study. Menopause 2015;22(10):1035–44.
[12] Shadyab AH, MacEra CA, Shaffer RA, Jain S, Gallo LC, Gass MLS, et al. Ages at menarche and menopause and reproductive lifespan as predictors of exceptional longevity in women: The Women's Health Initiative. Menopause 2017;24(1):35–44.
[13] CDC/NCHS. CDC/NCHS National Vital Statistics Reports, 2013.
[14] Nichols HB, Trentham-Dietz A, Hampton JM, Titus-Ernstoff L, Egan KM, Willett WC, et al. From menarche to menopause: trends among United States women born from 1912 to 1969. Am J Epidemiol 2006;164(10):1003–11.
[15] Aso T. Demography of the menopause and pattern of climacteric symptoms in the East Asian region. First consensus meeting on menopause in the East Asian region. Geneva: Geneva Foundation for Medical Education and Research; 1997.
[16] Donnez J, Dolmans MM. Natural hormone replacement therapy with a functioning ovary after the menopause: dream or reality? Reprod Biomed Online 2018;37(3):359–66.
[17] Tao XY, Zuo AZ, Wang JQ, Tao FB. Effect of primary ovarian insufficiency and early natural menopause on mortality: a meta-analysis. Climacteric 2016;19(1):27–36.
[18] Bompoula MS, Valsamakis G, Neofytou S, Messaropoulos P, Salakos N, Mastorakos G, et al. Demographic, clinical and hormonal characteristics of patients with premature ovarian insufficiency and those of early menopause: data from two tertiary premature ovarian insufficiency centers in Greece. Gynecol Endocrinol 2020;36(8):693–7.
[19] Committee Opinion No. 605. Primary ovarian insufficiency in adolescents and young women. Obstet Gynecol 2014;20(5):245–7. Available from: http://content.wkhealth.com/linkback/openurl?sid = WKPTLP:landingpage&an = 01436319-201409000-00002.
[20] Nelson LM. Clinical practice. Primary ovarian insufficiency. N Engl J Med 2009;360(6):606–14. Available from: https://pubmed.ncbi.nlm.nih.gov/19196677.
[21] National Institutes of Health. Primary ovarian insufficiency: condition information. Available from: <https://www.nichd.nih.gov/health/topics/poi/conditioninfo/default>, 2016.
[22] National Institutes of Health. Primary ovarian insufficiency, 2017. Available from: <https://www.nichd.nih.gov/health/topics/factsheets/poi>.
[23] Nelson SM, Anderson RA. Prediction of premature ovarian insufficiency: foolish fallacy or feasible foresight? Climacteric 2021;1–10. Available from: https://doi.org/10.1080/13697137.2020.1868426.
[24] European Society of Human Reproduction and Embryology. Guideline on the management of premature ovarian insufficiency. Available from: <https://www.eshre.eu/Guidelines-and-Legal/Guidelines/Management-of-premature-ovarian-insufficiency.aspx>, 2015.
[25] Tsiligiannis S, Panay N, Stevenson JC. Premature ovarian insufficiency and long-term health consequences. Curr Vasc Pharmacol 2019;17(6):604–9.

[26] ACOG. ACOG practice bulletin no. 89. Elective and risk-reducing salpingo-oophorectomy. Obstet Gynecol 2008;111(1):231—41.
[27] ACOG. CO605: Primary ovarian insufficiency in adolescents and young women. Obstet Gynecol 2014;124(1):193—7.
[28] Qin Y, Jiao X, Simpson JL, Chen ZJ. Genetics of primary ovarian insufficiency: new developments and opportunities. Hum Reprod Update 2015;21(6):787—808.
[29] Fraison E, Crawford G, Casper G, Harris V, Ledger W. Pregnancy following diagnosis of premature ovarian insufficiency: a systematic review. Reprod Biomed Online 2019;39(3):467—76.
[30] Meyers CM, Boughman JA, Rivas M, Wilroy RS, Simpson JL. Gonadal (ovarian) dysgenesis in 46, XX individuals: frequency of the autosomal recessive form. Am J Med Genet 1996;63(4):518—24.
[31] Massanyi EZ, DiCarlo HN, Migeon CJ, Gearhart JP. Review and management of 46, XY disorders of sex development. J Pediatr Urol 2013;9(3):368—79. Available from: https://www.sciencedirect.com/science/article/pii/S1477513112002938.
[32] Kirshenbaum M, Orvieto R. Premature ovarian insufficiency (POI) and autoimmunity-an update appraisal. J Assist Reprod Genet 2019;36(11):2207—15.
[33] Domniz N, Meirow D. Premature ovarian insufficiency and autoimmune diseases. Best Pract Res Clin Obstet Gynaecol 2019;60:42—55.
[34] Zhu D, Chung HF, Pandeya N, Dobson AJ, Cade JE, Greenwood DC, et al. Relationships between intensity, duration, cumulative dose, and timing of smoking with age at menopause: a pooled analysis of individual data from 17 observational studies. PLoS Med 2018;15(11):e1002704.
[35] Patel S, Zhou C, Rattan S, Flaws JA. Effects of endocrine-disrupting chemicals on the ovary. Biol Reprod 2015;93(1):20.
[36] Tsiligiannis S, Panay N, Stevenson JC. Premature ovarian insufficiency: practical management approaches. In: Berga SL, Genazzani AR, Naftolin F, Petraglia F, editors. Menstrual cycle related disorders, volume 7: frontiers in gynecological endocrinology. Cham: Springer International Publishing; 2019. p. 143—53. Available from: https://doi.org/10.1007/978-3-030-14358-9_11.
[37] Rebar RW, Connolly HV. Clinical features of young women with hypergonadotropic amenorrhea. Fertil Steril 1990;53(5):804—10. Available from: https://www.sciencedirect.com/science/article/pii/S0015028216535134.
[38] Goldenberg RL, Grodin JM, Rodbard D, Ross GT. Gonadotropins in women with amenorrhea. The use of plasma follicle-stimulating hormone to differentiate women with and without ovarian follicles. Am J Obstet Gynecol 1973;116(7):1003—12.
[39] Jacoby VL, Grady D, Wactawski-Wende J, Manson JE, Allison MA, Kuppermann M, et al. Oophorectomy vs ovarian conservation with hysterectomy: cardiovascular disease, hip fracture, and cancer in the Women's Health Initiative Observational Study. Arch Intern Med 2011;171(8):760—8.
[40] Langrish JP, Mills NL, Bath LE, Warner P, Webb DJ, Kelnar CJ, et al. Cardiovascular effects of physiological and standard sex steroid replacement regimens in premature ovarian failure. Hypertension 2009;53(5):805—11.
[41] Bernini GP, Moretti A, Sgró M, Argenio GF, Barlascini CO, Cristofani R, et al. Influence of endogenous androgens on carotid wall in postmenopausal women. Menopause 2001;8(1):43—50.
[42] Gunning MN, Meun C, van Rijn BB, Maas A, Benschop L, Franx A, et al. Coronary artery calcification in middle-aged women with premature ovarian insufficiency. Clin Endocrinol 2019;91(2):314—22.
[43] Almeida M, Han L, Martin-Millan M, Plotkin LI, Stewart SA, Roberson PK, et al. Skeletal involution by age-associated oxidative stress and its acceleration by loss of sex steroids. J Biol Chem 2007;282(37):27285—97.
[44] Crofton PM, Evans N, Bath LE, Warner P, Whitehead TJ, Critchley HOD, et al. Physiological vs standard sex steroid replacement in young women with premature ovarian failure: effects on bone mass acquisition and turnover. Clin Endocrinol (Oxf) 2010;73(6):707—14.
[45] Drake MT, Clarke BL, Khosla S. Bisphosphonates: mechanism of action and role in clinical practice. Mayo Clin Proc 2008;83(9):1032—45.
[46] Lewis C, McEwen BS, Frankfurt M. Estrogen-induction of dendritic spines in ventromedial hypothalamus and hippocampus: effects of neonatal aromatase blockade and adult GDX. Brain Res Dev Brain Res 1995;87(1):91—5.
[47] Georgakis MK, Beskou-Kontou T, Theodoridis I, Skalkidou A, Petridou ET. Surgical menopause in association with cognitive function and risk of dementia: a systematic review and meta-analysis. Psychoneuroendocrinology 2019;106:9—19. Available from: https://www.sciencedirect.com/science/article/pii/S0306453018311478.
[48] Ross JL, Stefanatos GA, Kushner H, Bondy C, Nelson L, Zinn A, et al. The effect of genetic differences and ovarian failure: intact cognitive function in adult women with premature ovarian failure vs Turner syndrome. J Clin Endocrinol Metab 2004;89(4):1817—22. Available from: https://doi.org/10.1210/jc.2003-031463.
[49] Sarrel PM. Effects of hormone replacement therapy on sexual psychophysiology and behavior in postmenopause. J Womens Health Gend Based Med 2000;9(Suppl 1):25—32. Available from: https://doi.org/10.1089/152460900318830.
[50] Mishell DRJ, Nakamura RM, Crosignani PG, Stone S, Kharma K, Nagata Y, et al. Serum gonadotropin and steroid patterns during the normal menstrual cycle. Am J Obstet Gynecol 1971;111(1):60—5.
[51] Popat VB, Calis KA, Kalantaridou SN, Vanderhoof VH, Koziol D, Troendle JF, et al. Bone mineral density in young women with primary ovarian insufficiency: results of a three-year randomized controlled trial of physiological transdermal estradiol and testosterone replacement. J Clin Endocrinol Metab 2014;99(9):3418—26.
[52] Raudaskoski TH, Lahti EI, Kauppila AJ, Apaja-Sarkkinen MA, Laatikainen TJ. Transdermal estrogen with a levonorgestrel-releasing intrauterine device for climacteric complaints: clinical and endometrial responses. Am J Obstet Gynecol 1995;172(1 Pt 1):114—19.
[53] Cartwright B, Robinson J, Seed PT, Fogelman I, Rymer J. Hormone replacement therapy vs the combined oral contraceptive pill in premature ovarian failure: a randomized controlled trial of the effects on bone mineral density. J Clin Endocrinol Metab 2016;101(9):3497—505.
[54] Hubayter ZR, Popat V, Vanderhoof VH, Ndubizu O, Johnson D, Mao E, et al. A prospective evaluation of antral follicle function in women with 46, XX spontaneous primary ovarian insufficiency. Fertil Steril 2010;94(5):1769—74. Available from: https://doi.org/10.1016/j.fertnstert.2009.10.023.
[55] Nelson LM, Anasti JN, Kimzey LM, Defensor RA, Lipetz KJ, White BJ, et al. Development of luteinized Graafian follicles in patients with karyotypically normal spontaneous premature ovarian failure. J Clin Endocrinol Metab 1994;79(5):1470—5.
[56] Ovsyannikova TV, Kulikov IA. Hormonal contraception in women of reproductive age: endocrinological aspects. Gynecology 2019;21(1):65—8.
[57] Alper M, Jolly E, Garner P. Pregnancies after premature ovarian failure. Obstet Gynecol 1986;67(3 Suppl):59S—62S. Available from: https://journals.lww.com/greenjournal/Fulltext/1986/03001/Pregnancies_After_Premature_Ovarian_Failure.18.aspx.

[58] Rebar RW, Erickson GF, Yen SSC. Idiopathic premature ovarian failure: clinical and endocrine characteristics. Fertil Steril 1982;37(1):35–41. Available from: https://www.sciencedirect.com/science/article/pii/S001502821645973X.

[59] van Kasteren YM, Schoemaker J. Premature ovarian failure: a systematic review on therapeutic interventions to restore ovarian function and achieve pregnancy. Hum Reprod Update 1999;5(5):483–92. Available from: https://doi.org/10.1093/humupd/5.5.483.

[60] Surrey ES, Cedars MI. The effect of gonadotropin suppression on the induction of ovulation in premature ovarian failure patients. Fertil Steril 1989;52(1):36–41.

[61] Van Kasteren YM, Braat DDM, Hemrika DJ, Lambalk CB, Rekers-Mombarg LTM, Von Blomberg BME, et al. Corticosteroids do not influence ovarian responsiveness to gonadotropins in patients with premature ovarian failure: a randomized, placebo-controlled trial. Fertil Steril 1999;71(1):90–5.

[62] Grynberg M, Jacquesson L, Sifer C. In vitro maturation of oocytes for preserving fertility in autoimmune premature ovarian insufficiency. Fertil Steril 2020;114(4):848–53. Available from: https://doi.org/10.1016/j.fertnstert.2020.04.049.

[63] Committee P, Society A. Increased maternal cardiovascular mortality associated with pregnancy in women with Turner syndrome. Fertil Steril 2012;97(2):282–4. Available from: https://doi.org/10.1016/j.fertnstert.2011.11.049.

[64] van der Stege JG, Groen H, van Zadelhoff SJN, Lambalk CB, Braat DDM, van Kasteren YM, et al. Decreased androgen concentrations and diminished general and sexual well-being in women with premature ovarian failure. Menopause 2008;15(1):23–31. Available from: https://journals.lww.com/menopausejournal/Fulltext/2008/15010/Decreased_androgen_concentrations_and_diminished.8.aspx.

[65] Kingsberg SA, Larkin LC, Liu JH. Clinical effects of early or surgical menopause. Obstet Gynecol 2020;135(4):853–68. Available from: https://journals.lww.com/greenjournal/Fulltext/2020/04000/Clinical_Effects_of_Early_or_Surgical_Menopause.15.aspx.

[66] Dennerstein L, Koochaki P, Barton I, Graziottin A. Hypoactive sexual desire disorder in menopausal women: a survey of Western European women. J Sex Med 2006;3(2):212–22.

[67] Webber L, Anderson RA, Davies M, Janse F, Vermeulen N. HRT for women with premature ovarian insufficiency: a comprehensive review. Hum Reprod Open 2017;2017(2):1–11.

[68] Shifren JL, Braunstein GD, Simon JA, Casson PR, Buster JE, Redmond GP, et al. Transdermal testosterone treatment in women with impaired sexual function after oophorectomy. N Engl J Med 2000;343(10):682–8. Available from: https://doi.org/10.1056/NEJM200009073431002.

[69] Wierman ME, Arlt W, Basson R, Davis SR, Miller KK, Murad MH, et al. Androgen therapy in women: a reappraisal: an Endocrine Society clinical practice guideline. J Clin Endocrinol Metab 2014;99(10):3489–510.

[70] Nappi RE. To be or not to be in sexual desire: the androgen dilemma. Climacteric 2015;18(5):672–4. Available from: https://doi.org/10.3109/13697137.2015.1064268.

[71] Wåhlin-Jacobsen S, Pedersen AT, Kristensen E, Laessøe NC, Lundqvist M, Cohen AS, et al. Is there a correlation between androgens and sexual desire in women? J Sex Med 2015;12(2):358–73.

[72] de Almeida DMB, Benetti-Pinto CL, Makuch MY. Sexual function of women with premature ovarian failure. Menopause 2011;18(3):262–6.

[73] Gargus E, Deans R, Anazodo A, Woodruff TK. Management of primary ovarian insufficiency symptoms in survivors of childhood and adolescent cancer. J Natl Compr Canc Netw 2018;16(9):1137–49.

[74] Maciejewska-Jeske M, Szeliga A, Męczekalski B. Consequences of premature ovarian insufficiency on women's sexual health. Prz Menopauzalny 2018;17(3):127–30.

[75] Lethaby A, Ayeleke RO, Roberts H. Local oestrogen for vaginal atrophy in postmenopausal women. Cochrane Database Syst Rev 2016;(8):CD001500. Available from: https://doi.org/10.1002/14651858.CD001500.pub3.

[76] Machura P, Grymowicz M, Rudnicka E, Pięta W, Calik-Ksepka A, Skórska J, et al. Premature ovarian insufficiency—hormone replacement therapy and management of long-term consequences. Prz Menopauzalny 2018;17(3):135–8. Available from: https://pubmed.ncbi.nlm.nih.gov/30357030.

[77] Pacello PCC, Yela DA, Rabelo S, Giraldo PC, Benetti-Pinto CL. Dyspareunia and lubrication in premature ovarian failure using hormonal therapy and vaginal health. Climacteric. 2014;17(4):342–7.

[78] Bachelot A, Nicolas C, Gricourt S, Dulon J, Leban M, Golmard JL, et al. Poor compliance to hormone therapy and decreased bone mineral density in women with premature ovarian insufficiency. PLoS One 2016;11(12):e0164638.

[79] Rocca WA, Grossardt BR, Geda YE, Gostout BS, Bower JH, Maraganore DM, et al. Long-term risk of depressive and anxiety symptoms after early bilateral oophorectomy. Menopause 2018;25(11):1275–85.

[80] Hoekman EJ, Louwe LA, Rooijers M, van der Westerlaken LAJ, Klijn NF, Pilgram GSK, et al. Ovarian tissue cryopreservation: low usage rates and high live-birth rate after transplantation. Acta Obstet Gynecol Scand 2020;99(2):213–21.

[81] Man L, Lekovich J, Rosenwaks Z, Gerhardt J. Fragile X-associated diminished ovarian reserve and primary ovarian insufficiency from molecular mechanisms to clinical manifestations. Front Mol Neurosci 2017;10:1–17.

[82] Fritz R, Jindal S. Reproductive aging and elective fertility preservation. J Ovarian Res 2018;11(1):1–8.

[83] Donnez J, Dolmans M-M. Fertility preservation in women. Nat Rev Endocrinol 2013;9(12):735–49. Available from: http://www.nature.com/doifinder/10.1038/nrendo.2013.205.

[84] Sheikhansari G, Aghebati-Maleki L, Nouri M, Jadidi-Niaragh F, Yousefi M. Current approaches for the treatment of premature ovarian failure with stem cell therapy. Biomed Pharmacother 2018;102:254–62.

[85] Bos-Mikich A, Oliveira R De, Frantz N. Platelet-rich plasma therapy and reproductive medicine. J Assist Reprod Genet 2018;35(5):753–6.

CHAPTER

7

Reproductive and sexual health concerns for cancer survivors

Jessica R. Gorman[1] and Elizabeth K. Arthur[2]

[1]College of Public Health and Human Sciences, Oregon State University, Corvallis, OR, United States [2]College of Nursing and Comprehensive Cancer Center — Arthur G. James Cancer Hospital, Richard. J. Solove Research Institute, The Ohio State University, Columbus, OH, United States

Introduction

Life does not return to "normal" when cancer treatment ends. Alongside the financial, emotional, and physical burdens of cancer, exposure to cancer treatments such as chemotherapy, radiation, and surgery can pose significant risks to reproductive and sexual health (RSH). Cancer survivors navigate immediate as well as long-term and late effects of their treatment, which commonly include problems with sexual function, inability to have children, and challenges with intimacy [1–4]. When left unaddressed, these RSH concerns can negatively affect partner relationships and quality of life well after treatment ends [5–8].

RSH concerns are among the most common and distressing aspects of cancer survivorship [5,9,10]. Younger survivors have the hardest time adjusting to life after cancer, experiencing more unsupportive responses from family and friends, higher depressive symptoms, higher levels of avoidant coping, and more negative appraisal of the illness and its impact than older patients [11,12]. Younger survivors describe feeling that something has been "taken away" from them or that they are "missing out" because of forced and unexpected changes in their ability to have children and sexual relationships [13–15]. These concerns vary across the course of survivorship as they experience changes in life circumstances, relationships, family building goals, and health. Although breast and reproductive cancer survivors experience a more direct impact on their reproductive systems and functions, RSH concerns can affect all cancer survivors [4,16,17]. Better meeting survivors' RSH informational, medical, and supportive care needs over time could have a substantial positive impact on their relationships and quality of life. Attention to these concerns through comprehensive follow-up care is imperative [18–22].

In this chapter, we provide an overview of the RSH consequences of cancer as well as guidance for managing RSH concerns. We focus mainly on reproductive-aged cancer survivors, who are at a stage of life that is more likely to involve building intimate relationships and families [23,24]. Finally, we briefly discuss considerations for older adult, black, indigenous, and people of color (BIPOC) and lesbian, gay, bisexual, transgender, queer/questioning (LGBTQ +) survivors.

The reproductive and sexual health consequences of cancer and cancer treatment

The impact of cancer treatment on fertility

The possibility of having biological children is important to many reproductive-aged cancer survivors, but cancer treatments can threaten future fertility and have a distressing impact on their lives [7,24]. Although not all cancer treatments significantly increase infertility risk, high doses of alkylating chemotherapy and radiation treatment directed toward reproductive organs are associated with higher risk [25–27]. Individual risk is highly variable, dependent on age as well as the type and dose of the cancer treatment [28]. Endocrine therapy, common for breast cancer patients, can also affect childbearing as it commonly requires the patient to delay pregnancy for at least 5 years, resulting in further concomitant ovarian aging.

For reproductive-aged males, malignant disease can influence gonadal function and cancer treatment can result in anatomical defects, hormonal insufficiency, damage or depletion of the germinal stem cells, or absence of sperm [29,30]. As with females, the degree of impairment depends on cancer and treatment type, dosage, and pretreatment fertility [31]. For example, cisplatin-based chemotherapy results in sperm recovery of 55%–80%, while in male leukemia patients receiving regimens with cyclophosphamide or melphalan combined with total body irradiation, over 80% have permanent sterility [32,33]. Testicular cancer is the most common among young adult men and negatively impacts fertility for about a third of survivors [34].

Reproductive concerns after cancer

Regardless of cancer treatment, reproductive concerns are common among reproductive-aged cancer survivors and can continue for years after cancer treatment has ended [13,24,35,36]. Some survivors report that the potential loss of fertility is as painful as the cancer diagnosis itself [37]. Reproductive concerns extend beyond potential infertility to include a number of other worries: whether the patient's physical health will affect their capacity to parent; dealing with the emotional and practical barriers to achieving pregnancy; possible negative impacts of cancer on the health of their offspring; and disclosing possible infertility to a partner [13,38,39]. The high financial burden of cancer treatment faced by cancer survivors can compound worries about achieving parenthood goals, which may require additional expenses (i.e., via adoption or assisted reproductive technology) [40–43]. Psychosocial and financial burdens could also contribute to the observed lower rate of biological parenthood among cancer survivors as compared to the general population [44,45]. Even for those who do not desire a biological child, fertility can be important as it is often tied to a sense of femininity or masculinity, attractiveness, and self-esteem [38,46–48].

Although more research has focused on female cancer survivors, male survivors also experience reproductive concerns and have expressed a need for better reproductive-related information and support [36,49–51]. Men report a stigma about potential infertility, uncertainty about their fertility status, and concerns about disclosing infertility to their partners [49,52,53]. The financial burden of cancer can be a barrier to sperm banking and related treatments [40,41,54,55]. However, male survivors may also experience different and fewer reproductive concerns than female survivors [36]. For example, two studies have found that young adult males are most concerned about their future child's health (e.g., fear that child would get cancer someday), and least concerned about barriers to achieving pregnancy (e.g., it would take too much time and effort to father a child) [17,56]. The experience of infertility may also be fundamentally different for men and women, regardless of their cancer status [57–59]. Women may have more negative experiences related to identity, self-esteem, physical health, depression, stress, and anxiety [60], while men may be more concerned about aspects of control and their partner's response [61].

When these reproductive concerns are left unaddressed, they can contribute to poorer mental health and quality of life [8,62]. As these concerns arise and change throughout the course of survivorship, it is critical to provide the appropriate medical and supportive care. For example, cancer survivors may feel overwhelmed at the time of their cancer diagnosis, and unable to focus on fertility-related issues, even though having children might be a future goal. Later in survivorship, they may experience regret, be uncertain who to talk to about their reproductive concerns, be unsure about how to access needed RSH care, or be hesitant to seek medical care for fear of learning they are infertile [13,63].

Cancer's impact on sexual health

At least half of female survivors experience sexual health problems after cancer [1,64,65]. Sexual and intimacy concerns extend beyond the capacity to have sexual intercourse, and encompass both physical and psychological aspects, including physical discomfort, low desire, poor body image, loss of sexual self, and feelings of guilt and worries about partners' satisfaction [1,16,64–68]. Physical sexual concerns include those such as vaginal dryness and pain and psychological sexual concerns include worries about body changes and decreased sexual interest. These concerns can also lead to avoidance of sexual activity and new challenges for relationships. Breast cancer

TABLE 7.1 Common sexual health problems for women after cancer [64–66,77–83].

Type of sexual health problem	Percent of women with a cancer history who report this
Sexual dysfunction	31%–94%
Reduced sexual interest/desire	30%–85%
Difficulties with lubrication/arousal	5%–69%
Difficulties with orgasm	16%–43%
Experiencing pain with sex	8%–57%
Distress about sex	10%–43%
Being anxious about sex	3%–31%
Not finding sex pleasurable/enjoyable	12%–33%
Body image concerns	45%–55%

survivors commonly experience changes to their hormones and breasts that can negatively affect sexual activity and arousal [64,65]. Despite the fact that sexual health concerns are common, and that clinical guidelines are in place to encourage healthcare providers to discuss and manage these concerns with their patients [69–71], most women do not receive adequate information about sexual side effects or information about how to handle them [72–76]. Some common sexual problems are outlined in Table 7.1. Estimates of the prevalence of problems vary widely, in part due to variations in the samples, measurement tools used, and timing of assessments in relation to cancer treatment.

In younger men, testicular cancer is the most common cancer diagnosis, and also one of the most curable with guideline-concordant care [84]. Men treated for testicular cancer most commonly experience ejaculatory dysfunction [85], but may also experience decreased sexual enjoyment, decreased sexual desire, and erectile dysfunction that may last for some time after the completion of treatment. A recent study of 111 young men surveyed 2 years after treatment for testicular cancer showed 26% had persistent sexual dysfunction, primarily associated with dissatisfaction with sex life or lack of interest in sex, and not erectile dysfunction [17]. Partner status may relate to sexual function after testicular cancer, such that survivors without partners experience more erectile dysfunction and less sexual satisfaction [86]. Psychological sequelae of treatment, including anxiety, altered body image, and diminished sense of masculinity, have also been associated with sexual dysfunction after testicular cancer [86–89].

Prostate cancer is the most common cancer in older men, affecting genitourinary function. In older men, some of the most common sexual dysfunctions in cancer patients are erectile dysfunction and low libido or testosterone deficiency. These are likely due to a combination of physical and psychological factors. Erectile dysfunction is the most common complaint in older male cancer survivors. The treatments for prostate cancer often result in some degree of erectile dysfunction, although rates vary 25%–90% depending on treatment type [90]. Decreased libido can be the result of body image changes, treatment symptoms like fatigue, or cancer therapies that deplete testosterone [91]. Like younger men, the sexual side effects of cancer treatment in older men can cause decreased sense of masculinity, and increase symptoms of depression, anxiety, and relationship distress [92].

Managing reproductive and sexual health concerns after cancer

Despite the established importance of RSH in cancer survivorship and the related psychological concerns, medical and supportive RSH care often remain inadequate [7,19,59,93–97]. This may be particularly true for populations with poorer access to care and those living further from comprehensive cancer centers, where specialized services may be more readily available [98]. There is no "one-size-fits-all" strategy to address the range of RSH concerns that cancer survivors experience. Rather, a tailored approach to RSH care that takes into account the way their preferences and priorities change over time is important. Cancer survivors, and their partners, may need assistance in making decisions and obtaining referrals according to their current situation and goals [35]. For example, at the time of diagnosis, a discussion of the impact of cancer treatment on fertility and a consultation with a fertility specialist may be indicated [99,100]. However, ongoing conversations and family building plans are critical after treatment ends as well, regardless of earlier fertility preservation decisions. Additionally, many survivors (regardless of age) continue to need care and support for sexual health problems, which can also fluctuate over time. RSH care that addresses the physical and psychological concerns that survivors experience across the cancer continuum is needed [18–22].

Improving patient-provider communication about reproductive and sexual health

Effective communication about concerns and shared decision making about action steps are central to providing comprehensive RSH services and patient-centered care [101]. Although healthcare providers are responsible for raising the topic of RSH concerns after cancer and educating survivors about options for management, patients often find conversations with their providers unsatisfactory [24,76,102,103]. Survivors often feel that the RSH information offered by their healthcare providers is inadequate and desire repeated opportunities to discuss their concerns rather than a "one-time" conversation [19,103,104].

There are several known barriers to RSH communication in cancer settings, including insufficient time during appointments, healthcare providers lacking knowledge and training in how to respond to RSH concerns, misalignment between the provider's communication strategies and the patient's preferences, and providers making assumptions about their patients' sexual behavior, fertility, and family building plans [21,105–107]. Healthcare providers may also be less likely to discuss RSH concerns with younger and nonpartnered patients [8,108,109]. Embarrassment and stigma associated with sexuality pose additional challenges [110]. Cancer survivors may also be uncertain about what type of healthcare provider or service they need to address their RSH concerns, especially later in survivorship [110].

The way that cancer survivors perceive their relationships with their healthcare providers can influence their comfort and willingness to talk about their RSH concerns. Therefore one important strategy that healthcare providers can use to facilitate effective RSH conversations is to focus on building trust and rapport. This can contribute to creating a safe, comfortable space for open discussion of sensitive RSH topics [111,112]. There are many strategies that healthcare providers can use to improve RSH communication, including the following [35,72,110,112,113]:

1. Normalizing RSH topics by reminding patients that these are common challenges for many cancer survivors;
2. Encouraging patients to prepare for RSH conversations during their appointments by offering curated informational resources prior to the visit;
3. Initiating RSH conversations, rather than relying on patients to ask questions, and routinely asking about RSH concerns, such as with a standard questionnaire at each visit (see Fig. 7.1);

PROMIS Sexual Function Measure – 1 Item Screening Tool (187)
In the past 12 months, has there ever been a period of 3 months or more when you had any of the following problems or concerns? (check all that apply)
☐ You wanted to feel more interest in sexual activity
☐ Male: You had difficulty with erections (penis getting or staying hard)
☐ Female: Your vagina felt too dry
☐ You had pain during or after sexual activity
☐ You had difficulty having an orgasm
☐ You felt anxious about sexual activity
☐ You did not enjoy sexual activity
☐ Some other sexual problem or concern
☐ No sexual problems or concerns

Reproductive Concerns After Cancer: Fertility Potential Subscale (39, 188)
Thinking about how you feel right now about having (more) biological children someday, please say whether you strongly disagree, disagree, neither agree nor disagree, agree, or strongly agree with each statement. If you feel that a statement does not apply to you, please select "Neither Agree nor Disagree".
1. I am afraid I won't be able to have any (more) children.
2. I am worried about my ability to get pregnant [Female]/ biologically father [Male] a child (again).
3. I am concerned that I may not be able to have (more) children.

Follow-Up Questions
Would you like more information or resources about sexual/fertility issues?
Would you like to speak with someone about sexual/fertility issues?

FIGURE 7.1 Screening tools [39,114,115].

4. Conveying genuine caring and investment about the patient's life beyond cancer, and using active listening skills to create a warm, welcoming environment where sensitive topics can be discussed;
5. Facilitating access to RSH services after cancer, including for physical and mental health concerns, by integrating systems of referrals and offering dedicated appointments for RSH care specifically;
6. Increasing communication and coordination between providers on the care team (e.g., oncology and fertility specialists) to reduce the burden on patients;
7. Avoiding assumptions about a person's family building plans or sexual health based on age, relationship status, or other characteristics; and
8. Engaging partners and/or family members in RSH conversations and care decisions can be important aspect of care, if desired by the patient.

Guidance, online resources, and professional skills development are available to help healthcare providers better communicate with their patients about RSH concerns. The Enriching Communication Skills for Health Professionals in Oncofertility (ECHO) training program (echo.rhoinstitute.org/) is one such resource. The Oncofertility Consortium (oncofertility.northwestern.edu/), an international and interdisciplinary network of clinicians, scientists, and scholars, is another key resource for providers and survivors who are navigating fertility and family planning decisions after cancer. The Oncofertility Consortium has compiled helpful pocket guides and decision tools to facilitate conversations about fertility preservation options (http://www.savemyfertility.org/).

There are some frameworks available to help healthcare providers facilitate conversations about RSH concerns after cancer, including the Five A's framework and the Permission, Limited Information, Specific Suggestion, Intensive Therapy (PLISSIT) model [21,69,116].

Following the *Five A's* framework to discuss sexual health includes these steps:

1. *Ask*: Introduce the topic of sexual health and ask permission to discuss it
2. *Advise*: Provide brief information about the sexual health topic
3. *Assess*: Ask questions to help understand the individual's needs
4. *Assist*: Offer brief counseling and provide appropriate resources and referrals
5. *Arrange*: Schedule a follow-up appointment

Following the *PLISSIT* model involves:

1. Giving the individual *permission* to discuss and/or seek assistance for their sexual health concerns;
2. Offering *limited information* that is targeted to their concerns;
3. Offering *specific suggestions* to address those concerns; and
4. Referrals to other health professionals for *intensive therapy* to more fully address emotional and/or physical concerns (e.g., sex therapy).

Clinical guidelines for fertility consultation and preservation

According to guidelines set by the American Society of Clinical Oncology (ASCO), all reproductive aged patients should be advised about the potential impact of their cancer treatment on their fertility as early as possible before cancer treatment starts [117]. Those who are interested in fertility preservation, or who are ambivalent, should be referred by their oncology team to a fertility specialist for a fertility consultation. Another discussion may be needed after completion of treatment and/or if pregnancy is being considered. See Fig. 7.2 for a summary of options for fertility preservation. ASCO guidelines and more information can be found at: https://www.asco.org/research-guidelines/quality-guidelines/guidelines.

Management of infertility risk

During a consultation with a fertility specialist (reproductive endocrinologist), patients receive information about how their cancer treatment could affect their fertility and about fertility preservation options and resources if appropriate (i.e., patient is healthy enough), including costs, timing, potential delays in cancer treatment, and cultural and ethical considerations [118]. Examples of common fertility preservation modalities for female survivors include embryo and oocyte cryopreservation for women and cryopreservation of sperm for males (see Fig. 7.2). Discussions about infertility risk are an important aspect of high-quality cancer care for reproductive-

FEMALE
Embryo cryopreservation
Mature oocyte cryopreservation
Ovarian tissue cryopreservation
Ovarian transposition
Gonadal suppression (GnRH Analogs)[a]
Conservative surgical approaches
MALE
Sperm cryopreservation
Testicular tissue cryopreservation in prepubertal boys[b]

[a] Not an established modality
[b] Experimental only

FIGURE 7.2 Fertility preservation options [117].

aged patients [119] and the possibility of preserving fertility is an important aspect of coping with the burden of cancer for some survivors, providing a sense of hope and mitigating their infertility-related distress [49,50,59,120]. Having a fertility consultation has been associated with less decisional conflict, less regret, more satisfaction with life, and better quality of life among reproductive-aged survivors [37,121,122]. While consultation ideally occurs before cancer treatment, cancer survivors can also consult with a fertility specialist after their treatment is over. After completing treatment, consultations may include discussion of alternative family building options, such as adoption, as well as ovarian reserve monitoring and earlier or more aggressive fertility treatments to help women achieve their goals within a potentially shorter window of opportunity for having biological children [94].

There are a number of barriers to fertility consultation and fertility preservation utilization, including treatment-related time constraints, high cost, lack of access to specialist care, and patient characteristics (e.g., socioeconomic status, partner status). Healthcare providers may also lack training or have insufficient knowledge to adequately discuss fertility issues with their patients [42,43,123–128]. Oncology teams initiate discussions of fertility about half of the time [119], but there are inconsistent reports about how often patients receive information about the potential impact of cancer treatment on their fertility and how often they utilize fertility preservation options [129]. It is clear that survivors continue to experience unmet information needs, decision regret, and decision conflict about fertility preservation [24,121,122] and that suboptimal delivery of fertility care after cancer persists [130]. Furthermore, fertility consultation and the option to preserve fertility are commonly only provided at the time of cancer diagnosis and/or treatment, and do not adequately address the range of reproductive concerns that survivors experience later in survivorship [56,94,131].

When determining how best to support reproductive-aged cancer survivors during and after their cancer treatment, it is important to consider the emotional and practical barriers that survivors may face to accessing fertility-related care [42]. Making decisions about future family building plans and fertility preservation can be extremely challenging for those who are also confronted with cancer and cancer treatment [121]. The financial cost of these services poses a substantial barrier to access as well [42,43]. It is also important to note that although fertility consultation and preservation make important contributions to managing infertility risk, they represent only one aspect of comprehensive RSH care after cancer. For example, addressing survivors' and partners' fertility-related distress falls outside the scope of these services, and many survivors would also benefit from mental health and financial counseling. In many cases, fertility preservation is not possible or not accessible, which can also be distressing. Even when survivors do have access to fertility preservation options, uncertainty about whether they will achieve their future family building goals can be daunting. Routine, patient-centered assessment of family building goals and removing barriers to access for fertility consultation, fertility preservation, and supportive care services are important strategies for improving management of infertility risk after cancer.

Clinical guidelines for sexual health after cancer

Similar to guidelines for fertility consultation and preservation, ASCO recommends that a member of the healthcare team initiates a discussion regarding sexual health and dysfunction resulting from cancer or its treatment [132]. Psychosocial and/or psychosexual counseling should be offered to all individuals diagnosed with cancer. Counseling aims to improve sexual response, body image, intimacy and relationship issues, and overall sexual functioning and satisfaction. Medical and treatable contributing factors should be identified and addressed first. ASCO guidelines and more information can be found at: https://www.asco.org/research-guidelines/quality-guidelines/guidelines.

Management of women's sexual health problems

Initial conservative management of vaginal dryness and pain begins with lubricants (for timely needs related to sexual activity and vaginal penetration) and moisturizers (used regularly for maintenance of vaginal moisture). Management of vulvovaginal pain involves treatment of urogenital atrophy that results in thin vaginal tissue, decreased lubrication, and chronic vulvar irritation from estrogen deprivation [133–135]. Low-dose vaginal estrogen, oral estrogen, prasterone, and ospemifene could be considered depending on the patient's cancer and other medical history [133,136,137]. While vaginal estrogens may be effective for dryness, pain, and vaginal inelasticity, they are considered controversial for some cancer survivors with estrogen-sensitive tumors due to concern for systemic absorption [133,135]. Alternatively, women could be referred to a gynecologist for a detailed discussion of medication options.

Sexual desire, or libido, is a complex biopsychosocial phenomenon. Problems such as pain, anxiety, lack of enjoyment, or relationship problems might precipitate lack of desire and should be addressed first [138]. For patients with depression, anxiety, relationship or body image issues, a referral for psychotherapy should be considered [137]. For continued lack of desire, referral to a qualified sex therapist is recommended, as cognitive-behavioral therapy is efficacious for hypoactive sexual desire [139].

Nerve damage caused by chemotherapy or pelvic tumors may cause female orgasmic dysfunction [140]. Treatment for difficulties with orgasm focuses on managing underlying problems when possible, educating patients and partners about female anatomy and clitoral stimulation, and self-stimulation and/or vibrator therapy [137]. Strategies that help facilitate arousal response by drawing blood flow and promoting circulation in the pelvic area (e.g., pelvic floor exercises, vacuum devices) may also be helpful [135,141]. For women with decreased vaginal elasticity from cancer treatments, vaginal dilators used with lubricants and moisturizers are recommended to reduce pain with vaginal penetration [133,135]. Pelvic floor physical therapists can address dyspareunia (vaginal pain with penetration), as well as provide instruction on dilator use and pelvic floor muscle control [135]. Both women and men experiencing vasomotor symptoms such as hot flushes or night sweats should be offered interventions for symptomatic improvement, including behavioral options such as cognitive-behavioral therapy, slow breathing and hypnosis, and medications such as venlafaxine and gabapentin [132].

Management of men's sexual health problems

Treatment options for erectile dysfunction in men vary, and can include oral medications, injections, vacuum devices, and penile prosthesis [132,138]. Studies have shown improvement in erectile function recovery with the use of phosphodiesterase type 5 inhibitors (PDE5i) in the first year of recovery [142]. In the case of low testosterone, testosterone can be replaced with medication (oral, transdermal, subcutaneous, intramuscular, and nasal). Because of the psychological components of sexual function and satisfaction, including a psychosocial expert in the treatment plan is recommended when addressing sexual function changes in men with cancer.

Improving partner communication about reproductive and sexual health concerns

Although research on illness and symptom management largely focuses on individual health outcomes [143], many cancer survivors navigate life after cancer with a partner and can benefit from help communicating with them about their RSH concerns [13,15].

Couple communication is emerging as an important predictor of relationship health and sexual functioning after cancer [15,68,144,145]. There is scant research on couple communication about infertility after cancer, but in the general population couples who cope together and communicate effectively have more positive relationship and mental health outcomes [146,147]. Open communication after cancer is associated with lower distress, higher marital satisfaction, effective coping, and relationship closeness [148–151]. More broadly, partners who are able to engage in open communication and active collaboration while navigating through illness have more positive physical and mental health outcomes [152–154]. Strong relationships are also protective for family functioning, which can improve health and quality of life for both partners. However, couples experiencing stressful experiences, such as cancer, are more likely to exhibit ineffective communication skills [68,155,156]. Partner communication may be particularly important for navigating sexual difficulties and infertility, which can have a significant negative impact on relationships [68,144–146].

In a recent qualitative study of reproductive-aged breast cancer survivors and their partners, open communication was endorsed as the most important aspect of maintaining a healthy relationship and sex life after cancer [15]. More challenges arose when partners "held back" in an effort to prevent distress (protective buffering) instead of talking openly [148,156,157]. Those who disengaged reported feeling pulled apart and isolated from their partners. In contrast, those who worked through their problems as a team were able to find a "new intimacy" and renegotiate their sexual relationship together. Other helpful strategies include use of humor and avoidance of unwanted advice or solutions [149,158]. Importantly, self-care for both partners can also be an important contributor to couples' capacity to overcoming RSH challenges as a team. Support and education for couples navigating the RSH challenges of cancer are lacking and needed [68,144].

Special considerations

Assumptions about sexual health

Healthcare providers sometimes make assumptions about the sexual health of their patients. They may assume that only those with sexual organ cancer are at risk for sexual dysfunction. Though much of the research has focused on breast, gynecological and prostate cancer, survivors of any kind of cancer can have sexual problems [89,145]. Second, some may assume that heteronormative, vaginal penetrative "sexual intercourse" is the survivor's "normal sex" or goal of sexual health. As mentioned before, there are many ways to be sexually active, including alone, and some older adults may be satisfied with intimate activity and companionship that excludes coitus. Healthcare providers should not assume that singles are not having sex, or that healthy sexual activity is limited to partnered sexual intercourse. Sexual activity may include a range of activities, including masturbation (alone or partnered), oral sex, sexual intercourse, kissing, hugging, and touching. Many couples who have significant impacts on their ability to perform coitus find alternate ways to be intimate. Many couples renegotiate sex and intimacy after the effects of cancer treatment affect their sexual functioning and desire [159]. It is also important to avoid making assumptions about survivors' sexual orientation or gender identity. It is common for LGBTQ+ individuals to not disclose their sexual orientation and gender identity to their healthcare provider, and to avoid discussing sexual health [160]. And finally, healthcare providers should not assume that because the patient has cancer or because they are over 65 they are not having sex (or interested in having sex), even while on treatment. Studies of individuals with advanced cancer, on clinical trials, or receiving palliative care indicate survivors value sexual activity and intimacy with their partner [161,162].

LGBTQ+ cancer survivors

Existing research suggests a pattern of disparities in mental and physical health outcomes for LGBTQ+ survivors. When compared to heterosexual women, research suggests that sexual minority women are affected by breast cancer at younger ages and may respond differentially to treatment [163], experience more symptoms of psychological distress, experience lower satisfaction and patient-centered cancer care [164–166], and experience discrimination, gaps in care, and insufficient social support [167]. LGBTQ+ survivors appear to have significant unmet psychological and sexual health needs [168]. A recent qualitative study highlighted the need for recognition and support for partners of LGBTQ+ survivors, and found that the most commonly reported long-term impact of breast cancer was the devastating impact on their relationships and sexual intimacy [169].

Sexual wellbeing in LGBTQ+ individuals is complex and evidence in the literature is sometimes conflicting, for a number of possible reasons, including: changes in culture and acceptance over the decades [170]; variability among sexual orientation and gender identity groups [171]; a focus on HIV and substance abuse research; and how sexual activity is defined in studies [172]. Assessments of sexual function are not often validated in LGBTQ+ populations; asking "how often do you have sex" may have heteronormative connotations not inclusive of other ways of having sex [173]. Studies show the complexity of human sexuality and relationships, often conflating the effects of gender, gender of the partner [174], and sexual orientation. When examining how relationship factors influence sexual satisfaction and wellbeing, results are often similar to heterosexual couples [175]. In both groups, sexual function, sexual frequency, sexual communication, relationship satisfaction, and psychological health are all positively linked to sexual satisfaction [176].

In a healthy (noncancer) sample of men and women, the authors of one study compared sexual symptoms reported by heterosexual and LGB individuals, including oral and anal symptoms not typically assessed in sexual health studies [171]. Among United States men (heterosexual, gay, and bisexual) who reported any sexual activity in the past 30 days, there were no differences in erectile function or orgasm ability. However, sexual minority men reported worse symptoms such as oral dryness, anal discomfort, and lower orgasm pleasure and satisfaction. Among sexually active women (heterosexual, lesbian, and bisexual), there were no differences in vulvar/clitoral discomfort, orgasm pleasure, or satisfaction; however, sexual minority women reported worse oral dryness. Lesbian women reported lower vaginal discomfort than other women, and higher lubrication and orgasm ability than heterosexual women. Bisexual women reported higher interest, higher vulvar/labial discomfort and higher anal discomfort than other women. As illustrated in this study, sexual minority men and women may have diminished aspects of sexual function that have not traditionally been included in multidimensional self-report measures, such as oral and anal symptoms. Oncology clinicians should be aware of their patients' sexual concerns and recognize that LGBTQ+ patients may be more vulnerable to certain sexual difficulties than heterosexual patients. Regardless, sexual and gender minorities should have access to culturally sensitive and competent support services; see (http://www.lgbtcancer.org).

Black, indigenous, and people of color (BIPOC) cancer survivors

For BIPOC cancer survivors, changes in sexual health, experiences with sexual communication, and discussions of sexual health with healthcare providers are often shaped by their minority experiences. Women of color may experience poorer sexual function than non-Hispanic white women, citing more hot flashes, vaginal dryness, sexual dysfunction, and negative fertility outcomes [177–179]. Current research and clinical practice recommendations surrounding cancer survivorship [180], and sexual wellbeing specifically [132], are based on studies that overrepresent partnered, well-educated, non-Hispanic white women. Despite experiencing negative sexual health sequelae of treatment, women of minority groups are less likely to seek care for fertility concerns, have less successful outcomes of fertility treatment [4,177,181] and are less likely to seek help for sexual or relationship problems [182]. It is imperative that sexual wellbeing is addressed equitably and comprehensively for all cancer survivors, as an integral part of cancer survivorship care [132,183].

Older adult cancer survivors

Despite being the majority of cancer survivors, older adults (≥65 years) and their cancer survivorship needs are greatly understudied. In geriatric oncology survivors, sexual functioning after cancer treatment can be the most compromised health-related quality of life issue [184]. Despite this, much of what we know about sexual health in older adults comes from nononcology research. In a national study of sexuality and health in 3000 older men and women, the authors found that the prevalence of sexual activity declined with age [185]. However, 73% of the "young old" (57–64 years) and 53% of the old (65–74 years) were sexually active with a partner. Of those who report having sex, approximately half have at least one bothersome sexual problem. Older women commonly experience low desire, lack of lubrication, and inability to climax while men most often reported erectile difficulties. Aging can impact sexual wellbeing with loss of desire or function, cognitive impairment, comorbidities, and simultaneous use of multiple medications, which can affect physical function and mood [138]. Older adults are also more likely to experience loss of a spouse or partner, or diminished sexual activity due to their partner's health or sexual problems. Oncology healthcare professionals should routinely ask older adult survivors about sexual concerns, and not make assumptions about the desire for a healthy sex life based on age or partner status.

Key points and recommendations

- Cancer and cancer treatment can have a devastating impact on many aspects of life, including RSH.
- Based on professional society guidelines, healthcare providers have an obligation to discuss the impact of cancer and cancer treatment on fertility and sexual health. While these conversations most commonly occur at the time of cancer diagnosis, survivors and their partners can experience a variety of RSH concerns that evolve and persist throughout the course of survivorship.

- RSH care and support needs to be tailored to address these evolving concerns. There is no "one-size-fits-all" approach. Rather, a patient-centered approach with a long-term goal of achieving equity in access to RSH information and care across the cancer continuum (i.e., from the time of diagnosis onward) holds promise for improving outcomes.
- There are a number of tools and educational resources to help healthcare providers have more effective conversations with their patients about RSH concerns. Creating opportunities for ongoing discussions about both physical and psychological RSH concerns can improve capacity to recognize and addressing these concerns as they arise, ultimately reducing distress and improving quality of life.
- For partnered cancer survivors, supporting couples toward effective, open communication about their RSH concerns after cancer can improve relationship health and lead to more positive health outcomes.
- It is important for healthcare providers to avoid making assumptions based on age, partner status, sexual orientation, or other characteristics, when considering an individual's sexual health, fertility, or plans for future family building. Discussions and materials that are compatible with patients' beliefs, culture, gender identity, and sexual orientation, are paramount to ensuring equitable, patient-centered RSH care for all survivors.

References

[1] Wettergren L, Kent EE, Mitchell SA, Zebrack B, Lynch CF, Rubenstein MB, et al. Cancer negatively impacts on sexual function in adolescents and young adults: the AYA HOPE study. Psychooncology 2017;26(10):1632–9.

[2] Carter J, Chi DS, Brown CL, Abu-Rustum NR, Sonoda Y, Aghajanian C, et al. Cancer-related infertility in survivorship. Int J Gynecol Cancer 2010;20(1):2–8.

[3] Walshe JM, Denduluri N, Swain SM. Amenorrhea in premenopausal women after adjuvant chemotherapy for breast cancer. J Clin Oncol 2006;24(36):5769–79.

[4] Schover LR, van der Kaaij M, van Dorst E, Creutzberg C, Huyghe E, Kiserud CE. Sexual dysfunction and infertility as late effects of cancer treatment. EJC Suppl 2014;12(1):41–53.

[5] Levin AO, Carpenter KM, Fowler JM, Brothers BM, Andersen BL, Maxwell GL. Sexual morbidity associated with poorer psychological adjustment among gynecological cancer survivors. Int J Gynecol Cancer 2010;20(3):461–70.

[6] Vaz AF, Pinto-Neto AM, Conde DM, Costa-Paiva L, Morais SS, Pedro AO, et al. Quality of life and menopausal and sexual symptoms in gynecologic cancer survivors: a cohort study. Menopause 2011;18(6):662–9.

[7] Canada AL, Schover LR. The psychosocial impact of interrupted childbearing in long-term female cancer survivors. Psychooncology 2012;21(2):134–43.

[8] Patterson P, Perz J, Tindle R, McDonald FEJ, Ussher JM. Infertility after cancer: how the need to be a parent, fertility-related social concern, and acceptance of illness influence quality of life. Cancer Nurs 2021;44(4):E244–51.

[9] Robertson EG, Sansom-Daly UM, Wakefield CE, Ellis SJ, McGill BC, Doolan EL, et al. Sexual and romantic relationships: experiences of adolescent and young adult cancer survivors. J Adolesc Young Adult Oncol 2016;5(3):286–91.

[10] Ljungman L, Ahlgren J, Petersson LM, Flynn KE, Weinfurt K, Gorman JR, et al. Sexual dysfunction and reproductive concerns in young women with breast cancer: type, prevalence, and predictors of problems. Psychooncology 2018;27(12):2770–7.

[11] Arndt V, Merx H, Sturmer T, Stegmaier C, Ziegler H, Brenner H. Age-specific detriments to quality of life among breast cancer patients one year after diagnosis. Eur J Cancer 2004;40(5):673–80.

[12] Bidstrup PE, Christensen J, Mertz BG, Rottmann N, Dalton SO, Johansen C. Trajectories of distress, anxiety, and depression among women with breast cancer: looking beyond the mean. Acta Oncol 2015;54(5):789–96.

[13] Gorman JR, Bailey S, Pierce JP, Su HI. How do you feel about fertility and parenthood? The voices of young female cancer survivors. J Cancer Surviv 2012;6(2):200–9.

[14] Gorman JR, Usita PM, Madlensky L, Pierce JP. Young breast cancer survivors: their perspectives on treatment decisions and fertility concerns. Cancer Nurs 2011;34(1):32–40.

[15] Gorman JR, Smith E, Drizin JH, Lyons KS, Harvey SM. Navigating sexual health in cancer survivorship: a dyadic perspective. Support Care Cancer 2020;28(11):5429–39.

[16] Karabulut N, Erci B. Sexual desire and satisfaction in sexual life affecting factors in breast cancer survivors after mastectomy. J Psychosoc Oncol 2009;27(3):332–43.

[17] Ljungman L, Eriksson LE, Flynn KE, Gorman JR, Stahl O, Weinfurt K, et al. Sexual dysfunction and reproductive concerns in young men diagnosed with testicular cancer: an observational study. J Sex Med 2019;16(7):1049–59.

[18] Rubinsak LA, Christianson MS, Akers A, Carter J, Kaunitz AM, Temkin SM. Reproductive health care across the life course of the female cancer patient. Support Care Cancer 2019;27(1):23–32.

[19] Murphy D, Klosky JL, Termuhlen A, Sawczyn KK, Quinn GP. The need for reproductive and sexual health discussions with adolescent and young adult cancer patients. Contraception 2013;88(2):215–20.

[20] Huffman LB, Hartenbach EM, Carter J, Rash JK, Kushner DM. Maintaining sexual health throughout gynecologic cancer survivorship: a comprehensive review and clinical guide. Gynecol Oncol 2016;140(2):359–68.

[21] Park ER, Norris RL, Bober SL. Sexual health communication during cancer care: barriers and recommendations. Cancer J 2009;15(1):74–7.

[22] Benedict C, Hahn AL, McCready A, Kelvin JF, Diefenbach M, Ford JS. Toward a theoretical understanding of young female cancer survivors' decision-making about family-building post-treatment. Support Care Cancer 2020;28(10):4857–67.

[23] Stanton AM, Handy AB, Meston CM. Sexual function in adolescents and young adults diagnosed with cancer: a systematic review. J Cancer Surviv 2018;12(1):47–63.

[24] Logan S, Perz J, Ussher JM, Peate M, Anazodo A. A systematic review of patient oncofertility support needs in reproductive cancer patients aged 14 to 45 years of age. Psychooncology 2018;27(2):401–9.

[25] van der Kaaij MA, Heutte N, Meijnders P, Abeilard-Lemoisson E, Spina M, Moser EC, et al. Premature ovarian failure and fertility in long-term survivors of Hodgkin's lymphoma: a European Organisation for Research and Treatment of Cancer Lymphoma Group and Groupe d'Etude des Lymphomes de l'Adulte cohort study. J Clin Oncol 2012;30(3):291–9.

[26] Su HI, Kwan B, Whitcomb BW, Shliakhsitsava K, Dietz AC, Stark SS, et al. Modeling variation in the reproductive lifespan of female adolescent and young adult cancer survivors using AMH. J Clin Endocrinol Metab 2020;105(8):2740–51.

[27] Trivers KF, Fink AK, Partridge AH, Oktay K, Ginsburg ES, Li C, et al. Estimates of young breast cancer survivors at risk for infertility in the United States. Oncologist. 2014;19(8):814–22.

[28] Irene Su H, Lee YT, Barr R. Oncofertility: meeting the fertility goals of adolescents and young adults with cancer. Cancer J 2018;24(6):328–35.

[29] Fossa SD, Dahl AA. Fertility and sexuality in young cancer survivors who have adult-onset malignancies. Hematol Oncol Clin N Am 2008;22(2):291–303.

[30] van Casteren NJ, Boellaard WP, Romijn JC, Dohle GR. Gonadal dysfunction in male cancer patients before cytotoxic treatment. Int J Androl 2010;33(1):73–9.

[31] Dohle GR. Male infertility in cancer patients: review of the literature. Int J Urol 2010;17(4):327–31.

[32] Anserini P, Chiodi S, Spinelli S, Costa M, Conte N, Copello F, et al. Semen analysis following allogeneic bone marrow transplantation. Additional data evidence-based counselling. Bone Marrow Transplant 2002;30(7):447–51.

[33] Trottmann M, Becker AJ, Stadler T, Straub J, Soljanik I, Schlenker B, et al. Semen quality in men with malignant diseases before and after therapy and the role of cryopreservation. Eur Urol 2007;52(2):355–67.

[34] Huyghe E, Matsuda T, Daudin M, Chevreau C, Bachaud JM, Plante P, et al. Fertility after testicular cancer treatments: results of a large multicenter study. Cancer 2004;100(4):732–7.

[35] Crawshaw M. Psychosocial oncofertility issues faced by adolescents and young adults over their lifetime: a review of the research. Hum Fertil (Camb) 2013;16(1):59–63.

[36] Ussher JM, Perz J. Infertility-related distress following cancer for women and men: a mixed method study. Psychooncology 2019;28 (3):607–14.

[37] Letourneau JM, Ebbel EE, Katz PP, Katz A, Ai WZ, Chien AJ, et al. Pretreatment fertility counseling and fertility preservation improve quality of life in reproductive age women with cancer. Cancer 2012;118(6):1710–17.

[38] Carpentier MY, Fortenberry JD, Ott MA, Brames MJ, Einhorn LH. Perceptions of masculinity and self-image in adolescent and young adult testicular cancer survivors: implications for romantic and sexual relationships. Psychooncology 2011;20(7):738–45.

[39] Gorman JR, Drizin JH, Malcarne VL, Hsieh TC. Measuring the multidimensional reproductive concerns of young adult male cancer survivors. J Adolesc Young Adult Oncol 2020;9(6):613–20.

[40] Ketterl TG, Syrjala KL, Casillas J, Jacobs LA, Palmer SC, McCabe MS, et al. Lasting effects of cancer and its treatment on employment and finances in adolescent and young adult cancer survivors. Cancer. 2019;125(11):1908–17.

[41] Zheng Z, Jemal A, Han X, Guy Jr. GP, Li C, Davidoff AJ, et al. Medical financial hardship among cancer survivors in the United States. Cancer 2019;125(10):1737–47.

[42] Gorman JR, Drizin JH, Mersereau JE, Su HI. Applying behavioral theory to understand fertility consultation uptake after cancer. Psychooncology 2019;28(4):822–9.

[43] Benedict C, McLeggon JA, Thom B, Kelvin JF, Landwehr M, Watson S, et al. "Creating a family after battling cancer is exhausting and maddening": exploring real-world experiences of young adult cancer survivors seeking financial assistance for family building after treatment. Psychooncology. 2018;27(12):2829–39.

[44] Magelssen H, Melve KK, Skjaerven R, Fossa SD. Parenthood probability and pregnancy outcome in patients with a cancer diagnosis during adolescence and young adulthood. Hum Reprod 2008;23(1):178–86.

[45] Pivetta E, Maule MM, Pisani P, Zugna D, Haupt R, Jankovic M, et al. Marriage and parenthood among childhood cancer survivors: a report from the Italian AIEOP Off-Therapy Registry. Haematologica. 2011;96(5):744–51.

[46] Crawshaw MA, Sloper P. 'Swimming against the tide'—the influence of fertility matters on the transition to adulthood or survivorship following adolescent cancer. Eur J Cancer Care (Engl) 2010;19(5):610–20.

[47] Penrose R, Beatty L, Mattiske J, Koczwara B. Fertility and cancer—a qualitative study of Australian cancer survivors. Support Care Cancer 2012;20(6):1259–65.

[48] Dryden A, Ussher JM, Perz J. Young women's construction of their post-cancer fertility. Psychol Health 2014;29(11):1341–60.

[49] Crawshaw M. Male coping with cancer-fertility issues: putting the 'social' into biopsychosocial approaches. Reprod Biomed Online 2013;27(3):261–70.

[50] Chapple A, Salinas M, Ziebland S, McPherson A, Macfarlane A. Fertility issues: the perceptions and experiences of young men recently diagnosed and treated for cancer. J Adolesc Health 2007;40(1):69–75.

[51] Nahata L, Caltabellotta NM, Yeager ND, Lehmann V, Whiteside SL, O'Brien SH, et al. Fertility perspectives and priorities among male adolescents and young adults in cancer survivorship. Pediatr Blood Cancer 2018;65(7):e27019.

[52] Crawshaw MA, Glaser AW, Hale JP, Sloper P. Male and female experiences of having fertility matters raised alongside a cancer diagnosis during the teenage and young adult years. Eur J Cancer Care (Engl) 2009;18(4):381–90.

[53] Peddie VL, Porter MA, Barbour R, Culligan D, MacDonald G, King D, et al. Factors affecting decision making about fertility preservation after cancer diagnosis: a qualitative study. BJOG 2012;119(9):1049–57.

[54] Girasole CR, Cookson MS, Smith Jr. JA, Ivey BS, Roth BJ, Chang SS. Sperm banking: use and outcomes in patients treated for testicular cancer. BJU Int 2007;99(1):33–6.

[55] Huang IC, Bhakta N, Brinkman TM, Klosky JL, Krull KR, Srivastava D, et al. Determinants and consequences of financial hardship among adult survivors of childhood cancer: A report from the St. Jude Lifetime Cohort Study. J Natl Cancer Inst 2019;111(2):189–200.

[56] Drizin JH, Whitcomb BW, Hsieh TC, Gorman JR. Higher reproductive concerns associated with fertility consultation: a cross-sectional study of young adult male cancer survivors. Support Care Cancer 2021;29(2):741–50.
[57] Gardino S, Rodriguez S, Campo-Engelstein L. Infertility, cancer, and changing gender norms. J Cancer Surviv 2011;5(2):152–7.
[58] Greil AL, Slauson-Blevins K, McQuillan J. The experience of infertility: a review of recent literature. Sociol Health Illn 2010;32(1):140–62.
[59] Armuand GM, Wettergren L, Rodriguez-Wallberg KA, Lampic C. Women more vulnerable than men when facing risk for treatment-induced infertility: a qualitative study of young adults newly diagnosed with cancer. Acta Oncol 2015;54(2):243–52.
[60] Ying LY, Wu LH, Loke AY. Gender differences in experiences with and adjustments to infertility: a literature review. Int J Nurs Stud 2015;52(10):1640–52.
[61] Hjelmstedt A, Andersson L, Skoog-Svanberg A, Bergh T, Boivin J, Collins A. Gender differences in psychological reactions to infertility among couples seeking IVF- and ICSI-treatment. Acta Obstet Gynecol Scand 1999;78(1):42–8.
[62] Gorman JR, Su HI, Roberts SC, Dominick SA, Malcarne VL. Experiencing reproductive concerns as a female cancer survivor is associated with depression. Cancer. 2015;121(6):935–42.
[63] Kadan-Lottick NS, Robison LL, Gurney JG, Neglia JP, Yasui Y, Hayashi R, et al. Childhood cancer survivors' knowledge about their past diagnosis and treatment: childhood cancer survivor study. JAMA 2002;287(14):1832–9.
[64] Fobair P, Stewart SL, Chang SB, D'Onofrio C, Banks PJ, Bloom JR. Body image and sexual problems in young women with breast cancer. Psychooncology 2006;15(7):579–94.
[65] Jing L, Zhang C, Li W, Jin F, Wang A. Incidence and severity of sexual dysfunction among women with breast cancer: a meta-analysis based on female sexual function index. Support Care Cancer 2019;27(4):1171–80.
[66] Burwell SR, Case LD, Kaelin C, Avis NE. Sexual problems in younger women after breast cancer surgery. J Clin Oncol 2006;24(18):2815–21.
[67] Gilbert E, Ussher JM, Perz J. Sexuality after breast cancer: a review. Maturitas 2010;66(4):397–407.
[68] Loaring JM, Larkin M, Shaw R, Flowers P. Renegotiating sexual intimacy in the context of altered embodiment: the experiences of women with breast cancer and their male partners following mastectomy and reconstruction. Health Psychol 2015;34(4):426–36.
[69] Bober SL, Reese JB, Barbera L, Bradford A, Carpenter KM, Goldfarb S, et al. How to ask and what to do: a guide for clinical inquiry and intervention regarding female sexual health after cancer. Curr Opin Support Palliat Care 2016;10(1):44–54.
[70] Ligibel JA, Denlinger CS. New NCCN Guidelines® for survivorship care. J Natl Compr Cancer Netw 2013;11(5S):640–4.
[71] Runowicz CD, Leach CR, Henry NL, Henry KS, Mackey HT, Cowens-Alvarado RL, et al. American Cancer Society/American Society of Clinical Oncology Breast Cancer Survivorship Care guideline. J Clin Oncol 2016;34(6):611–35.
[72] Flynn KE, Reese JB, Jeffery DD, Abernethy AP, Lin L, Shelby RA, et al. Patient experiences with communication about sex during and after treatment for cancer. Psychooncology 2012;21(6):594–601.
[73] Cox A, Jenkins V, Catt S, Langridge C, Fallowfield L. Information needs and experiences: an audit of UK cancer patients. Eur J Oncol Nurs 2006;10(4):263–72.
[74] Hilarius D, Kloeg P, Gundy C, Aaronson N. Use of health-related quality-of-life assessments in daily clinical oncology nursing practice: a community hospital-based intervention study. Cancer 2008;113(3):628–37.
[75] Lewis PE, Sheng M, Rhodes MM, Jackson KE, Schover LR. Psychosocial concerns of young African American breast cancer survivors. J Psychosoc Oncol 2012;30(2):168–84.
[76] Reese JB, Sorice K, Beach MC, Porter LS, Tulsky JA, Daly MB, et al. Patient-provider communication about sexual concerns in cancer: a systematic review. J Cancer Surviv 2017;11(2):175–88.
[77] Aerts L, Enzlin P, Verhaeghe J, Vergote I, Amant F. Sexual and psychological functioning in women after pelvic surgery for gynaecological cancer. Eur J Gynaecol Oncol 2009;30(6):652–6.
[78] Carter J, Stabile C, Seidel B, Baser RE, Gunn AR, Chi S, et al. Baseline characteristics and concerns of female cancer patients/survivors seeking treatment at a Female Sexual Medicine Program. Support Care Cancer 2015;23(8):2255–65.
[79] Damast S, Alektiar K, Eaton A, Gerber NK, Goldfarb S, Patil S, et al. Comparative patient-centered outcomes (health state and adverse sexual symptoms) between adjuvant brachytherapy vs no adjuvant brachytherapy in early stage endometrial cancer. Ann Surg Oncol 2014;21(8):2740–54.
[80] Dizon DS, Suzin D, McIlvenna S. Sexual health as a survivorship issue for female cancer survivors. Oncologist. 2014;19(2):202–10.
[81] Jensen PT, Groenvold M, Klee MC, Thranov I, Petersen MA, Machin D. Longitudinal study of sexual function and vaginal changes after radiotherapy for cervical cancer. Int J Radiat Oncol Biol Phys 2003;56(4):937–49.
[82] Lindau ST, Gavrilova N, Anderson D. Sexual morbidity in very long term survivors of vaginal and cervical cancer: a comparison to national norms. Gynecol Oncol 2007;106(2):413–18.
[83] Oberguggenberger A, Martini C, Huber N, Fallowfield L, Hubalek M, Daniaux M, et al. Self-reported sexual health: breast cancer survivors compared to women from the general population—an observational study. BMC Cancer 2017;17(1):599.
[84] Gilligan T, Lin DW, Aggarwal R, Chism D, Cost N, Derweesh IH, et al. Testicular cancer, version 2.2020, NCCN Clinical Practice Guidelines in Oncology. J Natl Compr Cancer Netw 2019;17(12):1529–54.
[85] Jankowska M. Sexual functioning of testicular cancer survivors and their partners—a review of literature. Rep Pract Oncol Radiother 2011;17(1):54–62.
[86] Carpentier MY, Fortenberry JD. Romantic and sexual relationships, body image, and fertility in adolescent and young adult testicular cancer survivors: a review of the literature. J Adolesc Health 2010;47(2):115–25.
[87] Dahl AA, Mykletun A, Fossa SD. Quality of life in survivors of testicular cancer. Urol Oncol 2005;23(3):193–200.
[88] Rossen P, Pedersen AF, Zachariae R, von der Maase H. Sexuality and body image in long-term survivors of testicular cancer. Eur J Cancer 2012;48(4):571–8.
[89] Sadovsky R, Basson R, Krychman M, Morales AM, Schover L, Wang R, et al. Cancer and sexual problems. J Sex Med 2010;7(1 Pt 2):349–73.
[90] Jenkins L, Mulhall J. Impact of prostate cancer treatments on sexual health. In: Mydlo J, Godec C, editors. Prostate cancer. 2nd ed. Philadelphia, PA: Elsevier; 2016.

[91] Xu P, Choi E, White K, Yafi FA. Low testosterone in male cancer patients and survivors. Sex Med Rev 2021;9(1):133–42.

[92] Twitchell DK, Wittmann DA, Hotaling JM, Pastuszak AW. Psychological impacts of male sexual dysfunction in pelvic cancer survivorship. Sex Med Rev 2019;7(4):614–26.

[93] Armuand GM, Rodriguez-Wallberg KA, Wettergren L, Ahlgren J, Enblad G, Hoglund M, et al. Sex differences in fertility-related information received by young adult cancer survivors. J Clin Oncol 2012;30(17):2147–53.

[94] Kim J, Mersereau JE, Su HI, Whitcomb BW, Malcarne VL, Gorman JR. Young female cancer survivors' use of fertility care after completing cancer treatment. Support Care Cancer 2016;24(7):3191–9.

[95] Murphy D, Orgel E, Termuhlen A, Shannon S, Warren K, Quinn GP. Why healthcare providers should focus on the fertility of AYA cancer survivors: it's not too late!. Front Oncol 2013;3:248.

[96] Ruddy KJ, Gelber SI, Tamimi RM, Ginsburg ES, Schapira L, Come SE, et al. Prospective study of fertility concerns and preservation strategies in young women with breast cancer. J Clin Oncol 2014;32(11):1151–6.

[97] Logan S, Perz J, Ussher JM, Peate M, Anazodo A. Systematic review of fertility-related psychological distress in cancer patients: informing on an improved model of care. Psychooncology 2019;28(1):22–30.

[98] Tesauro GM, Rowland JH, Lustig C. Survivorship resources for post-treatment cancer survivors. Cancer Pract 2002;10(6):277.

[99] Coccia PF, Pappo AS, Altman J, Bhatia S, Borinstein SC, Flynn J, et al. Adolescent and young adult oncology, version 2.2014. J Natl Compr Cancer Netw 2014;12(1):21–32.

[100] Metzger ML, Meacham LR, Patterson B, Casillas JS, Constine LS, Hijiya N, et al. Female reproductive health after childhood, adolescent, and young adult cancers: guidelines for the assessment and management of female reproductive complications. J Clin Oncol 2013;31(9):1239–47.

[101] Levit L, Balogh E, Nass S, Ganz PA, editors. Delivering high-quality cancer care: charting a new course for a system in crisis. Washington, D.C.: The National Academies Press; 2013.

[102] Barlevy D, Wangmo T, Elger BS, Ravitsky V. Attitudes, beliefs, and trends regarding adolescent oncofertility discussions: a systematic literature review. J Adolesc Young Adult Oncol 2016;5(2):119–34.

[103] Scanlon M, Blaes A, Geller M, Majhail NS, Lindgren B, Haddad T. Patient satisfaction with physician discussions of treatment impact on fertility, menopause and sexual health among pre-menopausal women with cancer. J Cancer 2012;3:217–25.

[104] Mazor KM, Beard RL, Alexander GL, Arora NK, Firneno C, Gaglio B, et al. Patients' and family members' views on patient-centered communication during cancer care. Psychooncology 2013;22(11):2487–95.

[105] Quinn GP, Vadaparampil ST. Fertility preservation and adolescent/young adult cancer patients: physician communication challenges. J Adolesc Health 2009;44(4):394–400.

[106] Park ER, Bober SL, Campbell EG, Recklitis CJ, Kutner JS, Diller L. General internist communication about sexual function with cancer survivors. J Gen Intern Med 2009;24(Suppl 2):S407–11.

[107] Bober SL, Recklitis CJ, Campbell EG, Park ER, Kutner JS, Najita JS, et al. Caring for cancer survivors: a survey of primary care physicians. Cancer. 2009;115(18 Suppl):4409–18.

[108] Bibby H, White V, Thompson K, Anazodo A. What are the unmet needs and care experiences of adolescents and young adults with cancer? A systematic review. J Adolesc Young Adult Oncol 2017;6(1):6–30.

[109] Ussher JM, Cummings J, Dryden A, Perz J. Talking about fertility in the context of cancer: health care professional perspectives. Eur J Cancer Care (Engl) 2016;25(1):99–111.

[110] Gorman JR, Drizin JH, Smith E, Flores-Sanchez Y, Harvey SM. Patient-centered communication to address young adult breast cancer survivors' reproductive and sexual health concerns. Health Commun 2020;1–16.

[111] McCormack LA, Treiman K, Rupert D, Williams-Piehota P, Nadler E, Arora NK, et al. Measuring patient-centered communication in cancer care: a literature review and the development of a systematic approach. Soc Sci Med 2011;72(7):1085–95.

[112] Epstein R, Street RJ. Patient-centered communication in cancer care: promoting health and reducing suffering. Bethesda, MD: National Cancer Institute; 2007.

[113] Stabile C, Goldfarb S, Baser RE, Goldfrank DJ, Abu-Rustum NR, Barakat RR, et al. Sexual health needs and educational intervention preferences for women with cancer. Breast Cancer Res Treat 2017;165(1):77–84.

[114] Flynn KE, Lindau ST, Lin L, Reese JB, Jeffery DD, Carter J, et al. Development and validation of a single-item screener for self-reporting sexual problems in United States adults. J Gen Intern Med 2015;30(10):1468–75.

[115] Gorman JR, Pan-Weisz TM, Drizin JH, Su HI, Malcarne VL. Revisiting the Reproductive Concerns After Cancer (RCAC) scale. Psychooncology 2019;28(7):1544–50.

[116] Annon JS. The PLISSIT model: a proposed conceptual scheme for the behavioral treatment of sexual problems. Am J Sex Educ Ther 1976;2(1):1–15.

[117] Oktay K, Harvey BE, Partridge AH, Quinn GP, Reinecke J, Taylor HS, et al. Fertility preservation in patients with cancer: ASCO Clinical Practice Guideline update. J Clin Oncol 2018;36(19):1994–2001.

[118] Lockart BA. The fertility preservation (FP) consult. In: Woodruff TK, Shah DK, Vitek WS, editors. Textbook of oncofertility research and practice: a multidisciplinary approach. Switzerland: Springer; 2019. p. 265–71.

[119] Ussher JM, Parton C, Perz J. Need for information, honesty and respect: patient perspectives on health care professionals communication about cancer and fertility. Reprod Health 2018;15(1):2.

[120] Trèves R, Grynberg M, Parco S, Finet A, Poulain M, Fanchin R. Female fertility preservation in cancer patients: an instrumental tool for the envisioning a postdisease life. Future Oncol 2014;10(6):969–74.

[121] Mersereau JE, Goodman LR, Deal AM, Gorman JR, Whitcomb BW, Su HI. To preserve or not to preserve: how difficult is the decision about fertility preservation? Cancer. 2013;119(22):4044–50.

[122] Deshpande NA, Braun IM, Meyer FL. Impact of fertility preservation counseling and treatment on psychological outcomes among women with cancer: a systematic review. Cancer. 2015;121(22):3938–47.

[123] Goodman LR, Balthazar U, Kim J, Mersereau JE. Trends of socioeconomic disparities in referral patterns for fertility preservation consultation. Hum Reprod 2012;27(7):2076–81.

[124] Niemasik EE, Letourneau J, Dohan D, Katz A, Melisko M, Rugo H, et al. Patient perceptions of reproductive health counseling at the time of cancer diagnosis: a qualitative study of female California cancer survivors. J Cancer Surviv 2012;6(3):324–32.

[125] Shimizu C, Bando H, Kato T, Mizota Y, Yamamoto S, Fujiwara Y. Physicians' knowledge, attitude, and behavior regarding fertility issues for young breast cancer patients: a national survey for breast care specialists. Breast Cancer 2013;20(3):230–40.

[126] Letourneau JM, Smith JF, Ebbel EE, Craig A, Katz PP, Cedars MI, et al. Racial, socioeconomic, and demographic disparities in access to fertility preservation in young women diagnosed with cancer. Cancer. 2012;118(18):4579–88.

[127] Quinn GP, Vadaparampil ST, Bell-Ellison BA, Gwede CK, Albrecht TL. Patient-physician communication barriers regarding fertility preservation among newly diagnosed cancer patients. Soc Sci Med 2008;66(3):784–9.

[128] Schover LR, Rybicki LA, Martin BA, Bringelsen KA. Having children after cancer. A pilot survey of survivors' attitudes and experiences. Cancer. 1999;86(4):697–709.

[129] Flink DM, Sheeder J, Kondapalli LA. A review of the oncology patient's challenges for utilizing fertility preservation services. J Adolesc Young Adult Oncol 2017;6(1):31–44.

[130] Logan S, Perz J, Ussher J, Peate M, Anazodo A. Clinician provision of oncofertility support in cancer patients of a reproductive age: a systematic review. Psychooncology 2018;27(3):748–56.

[131] Young K, Shliakhtsitsava K, Natarajan L, Myers E, Dietz AC, Gorman JR, et al. Fertility counseling before cancer treatment and subsequent reproductive concerns among female adolescent and young adult cancer survivors. Cancer 2019;125(6):980–9.

[132] Carter J, Lacchetti C, Rowland JH. Interventions to address sexual problems in people with cancer: American Society of Clinical Oncology Clinical Practice Guideline adaptation summary. J Oncol Pract 2018;14(3):173–9.

[133] Chism LA, Magnan MA. Talking to cancer survivors about dyspareunia and self-management. Nursing. 2017;47(10):24–9.

[134] Calleja-Agius J, Brincat MP. Urogenital atrophy. Climacteric 2009;12(4):279–85.

[135] Carter J, Goldfrank D, Schover LR. Simple strategies for vaginal health promotion in cancer survivors. J Sex Med 2011;8(2):549–59.

[136] Pinkerton JV. Hormone therapy: key points from NAMS 2017 position statement. Clin Obstet Gynecol 2018;61(3):447–53.

[137] ACOG. Female sexual dysfunction: ACOG Practice Bulletin Summary, NUMBER 213. Obstet Gynecol 2019;134(1):203–5.

[138] Arthur E, Worly B, Carpenter K, Postl C, Rosko A, Krok-Schoen J, et al. Let's get it on: Addressing sex and intimacy in older cancer survivors. J Geriatr Oncol 2021;12(2):312–15.

[139] Frühauf S, Gerger H, Schmidt HM, Munder T, Barth J. Efficacy of psychological interventions for sexual dysfunction: a systematic review and meta-analysis. Arch Sex Behav 2013;42(6):915–33.

[140] DeSimone M, Spriggs E, Gass JS, Carson SA, Krychman ML, Dizon DS. Sexual dysfunction in female cancer survivors. Am J Clin Oncol 2014;37(1):101–6.

[141] Lowenstein L, Gruenwald I, Gartman I, Vardi Y. Can stronger pelvic muscle floor improve sexual function? Int Urogynecol J 2010;21(5):553–6.

[142] Bannowsky A, Schulze H, van der Horst C, Hautmann S, Jünemann KP. Recovery of erectile function after nerve-sparing radical prostatectomy: improvement with nightly low-dose sildenafil. BJU Int 2008;101(10):1279–83.

[143] Lyons KS, Lee CS. The theory of dyadic illness management. J Fam Nurs 2018;24(1):8–28.

[144] Keesing S, Rosenwax L, McNamara B. A dyadic approach to understanding the impact of breast cancer on relationships between partners during early survivorship. BMC Womens Health 2016;16(1):57.

[145] Perz J, Ussher JM, Gilbert E, The Australian Cancer and Sexuality Study Team. Feeling well and talking about sex: psycho-social predictors of sexual functioning after cancer. BMC Cancer 2014;14:228.

[146] Cousineau TM, Domar AD. Psychological impact of infertility. Best Pract Res Clin Obstet Gynaecol 2007;21(2):293–308.

[147] Pasch LA, Sullivan KT. Stress and coping in couples facing infertility. Curr Opin Psychol 2017;13:131–5.

[148] Kayser K, Watson LE, Adnrade JT. Cancer as a "we-disease": examining the process of coping from a relational perspective. Fam Syst Health 2007;25(4):404–18.

[149] Manne S, Ostroff J, Winkel G, Goldstein L, Fox K, Grana G. Posttraumatic growth after breast cancer: patient, partner, and couple perspectives. Psychosom Med 2004;66(3):442–54.

[150] Manne SL, Ostroff JS, Norton TR, Fox K, Goldstein L, Grana G. Cancer-related relationship communication in couples coping with early stage breast cancer. Psychooncology 2006;15(3):234–47.

[151] Badr H, Acitelli LK, Taylor CL. Does talking about their relationship affect couples' marital and psychological adjustment to lung cancer? J Cancer Surviv 2008;2(1):53–64.

[152] Berg CA, Upchurch R. A developmental-contextual model of couples coping with chronic illness across the adult life span. Psychological Bull 2007;133(6):920–54.

[153] Lee CS, Vellone E, Lyons KS, Cocchieri A, Bidwell JT, D'Agostino F, et al. Patterns and predictors of patient and caregiver engagement in heart failure care: a multi-level dyadic study. Int J Nurs Stud 2015;52(2):588–97.

[154] Lyons KS, Lee CS, Bennett JA, Nail LM, Fromme EK, Hiatt SO, et al. Symptom incongruence trajectories in lung cancer dyads. J Pain Symptom Manag 2014;48(6):1031–40.

[155] Manne SL. Intrusive thoughts and psychological distress among cancer patients: The role of spouse avoidance and criticism. J Consult Clin Psychol 1999;67(4):539–46.

[156] Manne SL, Dougherty J, Veach S, Kless R. Hiding worries from one's spouse: protective buffering among cancer patients and their spouses. Cancer Res Ther Control 1999;8:175–88.

[157] Kuijer RG, Ybema JF, Buunk BP, De Jong GM, Thijs-Boer F, Sanderman R. Active engagement, protective buffering, and overprotection: three ways of giving support by intimate partners of patients with cancer. J Soc Clin Psychol 2000;19(2):256–75.

[158] Baucom DH, Porter LS, Kirby JS, Gremore TM, Keefe FJ. Psychosocial issues confronting young women with breast cancer. Breast Dis 2005;23:103–13.

[159] Ussher PJ, Gilbert E, Wong WKT, Hobbs K. Renegotiating sex and intimacy after cancer: resisting the coital imperative. Cancer Nurs 2013;36(6):454–62.

[160] Flynn KE, Whicker D, Lin L, Cusatis R, Nyitray A, Weinfurt KP. Sexual orientation and patient-provider communication about sexual problems or concerns among United States adults. J Gen Intern Med 2019;34(11):2505–11.

References

[161] Rouanne M, Massard C, Hollebecque A, Rousseau V, Varga A, Gazzah A, et al. Evaluation of sexuality, health-related quality-of-life and depression in advanced cancer patients: a prospective study in a Phase I clinical trial unit of predominantly targeted anticancer drugs. Eur J Cancer 2013;49(2):431–8.

[162] Shell JA. Sexual issues in the palliative care population. Semin Oncol Nurs 2008;24(2):131–4.

[163] Boehmer U, Glickman M, Winter M, Clark MA. Long-term breast cancer survivors' symptoms and morbidity: differences by sexual orientation? J Cancer Surviv 2013;7(2):203–10.

[164] Hulbert-Williams NJ, Plumpton CO, Flowers P, McHugh R, Neal RD, Semlyen J, et al. The cancer care experiences of gay, lesbian and bisexual patients: a secondary analysis of data from the UK Cancer Patient Experience Survey. Eur J Cancer Care (Engl) 2017;26(4).

[165] Jabson JM, Kamen CS. Sexual minority cancer survivors' satisfaction with care. J Psychosoc Oncol 2016;34(1–2):28–38.

[166] Desai MJ, Gold RS, Jones CK, Din H, Dietz AC, Shliakhtsitsava K, et al. Mental health outcomes in adolescent and young adult female cancer survivors of a sexual minority. J Adolesc Young Adult Oncol 2021;10(2):148–55.

[167] Hill G, Holborn C. Sexual minority experiences of cancer care: a systematic review. J Cancer Policy 2015;6:11–22.

[168] Seay J, Mitteldorf D, Yankie A, Pirl WF, Kobetz E, Schlumbrecht MP. Survivorship care needs among LGBT cancer survivors. J Psychosoc Oncol 2018;36(4):393–405.

[169] Brown MT, McElroy JA. Unmet support needs of sexual and gender minority breast cancer survivors. Support Care Cancer 2018;26(4):1189–96.

[170] Cohen JN, Byers ES. Beyond lesbian bed death: enhancing our understanding of the sexuality of sexual-minority women in relationships. J Sex Res 2014;51(8):893–903.

[171] Flynn KE, Lin L, Weinfurt KP. Sexual function and satisfaction among heterosexual and sexual minority United States adults: a cross-sectional survey. PLoS One 2017;12(4):e0174981.

[172] Tracy JK, Junginger J. Correlates of lesbian sexual functioning. J Womens Health (Larchmt) 2007;16(4):499–509.

[173] Scott SB, Ritchie L, Knopp K, Rhoades GK, Markman HJ. Sexuality within female same-gender couples: definitions of sex, sexual frequency norms, and factors associated with sexual satisfaction. Arch Sex Behav 2018;47(3):681–92.

[174] van Rosmalen-Nooijens KAWL, Vergeer CM, Lagro-Janssen ALM. Bed death and other lesbian sexual problems unraveled: a qualitative study of the sexual health of lesbian women involved in a relationship. Women Health 2008;48(3):339–62.

[175] Henderson AW, Lehavot K, Simoni JM. Ecological models of sexual satisfaction among lesbian/bisexual and heterosexual women. Arch Sex Behav 2009;38(1):50–65.

[176] Fleishman JM, Crane B, Koch PB. Correlates and predictors of sexual satisfaction for older adults in same-sex relationships. J Homosex 2020;67(14):1974–98.

[177] Butts SF, Seifer DB. Racial and ethnic differences in reproductive potential across the life cycle. Fertil Steril 2010;93(3):681–90.

[178] Thurston RC, Bromberger JT, Joffe H, Avis NE, Hess R, Crandall CJ, et al. Beyond frequency: who is most bothered by vasomotor symptoms? Menopause 2008;15(5):841–7.

[179] Huang AJ, Moore EE, Boyko EJ, Scholes D, Lin F, Vittinghoff E, et al. Vaginal symptoms in postmenopausal women: self-reported severity, natural history, and risk factors. Menopause 2010;17(1):121–6.

[180] Denlinger CS, Sanft T, Baker KS, Baxi S, Broderick G, Demark-Wahnefried W, et al. Survivorship, version 2.2017, NCCN Clinical Practice Guidelines in oncology. J Natl Compr Cancer Netw 2017;15(9):1140–63.

[181] Jain T, Hornstein MD. Disparities in access to infertility services in a state with mandated insurance coverage. Fertil Steril 2005;84(1):221–3.

[182] Bradford A, Fellman B, Urbauer D, Gallegos J, Meaders K, Tung C, et al. Assessment of sexual activity and dysfunction in medically underserved women with gynecologic cancers. Gynecol Oncol 2015;139(1):134–40.

[183] Lindau ST, Abramsohn EM, Matthews AC. A manifesto on the preservation of sexual function in women and girls with cancer. Am J Obstet Gynecol 2015;213(2):166–74.

[184] Krok J, Baker T, McMillan S. Sexual activity and body image: examining gender variability and the influence of psychological distress in cancer patients. J Gend Stud 2013;22(4):409–22.

[185] Lindau ST, Schumm LP, Laumann EO, Levinson W, O'Muircheartaigh CA, Waite LJ. A study of sexuality and health among older adults in the United States. N Engl J Med. 2007;357(8):762–74.

PART III

Additional considerations

CHAPTER

8

Lesbians pursuing parenthood: pathways, challenges, and best practices

Marie Hayes and Julia T. Woodward

Departments of Psychiatry and Behavioral Sciences, Department of Obstetrics and Gynecology, Duke University Health System, Durham, NC, United States

Case example

Note: Names and clinical details have been altered to protect patient confidentiality.

Sarah (higher education administration; age 36) and Anne (social worker, age 32) began dating 2 years ago and legally married 1 year ago. Both identify as female and lesbian. They expressed relief at the protections legal marriage affords their family. Each described the unique bond they share and their excitement about having found a stable, loving relationship in which to pursue family building. The couple considered multiple pathways to parenthood, researching adoption and fertility treatment most carefully. They ultimately ruled out adoption due to its expense and potential for discrimination by agencies and birth mothers. Through these discussions, Sarah's initial ideas about experiencing pregnancy and breastfeeding crystallized into a clear desire; conversely, Anne expressed discomfort with either of these roles. Anne identifies as female, but embodies a more gender-neutral expression, choosing to wear her hair short, flatten her breasts with a sports bra, and wear more gender-neutral clothing. As such, the decision about who would carry the pregnancy was relatively easy and the couple decided to move forward with finding a supportive fertility clinic.

Anne's university employer had a fertility clinic and because she had been an employee for 2 years, they had some insurance coverage for fertility services so the couple started there. Looking at the clinic's website, they found inclusive language and images. When filling out the clinic's intake forms, they were comforted by references to "patient/partner" rather than "wife/husband." They recall that their reproductive endocrinologist asked about their preferred pronouns, but the billing specialist did not. Their doctor recommended that they begin with donor insemination (intrauterine insemination or IUI) and referred them to the team's psychologist for a consultation about using donor sperm. They reported feeling anxious about meeting with the psychologist, worried that this appointment would act as a barrier to their dreams and frustrated at an additional step in the process. Afterward, Sarah and Anne reported that this consult was not what they expected, affirmed their family type, and provided answers to many of the questions they had been discussing at home. They were glad to learn it was equally required of everyone using donor sperm and not just of them because they were lesbians.

Sarah and Anne found that choosing a sperm source was harder than choosing who would carry the pregnancy. They talked to friends, considered potential known donors, and even discussed the possibility of known sperm donation with one gay friend. Through these discussions, their gay friend realized that if he helped Sarah and Anne to have a baby, he likely would want to play a larger role in the life of the child, potentially assuming the role of father. Sarah and Anne knew they were looking for less involvement from a known donor. They wanted to raise a baby within the context of their loving marriage and without incorporating a third person in decision making or physical custody. As a result, they decided to choose a donor from a sperm bank instead. They purchased several vials of sperm from a donor they both liked, paid for medications to support Sarah's egg production, and scheduled their IUI cycle. At this juncture in their family-building journey, Sarah and Anne reflected on the multiple logistical and decision-making steps they had needed to complete already. They expressed relief at finally starting fertility treatment.

Unfortunately, Sarah's first two IUI cycles were unsuccessful. Sarah had felt fine emotionally after the first cycle, but the second negative result was both surprising and very disappointing to her. Anne reported feeling disappointed as well as helpless, given that she was not the one undergoing treatment. They briefly considered choosing a new sperm donor, but felt daunted by the prospect of repeating the search process and finding another donor about whom they felt as excited. They also considered whether to switch gears and have Anne undergo the next IUI procedure, but Anne felt conflicted about this option. She expressed a strong desire for parenthood, the wish to achieve success and thus relief from more treatment cycles, and frustration at the amount of time passing. At the same time, she felt significant unease with the idea of living in a female body blooming in pregnancy.

Happily, changing gears became unnecessary when Sarah's third IUI cycle was successful. Sarah and Anne both reported great excitement and relief at the positive news. After two ultrasounds confirming a heartbeat and good fetal development at the fertility center, they graduated to receiving prenatal care at an obstetrical (OB) clinic. LGBTQ+ friends who had become parents 2 years earlier recommended the OB practice and pediatrician they chose. Sarah and Anne felt relieved in using their friends' suggestions and thus not needing to embark on another research project to identify medical providers for the next steps in their journey. They contacted a LGBTQ+-friendly reproductive attorney from the list provided by their fertility center to find out more about how to establish and protect Anne's parental rights. They enjoyed watching Sarah's body change as the pregnancy developed and picked a paint color for the nursery.

Tragically, at 25 weeks, Sarah experienced premature rupture of the amniotic membrane. Their baby boy, whom they named Bennett, was delivered prematurely and did not survive. Both Sarah and Anne reported feelings of disbelief, shock, horror, and intense grief. Sarah's OB recommended that she seek supportive counseling and Sarah reached back out to the psychologist at the fertility center for grief counseling and treatment of Post-traumatic Stress Disorder (PTSD). The psychologist identified that Anne had not been offered supportive counseling to cope with her grief and provided referral to another mental health provider. The couple remained committed to having a baby but worn down by their experiences and terrified to try again.

Sarah and Anne wanted a subsequent pregnancy to end differently and thus reconsidered all their previous choices. Should they choose a new sperm donor? Should they have Anne carry the pregnancy? Should they switch to *in vitro fertilization* (IVF) or another clinic? Allowing the couple to explore their options in psychotherapy and identifying their efforts to exert control in a largely uncontrollable terrain was helpful. Sarah learned alternate coping strategies more suited to coping with uncertainty; she and Anne began to recover emotionally. Sarah's medical team recommended a cerclage after her next successful cycle, a surgical stitch placed around the cervix at the end of the first trimester to prevent premature rupture of the amniotic membrane. They felt comforted that this procedure should prevent another similar pregnancy loss and decided to have Sarah undergo one additional IUI procedure. Of note, the couple had been counseled early in treatment to pay attention to donor cutoffs and the reality that multiple treatment cycles might be necessary to bring home a baby. As a result, Sarah and Anne had purchased several vials of their donor's sperm and had enough supply to do another cycle.

Sarah got pregnant immediately, but this news triggered intense anxiety and fears of another miscarriage. She addressed these reactions in weekly therapy and worked to accept that this anxiety would not cause another miscarriage. She hoped this pregnancy would be a girl, both because it would feel different and thus potentially "safer" and also because she worried that having a boy would erase Bennett's place in the family. Like many women who have experienced pregnancy loss and are pregnant again, she expressed worry that emotionally bonding with the new baby would be disloyal to the lost child. Sarah felt significantly better once the cerclage was placed at 14 weeks and again once she passed the milestone of 25 weeks, the gestational age at which she had lost Bennett. Anne reported her own complex emotional journey: excitement at the growing pregnancy, fears for Sarah's safety, a sense of being less central in the pregnancy, and some delayed bonding with the baby as a result.

At 39 weeks, Sarah had an uneventful delivery of a healthy baby girl, whom she and Anne named Avery. Because the couple had secured a prebirth order, both Anne and Sarah were listed on the birth certificate and they had plans to pursue second-parent adoption for Anne once life settled down. As they entered the postpartum period, Sarah and Avery got off to good start with breastfeeding, an experience that Sarah described as exhausting but emotionally rewarding. She felt strongly bonded to Avery and confident in her ability as a parent. Anne's emotional experience was more complex. She sometimes felt like an outsider when watching the physical bond between Sarah and Avery. Anne had not contributed to the child's genetics, did not carry the pregnancy, was not able to feed the baby who was not yet taking a bottle, and thus was not as able to soothe her. Anne knew she loved Avery, but sometimes wondered where she fit in. Sarah reported feeling a combination of sadness that Anne felt disconnected and guilt that she had such a strong tie to Avery. In therapy, Sarah was encouraged to communicate openly about these feelings and to create opportunities for Anne to care for Avery independently to strengthen their emotional bond.

Six months later, Avery was thriving and both Sarah and Anne had adjusted to family life. Avery was now taking a bottle, allowing Anne to participate in all aspects of caring for her. Anne and Avery now had their own unique relationship that increased Anne's sense of confidence and importance. Sarah and Anne described their journey to parenthood as exhausting and stressful, but ultimately redemptive. They felt that their investment of time, energy, money, and emotion had been worth it, but they expressed the need for a period of recovery before thinking about bringing a second child into the world.

Introduction

A generation ago, the only lesbians experiencing the joys and challenges of parenthood were those who had conceived their children in a previous heterosexual relationship. Thankfully, the world has changed dramatically in the past several decades and now lesbians are building their families in unprecedented numbers. This chapter seeks to elucidate the unique family-building experiences of these women. We begin by describing the history of overt as well as subtle discrimination faced by lesbians seeking parenthood and the barriers that still exist today. We outline multiple pathways to parenthood for lesbians and detail their relative advantages and disadvantages. We discuss the myriad decisions lesbians must tackle as they prepare for parenthood, including whose eggs, uterus, and sperm will be used to bring their baby into the world. We examine the data on the pregnancy, childbirth, and postpartum experiences of lesbians giving birth and their nongestating partners. Finally, we explore important legal, educational, and policy recommendations aimed at improving the clinical care provided to lesbians pursuing parenthood. Providers caring for lesbian patients have a special duty to seek training and learn best practices for supporting their distinct needs.

Clarifying terminology is an important first step when providing care to patients with diverse sexual orientations and gender identities. The LGBTQ+ umbrella includes patients who identify as lesbian, gay, bisexual, transgender, questioning, queer, intersex, pansexual, two-spirit (2S), androgynous, and asexual. In this chapter, we will focus on lesbians planning family building. The nonprofit organization GLAAD defines a lesbian as "a woman whose enduring physical, romantic, and/or emotional attraction is to other women" [1]. It is important to note that gender identity (a person's concept of themselves as male, female, both, or neither) and sexual orientation (a person's enduring pattern of attraction to others) are independent. Not all lesbians identify as female and may fall elsewhere on the gender-identity spectrum (e.g., identify as gender nonbinary or neither wholly female nor male). To acknowledge this range of experiences among lesbian individuals, we use the term "parent" rather than "mother" here, as "mother" presumes female gender identity.

The majority of existing research and bulk of clinical services provided have focused on partnered lesbians seeking parenthood. As a result, literature reviewed here often focuses on lesbian dyads rather than single lesbians seeking parenthood or coparenting arrangements between a lesbian couple and a man or gay couple. This focus reflects the data available rather than a bias favoring lesbian couples over single or coparenting lesbians.

Historical context

Historically, Western cultural traditions have favored heterosexual, two-parent families and viewed nontraditional families, including those comprised of same-sex individuals, as aberrant. Decisions about both custody of children and access to fertility treatment were made considering "the best interest of the child," a standard often used in adoption or child custody cases. Experts using this lens cited fears that children raised in lesbian households would be psychologically damaged and that their sexual orientation or gender identity would be atypical [2]. As recently as the 1990s, the prevailing attitude in Western societies was that a family structure that might influence a child to grow up to be gay or lesbian was an influence to be avoided at all costs. As a result of these biases, lesbians frequently were viewed as unfit parents and unsuitable candidates for care in reproductive medicine clinics. Lesbians who sought to build their family using donor sperm were met with resistance or refused care altogether. Legal access to adoption by same-sex couples in the United States was determined at the state level, and in many places was either limited to one lesbian parent adopting as a single person or banned altogether [3]. States banning adoption by same-sex couples falsely argued that these families had higher rates of alcohol and drug use than heterosexual couples and that these substance use issues would interfere with good parenting practices [4]. Lesbian mothers who had borne children within a previous heterosexual marriage faced the unthinkable choice of having to either hide their sexual orientation and associated romantic relationships or relinquish custody of their children.

To better understand who was being allowed access to assisted reproductive technology (ART), Gurmankin and colleagues [5] polled fertility clinics across the United States about their policies on providing fertility care to various patient groups. The authors got responses from 210 clinics. The data revealed that 17% of fertility clinics were very likely to turn away lesbians seeking donor insemination. Fertility clinics might enact their resistance to providing care to lesbians by denying an initial consultation appointment to women identifying as lesbian, erecting multiple "procedural barriers" once sexual orientation was discovered, or refusing to receive donor sperm for patients who were not heterosexual [6]. Some clinics required prospective lesbian patients to request access to reproductive medicine services by writing a letter that included a description of their motivation for parenthood as well as evidence of their fitness to parent [7].

Johnson also explored clinics' openness to treating lesbian patients as indicated by information on their websites [8]. This 2012 study coded data obtained from all of the 402 fertility clinics who reported to the Center for Disease Control (CDC) and the Society for Assisted Reproductive Technology (SART) from 2005 to 2007. Of the 10.2% of clinics rated unaccepting of lesbian patients based on website information, implicit (rather than explicit) gatekeeping was most commonly identified. For example, websites would refer to infertility as a heterosexual couple's issue, define the husband as the sperm source, or mention only male-factor infertility when discussing donor sperm [8]. Some clinics demonstrated more explicit barriers such as calling insemination procedures AIH, which stood for "Artificial Insemination with Husband's Sperm." Only approximately one-third of clinics explicitly discussed alternative family-building opportunities for nontraditional couples. Although many websites did not obviously discriminate against same-sex patients, they often failed to communicate openness and inclusivity [8].

In an effort to either justify or challenge these discriminatory practices, psychologists and social science researchers, led by pioneer Susan Golombok in the United Kingdom, began to test beliefs about the negative impact of lesbian parenting. Golombok and her colleagues [9] first conducted research examining the psychological functioning of children born into heterosexual families whose parents divorced when the mother embraced her lesbian identity. The researchers found that these children experienced no more psychological distress or behavioral problems than children being raised after divorce by heterosexual parents. These findings flew in the face of prevailing wisdom and were met with skepticism. Critics were concerned that the results were not generalizable to children who were raised from birth by lesbian parents, as the study only included those children whose early childhoods were spent in heterosexual households [10]. Over time, as the number of lesbians having children through assisted reproduction rose and thus the number of children raised from birth without an opposite-sex parent increased, researchers were able to investigate this family type more fully. Studies conducted by multiple research teams and employing longitudinal designs confirmed earlier findings that children raised by same-sex parents are not more likely to have negative mental health or behavioral outcomes than their peers raised by heterosexual parents [11]. Studies comparing children adopted by same-sex couples to those adopted by heterosexual couples also found no evidence of psychological impairment or greater suffering associated with parents' sexual orientation [3].

In 2005 influenced by the growing body of empirical literature debunking myths about the dangers of same-sex parenting, the American Psychological Association [12] released a publication formally noting the lack of evidence that sexual orientation negatively impacts parenting effectiveness. In 2013 the Ethics Committee of the American Society for Reproductive Medicine (ASRM) issued an official statement encouraging equal access to fertility services regardless of patients' marital status or sexual orientation [13]. These policy changes soon began to influence clinical services offered to lesbian families. Data collected by SART in 2014 revealed that approximately 60% of fertility clinics in the United States had begun providing care to lesbians [14].

The landmark 2015 legal case of Obergefell v. Hodges arguably had the greatest impact on access to services for prospective lesbian parents. In this case, the United States Supreme Court ruled that bans on same-sex marriages passed in some states were unconstitutional, thereby allowing same-sex individuals to get legally married. This ruling went beyond simply permitting same-sex marriage; it provided legal standing to same-sex couples and thus legitimized same-sex families. As a result, fertility clinics in the United States were now legally required to treat all married couples seeking treatment, regardless of their sexual orientation or identity [14]. States also could no longer legally prevent married same-sex couples from pursuing adoption. This monumental court case allowed for legal access to family-building services for all family types, including lesbians. As we will discuss later in this chapter, much work remains to make fertility-related care accessible and friendly to LGBTQ+ patients, but these scientific, legal, and policy advancements signaled the arrival of a new era.

Decisions, decisions: preparing for pregnancy

As a result of this legal and cultural evolution, much like heterosexual couples, a growing number of lesbian couples now seek to bring a biological child into their union. Kleinert and colleagues [15] found that age and the desire to establish family roots or increase meaning in life were critical factors driving decisions about when to pursue parenthood in same-sex couples. Boye and Evertsson [16] found that lesbian couples with higher household income and education levels were more likely to become parents. These sociodemographic factors would predict having both the financial resources and procedural expertise needed to navigate the more complex family-building process faced by lesbians. Perhaps surprisingly, Kleinert and colleagues [15] found that neither internalized stigma of one's own sexual orientation nor negative experiences as a result of sexual orientation negatively impacted the decision to pursue parenthood for those in a same-sex relationship. We might hypothesize that lesbians who pursue parenthood have done more work to resolve internalized stigma or cope with discriminatory experiences. The powerful desire to experience parenthood may trump past negative emotions and social interactions. Perhaps lesbians wish to give their child a more inclusive and accepting environment than the one in which they were raised. Clearly, additional research is needed to fully understand factors that influence a lesbian couple's decision about when to begin family building.

Once ready and in contrast to heterosexual couples, lesbians considering parenthood must collaborate on a series of decisions and involve outsiders in an intimate experience. Lesbian pregnancies are intentional and never unplanned. Substantial resources must be allocated to the "project" of having a child. Lesbians sometimes liken the experience of family building to pushing a ball up a hill: if they stop pushing at any time, the ball rolls backward and the dream of parenting is now farther away. They may express jealousy of a heterosexual couple who can just stop using birth control and often soon be on their way to parenthood.

The lesbian couple planning for parenthood must grapple with a host of emotional, physical, logistical, social, and financial questions. First, the couple must decide which family building strategy to use—home insemination, fertility treatment, foster care, or adoption? How much do each of these options cost? How long does it take to achieve pregnancy this way and how does that align with their desired timeline? Which partner will carry the pregnancy? Whose eggs will be used? Where will the sperm come from? What financial resources are available and will insurance provide any coverage? And, finally, what do their family and friends think? Will they be accepting and supportive of this family-building process and the hoped-for future child? These questions will be weighed and reviewed before a lesbian couple has their first interaction with a healthcare professional. Of note, for lesbians who ultimately choose to pursue care at a fertility center, providing data to support developing answers to these important questions is the specific purpose of the consultations with medical and mental health professionals.

Clinical conversations and a select body of literature shed light onto the decision-making process for lesbians deciding which partner will contribute their eggs and which will carry the pregnancy. Patients will often discuss considering factors such as each partner's age, professional role or commitments, insurance coverage, and/or personal desire to have a genetic connection. Other factors influencing this decision include perceptions of job security and reproductive health [17–19]. Gender identity and expression can also be an important factor influencing these choices. It is not uncommon for one member of the lesbian couple to express that they have always wanted to experience pregnancy and/or breastfeeding. These biological processes may feel more comfortable and in line with this partner's (typically female) gender identity and expression. Individuals who identify as gender nonconforming or nonbinary often express discomfort or even distress at the idea of carrying a pregnancy, as was described in the case example [20]. Finally, some lesbian couples might decide to switch roles when pursuing a second pregnancy, offering the other parent the opportunity to experience a genetic or gestational tie to the next child. There is some data that this pattern may be most likely to occur when both partners are highly educated [16]. It is important to note that there are no rules for how a couple might determine which partner fulfills which roles. Each partnership is unique and each lesbian couple must navigate these decisional conversations in their own way.

Pathways to parenthood

There are a number of pathways that lesbians seeking parenthood may consider. These include adoption or foster care, at-home insemination, and/or pursuing fertility treatment. Each option is characterized by unique benefits and challenges. It is important for providers treating lesbians to understand the diversity of choices they must navigate.

Adoption

In a study done in 2007, Gates [21] reported that roughly 2 million gay and lesbian couples were interested in adoption and later found that same-sex couples are four times more likely to become parents via adoption than their opposite-sex peers. Adoption appeals to these couples because it bypasses medically invasive ART interventions, which may or may not produce a healthy child. Further, lesbians pursuing adoption celebrate the beauty of a process which brings together a child who has no parents and parents who have no child. For lesbian couples, adoption allows both parents to feel equally connected to their child because neither has a genetic or gestational tie. Finally, the adoption process legally recognizes both parents from the start. This is in contrast to assisted reproduction, where the nonbiological parent seeking legal standing often must complete a second-parent adoption to secure their parental rights, even if the child was conceived within their same-sex marriage.

Pursuing adoption is not without challenges, however. Domestic adoption is expensive: it typically costs tens of thousands of dollars compared to a few thousand dollars to pursue insemination with donor sperm in a fertility center. Adoption is often a lengthy process that includes formal evaluation of the adopting couple and their home. A criminal background check, fingerprinting, review of financial resources, submission of recommendations, and a home study with a licensed mental health professional are standard aspects of this state-regulated process of placing children for adoption. Adopting couples almost universally describe feeling worried about presenting themselves in the best light and being deemed "good enough" to become parents. For lesbians with a history of experiencing discrimination, this evaluation process is often even more daunting.

At-home insemination

Some lesbians will try at-home insemination prior to or instead of seeking care at a fertility clinic. Because this method of family building is not regulated or tracked, exact prevalence rates are hard to come by. The process of at-home insemination involves placing sperm inside the vagina of the partner planning to carry the pregnancy using a small cup or syringe. Sperm can come from either a sperm bank (a deidentified sperm donor) or acquaintance, friend or family member (a known sperm donor). In recent years, lesbians seeking sperm also have turned to Facebook groups, web pages, and apps aimed at connecting women needing sperm with men willing to provide it [22]. These men can indicate preferences such as whether they are willing to provide sperm for later at-home insemination or through sexual intercourse, whether sperm will be given for free or at a cost, and whether they would like to communicate with the child in the future or not.

Lesbians who choose at-home insemination highlight the greater degree of autonomy and privacy this option affords [19,23]. Pursuing at-home insemination does not require presenting at a fertility center, explaining the desire for parenthood, involving medical providers, and ultimately receiving a bill for the care received. As such, at-home insemination may be less expensive and involve a shorter timeline than traditional fertility treatment. Because the barrier to parenthood is not infertility but rather not having a partner who produces sperm, at-home insemination more closely mirrors the intimate process of conception enjoyed by heterosexual couples. Frequently, lesbian couples choosing this pathway seek to create a romantic, intimate sexual experience and inseminate as part of the sexual act. Although not supported by the data, the couple also may prioritize the inseminated partner experiencing an orgasm after the introduction of sperm to increase the likelihood of achieving pregnancy.

While there are advantages to at-home insemination, especially for supporting autonomy and sense of agency over one's body, this unregulated process also involves some important risks. First, men providing sperm for at-home insemination typically have not undergone any evaluation which would screen for sexually transmitted diseases, genetic disorders, or psychiatric conditions, among other factors. Insemination with unscreened donor sperm has resulted in women acquiring sexually transmitted infections that required treatment before additional conception cycles can be attempted. Men providing sperm in this unfettered climate face no limits on the number of children they may produce, and instances of dozens or even hundreds of children being born from one man have already been documented [22]. These "supergroups" of donor-conceived children raise the specter of one man passing a genetic condition to a large number of offspring as well as the risk of accidental incest if donor-conceived children meet and begin a relationship. A large number of donor-conceived offspring from a single man was a phenomenon previously identified in the practice of commercial sperm banks and led to the creation of limits on the number of families that could be created from one donor [24].

From a practical standpoint, appropriately timed and targeted insemination is a skill. The ability to perform it improves with practice, something inexperienced couples attempting at-home insemination do not yet have. As a result, time to conception with this method could be longer than if the couple were receiving care from an experienced provider at a fertility center. Additionally, lesbians pursuing at-home insemination do not have access to the specialized guidance about sperm donors and sperm banks that should be a standard part of patient counseling at fertility centers. All individuals using donor sperm, including women in lesbian relationships, benefit from the opportunity to learn about the advantages and disadvantages of deidentified versus known sperm donation, adjustment, and common informational needs of donor-conceived children, and guidance on when and how to talk to a future child about their donor-conception origins. A detailed description of this psychological consultation is given later in this chapter.

Lesbians planning at-home insemination with sperm from a known donor face several additional risks. When considering personal and family history of psychopathology or substance use, it may be difficult for the lesbian couple to press a donor with whom they have a relationship for sensitive details (e.g., "Exactly how much alcohol did you drink during that difficult period? Did your uncle have typical social struggles...or was it Asperger's?"). Because many psychiatric and substance use disorders have a genetic component and thus may be transmitted to a child, careful review of the donor's history is critical. The lesbian couple and sperm donor also must tackle sensitive issues such as what role the donor will play in the life of the child (if any), whether he will be identified as the donor to the child, and whether and how future contact will occur. In a fertility center, mental health professionals trained in the psychosocial aspects of known donor arrangements facilitate discovery and consensus in these crucial conversations between all parties. In an at-home insemination, the lesbian couple must rely on their own informal research to identify all important issues to address with their donor (and his partner) and may feel unprepared for the complexities revealed.

Finally, and very significantly, lesbians seeking at-home insemination with known donor sperm may not be informed about the legal rights of the sperm donor in their state. Overwhelmingly in the United States, the only way to terminate the parental rights of a sperm donor is to have the sperm pass through the hands of a medical provider. At-home insemination bypasses that mechanism and thus preserves the donor's parental rights. A lesbian couple initially thrilled about using the sperm of a male friend may be dismayed to see that friend change his mind about his level of involvement once an adorable child is born. If they did not terminate his parental rights through a formal legal contract prior to the insemination, they may now be forced to share decision making and custody. Being uninformed about these legal nuances, seeing legal consultation as onerous and optional, and bypassing formal legal contracting with known sperm donors is more likely in the unstructured at-home insemination environment.

Assisted reproductive technology

The rise in the number of LGBTQ+ families over the past several decades has been driven in large part by ART. Lesbians creating families through fertility treatment cite a number of benefits to formal ART. First, success rates are likely to be higher for women building their families with the help of fertility experts, especially for women of advanced maternal age and those with underlying fertility challenges like endometriosis, polycystic ovarian syndrome or premature ovarian insufficiency. Prospective parents have access to more comprehensive services through a fertility clinic, including advanced diagnostic testing, prescription medications, surgery, IVF, and genetic testing of embryos.

Although the most common fertility treatment elected by lesbians in a fertility center is donor insemination, couples may also choose to pursue IVF where one partner contributes the egg (creating a genetic tie to the baby) and the other partner carries the pregnancy (creating a gestational tie to the baby). These cycles are appropriately called "reciprocal IVF" or "shared IVF." They should not be referred to as a "donor IVF cycle" and donor gamete consent forms should not be signed. Procedurally, a donor is not intended to play a parental role or be involved in the life of a child. Using donor language is an example of heteronormative bias and is often insulting to the lesbian couple creatively establishing a unique connection between each woman and the child. Additionally, if the couple's relationship were to end in the future, it can put the parent listed as a "donor" in a dangerous legal position with regard to parental rights.

Importantly, because women having lesbian sex do not face risk of pregnancy, they may mistakenly assume they are fertile and that pregnancy will occur as soon as attempts at conception begin. This false confidence may cause lesbians to defer medical evaluation as well as delay family-building efforts, choices which can both delay diagnosis of underlying medical conditions that impact fertility and increase the risk of facing age-related infertility. Reproductive endocrinologists may also fail to evaluate for underlying infertility issues because of the presumption that pregnancy has not occurred only because the woman has not been exposed previously to sperm.

In addition to more advanced medical services, lesbians seeking parenthood in a fertility clinic should have access to supportive psychological services. Lesbians pursuing ART are inherently different from heterosexual patients in that they likely have not experienced the grief associated with infertility or pregnancy loss. Their clinical care must reflect that. Unfortunately, they may go on to experience these fertility challenges and, regardless of treatment success, they must cope with the intensity of fertility treatment and risk of pregnancy loss. Additionally, as noted before, lesbians face greater discrimination and cultural bias which constitute unique stressors. Mental health professionals affiliated with or integrated into fertility centers should be knowledgeable about these multiple challenges and can offer targeted support interventions. In addition to supportive counseling, standard of practice involves a psychological consult for all patients using donor sperm, including lesbians. While it is possible for lesbian patients to seek out these kinds of support when doing at-home insemination, referral to a qualified mental health provider is more routine within the fertility clinic setting.

A final advantage to family building within a fertility center is standardized referral of lesbians using donor sperm to an attorney. Although Obergefell v. Hodges legalized same-sex marriage in the United States, the legal presumption of parenthood for a child conceived within a same-sex marriage has not yet been tested and affirmed in most states. Fertility center providers should not offer legal advice, but they can highlight the protections offered by legal contracts, prebirth parentage orders and second-parent adoptions and refer to qualified local attorneys.

Pursuing formal fertility treatment involves several important challenges that must be navigated by the lesbian couple. First, fertility treatment is typically viewed as stressful, even for patients without a history of unsuccessful attempts at conception [25]. Treatment cycles typically involve hope and excitement as well as worry, future focus, and a paradoxical desire to be stress-free to achieve success. Second, ART represents a significant financial burden for patients, which is exacerbated by a lack of insurance coverage. While coverage varies by state and employer, insurance companies typically view fertility treatment as unrelated to illness, not medically necessary, and therefore elective. As of 2020, only 19 states in the United States mandated insurance coverage for fertility treatment and only 13 mandated coverage of expensive IVF treatment [26].

The medical definition of infertility can interfere with a lesbian couple's ability to use insurance benefits, even if they live in a state that mandates insurance coverage of fertility treatment. Specifically, infertility is defined as the inability to successfully conceive after 12 months of unprotected intercourse (or, 6 months if over the age of 35) [27]. This definition is inherently problematic if you are a woman who is not engaging in intercourse with an individual who produces sperm. The inability to conceive within a lesbian relationship is the result of the preferred absence of a male partner, rather than evidence of physiological impediment or medical disorder. As a result of this heteronormative definition of infertility, lesbians may be denied insurance coverage for fertility services and left to pay for care out of pocket. Additionally, insurance company policies may extend fertility coverage only to couples who are legally married (only recently an option for lesbians) and may deny coverage if donor gametes are used. At present, reproductive endocrinologists providing fertility treatment to lesbians may use diagnoses like "female infertility due to male factor" to circumnavigate these insurance barriers. This diagnosis may be welcomed if it allows insurance benefits to be used as well as resented because it implies medical dysfunction.

The cost of fertility treatment is especially problematic when sexism and unequal pay are considered. Women continue to be paid less than their male counterparts in comparable jobs. With the current gender pay gap, a woman makes only 81 cents to every dollar made by a man [28]. Lesbian relationships are by definition comprised of two women, likely resulting in a lower net income and greater financial barriers to ART as compared to heterosexual or same-sex male couples. The differential financial burden of ART on lesbians may cause them to delay seeking fertility care until they are more financially secure and can better afford care. Unfortunately, advancing maternal age is associated with lower pregnancy rates and higher miscarriage and pregnancy complication risks. Demographic factors like race also can intersect with sexual orientation to impact access to fertility treatment. For example, women of color are less likely to receive medical support for fertility compared to white women [29] and often face the stereotype of being hyperfertile. Consequently, it may be most difficult for lesbians of color-seeking parenthood to access fertility treatment. In sum, the systemic barriers to accessing fertility care uniquely faced by couples comprised of two women may slow a lesbian couple's progression to ART. Sadly, this delay may complicate their family-building efforts even more, especially if they desire multiple children.

Psychological consultation for patients using donor sperm

A medical or nursing provider treating a lesbian describing her fears about starting IVF after multiple failed donor IUI cycles is likely to grasp the importance of making a referral for supportive counseling. The provider also is likely to refer a lesbian who has just experienced a pregnancy loss or who reports that she and her partner are not aligned with regard to next treatment steps. In each of these instances, it is notable that the provider demonstrates awareness that a lesbian may face infertility challenges in addition to needing to navigate third-party reproduction. In these encounters, the patient is expressing distress and is likely to appreciate acknowledgment of her emotions by the medical team and access to psychological care with a knowledgeable mental health provider.

However, many lesbians arriving at a fertility center to initiate care are not in distress—they just need safe access to screened donor sperm. Many fertility clinics suggest or require lesbians using donor sperm to complete a psychological consultation with a mental health provider. When the fertility provider makes this referral, lesbians often perceive this as another example of bias and discrimination against them from a system that does not accept them. Fertility providers themselves may not understand what occurs in this consult and may refer to the appointment as an "evaluation," a term which implies determining fitness to parent or establishing whether a patient can proceed with treatment. Using this inaccurate language, especially with patients from a traditionally marginalized group, leads to questions like: "Who will be judging me? What if I fail this test? Will I be able to access fertility treatment if I do?."

Fertility providers need to understand that gamete *donors* need a psychological *evaluation*; gamete *recipients* need a psychoeducational *consultation*. As such, the appointment offered to lesbians planning to use donor sperm is appropriately called a consultation, with the primary goals being education and support. This one-time consult should be standard of care for all patients who are using donor sperm, donor eggs, or donor embryos to create their families. It should be equally required of all family types using donor gametes and not differentially required of same-sex couples. The goal of this section is to elucidate exactly what issues are explored in this consult for the benefit of providers and their future patients alike.

Because the mental health consult for donor gamete recipients is often poorly understood by the medical team and poorly described in the referral, and because of the discrimination they commonly face, lesbians presenting for this consult often report feeling anxious at the outset. Once they learn that the purpose of the meeting is to provide answers to many of the questions they have been discussing at home; however, same-sex couples often report a significant sense of relief and engagement in the visit. They often report feeling appreciative of the opportunity to learn information they could not find online from a provider whose expertise is in working with donors and recipients. Occasionally, a couple will present in the consult with obvious psychological dysfunction, untreated substance abuse, or severe partner discord; in these rare cases, referral should be made for treatment and resolution of those issues before proceeding with care. However, the intent of the consult is not to probe about the couples' functioning, but rather to provide critical information to aid them in their family-building journey.

Couples using donor sperm, regardless of their sexual orientation or gender identity, typically have a whole host of questions that have not been covered in appointments with their medical providers; these are the focus of the psychoeducational consult. For example, couples wonder: "Why do some men decide to become sperm donors? How are they screened by the sperm banks? Do sperm donors learn about the children they help produce? What are the best resources for telling my child about how they were brought into the world?." In the psychoeducational consult, lesbian patients should be given information about sperm donor characteristics and common motivations for donation. They should be informed about the screening protocols of sperm banks affiliated with their fertility clinic and how those differ between banks. For example, although many banks have a similar process for medical evaluation and genetic testing of donors, they vary widely in whether and how they conduct a psychological evaluation of donors. Prospective parents are frequently surprised to learn that comprehensive screening for psychiatric conditions like Schizophrenia, Bipolar disorder, and Autism currently is offered by only a very limited number of sperm banks. Patients should be helped to parse the multiple technical terms used on sperm bank websites (e.g., "What is the difference between an anonymous donor and an identity-release donor?"). Prospective parents are often surprised to learn that choosing an identity-release donor affords a mechanism for accessing critical medical or psychological information for their child in the future, rather than exposing them to interference from an outsider as they are raising their child. Couples should be informed about how sperm banks limit the number of children born from a single donor, the industry variability in those cutoffs, and the associated benefits in reporting the birth of their child back to the bank.

The psychological consultation also provides an opportunity for the couple to consider a wide range of additional issues, some with immediate implications and some more long term. For example, couples have an opportunity to discuss what characteristics they each prioritize in their sperm donor and how much these desires overlap or diverge. For example, are they looking for physical features similar to the nonbiological lesbian partner? Or, possibly personality traits or other idiosyncratic details that might increase a sense of connection between the nonbiological parent and their child? Couples can benefit from hearing how others approach the sometimes-daunting task of selecting a donor. Other questions explored in this consult include: What does their support system think of their plan to have a child? If there are any unsupportive or disapproving family members, what might be done to navigate this difficulty? If others express concern about how being raised by lesbian parents might impact the child, what data can be provided to reassure them about the positive outcomes for children in these families? What parent name will each partner choose (e.g., one deciding to be called "mom" and the other "mama," if they both identify as female)? When should the couple inform their child about the sperm donor and what resources are available to support those conversations? Patients should be given the opportunity to review children's books addressing donor sperm origins and given resources about books and websites aimed at supporting lesbian parents that can be accessed after the consult is complete. Some of these issues may be familiar to the couple; some often have not been considered previously.

Finally, the psychological consult provides an opportunity to acknowledging the unique perspective of the nongenetic, nongestating parent. This partner can feel displaced or ignored in the fertility treatment process. She can express fear about being seen as a less central or less important parent due to the fact that she does not play a biological role in creating the child. Naming and normalizing these feelings at the preconception stage is helpful, as is sharing research that shows these fears often seem inconsequential once the child is born and the parent-child relationship is established. Broadly speaking, having a specialized provider who is skilled in navigating these conversations is critical. Because lesbians are more likely to have encountered barriers in accessing ART and experience higher levels of stigma, sexism, and prejudice than heterosexual couples, it is important for mental health providers providing this psychological consultation to lesbians to navigate conversations with sensitivity.

Most mental health providers conduct these consults in an individual format. In our center, these consults typically are offered in a small-class format for a maximum of three lesbian couples. The consult is specifically tailored to the needs and perspectives of lesbian patients, and thus, for example, does not include reference to feelings of grief about trying to conceive unsuccessfully for a long period of time. Benefits to the patient of this group approach include connecting with other lesbians pursuing parenthood through donor sperm, enhancing a sense of community, and learning from the experiences of and questions asked by other attendees. Patients can request an individual consult if desired and confidentiality of the consult is discussed at the outset. In the group consult, patients frequently swap reactions to various sperm bank websites, experiences of friends who have already become parents through donor sperm, and recommendations for LGBTQ+-friendly OBGYN practices. They validate each other's frustration at needing to involve a third person in creating their child or offer ideas about how to talk to a conservative, disapproving family member. Both the individual and the group format are appropriate to support the family-building journey of lesbians using donor sperm.

Psychological preparation for lesbians working with a known sperm donor

As noted before, some lesbians embarking upon family building have a relationship with someone they would like to use as their known sperm donor. Working with a known sperm donor confers a number of significant advantages to lesbians and their children. First, even initiating this conversation with a potential donor can have a positive impact on the relationship with him. Donors often report feeling honored and flattered to be considered for this important role, regardless of their final decision. Second, rather than learning about a donor through a static and circumscribed online profile, the lesbian couple will have more complete knowledge of their known donor's characteristics, a knowledge developed through repeated interactions with him. Working with a known donor makes it simpler to access updated medical or psychological information about him over time. When the couple wonders how his health may have changed over a period of years, they can reach out to him directly for an update. When these common questions arise for parents who used a donor from a sperm bank, the couple must have originally selected an identity-release donor, wait until the child is 18, and have the child be the one to initiate contact with the bank. The bank or the adult child must then be able to find the donor and solicit his responses. It is easy to see how multiple logistical barriers can impede this flow of information. Alternatively, using a known donor makes it easier to satisfy the child's natural curiosity about his or her sperm donor. Finally, because it is rare for a man to serve as the known sperm donor to multiple families, children born through known sperm donation are likely to have fewer genetic half-siblings. Commercial sperm banks typically use a cutoff of 25 families who can purchase sperm from the same donor. If those families have an average of 1–2 children, a desirable donor is likely to produce 25–50 children, who are the genetic half-siblings of the lesbian couple's child. The known sperm donor is likely to have a substantially smaller number of his own children, a fact that is often a comfort to the lesbian couple evaluating their options.

Working with a known sperm donor also involves several potential drawbacks. First, it necessitates a longer timeline. Vials of sperm at a sperm bank are available for immediate purchase and come from donors who have already had medical evaluation, genetic testing, sexually transmitted disease testing, and sometimes psychological screening. As required by the Federal Drug Administration (FDA) (who regulates use of donor tissue) and the ASRM, known sperm donors must complete each of these evaluation steps, appointments which take time to schedule and complete. The FDA requires that vials of sperm be quarantined for a minimum of 35 days before they can be used in a treatment cycle, creating another delay for the lesbian couple trying to build their family. Secondly, each of these evaluation appointments costs money, an expense typically borne by the lesbian couple planning pregnancy, not the donor himself. Finally, as noted before, lesbians working with a known sperm donor who wish to be the sole legal parents must hire an attorney to execute a contract terminating the donor's parental rights. This represents yet another logistical step and expense in an already complex process.

When using known donor sperm in a fertility center, lesbians should be referred for the psychological consult described above, and their donor should be referred for a psychological evaluation. If the donor has a partner, s/he should be separately interviewed to assess comfort with the donation. A final joint meeting between the lesbian couple, donor, and donor's partner and the mental health professional allows an opportunity to reach consensus on any areas of discrepancy identified. The goal of these meetings is to ensure that all parties feel well-prepared and supported in this process and to prevent problems that can arise from failure to consider nuances and details. Experienced mental health professionals can share the lessons learned from previous known donor arrangements to strengthen and support the current arrangement. The lesbian couple's psychological consult should be tailored to include information specifically relevant to known donation and this particular known donor. As such, the group consultation model described before is not appropriate in these cases.

During these meetings, a qualified mental health provider should discuss considerations relevant to all parties in the donation process, including topics that might be difficult to broach or otherwise overlooked. Topics may include the donor's response to being asked to donate (i.e., flattered, excited vs coerced, uncomfortable), his perception of being able to decline the request, his understanding of the donation process, any personal and family history of medical and psychological disorders which may be genetically transmissible, the joint decision-making process used by the recipient couple to select this (vs another) known donor, the impact of the donation on the relationship between the donor and recipient couple, whether the donor will provide input in future decisions (e.g., medical management of a birth defect or timing of pediatric vaccinations), whether the donor will be identified to the future child and when, whether the child will be identified to the known donor's own children or family members, and what expectations all parties have regarding contact between the future child and the donor. Of note, a known donor with a history of genetically transmissible medical or psychiatric conditions may still be an excellent match for the lesbian couple. The goal of evaluating for these disorders is to ensure full knowledge on the part of the recipient couple, rather than reflecting an expectation that the donor be "perfect." Finally, the mental health professional should offer referral to qualified local attorneys with expertise in known sperm donation to assist all parties in finalizing a legal contract that codifies the consensus achieved in the joint meeting.

Understanding the fertility clinic experience for lesbians seeking parenthood

Given the tremendous legal, societal, and medical barriers faced by this population, it should not be surprising that lesbians report being careful about their selection of a fertility clinic. Barriers to accessing fertility care can be implicit and explicit. Medical and mental health professionals providing specialized fertility care must develop an awareness of the discrimination lesbians face and concerns they have about treatment in the clinic. A growing body of work is helping to better understand lesbians' experiences in fertility clinic settings [30–32]. Researchers have used both qualitative and quantitative methods to evaluate patient experiences, clinic practices, and website content; findings are relatively consistent across studies. In this section, we will outline major findings from this research to educate fertility clinic providers about best practices in supporting lesbians seeking parenthood.

Because fear of judgment and discrimination is an important barrier to accessing care for these patients, lesbians often report scanning fertility clinic websites and waiting rooms in an effort to determine how LGBTQIA + -friendly the practice is likely to be. In 2017 Wu and colleagues analyzed fertility clinic websites in the United States and found that only 53% contained LGBTQ-friendly content [32]. Websites were rated LGBTQ-friendly if they had at least one LGBTQ-inclusive keyword (e.g., lesbian, bisexual, homosexual, LGBTQ, same-sex, etc.) or "homepage cue" (e.g., rainbow flags, photos, including same-sex couples, or statements discussing nondiscrimination policies for LGBTQ patients). When looking at differences by region, clinics in the Northeast were found to be the most LGBTQ-inclusive, with 72%, including LGBTQ references in their websites. About 66% of West Coast clinics included this content. The Midwest and South were found to be least inclusive, with only 39% of clinics displaying LGBTQ-friendly material on their websites. When looking at clinic-specific variables, larger clinic size was associated with more LGBTQ-friendly website content, whereas practice type and state-mandated fertility insurance coverage did not play a role [32].

Lesbian patients' efforts to evaluate how welcomed they will be at a particular clinic do not stop at a review of fertility clinic's website. Lesbians report seeking symbolic representations of inclusiveness once they arrive to the clinic. These may include rainbow flags on entry doorways or in waiting rooms, same-sex images in brochures, and nonheteronormative language on new patient paperwork. Additionally, there are many communication practices that impact the lesbian couples' perception of inclusion. Does the medical team ask about both patients preferred gender pronouns? Does the team know that the patient is in a same-sex relationship and the other person present in the room is also an intended parent, rather than a friend or support person? How much do they interact with the nonbiological female partner? Do they use the appropriate terminology such as wife or partner? Do they afford her the same status as heterotypical male partners, equally informing her about treatment options and including her in decision-making? Providing sensitive and supportive care to lesbians requires attention to language choice and communication practices. Being uninformed about the unique perspective of lesbians and failing to tailor communication to their family type can result in providers enacting microaggressions against these patients, whether intended or not.

Pregnancy and childbirth

Sadly, once pregnant, lesbian parents are not protected from the negative pregnancy outcomes experienced by heterosexual couples. Pregnancy loss is an all-too-common event, experienced by approximately one in four women who have been pregnant [33]. Experiencing a miscarriage may be the first time the lesbian couple has faced a fertility complication and may trigger the feelings of confusion and grief so familiar to infertile heterosexual couples. It can feel even more devastating to lose a pregnancy achieved after the effort and expense of ART, when it is not possible to easily attempt conception again at home. Lesbian couples going through miscarriage report greater loss of control over their body and their future when compared to heterosexual couples [34].

Once the risk of early miscarriage has passed, it is common for lesbians to express joy in leaving a medicalized process behind and focusing on the natural process of pregnancy. Of note, lesbian parents report more positive feelings during pregnancy compared to heterosexual or gay parents conceiving through ART, especially in the early stages [35]. This greater positive affect during early pregnancy may be explained by the fact that the lesbian couple is less likely to have experienced the stress of infertility. Unlike a heterosexual woman trying to conceive unsuccessfully, the lesbian woman may never have seen her body as "broken," endured months of disappointing sex, or viewed getting her period as a sign of failure. Having been spared the impact of coping with infertility and its associated impacts on mood, her emotional experience of pregnancy after ART can be more positive and less anxious.

Regardless of the means used to achieve pregnancy, lesbians must continue to navigate a healthcare system geared toward heterosexual patients. First, they must find an LGBTQ + -friendly obstetrician and pediatrician. Lesbians describe using similar strategies to evaluate how accepting an OBGYN or pediatric practice will be as they did to evaluate a fertility practice. They note fears about being less welcomed than heterosexual couples at these practices and frustration at waiting room images and intake forms that exclude nontraditional family types. They report feeling out of place in childbirth classes, the one lesbian couple in a room of heterosexual couples. They notice "Daddy Boot Camp" prenatal classes aimed at teaching fathers skills like how to change a diaper or how to bond with a newborn and the absence of a comparable class for the nonbiological lesbian parent. Sadly, some lesbian parents are not offered any childbirth or parent education [36].

Like heterosexual fathers, nonbiological lesbian parents can feel sidelined [37,38]. The woman carrying the pregnancy has immediate status and is the focus of prenatal care visits. Her body is changing weekly and as the pregnancy progresses, she experiences regular interaction with the baby in the form of movement. Like all mothers, pregnant lesbian parents will begin to attribute personality characteristics to their baby based on these movements (e.g., "She's so strong and active"; "He likes jazz music"; and "She is a night owl"). The nonbiological lesbian parent does not have these interactions and cannot participate in this type of conversation about the baby. She may be ignored in prenatal visits and can feel invisible. As a result, like heterosexual fathers, it is not uncommon for the nonbiological lesbian parent to express anxiety and concern about feeling unprepared for or less connected to the baby. When considering the childbirth experience itself, some nonbiological lesbian parents report a positive experience at the hospital whereas others report feeling they are ignored by hospital staff or that the labor and delivery nurses are not comfortable with their presence as a coparent [38].

Receiving care from diverse healthcare providers may be a high priority for lesbians during pregnancy. In some instances, lesbian parents-to-be will opt to go out-of-network to see a physician who has a nontraditional sexual orientation or gender identity to increase their sense of acceptance and support [39]. Similarly, lesbian parents-to-be may choose a hospital or provider that they know has a diverse team member on staff [40]. Fear of not being accepted or supported may even influence some parents to give birth at home rather than visit heteronormative delivery wards in the hospital [39,40]. Home births can be intimate and beautiful, but also are associated with greater risks to parent and baby if there are complications. Interestingly, lesbian parents in one Canadian study noted that the care they received from midwives and doulas was more affirming and sensitive than the care they received from OB nursing staff [41]. Evaluating the clinical experiences and training of these midwives and doulas that resulted in greater sensitivity could allow health systems to design training for other healthcare providers to ensure better care for nontraditional patients.

Postpartum phase: benefits and challenges

The period after giving birth and meeting a new child is an exciting time for any family. In addition to this joy, parents of newborns are often tired, overwhelmed by the demands of care, and unsure in their new role. In this regard, lesbian parents share much in common with heterosexual parents. Some new parents experience more significant emotional difficulties. Postpartum depression, defined as major or minor depression within 3 months of giving birth, is experienced by roughly 20% of new mothers [42]. There is mixed evidence about whether lesbian parents experience differential rates of postpartum depression. Rubio and colleagues found similar rates of postpartum depression when comparing lesbian parents to their heterosexual or gay peers [35]. Conversely, Ross and colleagues found that, likely because of experiencing greater previous victimization and discrimination, lesbian parents were at a higher risk for postpartum depression than heterosexual parents [43]. It is important to note that similar to new fathers, nonbiological lesbian parents are also at risk for depression in the postpartum period. Additionally, like new fathers, many nonbiological lesbian parents report feeling as though their emotional needs are ignored in the postpartum period [38,44].

Social support is a major predictor of postpartum adjustment and lesbians may be at risk for receiving less support for a number of reasons [19,45,46]. The lesbian couple might receive less support from judgmental family members not comfortable with their sexual orientation and fearful about the impact of a nontraditional family structure on the adjustment of the child. Some lesbians are not "out" with family prior to having a child and a romantic relationship previously left undefined is now in full view.

Additionally, lesbian parents may find that they now live at the intersection of two worlds: the gay community and the parenting community; they may find they no longer fit completely in either place [34,46]. Lesbians may find that their friends in the gay community are baffled by or unsupportive of their family building efforts [19]. They might receive less support from their gay friends who do not have an interest in having children and cannot relate to the day-to-day challenges of parenthood. The couples' social support network may shift to include more heterosexual families similarly in the throes of raising children and therefore mourn the loss of closeness with gay friends engaged in very different activities. These new heterosexual friends may relate quickly to the lesbian couple's parenting experiences, but not understand their LGBTQ+-perspective and associated challenges.

Lesbians navigating a heterotypical healthcare system might be slower to share difficulties they are experiencing in the postpartum period, feeling the need to "put on a brave face" or else reaffirm bias held by the healthcare team. This reluctance to express when difficulties are mounting may impede the lesbian couple's referral to appropriate support resources, like lactation consultants, pelvic physical therapy specialists, and mental health professionals. Finally, obstetricians caring for lesbian parents in the postpartum window may be less likely to provide specific recommendations about resumption of sex than they would for heterosexual couples, leaving the lesbian couple to figure it out on their own. Stigmatization and internalized homophobia can leave the lesbian couple unsure how and when to proceed with sex and uncomfortable discussing it with their OB. Clearly, more research is needed to better understand the postpartum experiences of lesbian parents and develop appropriate policy and programmatic supports.

Legal considerations

At some point during preconception planning, pregnancy, or following the birth of their child, lesbian families must take additional legal steps to secure equal parental rights for the nonbiological lesbian parent and define or terminate the rights of a known sperm donor, if applicable. Currently, in most parts of the United States, the presumption that a child born within a marriage is the legal child of both parents protects only heterosexual families and does not apply automatically to lesbian families. Nonbiological lesbian parents who do not secure their parental rights through a legal mechanism cannot make healthcare or schooling decisions for their child. If their relationship were to end, the nonbiological lesbian parent could lose custody and visitation with the child.

To address this vulnerability, in some states, the nongestating lesbian parent can apply for a prebirth order. This is a document signed by a judge that legally establishes the parentage of a child. With this document, the nonbiological lesbian parent can be listed on the child's birth certificate, ensuring immediate and unrestricted access to the baby and the ability to make medical decisions. If lesbian parents are not able to obtain a prebirth order, they might be able pursue the legal mechanism of second-parent adoption to ensure equal parental rights. Second-parent adoption (also called "step-parent" adoption in some states) confers to the nonbirth parent the same legal rights and recognition as the birth parent. Importantly, some states granting second-parent adoptions require that the parties be legally married for some period of time to complete the adoption. This marital requirement represents another example of heteronormative standards being applied to nontraditional families and can represent another logistical and financial hurdle to overcome. Both prebirth orders and second-parent adoptions grant the nonbiological lesbian parent equal status in the eyes of the law, but are not available in all 50 states and thus cannot protect all lesbian families.

Securing these legal documents represents another financial and logistical barrier to parenthood not experienced by heterosexual couples. The lesbian couple must engage in more coordination and planning, finding and paying for an attorney with expertise in supporting LGBTQ+ family building. The term "second-parent" often feels demeaning, seemingly deprioritizing the nongestating partner who may already feel slighted. Undergoing a second-parent adoption home study can feel offensive to the lesbian couple who has lovingly and intentionally brought their baby into the world.

Access to paid maternity leave is a second major legal issue for lesbian parents. In the United States, paid maternity leave is not federally regulated, resulting in substantial variability in access to leave, duration of leave, and whether it is paid or unpaid. The majority of states lack any specific family leave laws and defer to the federal Family and Medical Leave Act (FMLA), which requires that parents be given 12 weeks per year of unpaid time off following the adoption or birth of a child. In 2015 the United States Department of Labor issued a statement clarifying that the nonbiological parent in a same-sex relationship is eligible for FMLA leave, even if she is not yet the legal adoptive parent of the child, provided the lesbian couple is considered legally married through marriage or common law [47]. Despite this legal protection, employers vary in how accepting they are of lesbians generally and lesbians pursuing parenthood specifically. Lesbians may find that their need to apply for parental leave requires them to become more "out" at work, a process which can feel scary and may even trigger frank discrimination. The workplace culture regarding same-sex parenting also can impact how accepted and supported she feels as a new parent.

A final legal factor to be considered by new parents in lesbian families is their last name. The lesbian couple must decide if they will each keep their last name, take the name of one partner, or hyphenate their last names. Further, they must decide which last name to give their child. Choosing to share the same last name can communicate family standing and unity to the outside world. A lesbian parent who shares the same last name as her child may find she is afforded greater acceptance when communicating with the child's school system or pediatrician's office. Some lesbian parents choose to give their child the last name of the nonbirth parent, a step that can increase sense of joining and connection between the child and that parent [48].

Policies, procedures, and practices to support lesbians pursuing parenthood

Given the implicit bias and explicit discrimination often faced by lesbians, we outline a number of recommended policies and procedures here. These recommendations are aimed at improving patient care, satisfaction with care, and ultimately healthcare outcomes of all LBGTQ+ families.

Recommendations for individual providers

- Seek training in providing culturally sensitive care to LGBTQ+ families. In addition to reading relevant literature, investigate training that may be offered online or through your institution. The Mental Health Professional Group of the ASRM offers an online Certificate Course for mental health professionals with a section on LGBTQ-specific family-building issues. The Family Equality Council also offers an excellent online professional training program, called Open Door, aimed at educating providers working with nontraditional families of multiple types.
- Become familiar with various routes to parenthood for LGBTQ+ patients and the risks and benefits associated with each option.
- Develop knowledge about relevant educational resources and community supports for LGBTQ+ patients planning and experiencing parenthood. These resources should include best books, websites, and social media groups, support groups (local or online; e.g., "Dykes and Tykes"; "Mombian: Sustenance for Lesbian Moms") and community centers as well as most supportive local medical practices, adoption agencies, and family law attorneys. The LGBTQ Parenting Network is a nonprofit organization that supports education, networking, research, and community events and is an excellent resource for providers and parents alike.
- Choose language carefully. Use the language used by patients: do they call their significant other "partner," "wife," or something else? Do they refer to becoming a "parent" rather than a "mother"?
- Ask about sexual orientation and gender identity. Ask about preferred pronouns. Ask about which partner will assume which role (e.g., egg source, person carrying the pregnancy), rather than making assumptions based on outward appearance or clothing choice. Approach conversations with openness and curiosity.
- Be alert for heteronormative assumptions and biases, including assuming that a woman has a male partner or that the other woman at an appointment is a support person rather than a romantic partner.
- For lesbian couples planning reciprocal IVF, do not use the heteronormative terms or paperwork that refer to "donor" and "recipient."
- Being mindful of lesbians' likely history of experiencing discrimination and potential to feel marginalized, recognize and engage the nonbiological lesbian parent in all discussions about family-building options. Remember that they will be actively engaged in parenting the future child and thus should be equally involved in the preconception process.
- Use accurate and sensitive language when referring patients using donor sperm to psychological consultation. Do not use the term "evaluation" and include a brief description of what the couple can expect (e.g., an educational meeting to discuss issues like donor selection, donor screening, how and when to disclose to a future child, mechanisms for getting more information about the donor should questions come up in the future, etc.).
- Screen for postpartum depression in new lesbian parents (both biological and nonbiological) just as should be done for heterosexual parents.
- Provide specific guidance about when sex can resume after delivery, just as would be done for heterosexual couples.

Recommendations for clinics and programs

Although individual providers must take personal responsibility for providing sensitive and inclusive care to LGBTQ+ patients, they must be aided by sensitive and inclusive practices in the places where they work.

- Offer staff at fertility centers, OBGYN practices, and pediatric practices training in providing care to LGBTQ+ patients. Assist providers in developing expertise in understanding the experience and needs of both lesbian parents. Training could include topics such as patients' life experiences, history of discrimination and bias, examples of unconscious bias, patients' psychological outcomes, family outcomes, and communication expectations/needs. Training should include not just providers but also appointment schedulers, medical support staff, nurses, billing and laboratory staff. Increasing the team's knowledge about diverse family types can increase not only their sensitivity but also their confidence in providing excellent clinical care.
- Include diverse images on clinic websites and in waiting rooms to create a more welcoming environment for LGBTQ+ patients.
- Review consent forms and intake paperwork for heteronormative language. Edit forms and electronic medical records to allow for a variety of gender identities and sexual orientations and to highlight preferred pronouns. These modifications allow staff to quickly recognize a patient's preferred identity in a greeting and thus make a good first impression.
- Offer LGBTQ+-inclusive centering pregnancy groups, childbirth, and new parent classes to improve the pregnancy experience of lesbian parents and increase their confidence with the transition to parenthood.
- To the extent possible, hire a diverse staff. Can LBGTQ+ patients see their own family types or identities in staff members? Do they feel represented in the clinic?

Conclusion

A series of positive changes have come together to make parenthood for lesbians more accessible than ever. Cultural evolution, scientific evidence of positive child and family outcomes, ART, and new legal protections now allow lesbians significantly greater access to family building. Despite these advances, the journey for lesbian parents-to-be continues to be more arduous, complex, expensive, and controversial than it is for heterosexuals. Significant work remains to be done to eliminate barriers, both obvious and subtle, for lesbians pursuing parenthood. The aim of this chapter is to outline the unique experiences and needs of lesbians becoming parents, identify barriers to care, and highlight strategies to address them. As with many systemic and cultural prejudices laid bare during the COVID-19 pandemic, the first steps in transforming care for lesbian parents begin with listening, asking questions, and building understanding. Well-informed and culturally sensitive providers engaging in this process of transformation can better respond to the needs of all families, creating a more inclusive healthcare environment for all.

Key takeaways

- Lesbian parents have similar positive adjustment to parenting when compared to heterosexual parents. Those who became parents after ART may even evidence greater positive affect than other families created through ART.
- Extensive research has debunked the myth that children raised in lesbian families show higher rates of psychopathology or difficulty with adjustment. Further, children raised by lesbian parents are not more likely to choose same-sex romantic relationships in adolescence or adulthood.
- The family-building journey is significantly more challenging for lesbian couples than for heterosexual couples. Lesbians must cope with overt and subtle discrimination and prejudice in society generally and in healthcare specifically. They must engage in a multifaceted decision-making process, navigate a more complex logistical process, and cope with greater financial expense.
- Interdisciplinary care of lesbians pursuing parenthood is critical and may include medical and nursing providers, mental health professionals, adoption coordinators, sperm bank employees, and legal representatives.
- Providers serving lesbians must seek training to become educated about their unique challenges and needs. Fertility clinics, OBGYN practices, and pediatric offices should enact systemic changes to explicitly welcome and appropriately support lesbians pursuing parenthood.

References

[1] GLAAD. GLAAD media reference guide—lesbian/gay/bisexual glossary of terms [Internet]. Available from: <https://www.glaad.org/reference/lgbtq>; 2016 [cited January 28, 2021].

[2] Golombok S. We are family: what really matters for parents and children. Scribe; 2020.

[3] Averett P, Nalavany B, Ryan S. An evaluation of gay/lesbian and heterosexual adoption. Adopt Q 2009;12(3–4):129–51.

[4] United States News & World Report [Internet]. Available from: <http://www.usnews.com/articles>; November 25, 2008 [cited January, 2021].

[5] Gurmankin AD, Caplan AL, Braverman AM. Screening practices and beliefs of assisted reproductive technology programs. Fertil Steril. 2005;83(1):61–7.

[6] Nicol N. Politics of the heart: recognition of homoparental families in Quebec. In: Epstein R, editor. Who's your daddy? and other writings on queer parenting. Sumac Press; 2009. p. 180–96.

[7] Epstein R. Space invaders: queer and trans bodies in fertility clinics. Sexualities 2018;21(7):1039–58.

[8] Johnson KM. Excluding lesbian and single women? An analysis of United States fertility clinic websites. Womens Stud Int Forum 2012;35(5):394–402.

[9] Golombok S, Spencer A, Rutter M. Children in lesbian and single-parent households: psychosexual and psychiatric appraisal. J Child Psychol Psychiatry 1983;24(4):551–72.

[10] Golombok S, Tasker F. Children in lesbian and gay families: theories and evidence. Annu Rev Sex Res 1994;5(1):73–100.

[11] Chan RW, Raboy B, Patterson CJ. Psychosocial adjustment among children conceived via donor insemination by lesbian and heterosexual mothers. Child Dev 1998;69(2):443–57.

[12] American Psychological Association (APA). Lesbian and gay parenting [Internet]. Available from: <https://www.apa.org/pi/lgbt/resources/parenting-full.pdf>; 2005 [cited 2021].

[13] Ethics Committee of the American Society for Reproductive Medicine. Access to fertility treatment by gays, lesbians, and unmarried persons: a committee opinion. Fertil Steril. 2013;100(6):1524–7.

[14] Carpinello OJ, Jacob MC, Nulsen J, Benadiva C. Utilization of fertility treatment and reproductive choices by lesbian couples. Fertil Steril. 2016;106(7):1709–13.

[15] Kleinert E, Martin O, Brähler E, Stöbel-Richter Y. Motives and decisions for and against having children among nonheterosexuals and the impact of experiences of discrimination, internalized stigma, and social acceptance. J Sex Res 2015;52(2):174–85.

[16] Boye K, Evertsson M. Who gives birth (first) in female same-sex couples in Sweden? J Marriage Fam 2020;83(4):925–42.

[17] Bos HM, Van Balen F, Van den Boom DC. Planned lesbian families: their desire and motivation to have children. Hum Reprod 2003;18(10):2216–24.

[18] Bos HM, Van Balen F, Van, den Boom DC. Experience of parenthood, couple relationship, social support, and child-rearing goals in planned lesbian mother families. J Child Psychol Psychiatr 2004;45(4):755–64.

[19] Holley SR, Pasch LA. Counseling lesbian, gay, bisexual, and transgender patients. Fertility counseling: clinical guide and case studies. Cambridge University Press; 2015. p. 180–96.

[20] Ryan M. The gender of pregnancy: masculine lesbians talk about reproduction. J Lesbian Stud 2013;17(2):119–33.

[21] Gates GJ. LGBT parenting in the United States [Internet]. Williams Institute, UCLA School of Law. Available from: <https://williamsinstitute.law.ucla.edu/publications/lgbt-parenting-us/>; 2013 [cited January 31, 2021].

[22] Bowles N. The sperm kings have a problem: too much demand [Internet]. The New York Times. Available from: <https://www.nytimes.com/2021/01/08/business/sperm-donors-facebook-groups.html>; 2021 [cited January 31, 2021].

[23] Baetens P, Brewaeys A. Lesbian couples requesting donor insemination: an update of the knowledge with regard to lesbian mother families. Hum Reprod Update 2001;7(5):512–19.

[24] Nelson MK, Hertz R, Kramer W. Gamete donor anonymity and limits on numbers of offspring: the views of three stakeholders. J Law Biosci 2016;3(1):39–67.

[25] Beaurepaire J, Jones M, Thiering P, Saunders D, Tennant C. Psychosocial adjustment to infertility and its treatment: male and female responses at different stages of IVF/ET treatment. J Psychosom Res 1994;38(3):229–40.

[26] Discover infertility treatment coverage by US state [Internet]. Infertility coverage by state. RESOLVE. Available from: <https://resolve.org/what-are-my-options/insurance-coverage/infertility-coverage-state/#:~:text=As%20of%20August%202020%2C%2019,(medically%2Dinduced)%20infertility>; 2020 [cited January 19, 2021].

[27] Evers JL. Female subfertility. Lancet. 2002;360(9327):151–9.

[28] The United States Census Bureau. Income, poverty and health insurance coverage in the United States: 2019 [Internet]. The United States Census Bureau. Available from: <https://www.census.gov/newsroom/press-releases/2020/income-poverty.html>; 2020 [cited January 28, 2021].

[29] Blanchfield BV, Patterson CJ. Racial and sexual minority women's receipt of medical assistance to become pregnant. Health Psychol 2015;34(6):571.

[30] Marvel S, Tarasoff L, Epstein R, Green DC, Steele L, Ross L. Listening to LGBTQ people on assisted human reproduction: access to reproductive material, services, and facilities. In: Lemmens T, editor. Regulating creation: the law, ethics, and policy of assisted human reproduction. University of Toronto Press; 2016.

[31] Ross LE, Tarasoff LA, Anderson S, Epstein R, Marvel S, Steele LS. Sexual and gender minority peoples' recommendations for assisted human reproduction services. J Obstet Gynaecol Can 2014;36(2):146–53.

[32] Wu HY, Yin O, Monseur B, Selter J, Collins LJ, Lau BD, et al. Lesbian, gay, bisexual, transgender content on reproductive endocrinology and infertility clinic websites. Fertil Steril. 2017;108(1):183–91.

[33] Blohm F, Friden B, Milsom I. A prospective longitudinal population-based study of clinical miscarriage in an urban Swedish population. BJOG 2008;115(2):176–82.

[34] Wojnar D. Miscarriage experiences of lesbian couples. J Midwifery Womens Health 2007;52(5):479–85.

[35] Rubio B, Vecho O, Gross M, Van Rijn-van Gelderen L, Bos H, Ellis-Davies K, et al. Transition to parenthood and quality of parenting among gay, lesbian and heterosexual couples who conceived through assisted reproduction. J Family Stud 2020;26(3):422–40.

[36] Röndahl G, Bruhner E, Lindhe J. Heteronormative communication with lesbian families in antenatal care, childbirth and postnatal care. J Adv Nurs 2009;65(11):2337–44.

[37] Deave T, Johnson D. The transition to parenthood: what does it mean for fathers? J Adv Nurs 2008;63(6):626–33.

[38] Wojnar DM, Katzenmeyer A. Experiences of preconception, pregnancy, and new motherhood for lesbian nonbiological mothers. J Obstet Gynecol Neonatal Nurs 2014;43(1):50–60.

[39] Stewart M. "We just want to be ordinary": lesbian parents talk about their birth experiences. Midwifery Dig 2002;12(3):415–18.

[40] Buchholz SE. Experiences of lesbian couples during childbirth. Nurs Outlook 2000;48(6):307–11.

[41] Ross LE, Steele LS, Epstein R. Service use and gaps in services for lesbian and bisexual women during donor insemination, pregnancy, and the postpartum period. J Obstet Gynaecol Can 2006;28(6):505–11.

[42] Gavin NI, Gaynes BN, Lohr KN, Meltzer-Brody S, Gartlehner G, Swinson T. Perinatal depression: a systematic review of prevalence and incidence. Obstet Gynecol 2005;106(5 Part 1):1071–83.

[43] Ross LE, Steele L, Goldfinger C, Strike C. Perinatal depressive symptomatology among lesbian and bisexual women. Arch Womens Ment Health 2007;10(2):53–9.

[44] Melrose S. Paternal postpartum depression: how can nurses begin to help? Contemp Nurse 2010;34(2):199–210.

[45] O'hara MW, Swain AM. Rates and risk of postpartum depression—a meta-analysis. Int Rev Psychiatry 1996;8(1):37–54.

[46] Robertson E, Grace S, Wallington T, Stewart DE. Antenatal risk factors for postpartum depression: a synthesis of recent literature. Gen Hosp Psychiatry 2004;26(4):289–95.

[47] Kastrinsky HM. DOL: Proposed Rule to Change Definition of Spouse for FMLA Purposes; Persuader Rules Imminent• OFCCP: New Pay Reporting Rules for Federal Contractors; Directive Against Transgender Discrimination Restated• OSHA: MOU Reached with Federal Motor Carrier Safety Administration; Temporary Worker Initiative Stressed; Electronic Record-Keeping Proposal Delayed• Executive Orders: Federal Contractors Required to Self-Report Employment-Law Violations; Discrimination by Federal Contractors Prohibited Against LGBT Employees. Employ Relat Today 2015;41(4):67–76.

[48] Mason Bergen K, Suter EA, Daas KL. "About as solid as a fish net": symbolic construction of a legitimate parental identity for nonbiological lesbian mothers. J Family Commun 2006;6(3):201–20.

CHAPTER 9

Gay men, as individuals and as a community, overcoming reproductive challenges to have children

Guy Ringler[1] and Cyd Zeigler[2]

[1]California Fertility Partners, Los Angeles, CA, United States [2]Department of Journalism and Communication, University of Florida, Gainesville, FL, United States

Article

The conception of a human being that results from the sexual expression of love shared between a man and a woman is a beautiful idea that we are taught as young people as a goal. However, for many individuals the route to a family can take different paths.

The desire to reproduce is biologically instilled and can be ignited at an early age. Our culture teaches young men and women—through our families, our society, and the media [1]—that pregnancies should be planned and conceived through the intimate expression of our love for our life partners. While the messages we collectively send young people are expanding in this area, a perceived ideal continues to be messaged.

Young men who feel a desire to have children but who do not have a sexual attraction to women can experience distress and anxiety as they come to terms with their sexuality. About 40–50 years ago there were no options for gay men to have children unless they had sex with, and usually married, a woman to reproduce. The realization that one may not be able to have children of their own—at least through sexual intercourse—can increase the angst that often accompanies one's acceptance of their sexuality. This is true not just for the young gay or queer man but also for his family members who have dreams of grandchildren, or nieces and nephews.

The make-up of American families shifted in the latter half of the 20th century as more lesbian women and gay men were developing families of their own. In 1968 a gay man, Bill Jones, became the first single man to adopt a child in California and one of the first in the country. A decade later, in the late 1970s, New York became the first state to not reject adoption applications solely because of sexual orientation.

During the past two decades the family-building and reproductive options for gay men have significantly expanded, allowing men to have children and providing hope for young gay men faced with fears of being childless because of their sexuality. In this chapter we will discuss how gay men today are building families of their own.

Progress in acceptance and law for gay men

Over the last five decades gay men have achieved great progress in various parts of the world overcoming obstacles, including lack of acceptance of their sexual identity and lifestyle, the worldwide transmission of HIV, and laws against same-sex marriage. Each of these challenges has taken years of struggle and fight to achieve progress, and the end result is that gay men today—in many parts of the world—have greater freedoms, acceptance, and choices than ever before.

Of course, there is still a long way to go for the vast majority of gay men around the world to achieve sexual-orientation equality. While Americans have over the last decade argued over the right to marry, LGBT people in places like Iran and Jamaica fight for the right to simply live their lives openly [2]. Places like China are built on cultures that frown upon homosexuality and refuse to recognize relationships, even if their governments don't criminalize them.

Yet in much of Western culture, young gay men today can live freely, be accepted by their communities, date the men of their choice, and have the opportunity to marry or form a civil union if desired. Never before have so many gay men had the opportunity to pursue lives filled with personal fulfilment.

An additional freedom of LGBT people includes the option to have children and to build a family of their own. Since the 1970s many gay men have successfully adopted children despite facing numerous challenges, including legal blockades, most notably initiated by singer Anita Bryant's "Save our Children" campaign that resulted in a ban on adoption by "practicing homosexuals" in many jurisdictions in Florida. Several Supreme Court cases over the last decade, most notably *Pavan v. Smith* out of Arkansas, established a federal right for same-sex couples to marry and have their marriage treated equally [3]. Still, that right remains under attack as South Carolina was granted a waiver by the federal government in 2019 opening the door to discrimination [4].

For gay men who want to adopt children, the process involves contacting an adoption agency. Because lingering prejudices against the idea of gay men or same-sex male couples raising children persist, regardless of the law gay men are forced to navigate this dynamic in a way that straight people and opposite-sex couples often do not [5].

Emerging assisted reproductive technologies give gay men hope of a family

The development of assisted reproductive technologies (ART), such as in vitro fertilization (IVF) in which eggs are fertilized in a petri dish, has significantly changed the reproductive outlook for many individuals with fertility issues. Obstacles to getting pregnant such as blocked fallopian tubes, low sperm count, and pelvic adhesions can be bypassed by IVF, providing patients a previously unobtainable chance for pregnancy. One of the most important factors influencing the success rate of IVF is the age of the woman producing the eggs.

For patients with poor-quality eggs, low numbers of eggs, or without eggs, the use of donated eggs can provide an opportunity for conception. IVF with eggs from an egg donor allows gay or single men to create embryos for future transfer into a surrogate.

The first IVF baby was born in 1978 [6]. The use of donated eggs from a young woman to allow conception was first reported in 1980, and became clinically available in the early 1990s. The use of eggs recovered from healthy young egg donors, who are usually in their twenties, to create embryos provides very high pregnancy rates due to the high egg quality and high incidence of genetically normal (euploid) eggs obtained [7].

The emergence of gestational surrogacy, in which a genetically unrelated embryo is transferred into the uterus of an unrelated woman to allow conception, allows individuals without a uterus, patients with an abnormal uterine environment, or patients with systemic factors interfering with conception and development of a pregnancy, to have a child of their own.

In the mid-1990s, some bright, creative, and motivated gay men sought the assistance of fertility specialists to utilize the advances in reproductive medicine to help them have babies. Specifically, they wanted to create embryos using their sperm and the eggs of a selected egg donor, followed by embryo transfer into a gestational surrogate. The egg donor serves to bypass their lack of ovaries, and the surrogate gets around their inability to carry a pregnancy.

The issue of assisting gay men to have children was a question the medical community had not addressed before, and it was met with resistance from many medical professionals within the specialty. At the time, the field of reproductive medicine was still evolving and the availability of fertility services was considered to be inadequate to meet the needs of heterosexual individuals who needed fertility treatments to overcome their infertility. As a result, some fertility specialists felt that assisted reproductive procedures should be reserved for these patients [8].

I was first approached by a gay couple to help them have a baby through egg donation (a sister of one of the partners) and surrogacy (their neighbor) in the mid-1990s. Due to the resistance within the reproductive community at that time to treat gay couples, I sought the counsel of my former professor at the University of Pennsylvania as to whether or not my treating this couple could have a political impact on my medical career. He advised me to do what we were trained to do: help my patients with their medical needs and their desire to start a family. At that time there were several other open-minded and compassionate fertility specialists who also agreed to help gay men fulfill their dreams of having children.

In 2017 the Society for Assisted Reproductive Technology began tracking the gender of intended parents who were using gestational surrogates. That year they reported 1240 in the United States were men, and that number increased 38% to 1701 in 2018. [Oral communication, November 5, 2020, Mark Leondires, M.D., Reproductive Medicine Associates of Connecticut.]

Since the first cases in the mid-1990s, many gay men have made considerable efforts to pursue having children through surrogacy. While some fertility doctors have continued to avoid working with gay men—one 2017 study showed only 53% of fertility clinics in the United States marketed to the LGBTQ community on their websites—broader cultural and legal issues over the use of surrogacy abound [9]. In the United States there is a patchwork of legal hurdles to navigate. Some states, like California, have ideal laws for the intended parents, with compensation for surrogates fully legal and contract law recognizing the intended parents as the parents in a legal surrogacy arrangement. In one state—Michigan—compensated surrogacy is illegal. Other states have various levels of legal protections for the intended parents.

The evolving landscape of fertility treatments for gay men

Around the world, the legal issues are equally in flux. For years India had been an option for intended parents. Today, no foreigners can engage in commercial surrogacy in the country after the government banned surrogacy for anyone but residents of India [10]. In Italy, not only is surrogacy banned but marketing and conversation around the practice is banned as well. I've personally experienced protests and threats of arrest for simply discussing the topic in Italy, a combination of both legal issues and a culture founded in the Catholic Church. The basis for the Catholic Church's opposition to surrogacy oscillates, depending on the particular situation, from claiming concern for the bodies of impoverished women to an opposition to procreation without opposite-gender sex [11].

To be sure, both the cultural and legal acceptance of access to surrogacy by gay men—in addition to the increased acceptance of surrogacy access for everyone—seems to be building. It was only in 2020 that the State of New York made compensated surrogacy legal, after self-described feminists and political conservatives had joined together to stop its legalization for years. Ultimately a coalition of LGBTQ and non-LGBTQ people, led by State Senator Brad Hoylman, a gay man who had himself found fatherhood through surrogacy, was able to pass the Child-Parent Security Act of 2020 legalizing compensated surrogacy in the state.

This patchwork of acceptance has caused widespread problems beyond just access to surrogacy. Many gay men like Hoylman, who live in a jurisdiction with less-favorable surrogacy laws, will go elsewhere. I have personally helped men from across Europe, Asia, and North America become fathers in part because surrogacy is not legal where they live. Some of them face legal issues naturalizing their children, or even returning home with their baby, further complicating their struggles [12].

Although the social and legal aspects of gay family building have slowly evolved over the last few decades, the clinical science of reproductive medicine has made rapid advances resulting in higher pregnancy rates than ever before. Changes in embryo culture conditions, improvements in embryo freeze/thaw protocols, increased experience by embryologists in embryo biopsy for genetic testing, as well as improved sensitivity and accuracy of genetic screening tests, have all contributed to better outcomes for all patients undergoing IVF [13].

The pregnancy rates are very high because of the young age of the egg donors, and the highly receptive uterine environment for embryo implantation provided by the surrogate—preferably a woman with a history of proven fertility. Reports on genetic testing of embryos from egg donors under the age of 35 have shown that approximately 60%–70% are normal [14]. These high-quality embryos are then transferred into the optimal uterine environment provided by the gestational carrier. The chances for pregnancy increase if that surrogate has a history of proven reproductive success.

Over the past 25 years since the initial treatment cycles, advances in all aspects of IVF have served to improve overall pregnancy rates. In our practice we achieve approximately 70% live-birth rate per single-embryo transfer. In addition, the access to fertility care for the LGBT community has greatly improved as the reproductive medical community has opened its collective doors to gay men and lesbian women seeking fertility services. An editorial published in Fertility and Sterility in 2007 titled "Should we be treating gay patients?" [8] seems almost antiquated today. By 2013 the Ethics Committee of the American Society for Reproductive Medicine (ASRM) penned an opinion that gay men should have access to ART for their own reproductive interests, and the committee said there was "no scientific evidence" to support fears that gay men may not be able to parent children as effectively as their heterosexual counterparts [15]. In the 1990s there were only a handful of IVF programs accepting gay patients. Today prospective dads can find clinics across the country willing to help them with fertility treatments.

Still, various fiscal elements can present seemingly insurmountable hurdles for many. Given the high cost of IVF with surrogacy, gay men can expect to pay approximately 150–200 thousand dollars for the entire process, depending on various elements, including travel, selection of the egg donor, legal fees, and various concierge services. Medical complications during or after birth can double or triple those numbers. Today, more and more insurance plans—particularly those created for forward-looking companies, many of them in Silicon Valley—are designed to help cover some of these costs. In addition, there are organizations that work with intended parents to lower costs by creating discounts with providers and fundraising to build "scholarship" programs [16].

Despite these challenges, the approach many gay men take to the process is one of positivity that is often very different from the approach of heterosexuals to the process. Heterosexual intended parents often come into the field after many failed treatment cycles and are emotionally and physically broken down when they start treatment. Infertility treatment can make some individuals feel less attractive and less sexual by all of the medical investigations, probing, and attention [17]. Fertility treatment has been attributed as a potential cause or aggravator of sexual dysfunction for heterosexual couples [18]. Conversely, gay men often view surrogacy as an opportunity, as opposed to a last resort. As a result, many surrogates have found gay couples to be much more appreciative and easier to work with than heterosexual couples who approach the process only after many years of failed cycles.

The process of gestational surrogacy pregnancy in five steps

Family building for gay men—as well as others pursing third-party reproduction—takes a team of professionals to successfully coordinate these complex treatment cycles.

The team includes a fertility specialist, sperm providers (for gay men, usually an intended parent), an egg-donor agency, a surrogacy agency, and reproductive attorneys. The agencies provide egg donor and surrogate candidates, arrange preliminary screenings, and assist the intended parents with egg-donor selection and surrogate matches. All of that comes together through contracts and agreements written by lawyers with expertise in reproductive law.

Prospective parents planning their family through assisted reproduction should start the process by meeting with a respected fertility specialist working in an IVF program with extensive experience in third-party reproduction.

It is essential that LGBT individuals are treated with acceptance and respect within all levels of the medical practice, including the receptionists, phlebotomists, nurses, physicians, and other staff members. Fertility treatment is a very personal process for all patients, but especially for gay individuals who may have faced discrimination and prejudices during their development and coming out journeys. They deserve respect and tolerance during their treatment.

The process of family building for gay men is straightforward and can be broken down into five steps.

The first step is to have a semen analysis to assess the quantity and quality of the sperm. If the semen analysis is normal, one can freeze the sperm for use in the IVF cycle. For men with a severe defect in sperm quantity and/or quality, a referral to a reproductive urologist is given to evaluate the cause of the sperm abnormality, and to provide treatment. For these patients, a fresh semen specimen at the time of egg retrieval may be recommended. Most men take pride in finding out their sperm parameters are normal, and can be disappointed if not, though one study in the Asian Journal of Andrology argues that gay men are either unaffected, or may even be psychologically buoyed, by low sperm count [19]. If an intended father's sperm count is low, it's helpful to have a discussion about lifestyle changes and supplements that may improve their sperm and future embryo health.

Men providing sperm to create embryos for transfer into a surrogate must complete infectious-disease-screening tests, a physical exam, and a health-and-lifestyle questionnaire outlined by the United States Food and Drug Administration in the United States. The intended father also has blood drawn for genetic-carrier screening. Knowledge of mutations for recessive genetic disease is imperative before confirming an egg donor for the process to help prevent disease in the children.

Same-sex male couples have the unique option of having the choice to use the sperm from one or both prospective fathers to procreate their family. This important decision is based in part upon the individuals' desires to have a biological connection to their child or not. The count and quality of sperm from the two prospective fathers can also play a role in decision making. Many couples decide to split the eggs into two groups and inseminate half of the eggs with each intended parent's sperm. After embryos are created, they can decide whether to transfer one or two embryos, using one prospective father's sperm or one from each patient.

Some gay couples have asked if they can mix their sperm together before inseminating the eggs of their donor. It's possible, but this is not recommended for several reasons. Adding sperm of lower motility to a normal specimen can negatively impact the outcome by decreasing the ratio of highly motile sperm. In addition, a semen specimen with lower quality sperm could have substances present in the semen which could exert a negative impact on the higher quality sperm. Not knowing from which man the sperm came also hinders the ability of a doctor to assess sperm impact if there are suboptimal results, and it also precludes us from knowing the genetic identity of the child until after birth.

Today, most physicians recommend, and most couples opt for, a single-embryo transfer, to minimize the risk for twins, which increases the risk of many complications during the pregnancy. In this scenario the intended fathers need to decide which intended parent will be the first biological father, and who will delay their biological conception. Often this decision is based upon which intended dad feels the greatest desire to have a child, perhaps the person who initiated the process for the couple. Increasingly, gay men who want twins are urged to engage with two surrogates simultaneously. This allows the couple to have twins born usually days apart while avoiding potential medical complications often brought on by twins carried by the same woman [20].

The second step is selection of the egg donor. There are many egg-donor agencies in the United States today that provide candidates for the treatment process. The donors are healthy women, generally between the ages of 21 and 34, who offer to donate their eggs (usually for a price) from a menstrual cycle to the recipient or intended parent. The eggs then become the legal property of the intended parent. In the United States, these agencies provide the intended parents with photographs of prospective egg donors, personal background, and lifestyle information, as well as family medical history. The donors may be anonymous, known to the intended parents, or something in between. Once a candidate is selected, she completes medical screening that includes psychological evaluation, genetic testing, physical exam, ovarian reserve testing, infectious disease screening, and urine drug testing. Guidelines for the medical screening of egg donor candidates have been published by the American Society for Reproductive Medicine [21].

Once the donor has been medically cleared for treatment and has signed contracts and consents, and United States Food and Drug Administration-mandated medical tests are completed, the IVF treatment cycle begins, commencing the third step.

During the treatment cycle the donor takes daily injections of follicle-stimulating hormone and human-menopausal gonadotropins to stimulate the development of the eggs that her ovaries recruited for that month. The donor is monitored by serial ultrasounds and blood tests to determine the best time to retrieve the eggs. She is usually ready for the surgical procedure of egg retrieval approximately 11–12 days after starting the medications.

The egg retrieval is a short surgical procedure performed under intravenous sedation and takes about 20 minutes. The incidence of complications is low and most patients recover quickly over the few days after surgery [22].

On the day of egg retrieval, vials of sperm from the intended dads are thawed, and several hours after the egg retrieval, the eggs are inseminated. The fertilization rate of mature eggs is approximately 75%. Once fertilized, the embryos are cultured over the next 6–7 days until the blastocyst stage, when they can be frozen through vitrification, biopsied for preimplantation genetic testing (PGT), or transferred directly into the surrogate's hormonally prepared uterus. In most IVF programs today, all embryos are frozen and stored until transfer into the surrogate at a later date. With today's advanced vitrification protocols, pregnancy rates using frozen embryos are the same, or even higher, than using fresh embryos [23].

Although clinical studies have not yet demonstrated that PGT of embryos created with donor eggs can significantly improve live birth rates, most intended parents working with us elect to have their embryos tested, as a screen for Down's syndrome and other chromosomal abnormalities. PGT also reveals the gender of the embryos, which can be helpful for family planning.

Step four is to find a surrogate to carry the pregnancy. The United States is the world leader in gestational surrogacy due to the legal framework in many states and the high quality of reproductive medical care available today. There are many surrogacy agencies that provide gestational carriers for intended parents. These agencies conduct the initial recruitment and social screening of the surrogate candidates, and some preliminary medical screening to include collection of all prior pregnancy medical records.

Once a match is made, the surrogate is referred to an IVF clinic to complete her medical screening. The fertility specialist will review all of her prior pregnancy records and perform a physical exam, uterine evaluation, infectious disease screening, and urine drug screening. Clinical guidelines for the evaluation and screening of gestational carriers have been published by ASRM [24].

The medical screening includes evaluation by a mental-health professional to assess her suitability for the surrogacy process. After she is medically cleared, she receives consultation with a reproductive attorney. Once legal contracts between the surrogate and intended parents are complete, they proceed to step five: the embryo transfer.

To prepare the surrogate for the embryo transfer she is given hormones in amounts to mimic the natural menstrual cycle. She starts with 2 weeks of estrogen to thicken the endometrial lining, followed by progesterone to make the lining receptive to embryo implantation. On the sixth day of progesterone, in the middle of the window of implantation, an embryo is thawed and transferred into the uterine cavity under ultrasound guidance [25]. Once a pregnancy is established, she will be maintained on hormone supplementation until the placenta becomes functional, which usually occurs by the 11th week of pregnancy.

Sexualizing the gestational-surrogacy process for gay men

Making a baby for gay couples is not literally a sexual experience, as it is for heterosexual couples, but it can still evolve as an act of love for each other and their future family. My first gay couple wanted to use the eggs from one of the intended dad's sisters, with his partner's sperm, so the child would be a mixture of their family genetics and to them conceived as an act of love.

Because gay men use assisted reproduction to conceive their baby, they must plan personally and financially for the process. They cannot have a child through unplanned sex or after a wild weekend of sexual release. Gay men must investigate their treatment options, interview a team of professionals, and commit a significant amount of money before they can begin the process. For the intended fathers, each of these steps can be seen as an act of love for their future child, and for each other, in contrast to the heterosexual couple who have failed to conceive through their own love-making attempts and now are turning to assisted reproduction often with a sense of disappointment and failure. That sense of failure for opposite-sex couples can in turn lead to deeper issues in the sexual relationship [26].

To initiate the treatment process, men masturbate into a cup to assess their sperm quantity and quality, and for possible freezing. This sexual act is usually conducted in a doctor's office or laboratory, often with the visual assistance of pornography and not sexual stimulation provided by one's partner. It is not an act of love making, but rather a specimen-collection procedure.

Whether or not individuals attempt to make this experience a sexual expression of love for their partner and not just a physiologic act, has not been documented. A prospective dad recently told me that due to COVID-19, their doctor advised them to go to a local hotel to collect their specimens. Instead, they went to their car in a private office parking lot to give their specimens. They found the experience funny and turned it into an erotic adventure. They shared a memory that will be told to close friends for years to come of how they "conceived" their child.

Throughout the treatment process gay men are updated on the status of their sperm, eggs, and embryos, to keep them as an active participant in the process. The intended dads may have an open or closed agreement with their egg donor, but always meet and remain in contact with their surrogate during the process. Prior to the COVID-19 pandemic, intended parents were usually present in the embryo transfer room, which allowed them to share the intimate moment of conception with their surrogate. During the pandemic we ask the surrogates if they would like to use Facetime with the intended parents to have them virtually present for the transfer procedure. Most surrogates are happy to have them present, and former patients have told me how important this experience was for them. Although the embryo transfer is not a sexual experience it can be a very intimate and emotionally impactful day for both intended parents and gestational carriers.

Broader societal implications of gay men having children

The societal impact of gay men having children has both mirrored and contributed to increased cultural acceptance of same-sex couples. In 2013 a Gallup poll showed only 53% of Americans believed same-sex couples should have equal marriage rights to opposite-sex couples; just 5 years later that had increased to 67%. Also, via Gallup, in 2003 only 49% of Americans felt gay men should be allowed to adopt children. By 2019 that was 75%. Just recently it was reported that Pope Francis, the head of the Catholic Church, stated that he supports the civil union of gay couples and is supportive of gay family building [27]. While the church has made clear the Pope did not change Catholic doctrine, his statement is a dramatic shift from the positions of previous Popes.

Anecdotally, surrogates have shared with me how proud they are to help gay men have children, and they share that pride with their families, friends, and local communities. These women become ambassadors, of sorts, for the LGBTQ community, helping to normalize the idea of gay men having children often in smaller towns and rural areas that may not have a strong local LGBTQ community.

In China, where homosexuality is still widely rejected [28], we've noticed an interesting phenomenon. Multiple Chinese patients of mine have reported that they were afraid to share anything about their gay life, including their partner, with their parents. Yet once their surrogate was pregnant and a baby was on the way, they used that moment to introduce their partner and announce the arrival of a baby. In these cases, the instant love of a newborn in Chinese families has overcome any negative feelings they might have about their son's same-sex relationship. They are simply excited to be grandparents. It's been a powerful tool for many gay men in China to build open, honest relationships with their parents and help shift culture one family at a time.

All of this has been buoyed by research showing the success of gay men as parents. Susan Golombok, Professor of Family Research and director of the Centre for Family Research at the University of Cambridge, expanded this field of study by evaluating the quality of parent-child relationships, child adjustment, and child sex-typed behavior in adopted children raised in families headed by two gay men, two lesbian women, and two heterosexual people. She reported more positive parental wellbeing and parenting in gay-father families when compared to heterosexual families [29]. In addition, child-externalizing problems were greater in children in heterosexual families. These findings demonstrated the ability of gay fathers to successfully parent young children in a healthy, supportive environment.

There was no difference in sex-typed behavior between children with gay fathers and children with lesbian mothers or heterosexual parents. This is consistent with other studies and supports the conclusion that the sexual orientation of a parent does not influence the gender development of children.

An extensive longitudinal study published this year by Mazrekaj et al., analyzed all the children born in the Netherlands from 1998 to 2007 [30]. They followed the educational performance of 2971 children raised from birth with same-sex parents and over one million children from heterosexual parents. They found that the children raised by same sex parents performed better in both primary and secondary education than those raised in different-sex parent homes.

The increase in parenting interest among gay men has led to greater cultural acceptance, and that greater acceptance has generated more interest in parenthood. Once a distant dream, having biological children is now an achievable goal for many gay men who want to become parents. Young gay men who are struggling to accept their sexuality and balancing their desire to have children someday can find some peace knowing there is a way to achieve both—happy personal lives and becoming parents.

References

[1] Signiorielli N, Morgan M. Television and the family: the cultivation perspective. In: Bryant J, Bryant JA, editors. Television and the American family. 2nd ed. Mahwah, NJ: Lawrence Earlbaum Associates; 2001. p. 333–42.

[2] Yadegarfard M. How are Iranian gay men coping with systematic suppression under Islamic law? A qualitative study. Sex Cult 2019;23(4):1250–73. Available from: https://doi.org/10.1007/s12119-019-09613-7.

[3] Sanders S. Pavan v. Smith: Equality for gays and lesbians in being married, not just in getting married. 2016–2017 ACS Supreme Court Review 161, 2017.

[4] Tatum S, Flaherty A. Trump administration, South Carolina sued over gay couple turned away by religious foster care agency. ABC News, May 31, 2019.

[5] Massey SG, Merriwether AM, Garcia JR. Modern prejudice and same-sex parenting: shifting judgments in positive and negative parenting situations. J GLBT Fam Stud 2013;9(2):129–51. Available from: https://doi.org/10.1080/1550428X.2013.765257.

[6] Dow K. Now she's just an ordinary baby': the birth of IVF in the British Press. Sociology 2019;53(2):314–29.

[7] Wang YA, Farquhar C, Sullivan EA. Donor age is a major determinant of success of oocyte donation/recipient programme. Hum Reprod 2012;27(1):118–25.

[8] Greenfeld D. Gay male couples and assisted reproduction: should we assist? Fertil Steril 2007;88(1):18–20.

[9] Wu HY, Yin O, Monseur B, Selter J, Collins LJ, Lau BD, et al. Lesbian, gay, bisexual, transgender content on reproductive endocrinology and infertility clinic websites. Fertil Steril 2017;108(1):183–91.

[10] Huber S, Karandikar S, Gezinski L. Exploring Indian surrogates' perceptions of the ban on international surrogacy. Affilia 2018;33(1):69–84. Available from: https://doi.org/10.1177/0886109917729667.

[11] Aznar J, Martínez Peris M. Gestational surrogacy: current view. Linacre Q 2019;86(1):56–67. Available from: https://doi.org/10.1177/0024363919830840.

[12] Wendy N, Hudson N, Culley L. Gay men seeking surrogacy to achieve parenthood. Reprod Biomed Online J 2013;27(3):271–9. Available from: https://doi.org/10.1016/j.rbmo.2013.03.016.

[13] Eskew AM, Jungheim ES. A history of developments to improve in vitro fertilization. Mo Med 2017;114(3):156–9.

[14] Ovation Laboratory. Genetic statistics and laboratory performance report. Study examining normality of embryos at California Fertility Partners and other fertility clinics. Study examined 55 samples from January 2020 to June 2020.

[15] The Ethics Committee of the American Society for Reproductive Medicine. Access to fertility treatment by gays, lesbians, and unmarried persons: a committee opinion. Fertil Steril 2013;100(6):1524–7. Available from: https://doi.org/10.1016/j.fertnstert.2013.08.042.

[16] LGBTQ-friendly organizations offering grants and other financial assistance include The Family Formation Charitable Trust, Journey to Parenthood and Nest Egg Foundation. Men having babies offers assistance to gay and bisexual men specifically.

[17] Hasanpoor-Azghdy SB, Simbar M, Vedadhir A. The emotional-psychological consequences of infertility among infertile women seeking treatment: results of a qualitative study. Iran J Reprod Med 2014;12(2):131–8.

[18] Lara LA, Fuentealba-Torres M, dos Reis RM, Cartagena-Ramos D. Impact of infertility on the sexuality of couples: an overview. Curr Sex Health Rep 2018;10:353–9. Available from: https://doi.org/10.1007/s11930-018-0182-1.

[19] Wibowo E, Johnson TW, Wassersug RJ. Infertility, impotence, and emasculation—psychosocial contexts for abandoning reproduction. Asian J Androl 2016;18(3):403–8. Available from: https://doi.org/10.4103/1008-682X.173937.

[20] Gao L, Lyu SP, Zhao XR, Wu Y, Hua RY, Wang S, et al. Systematic management of twin pregnancies to reduce pregnancy complications. Chin Med J (Engl) 2020;133(11):1355–7. Available from: http://doi.org/10.1097/CM9.0000000000000808.

[21] Gorrill MJ, Johnson LK, Patton PE, Burry KA. Oocyte donor screening: the selection process and cost analysis. Fertil Steril 2001;75(2):400–4. Available from: https://doi.org/10.1016/s0015-0282(00)01711-8 PMID: 11172847.

[22] Bodri D, Guillén JJ, Polo A, Trullenque M, Esteve C, Coll O. Complications related to ovarian stimulation and oocyte retrieval in 4052 oocyte donor cycles. Reprod Biomed Online 2008;17(2):237–43. Available from: https://doi.org/10.1016/s1472-6483(10)60200-3.

[23] Pavone ME, Innes J, Hirshfeld-Cytron J, Kazer R, Zhang J. Comparing thaw survival, implantation and live birth rates from cryopreserved zygotes, embryos and blastocysts. J Hum Reprod Sci 2011;4(1):23–8. Available from: https://doi.org/10.4103/0974-1208.82356.

[24] Practice Committee of the American Society for Reproductive Medicine and the Practice Committee for the Society for Assisted Reproductive Technology. Recommendations for practices utilizing gestational carriers: an ASRM Practice Committee guideline. Fertil Steril 2012;97(6):1301–8.

[25] Practice Committee of the American Society for Reproductive Medicine and Practice Committee of the Society for Assisted Reproductive Technology. Recommendations for practices utilizing gestational carriers: a committee opinion. Fertil Steril 2017;107(2):e3–e10. Available from: https://doi.org/10.1016/j.fertnstert.2016.11.007.

[26] Tao P, Coates R, Maycock B. The impact of infertility on sexuality: a literature review. Australas Med J 2011;4(11):620–7.

[27] Povoledo E. Vatican clarifies Pope Francis's comments on same-sex unions. New York Times, November 2, 2020.

[28] Wang Y, Hu Z, Peng K, Rechdan J, Yang Y, Wu L, et al. Mapping out a spectrum of the Chinese public's discrimination toward the LGBT community: results from a national survey. BMC Public Health 2020;20(1):669. Available from: https://doi.org/10.1186/s12889-020-08834-y.

[29] Golombok S, Mellish L, Jennings S, Casey P, Tasker F, Lamb ME. Adoptive gay father families: parent-child relationships and children's psychological adjustment. Child Dev 2014;85(2):456–68. Available from: https://doi.org/10.1111/cdev.12155.

[30] Mazrekaj D, De Witte K, Cabus S. School outcomes of children raised by same-sex parents: evidence from administrative panel data. Am Sociol Rev 2020;85(5):830–56. Available from: https://doi.org/10.1177/0003122420957249.

C H A P T E R

10

Parenting in transgender and nonbinary individuals

Amanda R. Schwartz and Molly B. Moravek

Division of Reproductive Endocrinology and Infertility, Department of Obstetrics and Gynecology, University of Michigan, Ann Arbor, MI, United States

Introduction

According to population sampling research, it is estimated that 0.5%–1.3% of birth-assigned males and 0.4%–1.2% birth-assigned females identify as transgender. Extrapolating from these population samples with a conservative estimate of 0.5%, there are approximately 25 million transgender individuals worldwide [1]. In the United States, the number of individuals identifying as transgender has been rising with an estimation of 390 per 100,000 or 1.4 million transgender Americans in 2017 [2]. In discussion of transgender and nonbinary individuals and their family-building desires it is important first to distinguish between one's gender identity and sexual orientation. One's gender identity or internal experience of gender does not define one's sexual orientation, which refers to a person's emotional or sexual attraction to individuals of a specific or more than one gender. Cisgender people are individuals whose assigned sex at birth corresponds to their gender identity. Transgender people are individuals who experience an incongruity between one's assigned sex at birth and sense of self as a gendered person. Nonbinary individuals do not identify their gender as exclusively fitting into the categories of male or female, but rather experience their gender identity outside of this binary definition. Proper terminology is outlined in Table 10.1.

As understanding of sex and gender has evolved, so too has discussion in the scientific literature of individuals who identify as a gender that is different from their assigned sex at birth. The 1980 Diagnostic and Statistical Manual of Mental Disorders (DSM) III introduced diagnostic criteria for "transsexualism" which was defined by the persistent sense of discomfort and inappropriateness about one's anatomic sex and the persistent wish to be rid of one's genitals and live as a member of the opposite sex [3]. To be considered transsexualism, what was then labeled a "disturbance" could not be combined with another mental disorder or physical intersex condition, and it must have been present in the individual for at least 2 years. The 1987 DSM III-R noted two changes in the definition of transsexualism [4]. The first was striking the requirement that transsexualism could not exist with another mental health disorder or physical intersex condition, and the second was characterizing individuals who experienced gender dysphoria without a desire for sex reassignment as having a gender identity disorder of adolescence and nontranssexual type. The 1994 DSM IV replaced transsexualism with gender identity disorder, which described individuals whose gender-identity caused clinically significant distress or functional impairment [5]. Gender identity disorder was subsequently eliminated in the 2013 DSM V and replaced with gender dysphoria, defined as distress caused by a discrepancy between a person's gender identity and sex assigned at birth [6].

An important trend in the characterization of gender identity in the scientific literature is movement away from the understanding of transgender or nonbinary individuals as having a disorder or pathology that can be "fixed" according to a cisnormative view of gender expression. The 2013 change aimed to reduce social stigma and depathologize gender identity as a "disorder" while still supporting access to care for affected individuals. A

TABLE 10.1 Terminology.

Cisgender	A person whose gender identity is consistent with their sex assigned at birth.
Gender dysphoria	Distress caused by a discrepancy between a person's gender identity and sex assigned at birth. To meet DSM-V criteria must be clinically significant and cause impaired functioning.
Gender identity	An individual's internal experience of gender or internal sense of self from a gender perspective.
Gender-affirming hormone therapy	Feminizing and masculinizing hormone treatment aimed to align one's secondary sex characteristics with one's gender identity.
Gender-affirming surgery	Surgeries aimed to modify an individual's body to be more aligned with one's gender identity.
Nonbinary	Describes individuals whose gender identity is outside of the traditional binary definition of gender.
Sexual orientation	An individual's emotional or sexual attraction to individuals.
Transgender	Describes individuals who experience an incongruity between one's assigned sex at birth and sense of self as a gendered person.
Trans man/transgender man	A transgender individual whose gender identity is male.
Trans woman/transgender woman	A transgender individual whose gender identity is female.

Note: Definitions adapted from Fenway Institute National LGBTQIA + Health Education Center Glossary of Terms for Health Care Teams, 2020 and UCSF Transgender Care Terminology and Definitions, 2016.

critical component of the DSM V criteria for gender dysphoria is that the incongruence of assigned sex at birth and experienced gender identity causes clinically significant stress or impaired functioning. However, the debate continues as to whether this distress is brought about solely from the incongruence between experienced gender and one's assigned gender, or whether societal stigmatization, discrimination, targeted violence, and internalized transphobia is in fact the greater cause of clinically significant distress or impairment of functioning.

There is a wide spectrum of gender identities that may be experienced by individuals and this identity may be fluid. Individuals that identify as transgender or nonbinary may experience gender dysphoria and seek gender-affirming hormone therapy and/or gender-affirming surgery in an effort to align their physical appearance with their internal sense of self. The degree to which individuals pursue social or physical transition is highly varied and influenced by their own gender identity and desire for transition as well as financial, community/relationship, or healthcare barriers that they may face. To provide high-quality care for this community, healthcare providers need to be cognizant of the continuum along which individuals can identify and express their gender. We must recognize the diversity of this community to avoid cisnormative assumptions regarding preferences for family-building or parenting desires.

Transgender and nonbinary individuals represent an underserved population in medicine with a national survey reporting routine medical care in only 30%—40% of transgender individuals [7]. Discrimination on the basis of gender identity has negatively impacted the health and access to healthcare for this population. At the provider level, there is a lack of formal medical education specific to transgender patients and their unique healthcare needs which leads to variable provider comfort in treating transgender individuals and represents an additional barrier to providing high-quality healthcare for this population. As larger numbers of individuals identify as transgender and initiate gender-affirming care, there is greater need for literature to understand the effects of gender-affirming hormones on sexual and reproductive function, importance of fertility preservation counseling, and diversity of pregnancy and family-building experiences of transgender and nonbinary individuals.

Demographics of transgender parenting

There is limited research investigating the demographics and profile of parenting among transgender and nonbinary individuals. Studies of transgender and nonbinary individuals as parents are often restricted in sample size and the lack of inclusion of gender identity on most national surveys. A population-based survey of over 400 trans adults in Ontario, Canada found that 24.1% were parents. Among respondents, transgender parents were more likely to be assigned male at birth, older and with higher level of education completed and higher reported personal income as compared to non-parents. In this study, the majority of trans parents (77.9%) were biological parents, with 24.3% identifying as stepparents, 8.8% as partners of biological parents, and 3.6% as intentional nonbiological parents to their children [8].

In the United States, results of the National Transgender Discrimination Survey of over 6000 transgender and nonbinary adults found that 38% were parents. Respondents who transitioned later in life were more likely to be parents with 82% of those transitioning beyond age 55 being parents. Among gender identities, 41% of transgender individuals reported being parents as compared to 20% of nonbinary individuals. Similar to the Canadian survey, transgender women were more likely to be parents (52%) as compared to transgender men (17%) [9]. More recently, a study by Carone et al. using a United States national probability sample found that only 18.8% of transgender respondents were parents. Among parents, the majority identified as transgender women (52.5%), approximately one-third identified as nonbinary and only 11.7% as transgender men [10]. The variation in parenting demographics in studies of transgender and nonbinary individuals is likely influenced by region and method of population sampling which limit the generalizability of these findings and characterization of parenting along the gender spectrum.

Transgender parenting desires

Desire for parenting among transgender and nonbinary individuals is similarly poorly characterized in the scientific literature. Historically, transgender individuals in some countries were forced to choose between biological parenting and seeking gender-affirming care as sterilization was a precondition to pursue a legal gender change. As understanding of the spectrum of gender identity has evolved, many countries have removed such discriminatory jurisdiction increasing opportunity for parenthood among gender minorities and prompting investigation into the desire for parenting among transgender people. In the aforementioned population-based survey of transgender adults in Canada, 19.4% of current parents and 36.7% of nonparents reported a desire to have (more) children [8]. A cross-sectional multicenter study of 189 transgender adults in Germany found that among individuals that were about to start gender-affirming hormone care, 46% of trans men and 15% of trans women indicated having children was currently important to them and an additional 53% of trans men and 65% of trans women reported they could imagine having children in the future [11].

In a study of transgender adults in Belgium, 39% of survey respondents revealed a current or future desire to parent with younger people more likely to express a parenting desire. Potential barriers to fulfilling these desires included assumed difficulties with the process of adoption (41.3%), fear of their child being discriminated secondary to their parent's gender identity (38%), being discriminated against as a transgender parent (32.6%), and the cost of using their own gametes for reproduction (32.6%) [12]. An investigation of pathways to parenthood among transgender young adults found that approximately one-third planned to parent through adoption and 47% of respondents desired biologically related offspring. Trans women were more likely to desire adoption as compared to trans men [13].

Although interest in parenting has varied among studies, a systematic review of parenting goals among transgender young adults found that one-third to two-thirds desired to parent, biological or otherwise, at some point in their lifetime [14]. While limited studies investigating parental desires among transgender youth have shown a similar interest in becoming a parent, there appears to be less interest among transgender youth in fertility or having biologically related offspring. A cross-sectional survey of American transgender youth (mean age 16.8 years) revealed that only 20% of respondents felt it was important to have biological children [15]. In another survey of 156 transgender adolescents, only 36% reported interest in biologic parenthood while 71% expressed interest in parenting through adoption [16]. Similarly, a survey study of transgender youth and their parents found that while half of youth respondents endorsed a wish to parent in the future, less than a quarter desired a biological child. Although interest in fertility was low among transgender youth, over half of parents wished that their child would consider fertility preservation. Importantly, while the expressed interest in future fertility was low among transgender youth (24%), the majority wondered or were unsure if their desire for biologically related children may change over time [17]. The recognition among transgender youth that their fertility desires may be fluid highlights the potential for future regret and the importance of effective fertility counseling in this population.

Healthcare barriers

Historically transgender and nonbinary individuals have faced significant discrimination leading to socioeconomic limitations with negative consequences on the health of this underserved population. In the United States, transgender individuals are often targets of violence on the basis of gender identity with 35% reporting physical violence and 12% sexual violence [9]. Additionally, transgender and nonbinary people have double the poverty rate and nine times the rate of attempted suicide [18]. Many transgender individuals recognize an incongruence with their birth-assigned gender early in life and subsequent intolerance at home and in the education system leaves this population socially and economically vulnerable. In a 2015 survey of transgender young adults across the United States, 8% of the 27,000 respondents reported being estranged from their families on the basis of their gender identity, 30% reported having been homeless, and 17% reported such severe mistreatment that they left school [18].

While financial limitations restrict some from accessing medical care, discrimination on the basis of gender identity undoubtedly permeates the healthcare system creating further barriers to adequate healthcare for gender minorities, including reproductive care. Transgender and nonbinary individuals are much more likely to experience discrimination in the healthcare setting with one-third of transgender respondents in a national survey reporting a negative experience secondary to their gender identity [18]. This discrimination is not unique to the United States healthcare system as 22% of transgender respondents in the European Union Agency for Fundamental Rights Survey reported being personally discriminated against by healthcare personnel due to their identification as transgender [19]. Discrimination and violence in healthcare has justifiably lead to avoidance of healthcare with 23% of transgender individuals reporting that they did not see a doctor even when they needed to due to fear of mistreatment [18].

Barriers to parenting

Discrimination on the basis of gender identity likewise permeates the fertility and family-building spheres contributing to further obstacles to achieving parenthood for transgender and nonbinary individuals. In the field of reproductive endocrinology and infertility, providers have invoked personal bias and unfounded ethical concerns as justification to restrict transgender individuals from accessing assisted reproductive technologies [20]. In a qualitative study of transgender patients undergoing fertility treatment, one individual reported being denied access to all fertility services after disclosing that he was a trans man [21]. In an effort to combat such discrimination, a recent ethics committee opinion was published by the American Society for Reproductive Medicine which states "Professional autonomy, while a significant value in deciding whom to treat, is limited in this case by a greater ethical obligation, and in some jurisdictions, a legal duty, to regard all persons equally, regardless of their gender identity" [22]. While most fertility clinics do not overtly deny care to transgender individuals, access to fertility care is often restricted. An analysis of websites of over 300 fertility clinics in the United States revealed that only 53% contained content inclusive of LGBT people and only 32% specifically inclusive of transgender people [23]. Access to adoption services is likewise significantly restricted for transgender and nonbinary individuals. A survey investigating attitudes of adoption agencies toward gender minority people found that less than one-third of agencies had a nondiscrimination policy and only 16% actively recruited sexual and gender minority people as potential adoptive parents [24]. Transgender individuals are often highly excluded from mainstream and same-sex parenting resources creating further obstacles to achieving parenthood [25].

In many countries discriminatory legislation has represented a significant barrier to parenting for transgender and nonbinary individuals. Sterilization as a prerequisite for legal gender change has historically led many to conceptualize loss of fertility as the cost of achieving gender change. In 2014 the World Health Organization (WHO) released an interagency statement calling for the elimination of forced, coercive, and otherwise involuntary sterilization. In this statement, sterilization requirements for gender change were described as running "counter to respect for bodily integrity, self-determination, and human dignity" with the WHO calling for "revision of laws to remove any requirements for compulsory sterilization of transgender persons" [26]. Over the past 10 years, many countries, including Sweden, Germany, and Belgium have overturned laws requiring sterilization for legal gender change, but worldwide there is great variation with sterilization remaining a requirement for legal gender change in some countries such as Japan and certain states within the United States. Legal obstacles in the way of transgender parenting are not limited to sterilization requirements as gender transition has been used by courts as justification to deny or restrict custody of children. In a United States National Transgender Discrimination Study, 13% of respondents reported courts limiting or stopping relationships with their children on the basis of their gender identity [9]. Similarly, in a survey of over 400 Canadian transgender people, 18.1% reported no legal access to their child and 17.7% reported lost or reduced child custody because they were trans [8].

In pursuit of parenthood, the gynecology, primary care, or fertility clinic can be a source of discomfort for transgender and nonbinary people. Preconception or fertility care may be inherently dysphoric due to discussion of one's natal anatomy and reproductive potential. Pelvic examinations or procedures such as transvaginal ultrasounds or inseminations may potentiate this discomfort. While some challenges cannot be overcome, steps taken by providers, office staff, and clinics can significantly improve the experience of their transgender and nonbinary patients. Designing intake forms to ask all patients for their preferred name and pronouns and providing options beyond binary gender selection can allow patients to fill out the form correctly for themselves. Office staff and providers should be diligent regarding the use of patient's preferred names and pronouns, and work to avoid making assumptions regarding one's sexual identity or desired plans for parenthood. In interviews with transgender individuals that underwent fertility treatments, use of a patient's preferred name and pronouns greatly impacted their overall experience [21]. When pelvic examinations or procedures are necessary providers should be aware of any past trauma or testosterone use and use gender-neutral terminology to mitigate discomfort. Having gender neutral bathrooms, providing inclusive educational materials, and developing policies against gender-based discrimination, can create an environment that is both welcoming and affirming for transgender and nonbinary patients.

Impact of gender-affirming care on reproductive function

Transgender and nonbinary individuals represent a diverse population and experience varying levels of gender dysphoria. In response to this sense of incongruence, transgender and nonbinary individuals may take steps to better align their outward physical appearance with their internal self and gender identity. This can range from undergoing a social transition without gender-affirming treatments, pursuing a medical transition with gender-affirming hormones, undergoing minor surgical procedures and/or major gender-affirming surgeries. This range of lifestyle choices reflects the degree of emotional distress that the incongruity between self-identified gender and birth-assigned sex causes the individual as well as relationship factors, their economic status, medical comorbidities, and access to healthcare resources.

The impact of gender-affirming surgeries on an individual's reproductive potential is surgery-specific and depends upon the reproductive function of the natal organ. Many minor gender-affirming surgical procedures such as tracheal shave or feminizing facial procedures have no impact on reproductive function. Chest masculinization surgery, otherwise known as top surgery, does not affect one's ability to reproduce but may have consequences on one's future ability to breastfeed [27]. However, major gender-affirming surgery has a clear-cut impact on an individual's future reproductive potential. Transgender men who desire bottom surgery should consider future desires for genetic children as well as to carry a pregnancy prior to definitive surgery. A hysterectomy (with bilateral salpingectomy currently recommended to decrease future risk of ovarian cancer) eliminates a person's ability to carry a future pregnancy while a bilateral salpingooophorectomy removes a person's ability to provide gametes for biological-related children (unless reproductive tissues were previously cryopreserved or cryopreserved at the time of surgery). Transgender women or nonbinary individuals who pursue orchiectomy likewise eliminate their potential for future fertility unless semen was previously cryopreserved or testicular tissue frozen following removal.

While undergoing gender-affirming surgery has definitive implications on one's reproductive potential, the impact of gender-affirming hormone care on reproductive function is less clear. The current scientific literature pertaining to the impact of gender-affirming hormones on ovarian and testicular tissues is limited to observational studies with large variations in dose and duration of hormone therapy. The inconsistent results from these cohort studies and lack of robust multicenter findings create a challenge for fertility preservation counseling as the impact of gender-affirming hormones on future fertility is not well established.

Masculinizing hormones and fertility

Exogenous testosterone is the mainstay of hormone treatment for trans men and nonbinary individuals desiring masculinizing gender-affirming medical care. Testosterone can be administered as an intramuscular or subcutaneous injection or via a transdermal formulation in either a patch or gel. The goal of testosterone in gender-affirming care is to suppress traits of one's natal sex and induce secondary sexual characteristics congruent with an individual's gender identity. This is done through suppression of estradiol with the goal of increasing serum testosterone to physiologic male reference levels.

Testosterone as masculinizing therapy induces amenorrhea in the majority of transgender men and nonbinary individuals. This cessation of menses is likely achieved through a combination of ovulation suppression and endometrial atrophy [28]. In studies of testosterone therapy in trans men, the time to cessation of menses was variable with a reported range of 1–13 months, and the majority of patients became amenorrheic by 6 months of continuous treatment [29–31]. A recent prospective cohort of 267 transgender men initiating gender-affirming hormone therapy in the European Network for the Investigation of Gender Incongruence found that 82% achieved amenorrhea after 3 months and 91% achieved amenorrhea after 6 months of testosterone therapy [32].

Importantly, testosterone is not an effective form of contraception and patients can conceive while on masculinizing hormone therapy. Many trans men and nonbinary individuals incorrectly perceive testosterone as protective against pregnancy, which represents a failure in contraceptive counseling. In a survey of contraceptive use, 16% of transgender men reported testosterone as their method of birth control and 5.5% said healthcare providers had advised them that this was a reliable method. One individual in this study reported an unplanned pregnancy in the setting of irregular testosterone use [33]. In addition to concerns regarding the contraceptive efficacy of testosterone, pregnancy is an absolute contraindication to testosterone use due to potential teratogenic effects. Studies of testosterone exposure in pregnant rats have shown dose-dependent masculinization of female embryos [34,35]. A case report of transdermal testosterone exposure in a human pregnancy resulted in virilization of a female fetus [36]. Data extracted from cisgender pregnant females have shown an association between increased androgen levels and reduced birth weight raising further concerns for pregnancy in the setting of testosterone use [37]. In a survey of trans men who experienced pregnancy after gender-affirming therapy, the majority of patients were able to conceive within 6 months of testosterone discontinuation and 20% of patients conceived in the setting of testosterone-induced amenorrhea. Although obstetric data were limited to participant reports, pregnancy, delivery, and birth outcomes did not differ between those with or without prior testosterone exposure [38]. While testosterone can suppress ovulation, this suppression is likely incomplete, as demonstrated by pregnancies during testosterone-induced amenorrhea, and reversible, as demonstrated by reports of trans men conceiving after cessation of gender-affirming hormones.

The effect of prolonged testosterone exposure on ovarian histology is uncertain with analyses from specimens obtained at the time of gender-affirming surgery showing conflicting results. In an examination of ovaries obtained at time of gender-affirming surgery from 112 transgender men with an average of 3.7 years of androgen therapy, Grynberg et al. found that 79.5% had histological characteristics consistent with polycystic ovarian syndrome (PCOS) [39]. In a smaller prospective cohort of transgender men on testosterone, Loverro et al. similarly found that the majority of ovaries had an enlarged multifollicular appearance [40]. However, more recent histologic analysis of resected ovarian tissue in transgender individuals indicates that long-term androgen therapy does not appear to affect follicle number or distribution [41]. Additionally, a multicenter case series of ovarian pathology from trans men and gender nonbinary individuals provides evidence for persistent ovarian function on testosterone therapy with continued folliculogenesis in the majority of patients and average ovarian volume consistent with normative values in reproductive-aged women [42]. To further evaluate the role of testosterone on ovarian structure, Caanen et al. compared ultrasounds images from 56 trans men receiving gender-affirming hormone care with 80 cisgender female controls and found the prevalence of PCOS was similar between the groups [43].

Current research on the impact of testosterone on the maturation of oocytes and ovarian reserve is limited and further studies are needed before conclusions can be drawn. In an analysis of ovarian tissue from 40 transgender men with a mean androgen exposure of 58 weeks, De Roo et al. demonstrated promising in vitro maturation results with a high percentage of normal appearing spindles observed [41]. Other analyses of resected ovarian cortical tissue in transgender men have similarly found that androgen exposure does not appear to affect the in vitro developmental capacity of ovarian follicles [44,45]. The effect of testosterone on antimullerian hormone (AMH), a marker of ovarian reserve, has shown conflicting results. In one study of 22 transgender men, AMH was significantly lower after treatment with testosterone for 16 weeks. However, the ability to draw conclusions from the impact of testosterone is limited as individuals in the study protocol were also on a gonadotropin-releasing hormone agonist and aromatase inhibitor [46]. However, in a prospective cohort of 45 transgender adolescents receiving 6 months of masculinizing hormone treatment, no change in AMH was observed. In this cohort, transgender men were also treated with an androgenic progestin, lynestrenol, which may have influenced these findings [47]. The discrepancy in these findings may be secondary to the presence of additional hormone-modifying therapies which do not allow conclusions to be drawn regarding the isolated effect of testosterone therapy on AMH or ovarian reserve. In addition to limitations in sample size and potential confounding effects of additional hormonal medications, current research does not answer the question of whether the morphologic or laboratory changes observed with testosterone therapy directly affect an individual's fertility. Additionally, *if* fertility is impacted, the ultimate question is whether discontinuation of testosterone can reverse these changes?

Feminizing hormones and fertility

Gender-affirming hormone care for transgender women and nonbinary individuals desiring feminizing therapy typically includes estradiol in conjunction with an antiandrogen. Estradiol can be administered by many routes, including via an oral or sublingual tablet, transdermal patch or by injection. The most commonly administered antiandrogen in the United States is spironolactone which is an oral tablet typically dosed twice daily. The goal of this combination for gender-affirming hormone care is to minimize natal sex characteristics and to induce female secondary sexual characteristics such as breast development, reduction of body hair, and redistribution of facial and subcutaneous fat. This is done through suppression of testosterone levels with the goal of maintaining estradiol levels in the physiologic range for reproductive-age cisgender women.

There is some evidence that feminizing hormone therapy is associated with decreased semen parameters in transgender women; however, discontinuation of estradiol may lead to improved results. Early insights into the impact of hormonal therapy on spermatogenesis were extrapolated from studies of cisgender men taking male hormonal contraceptives. An analysis of sperm parameters in over 1500 eugonadal men using male hormonal contraceptives demonstrated that suppression of spermatogenesis was reversible with a 90% probability of full recovery by 12 months [48]. A study of the effect of estradiol on sperm parameters in a single transgender individual found a dose-dependent response with lower doses of estradiol having no effect on sperm motility while higher doses decreased sperm motility and total sperm count. When estradiol was discontinued sperm parameters recovered with sperm motility normalizing faster than sperm counts [49]. In a cohort of 28 transgender women at the time of fertility preservation, Adeleye et al. evaluated semen parameters according to prior hormone exposure. Of the 28 transgender women, 18 reported no prior hormone use, 3 had discontinued hormones prior to fertility preservation (with a mean discontinuation of 4.4 months), and 7 were receiving gender-affirming hormones at the time of specimen collection. The best semen parameters were observed in the hormone-naïve group. However, patients who had discontinued hormones prior to fertility preservation had semen parameters that remained within normal reference ranges [50]. These findings are in contrast to results of a retrospective cohort of 260 transgender women in the Netherlands in which semen quality at the time of fertility preservation was decreased as compared to reference values for the general population. Although only 12 transgender women had reported prior use of gender-affirming hormones, no correlation was found between prior exposure to feminizing hormones and diminished semen parameters [51].

Prolonged estradiol exposure has been associated with testicular damage and impaired spermatogenesis, but there is a large variation in reported findings and the potential reversibility of those findings. An analysis of testicular histology from 108 transgender women taking estrogens and antiandrogens prior to undergoing gender-affirming surgery found normal spermatogenesis in only 24% of patients with the majority of specimens showing varying degrees of impairment. Interestingly there was no correlation between spermatogenesis and gender-affirming treatment protocols. However, individuals who had discontinued hormone therapy prior to surgery had a higher average testicular weight as compared to those who continued hormone treatment until the time of surgery [52]. In a more recent study of testicular specimens from transgender women with prior hormone exposure, normal spermatogenesis was observed in only 11% of orchiectomy samples [53]. Kent et al. performed histologic analysis on orchiectomy specimens from 135 trans women receiving gender-affirming hormones with only 4% showing normal spermatogenesis. Although it was not significant, the results showed a trend toward poorer spermatogenesis with longer duration of feminizing hormone therapy received [54]. A comprehensive review of the influence of feminizing hormones on testicular morphology in transgender women found variable effects on structure and spermatogenesis. The impact of feminizing therapy on histological specimens ranged from no observable change with normal spermatogenesis and normal testicular morphology observed to complete cessation of spermatogenesis with decreased testicular volume and evidence of atrophy [55]. Given these inconsistent findings it is difficult to provide effective counseling on the impact of feminizing gender-affirming hormone care on future reproductive potential. Future research is necessary to better understand the effect of long-term estradiol on spermatogenesis and to determine if there is a dose-dependent relationship between estradiol exposure and impaired fertility. If there is clear evidence of impaired reproductive potential with feminizing hormone therapy, further studies are needed to ascertain whether these effects are reversible with discontinuation of treatment.

Fertility preservation

Transgender and nonbinary individuals access reproductive medicine either for fertility preservation and/or to fulfill parental desire, with fertility preservation often being the initial encounter. In the setting of the known effects of gender-affirming surgery and potential effects of gender-affirming hormones on an individual's fertility, there is consensus among major medical societies, including the American Society for Reproductive Medicine, the European Society of Human Reproduction and Embryology, and the World Professional Association for Transgender Health and the Endocrine Society, that transgender and nonbinary people should receive fertility preservation counseling prior to initiation of gender-affirming treatment. Many transgender individuals undergo transition during their reproductive years and express high interest in future parenting prior to transition [11,56]. Additionally, in a multicenter survey study of transgender individuals currently receiving gender-affirming treatment, one-fourth of respondents expressed a current desire for children, while 69.9% of trans women and 46.9% of trans men expressed interest in having children in the future [11]. The young age of many undergoing transition, as well as interest in parenting both prior to and following initiation of gender-affirming care, highlight the importance of fertility preservation counseling for transgender and nonbinary people.

Although there is consensus among major medical societies regarding fertility preservation counseling as standard of care prior to initiation of gender-affirming care, retrospective cohort and cross-sectional survey studies of transgender and nonbinary individuals indicate that in practice fertility preservation counseling is highly variable. A recent survey of transgender individuals in Belgium revealed that 37% of respondents had not received any information on fertility preservation. Only 36% of respondents had received fertility preservation information from healthcare workers with 14% reporting receiving it from an LGBT organization and 14% from their own research or through friends or acquaintances [12]. Similarly, in an Austrian survey of transgender individuals although 95% of respondents felt that fertility preservation counseling should be offered to all transgender and nonbinary people, 68% of respondents did not recall any prior fertility preservation counseling or advice [57]. Among transgender men who had previously undergone gender-affirming surgery, 19% of respondents reported that they considered freezing germ cells but had never spoken to a provider about it and 38% reported that they would have considered freezing germ cells if this option had been available [58]. This variation in fertility preservation counseling is likewise observed among transgender youths with a systematic review reporting rates of fertility preservation ranging from 12% to 100% [14]. More recently, in one study of fertility preservation among transgender adolescents, zero of the 79 transgender teens that received fertility preservation counseling chose to pursue fertility preservation services [59]. These studies demonstrate that fertility preservation counseling is incomplete for both transgender youth and adults and the standard of care is not being met for these patients.

Current research investigating fertility preservation among transgender and nonbinary individuals demonstrates a common theme of relatively low utilization of fertility preservation services as compared to interest in such services. The lack of awareness of the impact of gender-affirming care on reproductive function and understanding of fertility preservation options is likely a major contributing factor to the low uptake of fertility preservation among transgender and nonbinary individuals. In the aforementioned Austrian survey in which the majority of respondents did not recall receiving fertility preservation counseling, while 34% of respondents thought that sharing a genetic relationship with children was important, only 7% underwent fertility preservation. Among those that pursued fertility preservation the most cited reason was the desire to have the option available in the future [57]. In a multicenter study of transgender people in Germany, Auer et al. found that while 76% of respondents had thought about preserving germ cells prior to medical transition, only 9.6% of trans women and 3.1% of trans men had utilized fertility preservation services [11].

While incomplete fertility preservation counseling contributes to low uptake of fertility preservation services in the transgender and nonbinary community, the cost of fertility preservation as well as potential for hormone cessation and treatment to induce gender dysphoria represent additional obstacles to parenthood. Consideration of fertility preservation services forces transgender individuals to consider gametes and anatomy related to their birth-assigned sex which can be challenging to their gender identity. Fertility preservation can involve invasive procedures, such as transvaginal ultrasound or transvaginal oocyte retrieval, which can be highly dysphoric for transgender people. In one study of transgender individual's fertility desires, respondents cited prohibitive cost, no interest in genetically related offspring and the thought of children as inducing dysphoria as the most common reasons for declining fertility preservation [57].

In contemplating fertility preservation, transgender youth and young adults have the additional challenge of the maturity required to make decisions regarding future parenthood goals and potentially delaying initiation of gender-affirming hormones to achieve those future goals. In a study of attitudes toward fertility preservation among transgender youth (median age 15.2 years) prior to initiation of gender-affirming hormone care, Nahata et al. found that although 72 out of 73 patients received fertility preservation counseling only 3% utilized fertility preservation services. Reasons for declining to pursue fertility preservation included consideration for adoption, never wanting to have children, cost, discomfort with masturbating to produce a sample, and concern for potentially delaying hormone treatment [60]. Another survey of fertility preservation desires among American transgender youth and their parents revealed that the most common factor influencing fertility preservation decision making was discomfort with a body part that they do not identify with (69%) and over half of youth respondents felt that having children with their own gametes conflicted with their affirmed gender. Only 3% of youth, as compared to 33% of their parents, were willing to delay hormone treatment in the interest of fertility preservation [15].

Fertility preservation options for transgender men

Fertility preservation options for transgender men and nonbinary individuals assigned female at birth include oocyte cryopreservation, embryo cryopreservation using partner or donor sperm, and ovarian tissue cryopreservation (Table 10.2). Cryopreservation involves cooling of reproductive material to subzero temperatures with preservation of structural integrity so that gametes, embryo, or reproductive tissue can be used for later reproductive use. As compared to fertility preservation options for transgender women, fertility preservation procedures for transgender men or nonbinary individuals assigned female at birth can be laborious and dysphoric which may contribute to low uptake. In a survey of fertility preservation desires among transgender men only 9% of respondents had pursued fertility preservation, with an additional 16% considering fertility preservation in the future. Of the transgender men that did not pursue fertility preservation, reasons for declining included not feeling it was necessary (54%), feeling that having genetically related offspring is not important (23%), not wanting to take hormones to stimulate follicle development (28%), and high cost (28%). Among respondents considering future fertility preservation, prominent barriers identified included cost of freezing and storing gametes (74%), interrupting gender-affirming hormone care (61%), and the chance of conceiving from frozen oocytes (61%) [12]. In providing effective and complete fertility preservation counseling, providers should discuss the probability of a live birth, risks, and advantages or disadvantages as they pertain to each individual and their gender identity. Prepubertal transgender males are not candidates for oocyte or embryo cryopreservation due to the inability to retrieve mature eggs in this population, although there are case reports of mature eggs retrieved from youth who started puberty blockade at Tanner stage II or III. Therefore the only option for fertility preservation in prepubertal transgender males or nonbinary individuals would be ovarian tissue cryopreservation.

Ovarian tissue cryopreservation

Ovarian tissue cryopreservation is a procedure by which ovarian tissue is surgically resected, typically by a laparoscopic approach, and frozen for future use. It was originally used in female prepubertal cancer patients as a means to preserve fertility prior to gonadotoxic effects of chemotherapy or in women with highly aggressive malignancies in which there is felt to be insufficient time to complete oocyte cryopreservation. Ovarian tissue cryopreservation was previously considered an experimental technique, requiring research protocols at a finite number of institutions to be performed. However, in September 2019 the American Society for Reproductive Medicine no longer considers ovarian tissue cryopreservation to be experimental [61]. As of 2017 there have been over 130 reported live births following autotransplantation of previously cryopreserved ovarian tissue [62]. Results of a recent meta-analysis indicate that autologous ovarian tissue transplantation has an endocrine function restoration rate of 63.9% and live birth rate of 57.5% [63].

Ovarian tissue cryopreservation provides prepubertal transgender and nonbinary individuals with an option for preserving their reproductive potential prior to gender-affirming care. At institutions with necessary resources and protocols, ovarian tissue cryopreservation can be performed at the same time as gender-affirming surgery for adult transgender patients without the need for additional procedures [64]. Another advantage of this technique for transgender men is that it avoids the need for ovarian stimulation or invasive monitoring procedures. A disadvantage of ovarian tissue cryopreservation for trans men is that the autotransplantation of previously cryopreserved ovarian tissue and restoration of ovarian function may be undesirable or a cause of gender dysphoria. Additionally, transgender men, particularly those who have undergone a gender transition, may not wish to carry a pregnancy. In such a case future autotransplantation of cryopreserved ovarian tissue could be utilized to facilitate stimulation and retrieval of mature oocytes. To date there have not been any cases of nonautologous transplant of cryopreserved ovarian tissue or in vitro maturation of oocytes to achieve a pregnancy. With continued advances in oocyte maturation techniques this may represent a future pathway without the need for ovarian stimulation for transgender individuals [41].

TABLE 10.2 Fertility preservation options for transgender men and nonbinary individuals assigned female at birth.

Method	Description	Method of pregnancy	Advantages	Disadvantages
Oocyte cryopreservation	• Requires an approximately 2-week process of ovarian stimulation with ultrasounds and injectable medications followed by an oocyte retrieval procedure • Mature oocytes are frozen for future use	• Mature oocytes can be fertilized with partner or donor sperm • Resultant embryos may be transferred back to the individual, to a partner with a uterus (reciprocal IVF) or to a gestational carrier	• Established method for fertility preservation in transgender and nonbinary individuals • May be considered even after gender-affirming hormones have started • Does not require a reproductive partner at the time of fertility preservation • Provides the individual with full ownership over one's gametes • Generally well-tolerated outpatient procedure	• Ovarian stimulation may induce gender dysphoria (relating to the clinic environment, administration of hormones, ultrasounds, and oocyte retrieval process) • Oocyte retrieval is generally performed under IV sedation • Cost • Additional requirements if considering a gestational carrier
Embryo cryopreservation	• Same ovarian stimulation and oocyte retrieval procedure as before • Mature oocytes are fertilized with partner or donor sperm and resultant embryos frozen	Cryopreserved embryos may be transferred back to the individual, to a partner with a uterus (reciprocal IVF) or to a gestational carrier	• Established method for fertility preservation in transgender and nonbinary individuals • Option for genetic testing of embryos • Creation of embryos may provide more insight into the probability of future genetic parenting	• Same as oocyte cryopreservation • Potential concerns relating to embryo disposition
Ovarian tissue cryopreservation	• Surgical resection (typically via a laparoscopic approach) and cryopreservation of ovarian cortical tissue • Plan for future autologous ovarian tissue transplantation to achieve pregnancy or restore hormone function	• Autologous ovarian tissue transplantation to achieve future pregnancy via intercourse or • In vitro fertilization (IVF) with option for resultant embryos to be transferred to the individual, to a partner with a uterus (reciprocal IVF) or to a gestational carrier	• Fertility preservation option for prepubertal and postpubertal individuals • Successful pregnancies have resulted following autotransplantation of cryopreserved ovarian tissue • Does not require ovarian stimulation medication, monitoring procedures, or oocyte retrieval surgery • Does not require discontinuation of androgen therapy • May be performed at the time of gender-affirming surgery	• All pregnancies to date have involved autotransplantation • Autotransplantation of previously cryopreserved tissue may be undesirable or invoke gender dysphoria • Requirement of laparoscopic surgery • In vitro maturation is currently experimental

IV, Intravenous.

Oocyte cryopreservation

Transgender men and nonbinary individuals assigned female at birth that have initiated puberty are candidates for oocyte or embryo cryopreservation to preserve their fertility. The process of oocyte cryopreservation consists of pretesting labs in conjunction with a baseline ultrasound to determine likelihood of ovarian response and to inform counseling and dosing of stimulation medications. Individuals then undergo a process of ovarian stimulation with daily subcutaneous injections of gonadotropin medications. Throughout the stimulation process growth of ovarian follicles is monitored with regular ultrasounds until follicles reach a desired size indicating probability of oocyte maturity. Individuals then administer a "trigger" injection which is precisely timed to their oocyte retrieval procedure. The oocyte retrieval typically takes place under IV sedation and consists of transvaginal aspiration of follicular fluid containing oocytes. In the embryology lab the oocytes are isolated with vitrification of mature oocytes for future reproductive use. The typical timeline of the oocyte stimulation process is influenced by an individual's age, ovarian reserve, and stimulation protocol but is typically about 2 weeks.

An individual's probability of achieving a live birth from cryopreserved oocytes is influenced by their age at the time of oocyte retrieval and number of mature oocytes retrieved [65]. With improvements in cryopreservation and thawing techniques mature oocyte cryopreservation rates have steadily improved with success rates similar to those who pursue embryo cryopreservation [66,67]. As compared to embryo cryopreservation, advantages of oocyte cryopreservation include the ability to defer selection of donor or reproductive partner, avoidance of ethical dilemmas regarding embryo disposition, as well as control over one's individual gametes for future use.

Embryo cryopreservation

Embryo cryopreservation is another option for fertility preservation for transgender men and nonbinary individuals. Given the requirement for both oocytes and sperm for creation of embryos, embryo cryopreservation can be pursued by transgender men that have a committed partner who is capable of producing sperm and with whom they wish to reproduce or transgender men who are prepared to use donor sperm. Embryo cryopreservation involves the same process of ovarian stimulation and oocyte retrieval. The oocytes retrieved are then inseminated or injected in the laboratory with sperm from the individual's partner or sperm donor to create embryos. Advantages of embryo cryopreservation as compared to oocyte cryopreservation may include an ability to preserve fertility in conjunction with one's partner (if they are capable of producing sperm), improved counseling regarding the likelihood of success based on the number and quality of embryos created and the potential for genetic testing of the embryo.

While current technology does not allow for mature oocytes to be genetically tested, individuals that pursue embryo cryopreservation may elect to have their embryos genetically tested. Through a process known as preimplantation genetic testing for aneuploidies genetic testing can be performed to determine whether an embryo has the appropriate number of chromosomes to select for embryos with a higher likelihood of resulting in a successful pregnancy. Individuals with a high risk of passing a specific genetic condition to their offspring, such as breast of ovarian cancer (BRCA1 and 2), can elect to have preimplantation genetic testing for monogenic or single gene defects performed on cryopreserved embryos to select for unaffected embryos. A primary disadvantage of embryo cryopreservation in this population is that many transgender men pursue gender-affirming surgery and hormone care at a young age and therefore their desired partner (or donor) with whom to create embryos may be unknown or change with time. This has the potential to lead to conflict regarding embryo disposition and potentially less control over their cryopreserved gametes.

Fertility preservation outcomes for transgender men

Oocyte cryopreservation for fertility preservation in transgender individuals is a relatively new procedure. The first case report was of a 17-year-old transgender man undergoing oocyte cryopreservation prior to the initiation of testosterone which was published in 2014 [68]. Currently the outcomes data for fertility preservation among transgender men are limited to case reports and small case series. One retrospective cohort study comparing assisted reproductive technology outcomes of 12 transgender men (6 with prior testosterone treatment) to cisgender women found that there was no difference in the number of oocytes retrieved or oocyte maturity between transgender men without prior testosterone exposure, transgender men with prior testosterone use, and cisgender women. In this study the mean length of prior testosterone exposure was 77 months and the mean time of discontinuation of testosterone prior to ovarian stimulation was 9.3 months [69]. Similarly, in a series of 13 trans men (7 with prior testosterone treatment) undergoing ovarian stimulation to age and body mass index (BMI) matched cisgender women, there was no difference in the number of total oocytes retrieved and mature oocytes between groups. Among the transgender men, the authors reported that those with prior testosterone exposure had a lower number of oocytes retrieved as compared to those without prior gender-affirming hormone care. However, when the two outlier men with evidence of low initial ovarian reserve were removed from analysis, history of prior testosterone use did not portend a difference in oocytes retrieved [70]. In a larger investigation of 26 transgender men undergoing ovarian stimulation, more oocytes were retrieved in the transgender men as compared to age, BMI, and ovarian reserve matched controls [71]. Although larger prospective and multicenter trials are lacking, the outcomes from these early studies of ovarian stimulation in transgender men show promising results which are on par with cisgender women and support the use of assisted reproductive technology for fertility preservation in this population.

Qualitative studies of transgender men that have undergone ovarian stimulation provides insight into challenges unique to this population. In a prospective study of 17 transgender men undergoing oocyte cryopreservation in Sweden, the discontinuation of hormone therapy with resumption of menses was a particular challenge. On trans men stated "I felt a little bit in between being a woman and being a man, and one came back to square one again" and another perceived the return of his menses as the cause for relapse of self-harming behavior [72]. Another recurring theme was gender dysphoria triggered by stimulation hormones and the need for multiple pelvic examinations. One man described transvaginal ultrasounds as the most difficult part of the process reporting "for me it's genitals that I don't want to have and that I don't want to acknowledge" [72]. James-Abra et al. performed a qualitative analysis of 11 transgender individual's experience with assisted reproductive technology in Canada. The majority of individuals reported an overall negative experience with fertility care with one individual noting that they were "willing to let a whole lot slide ... the priority was having a kid" [21]. Emerging themes contributing to dissatisfaction with fertility care included problems with clinical documentation, heteronormative assumptions made by providers, and failure to use gender-neutral terminology as contributing to dissatisfaction with their care. In reference to frustration after being incorrectly identified as a cisgender woman one transgender man noted, "I think for some people ... it's just easier to revert to what they're familiar with, and their baseline is that women get pregnant and men give sperm" [21]. These incorrect assumptions made by healthcare providers highlight the need for increased provider education and awareness of the unique needs of transgender individuals seeking pregnancy.

In addition to creating a welcoming clinic environment and using desired names and pronouns, there are measures that fertility providers can take to minimize the dysphoria experienced by transgender individuals undergoing fertility preservation. Use of gender-neutral terminology for fertility preservation such as "gamete" rather than egg or oocyte and referring to patients as prospective parents rather than mothers can help to affirm patients' gender identity. If an individual's anatomy and body habitus will allow, attempts to use abdominal ultrasound in place of transvaginal imaging whenever feasible can help to mitigate patient discomfort. Aromatase inhibitors such as letrozole should be used during the ovarian stimulation process to limit physiologic rise of estradiol and thus limit hormone-induced feelings of dysphoria [73]. Consideration of random start stimulation protocols may be utilized to avoid waiting for menses to initiate an oocyte cryopreservation cycle. For transgender men who have already initiated gender-affirming hormone care prior to seeking fertility preservation, there are no data regarding how long testosterone needs to be discontinued—or if it needs to be discontinued at all—prior to initiating ovarian stimulation. A survey of transgender youth identified the need for discontinuation of gender-affirming hormones to undergo fertility preservation as a significant barrier with 34% reporting that they would pursue fertility preservation if it were possible to continue gender-affirming hormones during the process [15]. Limiting the duration of testosterone cessation or continuing testosterone through ovarian stimulation is an additional strategy that may help to improve the experience of transgender men undergoing oocyte cryopreservation.

Fertility preservation options for transgender women

Transgender women and nonbinary individuals assigned male at birth can pursue fertility preservation either through cryopreservation of sperm or testicular tissue (Table 10.3). Current research has demonstrated potential harmful effects of feminizing hormone therapy on testicular histology and spermatogenesis. Given the lack of data regarding whether this impact is dose or duration-dependent and whether these effects are reversible with

TABLE 10.3 Fertility preservation options for transgender women and nonbinary individuals assigned male at birth.

Method	Description	Method of pregnancy	Advantages	Disadvantages
Sperm cryopreservation	• Fresh sample typically obtained through masturbation • Number of collections needed influenced by semen parameters and desired future method to conceive • Penile vibratory stimulation and electroejaculation may be considered	• Cryopreserved sperm may be thawed and used for intrauterine insemination (IUI) or in vitro fertilization • IUI can be performed in a partner (if a uterus is present) or a gestational carrier • Can be used to fertilize mature eggs (either from a partner or donor) for in vitro fertilization with embryos transferred to a partner (if a uterus is present) or a gestational carrier	• Established method for fertility preservation • Does not require a reproductive partner at the time of fertility preservation • Provides the individual with full ownership over one's gametes • Avoidance of anesthesia • If semen parameters are adequate, may be used for intrauterine insemination • May be considered even after initiation of gender-affirming hormones • Relatively low cost	• Masturbation may induce gender dysphoria for some individuals • Decreased semen parameters found in some studies of transgender women even prior to initiation of gender-affirming hormones
Surgical sperm extraction	• Sperm retrieval either through aspiration or surgical extraction may be considered for individuals who are unable to produce an ejaculate or who have oligospermia or obstructive azoospermia	• Can be coordinated to an oocyte retrieval to fertilize fresh oocytes • Can be frozen and thawed in the future to fertilize mature oocytes (either from a partner or a donor) for in vitro fertilization with embryos transferred to a partner (if a uterus is present) or a gestational carrier	• Established method for fertility preservation • Does not require a reproductive partner at the time of fertility preservation • Provides the individual with full ownership over one's gametes • Avoids potential gender dysphoria related to ejaculation to produce a sperm sample	• May be cost prohibitive • Surgically retrieved sperm often can only be used for in vitro fertilization • Anesthetic needs are dependent upon technique utilized
Testicular tissue cryopreservation	• Testicular tissue is surgically extracted and cryopreserved for future reproductive use	• Dependent upon further advances in in vitro sperm maturation techniques or methods for autotransplantation. Theoretically, if sperm maturation was able to be accomplished in vitro, mature sperm could be utilized to inject mature eggs and form embryos	• *Experimental* fertility preservation option for prepubertal individuals (not experimental in postpubertal individuals) • May be performed at the time of gender-affirming surgery (gonadectomy)	• No pregnancies from cryopreserved prepubertal testicular tissue have been reported to date

discontinuation of hormones, the best option for fertility preservation is prior to initiation of hormone therapy. Transgender women pursuing gender-affirming surgery that includes bilateral orchiectomy will have complete loss of their potential for biologic parenthood unless reproductive tissue is frozen prior to or at the time of surgery. Prepubertal transgender females who have not undergone spermarche are unable to cryopreserve sperm and therefore their only option for fertility preservation is through experimental testicular tissue cryopreservation.

Sperm cryopreservation

Transgender women and nonbinary individuals that have undergone puberty are candidates for sperm cryopreservation. Advantages of sperm cryopreservation include a relatively straightforward process for collection, avoidance of anesthesia or medical treatment for most individuals, and the ability to have fertility preservation to be performed irrespective of partner status. Sperm can be obtained for cryopreservation through fresh ejaculate or through surgical extraction. Sperm cryopreservation with a semen sample typically obtained through masturbation represents the best option for fertility preservation for transgender women. However, producing a fresh sample for fertility preservation may be inherently challenging in this population. Survey studies of transgender adolescents and young adults describe the act of masturbating as triggering gender dysphoria for some individuals [60,74]. Consistent use of a patient's desired name and pronouns as well as gender-neutral terminology, avoidance of cisnormative assumptions, having a gender-neutral collection room and effective counseling can help create a more comfortable environment for collection for transgender women. Additionally, clinics may consider allowing patients to obtain a sample at home if that is feasible for an individual or couple.

In addition to causing dysphoria, transgender women may have difficulty with erection and ejaculation secondary to gender-affirming treatments or chronic medical conditions. Aids such as penile vibratory stimulation and electroejaculation, which have previously been used in for infertility treatments in men with spinal cord injuries, may be considered to assist trans women and nonbinary individuals in whom production of a fresh ejaculate may be challenging [75]. Phosphodiesterase type 5 (PDE-5) inhibitors, a medication typically used in the treatment of erectile dysfunction, may additionally be considered for as pharmacologic assistance for transgender individuals who have difficulty obtaining a sperm sample for cryopreservation [76]. Individuals who are unable to provide a sperm sample through ejaculation may consider surgical sperm collection, though this may be cost prohibitive for some. Surgical sperm retrieval is typically utilized for individuals who have severe infertility secondary to oligospermia or obstructive azoospermia in which a retrieval procedure represents the only means to obtain a quantity of sperm necessary for fertility preservation. Sperm retrieval can be performed via aspiration from the testes or epididymis or via surgical extraction with the retrieval technique selected dependent upon an individual's anatomy and sperm parameters. Surgical sperm extraction can be considered at the time of gender-affirming surgery for individuals that desire fertility preservation but are unable to otherwise produce a semen sample.

Sperm cryopreservation is ideally performed prior to initiation of gender-affirming care to avoid any potential deleterious impact on spermatogenesis. However, it can be performed at any point during an individual's gender transition and previous studies have demonstrated the ability to obtain samples adequate for fertility preservation from transgender women with a history of hormone treatment. Unfortunately, there is no consensus regarding how long feminizing hormone treatment should be discontinued prior to obtaining a sperm sample for fertility preservation. The quality and quantity of sperm obtained for cryopreservation informs future success rates and options for achieving biological parenthood. For transgender women with low sperm counts and prior exposure to gender-affirming hormone care, the use of a selective estrogen receptor modulator clomiphene citrate has been proposed as a potential method to expedite restoration of spermatogenesis [77]. Individuals considering future insemination (discussed in the next section) of a natal female partner or surrogate with cryopreserved specimen will need to cryopreserve a larger quantity of sperm to achieve a high probability of success. Depending upon one's semen analysis at the time of fertility preservation this may necessitate multiple collections to bank a desired quantity of cryopreserved sperm. Transgender women planning to use cryopreserved sperm for future in vitro fertilization with oocytes from a partner or donor will typically require a much smaller quantity of frozen sperm to achieve success. It is important to note that transgender women with severe infertility related to poor sperm quality or quantity would likely be unable to achieve pregnancy through inseminations and would be advised to use their cryopreserved specimen for in vitro fertilization with intracytoplasmic injection of the frozen sperm into oocytes if biologic parenthood was desired.

Embryo cryopreservation

As is the case with transgender men, embryo cryopreservation would also be an option for fertility preservation for transgender women and nonbinary individuals. Embryo cryopreservation should be pursued by transgender women only in cases where one is confident in their choice for an individual or donor with whom they wish to reproduce. For transgender individuals in committed relationships with an individual with whom they wish to parent (who may or may not be the desired source of alternate gametes), or who are certain of their desired donor for oocytes, cryopreservation of embryos allows for more specific estimations of the probability of achieving parenthood as well as the option for genetic testing of the embryo(s).

Testicular tissue cryopreservation

Testicular tissue cryopreservation is currently considered an experimental method of fertility preservation in prepubertal youth, but is the only fertility preservation option available to prepubertal transgender girls and nonbinary individuals assigned male at birth who are not yet capable of sperm production. Testicular tissue cryopreservation is a process by which testicular tissue is surgically extracted and frozen for future reproductive use. The ultimate goal for testicular tissue cryopreservation is to generate future mature sperm either through in vitro maturation techniques or through autotransplantation. Future advances in reproductive technologies are necessary in order for mature gametes to be obtained from testicular tissue cryopreservation and no pregnancies have been achieved through testicular tissue cryopreservation to date. For transgender women interested in gender-affirming surgery, testicular tissue cryopreservation could be performed from the orchiectomy specimen obtained without requiring additional surgical procedures, and is not considered experimental.

Fertility preservation outcomes for transgender women

Over the past 10 years, early outcome data from retrospective cohort studies have demonstrated sperm cryopreservation to be a feasible method for transgender and nonbinary individuals to maintain future reproductive potential prior to gender-affirming treatments. Multiple analyses of semen samples from transgender women have shown reduced sperm parameters even among women with no reported prior exposure to gender-affirming hormones. One such study of 29 transgender women with a mean age of 29 years and no prior feminizing hormone treatment found that motile sperm count at the time of cryopreservation was abnormal in almost 75% of individuals [78]. Another study of 78 healthy transgender women undergoing fertility preservation prior to initiation of gender-affirming hormone care found that compared to age-matched cisgender controls the transgender women had lower sperm concentration, total motile sperm count, and postthaw parameters, indicating increased cryosensitivity of samples. Specimens from 53% of transgender women in this cohort had sperm parameters diagnostic of oligozoospermia [79]. Reasons postulated for the decreased counts and quality of sperm at the time of fertility preservation include increased psychological stress faced by transgender individuals, potential underreporting for hormone therapy or body heat changes in the setting of tucking (a practice of moving natal male anatomy posteriorly to allow for a visibly smooth crotch contour) contributing to impaired spermatogenesis.

In an attempt to elucidate potential etiologies for depressed semen quality among transgender women without prior hormone exposure, Marsh et al. performed a case control study of 22 transgender women seeking fertility preservation prior to initiation of feminizing hormones. Semen samples from the transgender women were compared to fertile cisgender controls with the samples from transgender women demonstrating decreased sperm concentration, volume, and morphology. Transgender women were more likely to report symptoms of depression, anxiety, and stress compared to the control men with no difference in the frequency of ejaculation between groups. Additionally a significantly larger proportion of transgender women reported wearing tight undergarments or utilizing tucking, however, there was no correlation between tucking and sperm concentration or motility [80]. In a larger study of semen samples from 260 transgender women, the majority of whom reported no prior hormone use, the median values for all sperm parameters were significantly lower than WHO data for the general population and only 26% of thawed semen samples were determined to have quality that is high enough for intrauterine insemination (IUI). Known risk factors for poor semen quality such as BMI, alcohol use, and cannabis use were controlled for in this study with the authors suggesting that there may be factors specific to trans women that negatively impact their semen quality [51]. The reduced sperm counts and quality parameters observed in samples analyzed from transgender adults was not similarly demonstrated in a small prospective study of transgender adolescents and young adults. An analysis of semen parameters in young feminizing transgender patients, with a median age of 19 years, prior to gender-affirming hormone care median sperm counts and motility were within normal range with only a reduction in semen morphology observed [81]. Although limited by sample size, the higher quality of samples observed in this younger cohort as compared to adult studies may point to possible factors faced by transgender women, such as stress, tucking, or lifestyle choices that contribute negatively to their sperm quality over time. Further research is needed to elucidate potential causes for impaired sperm quality in transgender women, and whether any such causes are modifiable, to improve upon fertility counseling and parenting options for this population.

Surveys of attitudes toward fertility preservation provide insight into the experience and challenges of fertility care for transgender women and nonbinary individuals assigned male at birth. In a survey of trans women and nonbinary individuals assigned female at birth considering future fertility preservation, common fears listed included interruption or postponing of gender-affirming care (53%), high cost of care (47%), and having to masturbate to produce a sperm sample (27%) [82]. In a pattern similar to transgender men, the overall patient experience of trans women with assisted reproductive care is heavily impacted by the behaviors of their providers and culture of the clinic where they are receiving fertility care. A gender-affirming environment and culturally competent fertility providers were common themes in interviews with the minority of trans women who reported a positive experience. Trans women reporting a negative experience with assisted reproductive care commonly cited failure to use desired names and pronouns or inconsistencies in gender documentation as contributing to their discomfort with one trans woman noting, "there were tons of factual inaccuracies in all our documentation and everything. I mean, I had a health card that lists me as female, correctly, and on their charts they always had me as male" [21]. Incorrect heteronormative assumptions made by providers regarding desired methods of conception or conceiving "naturally" were additionally cited as common reasons for discomfort with one couple stating, "They were very interested in us making an effort to get pregnant at home [through intercourse] which wasn't anything that we had expressed interest in" [21].

Fertility care

Transgender or nonbinary people may wish to pursue fertility treatment for a multitude of reasons, including preservation of gametes prior to gender-affirming surgery or gender-affirming hormone care, personal or partner infertility, desire to reproduce in a partnership in which both sperm and oocytes are not available, desire to reproduce without a partner, plan for use of a surrogate, or desire for genetic testing of embryos. Reproductive options available for transgender individuals are influenced by their partner status and whether their partner wishes to provide reproductive gametes (Table 10.4). An individual's gender identity does not dictate their sexual identity and therefore couples in which one or both partners are transgender can have a variety of reproductive

TABLE 10.4 Methods for achieving biologic parenthood.

Method	Description	Timeline	Considerations
Intrauterine insemination (IUI)	• A sperm sample from a partner or donor is prepared in a laboratory and insemination timed with ovulation • The sperm sample is provided (or thawed) and prepared in the laboratory. Using a small catheter, the sperm sample is injected into the individual's uterus at the appropriate time in the cycle	• Insemination is timed with ovulation (mid-cycle) in order for the injected sperm sample to meet the ovulated oocyte(s) to achieve pregnancy • Time required for intrauterine insemination procedure is typically 5–10 minutes	• Clinic environment, ultrasound monitoring and IUI procedure may be dysphoric for some individuals • May be utilized in conjunction with ovulation medications to increase potential for fertilization • Some semen samples will not meet minimum criteria for IUI • Requirement of at least one patent fallopian tube to obtain pregnancy • Requires one partner to have a uterus/carry the pregnancy unless a genetic surrogate is utilized
In vitro fertilization (IVF)	• Sperm and oocytes may be obtained from an individual, partner or donor in any combination • Process by which oocytes are retrieved (or donor oocytes purchased) and fertilized in a laboratory with creation of embryos • Embryo are then implanted into an individual, partner (reciprocal IVF) or surrogate's uterus	• Ovarian stimulation with retrieval of oocytes is approximately a 10- to 4-day process • Mature oocytes can be fertilized following retrieval or thawed and fertilized with creation of embryos • Timing of embryo transfer is variable based upon embryo development and clinical protocols	• Clinic environment, ultrasound monitoring, retrieval and transfer procedures may invoke gender dysphoria • Reproductive option for individuals with poor semen parameters or surgically extracted sperm • Reciprocal IVF or use of a gestational carrier may be considered if the individual providing oocytes does not wish to or cannot carry a pregnancy
Surrogacy	(A) Traditional/genetic surrogate: individual assigned female at birth who provides the oocyte and carries the pregnancy (B) Gestational carrier: individual assigned female at birth who carries the pregnancy without any genetic contribution to the pregnancy	• In vitro fertilization is required for a gestational carrier with the timeline as before • Genetic surrogate may be achieved through intrauterine insemination or in vitro fertilization	• In the United States, laws regarding surrogacy fall under the jurisdiction of individual states with significant variation in legislation • If considering use of a surrogate in the future, specific FDA tests are required at the time that gametes are obtained

FDA, United States Food and Drug Administration.

options available. In a survey of transgender young adults desiring future parenthood, 25% reported that they planned to parent through sexual intercourse, 16% with the use of a surrogate, 9.4% with a known sperm donor, 9.4% with a sperm bank, and 3.1% using sperm donation from an unspecified source. For couples in which both oocytes and sperm are present and a partner with a uterus wishes to carry, reproduction through sexual intercourse represents an option. For all other couples, or those with one or both partners with infertility, fertility procedures should be discussed as potential routes to achieve parenthood. Selection of fertility treatments depends upon patient preferences, the quantity and quality of gametes available, underlying infertility diagnoses, access to care, and economic resources.

IUI, or therapeutic donor insemination if donor gametes are utilized, is a fertility procedure in which a sperm sample (either fresh or cryopreserved) is washed and processed to concentrate sperm. In a procedure timed to a natal female's ovulation, the sperm sample is then injected through a small catheter into that individual's uterus. In patients who are ovulatory this can be completed without medications while in anovulatory or otherwise interfile individuals oral or injectable medications can be used during one's cycle to increase probability of successful ovulation thereby increasing probability of pregnancy. An IUI is considered a relatively low-risk outpatient procedure that is tolerated similarly to a pap smear for most individuals. The likelihood of pregnancy from a single IUI procedure depends upon the age and fertility of both individuals producing gametes. In the absence of infertility or age-related fertility decline, an IUI is estimated to have approximately a 10%−15% probability of success with each cycle and therefore multiple cycles may be likely to achieve pregnancy [83]. Current research on success rates with IUI has demonstrated higher probability of success with sperm samples of at least 10 million motile, but reasonable pregnancy rates via IUI with sperm concentration between 5 million and 10 million motile sperm have been achieved [84].

Transgender women or nonbinary individuals assigned male at birth may wish to cryopreserve sperm prior to or during gender-affirming treatment to use for future IUI. At the time of fertility preservation, it is important that transgender individuals receive counseling regarding the probability of achieving pregnancy in the setting of the quantity and quality of their sperm sample. In light of research demonstrating reduced sperm counts and quality in trans women at the time of sperm cryopreservation, a significant portion of trans women desiring fertility preservation may have poor-quality sperm with sperm parameters that fall below recommendations for IUI. Banking additional sperm samples may help to overcome mildly reduced counts or allow for more trials of IUI. However, those with significantly reduced sperm quality would be unlikely to achieve pregnancy via IUI. Individuals with low sperm quantity and/or quality may consider in vitro fertilization with intracytoplasmic sperm injection as a means to achieve biologic parenthood if it is an economic option for them.

In a manner similar with cisgender individuals with infertility, in vitro fertilization can be considered as a means for transgender individuals to achieve parenthood of genetically related offspring. Success rates for in vitro fertilization vary widely based upon the quality of reproductive gametes involved with a natal female's age at which oocytes are harvested being a primary predictor. With improvements in assisted reproductive technology, success rates for achieving a live birth through in vitro fertilization have increased significantly over the past two decades. According to the 2017 National Society for Assisted Reproductive Technology (SART) data, the approximate live birth rate per oocyte retrieval for a woman with oocytes of age less than 35 is 55% [85]. In vitro fertilization represents the only current means by which transgender men can utilize cryopreserved oocytes to achieve pregnancy.

Counseling regarding pathways to biologic reproduction for transgender individuals would not be complete without discussion of surrogacy. A surrogate is a natal female who agrees prior to conception to carry a pregnancy with the intent to relinquish custody of the child to another person or couple following birth [86]. Surrogacy can be achieved by one of two routes, traditional surrogates and gestational carriers. A traditional surrogate, or genetic surrogate, is a natal woman who both provides the oocyte and carries the pregnancy. This is in contrast to a gestational carrier who carries the pregnancy without any genetic contribution to the offspring. While traditional surrogacy could be obtained through multiple routes, a gestational carrier requires in vitro fertilization. Legality of surrogacy varies greatly worldwide. In the United States, decisions regarding surrogacy fall under the jurisdiction of individual states. Some states, such as Michigan, explicitly deem surrogacy contracts unenforceable. States that do allow for legal use of gestational carriers have state-specific laws with restrictions such as maximum compensation that can be offered, restrictions in the role of planned parents in medical decision making and obligations for gestational carriers to abstain from drug use [87]. Although it can be challenging to conceptualize future reproductive plans at the time of fertility preservation counseling, transgender and nonbinary individuals that are considering use of a surrogate in the future in the United States will need to undergo additional testing at the time that their gametes are cryopreserved to comply with United States Food and Drug Administration regulations.

Pregnancy

Preconception and antepartum experience

The preconception experience of transgender men seeking pregnancy has been poorly characterized in current scientific literature. One survey study of 41 transgender men who experienced pregnancy after their transition found that one-third of reported pregnancies were unplanned. Among respondents, 61% reported prior use of testosterone and 88% of pregnancies were from the respondents' own oocytes. The majority of trans men conceived within 4 months of trying with only 15% receiving any preconception counseling and just 7% requiring the assistance of fertility drugs [38]. Despite over half of respondents reporting prior testosterone use, the lack of preconception counseling highlights the need for increased provider knowledge and resources to provide for the unique needs of transgender men desiring pregnancy. Qualitative studies of the preconception experience of transgender men reveal a common theme of conceptualizing pregnancy as a means to the desired outcome of parenthood [21,38,88]. For example, in consideration of pregnancy one transgender man stated "Even though I really hated the idea that I had to be seen as a woman in some places by some people to be pregnant, I really liked the idea of bringing life into this world ... I couldn't do it any other way" [88]. This emphasis on family building with focus on the goal of achieving parenthood represents a coping strategy used by some transgender men to deal with challenges in the preconception period.

Limited research has shown diversity in the experience of pregnancy for transgender men and nonbinary individuals. In interviews with transgender men who experienced pregnancy, the impact of pregnancy on their gender identity varied greatly. For many individuals, physiologic changes of pregnancy and antepartum interactions with healthcare providers led to internal conflict and worsening of gender dysphoria. One transgender man described pregnancy as an internal struggle noting "I really went through the pregnancies in a fog ... I knew there was something growing inside me but I wasn't connecting with it ... I wasn't thinking of myself as a mother who's pregnant at all" [88]. As was seen in the preconception period, some transgender men coped with these challenges by conceptualizing pregnancy as a necessary challenge to create their desired family as one trans man described "I looked at it as something to endure to have a child" [38]. On the other hand, some transgender men expressed an increased connection with their body and gender identity during pregnancy as one individual man described "the whole pregnancy and birth has made me more whole and more comfortable in my own skin, more comfortable with myself and my past" [88]. Similarly another transgender man noted "it was relieving to feel comfortable in the body I'd been born into" [38].

Interviews with transgender and nonbinary individuals that have experienced pregnancy identify loneliness as a common theme throughout the preconception and antepartum periods. Transgender and nonbinary individuals represent a marginalized group, with variable family and social support stemming from prejudice related to their gender identity, and the experience of pregnancy can contribute to further isolation. One transgender man described pregnancy as "lonely because I was the only one" [38]. These feeling of isolation were accentuated by a lack of support and lack of available resources for transgender men in pregnancy. Another transgender man described passing as not pregnant until the late third trimester due to his body habitus and "because people who don't assume that someone that looks like me could be pregnant" [38]. These interviews emphasize the need for development of inclusive educational materials and social support resources for transgender individuals in pregnancy. Continued training of healthcare providers and clinic staff is necessary to provide gender-affirming obstetric care and minimize the sense of disconnection and isolation experienced by transgender and nonbinary individuals in pregnancy.

Experience of pregnancy loss

The wide-ranging impact of pregnancy on gender identity as well as common feeling of isolation were likewise reflected in qualitative studies of transgender and nonbinary individuals that experienced pregnancy loss. An international qualitative study of 16 transgender men and nonbinary individuals' experience found dichotomous effects on gender identity. While the experience of pregnancy loss was distressing to all respondents, some transmasculine individuals viewed their ability to conceive as a sign that their body was working. One transgender man described, "it felt more positive than negative. I was sad but more like this can happen" [89]. On the other hand, some transgender and nonbinary individuals felt a disconnect from their body following pregnancy loss with one transgender man stating, "I felt betrayed-like I was supposed to be female and supposed to have babies and here I was trying to have a baby and we would get pregnant and then I would have a miscarriage" [88]. Interviews with transgender men experiencing miscarriage commonly revealed feelings of isolation and a lack of available support through the healthcare system. Following his miscarriage one individual noted, "there was no support for miscarriages at that time. I got sent away. There was no offer of counseling" and another individual stated that they "didn't feel like there was anything available" [89]. These interviews emphasize the importance of inclusive healthcare and the need for targeted support services for transgender individuals that experience miscarriage.

Intrapartum care

Labor and delivery can bring about additional challenges unique to transgender and nonbinary individuals. Aspects of childbirth such as cervical examinations, manual methods of cervical dilation and pushing require repetitive exposure of one's genitals and can evoke gender dysphoria and contribute to delivery preferences among transgender individuals. In the aforementioned survey of 41 transgender men, 44% delivered with nonphysician providers and 17% delivered at home [38]. This preference for nonphysician providers and for delivery outside of the hospital may reflect prior negative experiences and discrimination in the healthcare setting and/or poor access to care. In discussion of delivery planning, one transgender man said, "I never really wanted to do a home birth ... I was only going to have a home birth just out of fear of how the hospital wouldn't be able to deal with me" [90]. With regards to route of delivery one survey study reported 30% of transgender men delivered by cesarean section with one quarter of those being secondary to paternal request [38]. Interviews with transgender individuals in pregnancy reflecting varying preferences for method of delivery. For some transgender men, the exposure of a vaginal delivery can be unsettling with as one transgender man described his preference for a cesarean section stating, "I think that emotionally it was a better choice than having to push a baby out ... the thought of that part of my body being on display ... was just a little too much for me" [88]. This is in stark contrast to another transgender man's experience who described "pregnancy and childbirth were very male experiences for me. When I birthed my children, I was born into fatherhood" [38]. These diverse experiences of childbirth highlight the need for obstetric providers to avoid assumptions regarding delivery preferences or impact of delivery on a transgender person's identity as these experiences are unique to the individual. In the provision of gender-affirming care, providers should discuss the risks and benefits of different routes of delivery utilize a patient-centered approach to delivery planning.

Postpartum experience

The postpartum period has the similar challenge of isolation but introduces new concerns for transgender and nonbinary individuals, including consideration of chest feeding (i.e., breastfeeding) and discussion of initiating or restarting gender-affirming hormone care. Transgender and nonbinary individuals have higher baseline rates of depression and suicide and face increased discrimination and lack of familial support as compared to the general population. These findings in conjunction with the increase in loneliness and isolation reported during pregnancy contribute to an increased risk of postpartum depression among transgender and nonbinary individuals [38,88]. One transgender man described the postpartum experiences as a "heavy time, having a baby, not passing as male, all the changes and society telling me to just be happy" [38]. The increased potential for postpartum depression in this population warrants additional attention to risk factors and increased educational and counseling resources for transgender and nonbinary individuals in the months following delivery.

Chest feeding represents an option for some transgender and nonbinary men and providers should support individuals wishing to do so. In a survey study of transgender men who experienced pregnancy, approximately 51% reported chest feeding following delivery [38]. In another study of 22 transmasculine individuals, approximately 73% chose to chest feed with half of participants continuing to chest feed for over 1 year. The impact of chest feeding on gender dysphoria was highly variable with some individuals denying feelings of dysphoria associated with chest feeding, some reporting significant dysphoria inherent to the act of chest feeding and other reporting feelings of dysphoria triggered by social interactions. Gendered assumptions regarding their chest feeding desires as well as providers touching their chest without permission were triggers for gender dysphoria [27]. Healthcare providers should utilize gender-affirming terminology, respectful touch with permission, and limit exposure of one's chest postpartum to minimize the distress secondary to gender dysphoria that their transmasculine patients may experience with chest feeding. With the knowledge that the postpartum period and attempts to chest feed can trigger gender dysphoria in transmasculine patients, efforts should be made to avoid shared postpartum rooms when possible to limit patient discomfort. Interestingly nine of the individuals interviewed had undergone top surgery prior to conceiving. Although prior top surgery was associated with a difficulty obtaining infant latch, some individuals were still able to chest feed successfully despite prior surgery [27].

Providers should provide balanced counseling regarding the risks and benefits of chest feeding with an understanding that the decision to chest feed is highly personal. For transgender men and nonbinary individuals who do not wish to chest feed, providers should be well versed in recommendations regarding lactation suppression, including use of cool compresses, potential use of pumping to relieve discomfort and consideration of dopamine receptor antagonists in decreasing milk production [91]. Discussion of initiation or restarting of gender-affirming hormone care should also occur in the postpartum period. For individuals who do not wish to chest feed, masculinizing hormone therapy can be initiated or restarted in the postpartum period with many recommending to wait until 4- to 6-week postpartum to mitigate risk of venous thromboembolism. For individuals who do wish to chest feed, testosterone has been shown to suppress lactation, but there is limited rigorous data regarding the safety of testosterone therapy during lactation. Physicians should provide thorough counseling regarding the available research and potential risks of testosterone during lactation as well as the potential benefits of gender-affirming hormone care to the individual [91]. Some transgender men can experience significant mood changes and symptoms of depression in the postpartum period while waiting to restart testosterone therapy with one individual stating "that roller coaster was an insanity you cannot describe" [90]. For transmasculine individuals that experience significant gender dysphoria and mood symptoms, the benefits of gender-affirming hormone care may outweigh the risks of exposure during lactation [91]. Using a patient-centered approach, it is reasonable to resume testosterone treatment if necessary while chest feeding after an adequate milk supply has been established. It can also be helpful to have access to mental health providers well versed in these issues to help patients through their decision making.

Impact of parenting on children

Historically transgender individuals have been denied fertility services and other opportunities for parenthood on the basis of transphobic assumptions that parenting by a transgender individual would negatively impact the development of children [20,92]. A survey of attitudes toward transgender parenting found that American young adults were more likely to perceive a transgender couple as emotionally unstable and unfit to parent as compared to cisgender couples [93]. Transgender and nonbinary individuals face significant discrimination worldwide and as a result of their own experiences of transphobia some transgender individuals have expressed fear that becoming a parent would lead to stigmatization for their child [82,94]. However, multiple studies of children raised by transgender parents have debunked this myth that a parent's gender identity negatively impacts their children [95–99]. An early case series of 37 children raised by homosexual or transgender parent(s) found no difference in sexual or gender identity of the children as compared to those raised by cisgender heterosexual parents [95]. Freedman et al. performed a qualitative study on a clinical sample of 32 children with a transgender parent and found no effect on developmental milestones or evidence of gender identity disorder in the children [96].

Another study of 55 children found that the transgender identity of one parent does not negatively influence the sexual or gender identity development of a child. The authors found that younger age of the child at the time of parental gender transition predicted less family conflict and better adjustment for the child [97]. While gender transition can represent a parenting challenge, effective communication at the time of transition can positively impact parent-child relationships. In a study of 48 transgender parents, among parents that directly told their children about their decision to transition the majority of parent-child relationships improved or remained unchanged following transition [100]. More recently, Condat et al. performed a long-term follow up of children conceived by donor insemination in French couples with a cisgender woman and transgender man as compared to children raised by age and family-status matched cisgender couples. The authors found that transgender fatherhood did not impact on the mental health, cognitive development, or gender identity of the children [99]. These studies of child development in the context of transgender parenthood are reassuring and provide no evidence that having a transgender parent affects a child's gender identity, sexual orientation of development milestones. Additionally, the personal experiences of transgender individuals may uniquely allow them to role model authenticity and self-advocacy for their children [8]. These conclusions support actions to improve access to fertility care, foster care, and adoption services for transgender and nonbinary individuals considering parenthood.

Impact of parenting on gender identity and quality of life

There is limited research on the impact of parenting on gender identity or quality of life for transgender and nonbinary people. A United States national probability sample of transgender and cisgender respondents found no significant difference in mental health outcomes by gender identity among parents and nonparents [10]. Transgender parents report similar levels of transphobia and discrimination on the basis of gender identity as compared to nonparents. Despite facing similar societal stigmatization, a survey of transgender adults in Canada found that transgender parents were less likely to avoid public spaces due to transphobia as compared to nonparents [8]. While this may be secondary to parental responsibilities, the act of parenting may provide opportunities for new relationships with cisgender or other transgender parents. Achieving parenthood may be viewed by some transgender individuals as a triumph over the widespread message that they are not supposed to become parents contributing positively to their gender identity and sense of self [101]. An analysis of factors contributing to suicidal ideation among transgender adults, found that parenthood was a protective factor associated with decreased suicidal ideation among respondents [102]. In a survey of 50 transgender men, individuals with children scored higher on self-perceived mental health status and vitality measures as compared to age and relationship-matched controls [58]. Current literature supports a positive or negligible impact of parenthood on quality of life for transgender and nonbinary individuals. While further research is needed to further elucidate the role of parenting on quality of life measures, these early findings support improved access to parenting pathways for transgender and nonbinary people.

Conclusions

Transgender and nonbinary individuals have the same desires to parent as cisgender people, including the intent to nurture and build families. Despite this desire for parenthood transgender and nonbinary individuals face significant barriers to achieving parenthood, including societal stigmatization, discrimination in the healthcare setting, provider bias based in transphobia, and lack of access to fertility care. Unique to transgender and nonbinary individuals is the additional challenge of gender-affirming surgical and hormone treatments which can have significant negative consequences on their future reproductive potential. Given the known definitive impact of gender-affirming surgery on fertility and potential effects of gender-affirming hormones on future reproductive capacity, there is consensus among many international and national medical societies regarding the need for thorough fertility preservation counseling prior to initiation of gender-affirming treatments. However, many studies have demonstrated that this standard of care is not routinely met with fertility counseling failing to be universally offered to transgender individuals and when offered counseling may be incomplete. Even in the setting of effective fertility preservation counseling, additional barriers, including young age at time of transition without the maturity to consider future fertility goals, potential for fertility treatments and procedures to trigger gender dysphoria, prior discrimination in healthcare, and costs of treatment limit uptake of fertility treatment with the potential for reproductive regret.

There are multiple long-term studies of children raised by a transgender parent which debunk the transphobic assumption that the presence of a transgender parent negatively influences a child's development. Given these conclusions, the conversation regarding transgender and nonbinary individual's desire to parent needs to shift away from an ethical question of whether to support these desires to a pragmatic discussion of how to best support transgender individuals in their quest for parenthood. At the provider level there is a need for increased medical education regarding the unique needs of transgender and nonbinary individuals and the importance of using desired names and pronouns and avoiding cisnormative assumptions to adequately care for these individuals. Clinics need to evaluate their waiting rooms, intake forms, educational materials, and training of all staff to ensure that transgender and nonbinary individuals feel welcome and affirmed throughout their care. Fertility preservation for transgender and nonbinary individuals is an emerging field with many questions currently unanswered. Future research is needed to determine the impact of gender-affirming hormones on reproductive capacity and whether these effects are dose-dependent or reversible. Larger collaborative studies on the experience of transgender individuals receiving fertility care are needed to provide more effective fertility preservation counseling for transgender and nonbinary individuals.

References

[1] Winter S, Diamond M, Green J, Karasic D, Reed T, Whittle S, et al. Transgender people: health at the margins of society. Lancet 2016;388 (10042):390–400.

[2] Flores AR, Herman JL, Gates GJ, Brown TNT. How many adults identify as transgender in the United States? Los Angeles, CA: The Williams Institute; 2016.

[3] American Psychiatric Association. Diagnostic & Statistical Manual of Mental Disorders. Washington, DC: American Psychiatric Association; 1985.

[4] American Psychiatric Association. Revised Diagnostic and Statistical Manual of Mental Disorders: DSM-III-R. 3rd ed. Washington, DC: American Psychiatric Association; 1990. p. 567.

[5] American Psychiatric Association. Diagnostic and Statistical Manual of Mental Disorders: DSM-IV. Washington, DC: American Psychiatric Association; 1998. p. 886.

[6] American Psychiatric Association. Diagnostic and Statistical Manual of Mental Disorders: DSM-5. 5th ed. Washington, DC: American Psychiatric Publishing; 2013. p. 947.

[7] Feldman J, Bockting W. Transgender health. Minn Med 2003;86(7):25–32.

[8] Pyne J, Bauer G, Bradley K. Transphobia and other stressors impacting trans parents. J GLBT Fam Stud 2015;11(2):107–26.

[9] Grant JM, et al. Injustice at every turn a report of the National Transgender Discrimination Survey. Washington, DC: National Center for Transgender Equality, National Gay and Lesbian Task Force; 2011.

[10] Carone N, Rothblum ED, Bos HMW, Gartrell NK, Herman JL. Demographics and health outcomes in a United States probability sample of transgender parents. J Fam Psychol 2021;35(1):57–68.

[11] Auer MK, Fuss J, Nieder TO, Briken P, Biedermann SV, Stalla GK, et al. Desire to have children among transgender people in Germany: a cross-sectional multi-center study. J Sex Med 2018;15(5):757–67.

[12] Defreyne J, Van Schuylenbergh J, Motmans J, Tilleman KL, T'Sjoen GGR. Parental desire and fertility preservation in assigned female at birth transgender people living in Belgium. Fertil Steril 2020;113(1):149–157.e2.

[13] Tornello SL, Bos H. Parenting intentions among transgender individuals. LGBT Health 2017;4(2):115–20.

[14] Baram S, Myers SA, Yee S, Librach CL. Fertility preservation for transgender adolescents and young adults: a systematic review. Hum Reprod Update 2019;25(6):694–716.

[15] Persky RW, Gruschow SM, Sinaii N, Carlson C, Ginsberg JP, Dowshen NL. Attitudes toward fertility preservation among transgender youth and their parents. J Adolesc Health 2020;67(4):583–9.

[16] Chen D, Matson M, Macapagal K, Johnson EK, Rosoklija I, Finlayson C, et al. Attitudes toward fertility and reproductive health among transgender and gender-nonconforming adolescents. J Adolesc Health 2018;63(1):62–8.

[17] Strang JF, Jarin J, Call D, Clark B, Wallace GL, Anthony LG, et al. Transgender youth fertility attitudes questionnaire: measure development in nonautistic and autistic transgender youth and their parents. J Adolesc Health 2018;62(2):128–35.

[18] James SE, Herman JL, Rankin S, Keisling M, Mottet L, Anafi M. The report of the 2015 United States transgender survey. Washington, DC: National Center for Transgender Equality; 2016.

[19] European Union Agency for Fundamental Rights. Being trans in the European Union: comparative analysis of EU LGBT survey data. Luxembourg: European Union Agency for Fundamental Rights; 2014.

[20] Jones HW. Gender reassignment and assisted reproduction. Evaluation of multiple aspects. Hum Reprod 2000;15(5):987.

[21] James-Abra S, Tarasoff LA, Green D, Epstein R, Anderson S, Marvel S, et al. Trans people's experiences with assisted reproduction services: a qualitative study. Hum Reprod 2015;30(6):1365–74.

[22] Ethics Committee of the American Society for Reproductive Medicine. Access to fertility services by transgender persons: an Ethics Committee opinion. Fertil Steril 2015;104(5):1111–15.

[23] Wu HY, Yin O, Monseur B, Selter J, Collins LJ, Lau BD, et al. Lesbian, gay, bisexual, transgender content on reproductive endocrinology and infertility clinic websites. Fertil Steril 2017;108(1):183–91.

[24] Ross LE, Epstein R, Anderson S, Eady A. Policy, practice, and personal narratives: experiences of LGBTQ people with adoption in Ontario, Canada. Adopt Q 2009;12(3–4):272–93.

[25] Ryan D, Martin A. Lesbian, gay, bisexual and transgender parents in the school systems. Sch Psychol Rev 2000;29(2):207–16.

[26] World Health Organization. Eliminating forced, coercive and otherwise involuntary sterilization: an interagency statement. Geneva:: OHCHR, UN Women, UNAIDS, UNDP, UNFPA, UNICEF, WHO; 2014.

[27] MacDonald T, Noel-Weiss J, West D, Walks M, Biener M, Kibbe A, et al. Transmasculine individuals' experiences with lactation, chestfeeding, and gender identity: a qualitative study. BMC Pregnancy Childbirth 2016;16:106.

[28] Perrone AM, Cerpolini S, Maria Salfi NC, Ceccarelli C, De Giorgi LB, Formelli G, et al. Effect of long-term testosterone administration on the endometrium of female-to-male (FtM) transsexuals. J Sex Med 2009;6(11):3193–200.

[29] Nakamura A, Watanabe M, Sugimoto M, Sako T, Mahmood S, Kaku H, et al. Dose-response analysis of testosterone replacement therapy in patients with female to male gender identity disorder. Endocr J 2013;60(3):275–81.

[30] Deutsch MB, Bhakri V, Kubicek K. Effects of cross-sex hormone treatment on transgender women and men. Obstet Gynecol 2015;125 (3):605–10.

[31] Olson J, Schrager SM, Clark LF, Dunlap SL, Belzer M. Subcutaneous testosterone: an effective delivery mechanism for masculinizing young transgender men. LGBT Health 2014;1(3):165–7.

[32] Defreyne J, Vanwonterghem Y, Collet S, Iwamoto SJ, Wiepjes CM, Fisher AD, et al. Vaginal bleeding and spotting in transgender men after initiation of testosterone therapy: a prospective cohort study (ENIGI). Int J Transgend Health 2020;21(2):163–75.

[33] Light A, Wang L-F, Zeymo A, Gomez-Lobo V. Family planning and contraception use in transgender men. Contraception 2018;98 (4):266–9.

[34] Wolf CJ, Hotchkiss A, Ostby JS, LeBlanc GA, Gray LE. Effects of prenatal testosterone propionate on the sexual development of male and female rats: a dose-response study. Toxicol Sci 2002;65(1):71–86.

References

[35] Hotchkiss AK, Lambright CS, Ostby JS, Parks-Saldutti L, Vandenbergh JG, Gray LE. Prenatal testosterone exposure permanently masculinizes anogenital distance, nipple development, and reproductive tract morphology in female Sprague-Dawley rats. Toxicol Sci 2007;96(2):335–45.

[36] Patel A, Rivkees SA. Prenatal virilization associated with paternal testosterone gel therapy. Int J Pediatr Endocrinol 2010;2010(6):867471.

[37] Cho J, Su X, Phillips V, Holditch-Davis D. Association of maternal and infant salivary testosterone and cortisol and infant gender with mother-infant interaction in very-low-birthweight infants. Res Nurs Health 2015;38(5):357–68.

[38] Light AD, Obedin-Maliver J, Sevelius JM, Kerns JL. Transgender men who experienced pregnancy after female-to-male gender transitioning. Obstet Gynecol 2014;124(6):1120–7.

[39] Grynberg M, Fanchin R, Dubost G, Colau J-C, Brémont-Weil C, Frydman R, et al. Histology of genital tract and breast tissue after long-term testosterone administration in a female-to-male transsexual population. Reprod Biomed Online 2010;20(4):553–8.

[40] Loverro G, Resta L, Dellino M, Edoardo DN, Cascarano MA, Loverro M, et al. Uterine and ovarian changes during testosterone administration in young female-to-male transsexuals. Taiwan J Obstet Gynecol 2016;55(5):686–91.

[41] De Roo C, Lierman S, Tilleman K, Peynshaert K, Braeckmans K, Caanen M, et al. Ovarian tissue cryopreservation in female-to-male transgender people: insights into ovarian histology and physiology after prolonged androgen treatment. Reprod Biomed Online 2017;34(6):557–66.

[42] Grimstad FW, Fowler KG, New EP, Ferrando CA, Pollard RR, Chapman G, et al. Ovarian histopathology in transmasculine persons on testosterone: a multicenter case series. J Sex Med 2020;17(9):1807–18.

[43] Caanen MR, Schouten NE, Kuijper EAM, van Rijswijk J, van den Berg MH, van Dulmen-den Broeder E, et al. Effects of long-term exogenous testosterone administration on ovarian morphology, determined by transvaginal (3D) ultrasound in female-to-male transsexuals. Hum Reprod 2017;32(7):1457–64.

[44] Van Den Broecke R, Van Der Elst J, Liu J, Hovatta O, Dhont M. The female-to-male transsexual patient: a source of human ovarian cortical tissue for experimental use. Hum Reprod 2001;16(1):145–7.

[45] Lierman S, Tilleman K, Braeckmans K, Peynshaert K, Weyers S, T'Sjoen G, et al. Fertility preservation for trans men: frozen-thawed in vitro matured oocytes collected at the time of ovarian tissue processing exhibit normal meiotic spindles. J Assist Reprod Genet 2017;34(11):1449–56.

[46] Caanen MR, Soleman RS, Kuijper EAM, Kreukels BPC, De Roo C, Tilleman K, et al. Antimüllerian hormone levels decrease in female-to-male transsexuals using testosterone as cross-sex therapy. Fertil Steril 2015;103(5):1340–5.

[47] Tack LJW, Craen M, Dhondt K, Vanden Bossche H, Laridaen J, Cools M. Consecutive lynestrenol and cross-sex hormone treatment in biological female adolescents with gender dysphoria: a retrospective analysis. Biol Sex Differ 2016;7(1):14.

[48] Liu PY, Swerdloff RS, Christenson PD, Handelsman DJ, Wang CHormonal Male Contraception Summit Group. Rate, extent, and modifiers of spermatogenic recovery after hormonal male contraception: an integrated analysis. Lancet 2006;367(9520):1412–20.

[49] Lübbert H, Leo-Rossberg I, Hammerstein J. Effects of ethinyl estradiol on semen quality and various hormonal parameters in a eugonadal male. Fertil Steril 1992;58(3):603–8.

[50] Adeleye AJ, Reid G, Kao C-N, Mok-Lin E, Smith JF. Semen parameters among transgender women with a history of hormonal treatment. Urology 2019;124:136–41.

[51] de Nie I, Meißner A, Kostelijk EH, Soufan AT, Voorn-de Warem I AC, den Heijer M, et al. Impaired semen quality in trans women: prevalence and determinants. Hum Reprod 2020;35(7):1529–36.

[52] Schneider F, Neuhaus N, Wistuba J, Zitzmann M, Heß J, Mahler D, et al. Testicular functions and clinical characterization of patients with gender dysphoria (GD) undergoing sex reassignment surgery (SRS). J Sex Med 2015;12(11):2190–200.

[53] Jindarak S, Nilprapha K, Atikankul T, Angspatt A, Pungrasmi P, Iamphongsai S, et al. Spermatogenesis abnormalities following hormonal therapy in transwomen. BioMed Res Int 2018;2018(4):7919481.

[54] Kent MA, Winoker JS, Grotas AB. Effects of feminizing hormones on sperm production and malignant changes: microscopic examination of post orchiectomy specimens in transwomen. Urology 2018;121:93–6.

[55] Schneider F, Kliesch S, Schlatt S, Neuhaus N. Andrology of male-to-female transsexuals: influence of cross-sex hormone therapy on testicular function. Andrology 2017;5(5):873–80.

[56] Kreukels BPC, Haraldsen IR, De Cuypere G, Richter-Appelt H, Gijs L, Cohen-Kettenis PT. A European network for the investigation of gender incongruence: the ENIGI initiative. Eur Psychiatry 2012;27(6):445–50.

[57] Riggs DW, Bartholomaeus C. Fertility preservation decision making amongst Australian transgender and non-binary adults. Reprod Health 2018;15(1):181.

[58] Wierckx K, Van Caenegem E, Pennings G, Elaut E, Dedecker D, Van de Peer F, et al. Reproductive wish in transsexual men. Hum Reprod 2012;27(2):483–7.

[59] Chiniara LN, Viner C, Palmert M, Bonifacio H. Perspectives on fertility preservation and parenthood among transgender youth and their parents. Arch Dis Child 2019;104(8):739–44.

[60] Nahata L, Tishelman AC, Caltabellotta NM, Quinn GP. Low fertility preservation utilization among transgender youth. J Adolesc Health 2017;61(1):40–4.

[61] Practice Committee of the American Society for Reproductive Medicine. Electronic address: asrm@asrm.org. Fertility preservation in patients undergoing gonadotoxic therapy or gonadectomy: a committee opinion. Fertil Steril 2019;112(6):1022–33.

[62] Donnez J, Dolmans M-M. Fertility preservation in women. N Engl J Med 2017;377(17):1657–65.

[63] Pacheco F, Oktay K. Current success and efficiency of autologous ovarian transplantation: a meta-analysis. Reprod Sci 2017;24(8):1111–20.

[64] De Roo C, Tilleman K, T'Sjoen G, De, Sutter P. Fertility options in transgender people. Int Rev Psychiatry 2016;28(1):112–19.

[65] Cobo A, García-Velasco J, Domingo J, Pellicer A, Remohí J. Elective and onco-fertility preservation: factors related to IVF outcomes. Hum Reprod 2018;33(12):2222–31.

[66] Cobo A, García-Velasco JA, Coello A, Domingo J, Pellicer A, Remohí J. Oocyte vitrification as an efficient option for elective fertility preservation. Fertil Steril 2016;105(3):755–764.e8.

[67] Noyes N, Labella PA, Grifo J, Knopman JM. Oocyte cryopreservation: a feasible fertility preservation option for reproductive age cancer survivors. J Assist Reprod Genet 2010;27(8):495–9.
[68] Wallace SA, Blough KL, Kondapalli LA. Fertility preservation in the transgender patient: expanding oncofertility care beyond cancer. Gynecol Endocrinol 2014;30(12):868–71.
[69] Amir H, Yaish I, Samara N, Hasson J, Groutz A, Azem F. Ovarian stimulation outcomes among transgender men compared with fertile cisgender women. J Assist Reprod Genet 2020;37(10):2463–72.
[70] Adeleye AJ, Cedars MI, Smith J, Mok-Lin E. Ovarian stimulation for fertility preservation or family building in a cohort of transgender men. J Assist Reprod Genet 2019;36(10):2155–61.
[71] Leung A, Sakkas D, Pang S, Thornton K, Resetkova N. Assisted reproductive technology outcomes in female-to-male transgender patients compared with cisgender patients: a new frontier in reproductive medicine. Fertil Steril 2019;112(5):858–65.
[72] Armuand G, Dhejne C, Olofsson JI, Rodriguez-Wallberg KA. Transgender men's experiences of fertility preservation: a qualitative study. Hum Reprod 2017;32(2):383–90.
[73] Oktay K, Turan V, Bedoschi G, Pacheco FS, Moy F. Fertility preservation success subsequent to concurrent aromatase inhibitor treatment and ovarian stimulation in women with breast cancer. J Clin Oncol 2015;33(22):2424–9.
[74] Brik T, Vrouenraets LJJJ, Schagen SEE, Meissner A, de Vries MC, Hannema SE. Use of fertility preservation among a cohort of transgirls in the Netherlands. J Adolesc Health 2019;64(5):589–93.
[75] Kafetsoulis A, Brackett NL, Ibrahim E, Attia GR, Lynne CM. Current trends in the treatment of infertility in men with spinal cord injury. Fertil Steril 2006;86(4):781–9.
[76] Tur-Kaspa I, Segal S, Moffa F, Massobrio M, Meltzer S. Viagra for temporary erectile dysfunction during treatments with assisted reproductive technologies. Hum Reprod 1999;14(7):1783–4.
[77] Alford AV, Theisen KM, Kim N, Bodie JA, Pariser JJ. Successful ejaculatory sperm cryopreservation after cessation of long-term estrogen therapy in a transgender female. Urology 2020;136:e48–50.
[78] Hamada A, Kingsberg S, Wierckx K, T'Sjoen G, De Sutter P, Knudson G, et al. Semen characteristics of transwomen referred for sperm banking before sex transition: a case series. Andrologia 2015;47(7):832–8.
[79] Li K, Rodriguez D, Gabrielsen JS, Centola GM, Tanrikut C. Sperm cryopreservation of transgender individuals: trends and findings in the past decade. Andrology 2018;6(6):860–4.
[80] Marsh C, McCracken M, Gray M, Nangia A, Gay J, Roby KF. Low total motile sperm in transgender women seeking hormone therapy. J Assist Reprod Genet 2019;36(8):1639–48.
[81] Barnard EP, Dhar CP, Rothenberg SS, Menke MN, Witchel SF, Montano GT, et al. Fertility preservation outcomes in adolescent and young adult feminizing transgender patients. Pediatrics 2019;144(3):e20183943.
[82] Defreyne J, Van Schuylenbergh J, Motmans J, Tilleman K, T'Sjoen G. Parental desire and fertility preservation in assigned male at birth transgender people living in Belgium. Int J Transgend Health 2020;21(1):45–57.
[83] Schorsch M, Gomez R, Hahn T, Hoelscher-Obermaier J, Seufert R, Skala C. Success rate of inseminations dependent on maternal age? An analysis of 4246 insemination cycles. Geburtshilfe Frauenheilkd 2013;73(8):808–11.
[84] Starosta A, Gordon CE, Hornstein MD. Predictive factors for intrauterine insemination outcomes: a review. Fertil Res Pract 2020;6(1):23.
[85] Centers for Disease Control and Prevention, American Society for Reproductive Medicine, Society for Assisted Reproductive Technology. 2017 Assisted reproductive technology national summary report. Atlanta, GA: United States Department of Health and Human Services; 2019.
[86] ACOG. ACOG Committee Opinion No. 660: family building through gestational surrogacy. Obstet Gynecol 2016;127(3):e97–e103.
[87] Tsai S, Shaia K, Woodward JT, Sun MY, Muasher SJ. Surrogacy laws in the United States: what obstetrician-gynecologists need to know. Obstet Gynecol 2020;135(3):717–22.
[88] Ellis SA, Wojnar DM, Pettinato M. Conception, pregnancy, and birth experiences of male and gender variant gestational parents: it's how we could have a family. J Midwifery Womens Health 2015;60(1):62–9.
[89] Riggs DW, Pearce R, Pfeffer CA, Hines S, White FR, Ruspini E. Men, trans/masculine, and non-binary people's experiences of pregnancy loss: an international qualitative study. BMC Pregnancy Childbirth 2020;20(1):482.
[90] Hoffkling A, Obedin-Maliver J, Sevelius J. From erasure to opportunity: a qualitative study of the experiences of transgender men around pregnancy and recommendations for providers. BMC Pregnancy Childbirth 2017;17(Suppl 2):332.
[91] Patel S, Sweeney LB. Maternal health in the transgender population. J Womens Health (Larchmt) 2021;30(2):253–9.
[92] Green R, Money J. Transsexualism and sex reassignment. Baltimore, MD: John Hopkins Press; 1969.
[93] Weiner BA, Zinner L. Attitudes toward straight, gay male, and transsexual parenting. J Homosex 2015;62(3):327–39.
[94] Haines BA, Ajayi AA, Boyd H. Making trans parents visible: intersectionality of trans and parenting identities. Fem Psychol 2014;24(2):238–47.
[95] Green R. Sexual identity of 37 children raised by homosexual or transsexual parents. Am J Psychiatry 1978;135(6):692–7.
[96] Freedman D, Tasker F, di Ceglie D. Children and adolescents with transsexual parents referred to a specialist gender identity development service: a brief report of key developmental features. Clin Child Psychol Psychiatry 2002;7(3):423–32.
[97] White T, Ettner R. Adaptation and adjustment in children of transsexual parents. Eur Child Adolesc Psychiatry 2007;16(4):215–21.
[98] Chiland C, Clouet AM, Golse B, Guinot M, Wolf JP. A new type of family: transmen as fathers thanks to donor sperm insemination: a 12-year follow-up exploratory study of their children. Neuropsychiatr Enfance Adolesc 2013;61(6):365–70.
[99] Condat A, Mamou G, Lagrange C, Mendes N, Wielart J, Poirier F, et al. Transgender fathering: children's psychological and family outcomes. PLoS One 2020;15(11):e0241214.
[100] Veldorale-Griffin A. Transgender parents and their adult children's experiences of disclosure and transition. J GLBT Fam Stud 2014;10(5):475–501.
[101] Hafford-Letchfield T, Cocker C, Rutter D, Tinarwo M, McCormack K, Manning R. What do we know about transgender parenting? Findings from a systematic review. Health Soc Care Community 2019;27(5):1111–25.
[102] Moody C, Smith NG. Suicide protective factors among trans adults. Arch Sex Behav 2013;42(5):739–52.

CHAPTER 11

Trauma and its impact on reproduction and sexuality

Laura Covington

Shady Grove Fertility, Covington & Hafkin and Associates, Washington, DC, United States

Introduction

Infertility itself can be considered traumatic, and the infertility experience can also activate earlier trauma experiences. There are three elements to consider for trauma: the event, the experience, and the effect [1]. Considering the *event*, the American Psychiatric Association in the Diagnostic and Statistical Manual of Mental Disorders (DSM-5) defines a trauma as an exposure to "death, threatened death, actual or threatened serious injury, or actual or threatened sexual violence" through direct or indirect exposure, witnessing, or learning about a friend or relative who was exposed (p. 271) [2]. While it may seem a stretch to define infertility in this way, infertility and the subsequent experience can feel like an "actual or threatened serious injury," as one's body does not work the way anticipated, and is poked, prodded, and analyzed in treatment. Trauma can be a physical and/or a psychological injury. Multiple losses, real (i.e., early or late pregnancy losses, hysterectomy) and ambiguous [3] (i.e., the much hoped for child, trust in body), can be felt during infertility.

Trauma has a wide range of definitions and is relative based on one's *experience* of the event, meaning that what one person views as traumatic may not be traumatic to the next person [4,5]. Trauma also has varying adverse *effects* that include the psychological response to an "unbearable and intolerable" event, challenging a person's ability to cope (p. 1) [6]. It is the body's response to the experience.

Infertility can be viewed as a reproductive trauma which may challenge coping and alter perceived identity [7]. As research shows, infertility and fertility treatment can cause higher rates of anxiety and distress [8,9]. And when one experiences infertility, they also bring a history, which can include previous traumas. Formerly resolved and unresolved traumas can rearise in a variety of anticipated and unanticipated ways.

Trauma and infertility can impact the biological, psychological, and social wellbeing of the person, causing interruption and changes to sexual relationships. The purpose of this chapter is to understand how physical and psychological trauma can impact the infertility experience and the sexual relationship and provide tools to help a couple to navigate the infertility experience and improve their relationship, communication, and sexual connection. The chapter will use a case study to highlight how the trauma can impact infertility for the individuals and the couple.

Trauma and the sexual relationship

Trauma influences various areas of life. The trauma experience may also be felt and impact the linked lives of the trauma survivor, and conversely, previous and current relationships may impact how trauma is experienced. When one member of a couple experiences a trauma consequently the other is affected too. The reasons for this are multiple. The partner could experience their own trauma at hearing what happened (i.e., vicarious trauma), or the survivor may now relate to the partner differently due to the emotional fallout of the trauma, such as increased anger or withdrawal.

Bessel van der Kolk notes [6], when we experience a trauma, our body remembers not only psychologically but also physically and biologically. Both infertility and trauma can take a toll on the body and thus impact the sexual relationship. The sexual relationship can often be ignored, as fertility treatment takes precedent, but healing the sexual relationship can help the couple reconnect and offer a protective measure for dealing with the stress of infertility.

Sex can be an intrinsic trigger of trauma even when it takes place in a safe relationship. Research shows that traumatic events of both sexual and nonsexual nature can develop similar disruptions and problems with intimacy [10,11]. Some survivors may even seek sexual activity to try to combat the bad experience with a good one. After a trauma, intimacy is impacted by both psychological and biological factors, having a diffused effect on sexual function. Physiological causes of the sexual dysfunction can result in psychological distress and psychological distress can result in sexual dysfunction, impacting the interaction with the intimate partner [10]. The preexisting trauma histories can become more complicated with infertility as sex can lose some of its meaning and purpose in the absence of procreation through sexual intercourse.

The impact of trauma can alter the sexual relationship, the way the couple connects, as well as how a trauma survivor relates to the outside world and vice versa [11]. A "ripple effect" occurs, emphasizing the importance of including not just the individual but also the support network in recovery. When one partner experiences anxiety and stress in their sexual relationship, it can cause the same impact for the other person [12]. Addressing trauma and sex as a couple's issue is essential.

Grief at the core of trauma and infertility

Grief is tied to loss. Yet, even though grief and loss are often synonymous with death, grief is not confined to death. Grief can be at the core of both trauma and infertility, and there are several losses that happen with trauma and infertility. For trauma, there may be a loss of how the world was viewed, mourning for life before the trauma, a loss of trust in others, loss of a sense of self, loss of control, loss of a sense of safety and security, etc. For infertility, there may be a loss of the much wanted child (something that has never been), loss of control over the body, loss of opportunity, loss of time, loss of a pregnancy, loss of finances, etc. Loss of sexual identity can occur with both infertility and trauma. Sex brings new meaning and dynamics. With infertility, sex becomes about procreation and no longer enjoyable and fun. With trauma, sex may no longer feel safe and a way of connecting.

Infertility literature suggests that "failure to acknowledge and appropriately grieve losses of infertility has an impact on a couple's long-term adjustment to infertility as well as prospective decisions regarding treatment and family building alternatives" (p. 9) [13]. However, sharing grief with a partner can be difficult. To share your feelings, you need to know and identify how it is you feel. With the ambiguous losses of trauma and infertility, understanding emotions and finding the words to express them can present challenges. Even when you know your feelings, you need to be willing to share them, and one might not be willing to share for fear of overburdening a partner, not being understood, and/or protecting a partner. While a person may want to share the grief, loss, and experience, the desire to keep the trauma private as a safe haven conflicts with the longing to be deeply understood by a partner [14].

Grief is a process, not a state [15]; it is not a linear path nor is it time limited. Incorporating, understanding, and adapting to loss is an internal experience often expressed in varying outward emotional, cognitive, spiritual, and behavioral responses [16]. When we lose a loved one, the grief of losing them does not end after a certain amount of time. Different events, people, or thoughts can trigger grief feelings many years later and even when one has successfully assimilated the meaning and reality of the loss [15].

Trauma recovery is similar to grief. Even when it feels like the trauma has "been resolved," certain events, like experiencing infertility, can trigger that trauma response and bring up old feelings and memories. Understanding the trauma history is essential in providing care when a new "crisis" (i.e., infertility) arises.

Psychological trauma theory

Shattered assumption theory suggests that when a trauma is experienced it "shatters" our assumptions about the way we thought about ourselves, the world, and how we influence the world, often causing distress and disruption as we work to understand the trauma [17]. These assumptions can change the way we relate to others around us and can have psychological impacts which disrupt the sexual and intimate relationships. Examining and reevaluating these core beliefs and assumptions can aid in recovery, and positive change can grow from the trauma [18].

Jaffe and Diamond [19] frame the idea of a "reproductive trauma" around one's "reproductive story." The reproductive story explores a person's hopes and dreams about having a family, visions of what children will look like, and imaginings of being a parent. This technique assists to work through a reproductive trauma, understanding and changing previous assumptions, allowing for a new story to emerge. Reproductive trauma disrupts the conscious and unconscious written story. There may be previous assumptions about the self that need to be shifted and rewritten when experiencing infertility. These assumptions can include, "It's easy to get pregnant"; "Life is fair"; and "If I work hard, I will be rewarded (i.e., get pregnant)" [7]. Often few concrete answers exist to understand why the reproductive trauma occurred, and self-blame becomes an answer. This narrative which causes a decreased self-worth is a result of the trauma. Rewriting this narrative helps to work through the self-blame, more accurately define the experience, and find a new course to move forward.

How trauma impacts attachment

Bowlby suggests a biological basis for understanding the parent-infant relationship. Attachment theory proposes that attaching to a caregiver is a primary, biologically driven response, over a secondary-need satisfaction [20]. Attachment occurs before drives and instincts, contrary to Freud's drive theory. This early caregiving relationship makes for adaptation and maladaptation across the lifespan "from the cradle to the grave" [21]. Bowlby argues that across a lifetime, a person's mental health is deeply related to the early attachments who provide safety and support. Attachment provides a foundation for how we self-regulate. The reciprocal process with the primary attachments is a framework for a person's internal working model. The interactions and attachment from early life provide the foundation for value of the self, trust of others, and the self-interacting with the world.

Through her research building on Bowlby, Ainsworth describes three major styles of attachment: secure attachment, ambivalent-insecure attachment, and avoidant-insecure attachment [20]. Secure attachment happens when a primary caregiver appropriately attends to a child's needs, helping the child to use that person as a secure base where the child feels comfort and assurance when reunited with a caregiver after separation. Ambivalent-insecure attachment style shows suspicion to strangers and distress from separation of primary caregiver but refuses comfort when reunited. Avoidant-insecure attachment style does not necessarily seek nor reject comfort or interaction from a primary caregiver. Disorganized-insecure attachment type was added later to describe a fourth style where there is often a mixture of avoidance and resistance [22]. With early-childhood trauma while the brain is still developing, the internal working model is significantly impacted, illustrated through insecure attachment traits such as lack of confidence, self-loathing, and emotional dysregulation. Attachment theory provides a groundwork for how the brain and mind are organized, how personality characteristics originate, and achieve self-regulation [23].

Early-childhood attachment relationships are what might significantly impact a reaction to stress. What attachment theory does not fully address is the impact of trauma later in life, even when one has a secure attachment. The theory does suggest though that the development of a secure attachment may be a protective factor in the impact of later trauma, where with an insecure attachment a later trauma might reignite, exacerbate, or reinforce early attachment styles. Although even with secure attachment, later trauma can still fragment attachment styles and the internal working model. The trauma may challenge previous beliefs about relationships and how relationships work.

Early trauma can either impact how we develop secure or insecure attachments. Family of origin history can give insight to understand why couples are attaching and relating in certain ways. Early attachments may be a foundation for "relationship self-regulation" or "the ability of intimate partners to monitor relational processes and work on maintaining the relationship" through self-awareness (p. 130) [24]. Understanding early attachments helps to lay a foundation for understanding how a trauma may have altered or reaffirmed beliefs around relationships and attachments.

Trauma response theory

Research shows that there are different ways men and women express, process, and respond to stress and emotions, biologically and psychologically [25,26]. During stress, men tend to withdraw while women tend to engage in social supports [27]. The idea of "flight or fight" proposes that when faced with stress a primitive reaction activates either running from the stressor or staying to fight [28]. Yet other research suggests that many females, when faced with stress due to neuroendocrine and behavioral reasons, "tend and befriend" [29]. This concept suggests that women tend to their offspring, to reduce harm and neuroendocrine responses that may cause harm to health, and befriend, finding external social supports to reduce risk for mutual defense. While increased biological hormones, such as endorphins and oxytocin, might establish this difference for women, socialization may teach and maintain these gender differences.

Porges's polyvagal theory focuses on "approaches to healing that focus on strengthening the body's system for regulating arousal" (p. 80) [6]. One of the principles from the theory posits that trauma can impact human nervous system states and the body responds in three predictable reactions: (1) social engagement and connection (ventral vagal), (2) mobilization or "fight or flight" (sympathetic), and (3) immobilization or "freeze or collapse" (dorsal vagal) [30]. We initially turn to those around us for help and support. There is a feeling of safety and positive relationships at this level. As threat increases so does adrenaline. We move into the sympathetic nervous system with a more primitive need to mobilize and initiate defenses by fighting back or running for safety. Feelings include panic, fear, anger, and irritation. This level is also where "tend and befriend" appears as a defense with looking for protection and ways to diffuse conflict. Although there is a social engagement aspect, the motivations are driven by stress and a need to mobilize. These defenses can be helpful if we are successful in achieving safety, as there is resolution. However, when these strategies are unsuccessful or not possible and we cannot escape, we immobilize, shut down, or collapse. This stage includes dissociation and disconnection. The trauma can get stuck in our body at this level.

The most significant difficulties arise when immobilization occurs. However, mobilization and immobilization provide defensive reactions that can continue to play out in unhealthy ways after the trauma, particularly in relationships. The nervous system may activate at triggers of perceived threat that are actually nonthreatening. It is overactive and in overdrive, making it difficult to feel safe and causing a trauma response or a constant state of mobilization or immobilization. Consider the example of a soldier who has a history of multiple deployments that included a traumatic injury. Even when he is home and in a subjectively safe space, the nervous system has been altered and shaped by the history. A number of triggers could cause the neurological system to activate, such as a loud noise due to something falling to the ground or a person appearing unexpectedly. He may run out of the room (flight) or become extremely angry (fight). Let's say now, this man is experiencing infertility. His brain and nervous system have been altered by the previous trauma so his body more quickly tries to protect him from this stress by becoming angry, emotionally withdrawing from a partner, and/or losing interest in sex.

Biological and physical changes can occur with a trauma. The polyvagal theory illustrates certain ways the different nervous systems might impact the body when trauma occurs. Our body can provide signals when in crisis, such as shaking, increased heart rate, changes in body temperature, or feelings of nausea [31]. Understanding how the trauma impacts the body gives information to address these issues.

Trauma and relationships

Trauma can challenge our understanding of basic human relationship, making it hard to feel safe and engage in intimate relationships. Immobilization with fear, a physiological response, involves the body shutting down as a way of dealing with a trauma. To gain meaningful intimacy, there is a need for "immobilization without fear," but it can be difficult to understand the difference between safety and danger for a trauma survivor [30]. A loving embrace, a kiss, and a touch are examples of immobilization without fear. Beyond intimacy, this concept is also integral as one undergoes fertility treatment, experiencing procedures such as a genital examination for egg or sperm retrieval. To achieve "immobilization without fear," the central nervous system needs to return to a state to engage the ventral vagal, the part of the body that connects to social engagement, where trust within the relationship is established, returning connection, belonging, and thereby secure vulnerability.

How are trust and vulnerability rebuilt? Vulnerability is created through a safe environment. Critically, trauma treatment requires a compassionate, patient, and empathetic therapist who provides a safe space to explore the trauma and its effects. Empathy is considered a moderate positive indicator of therapeutic success [12,32]. Empathy can help to align the clinician and patient and begin to establish trust, laying the groundwork for vulnerability work.

A key ingredient of vulnerability is to understand, to accept, and to connect to oneself, building self-esteem. Acknowledging the self as a victim of trauma is an important part of vulnerability and moving toward being a survivor [33]. The clinician and trauma survivor relationship can serve as a place to create safety within this vulnerable relationship. However, because of the power differential, there is risk that it can mirror previous trauma experiences [34]. As a clinician it is important to be aware of the questions we engage the client in: why am I asking? Is there clinical use, or is it out of curiosity? The answer is that the clinician asks only questions of clinical use to treat the issues, particularly in the beginning as a therapeutic relationship is formed. Acknowledging the power differential and being careful not to take advantage of the client is essential to help with recovery. The clinician should practice neutrality to provide the client the opportunity to gain autonomy and power/control.

Vulnerability has negative and positive associations. At the core of the negative side of vulnerability is shame and guilt [35]. Shame and guilt can be a byproduct of trauma and are often seen with infertility patients [36–38]. Sex also breeds shame rooted in culture and community, and it can be hard to talk about because of the nature of privacy in sexual relationships. Shame causes avoidance and secrecy, and secrecy makes authentic trust impossible. Naming the shame and associated feelings, understanding where it comes from, having compassion for oneself, and connecting with others, namely, a partner, breaks down shame and builds resilience [35]. Shame can be fought by communicating feelings and thoughts. Vulnerability through emotional intimacy allows for a path to healthy physical intimacy [33]. It allows us to build trust and intimacy, empathy and understanding, and to take care of and be taken care of.

To understand trauma is to understand human vulnerability, where the core experience leads to disempowerment and disconnection [34]. To help a couple through the experience is to empower them individually to take control of their situations and thereby allowing a place for them to reconnect. However, when infertility occurs, autonomy can be removed as medical interventions are necessary to create a family.

To begin to repair the sexual relationship, safety must be established. Safety is built through an open, nonjudgmental space, which allows for trust. Trust is created through consistent words and actions in a safe environment, where positive vulnerability emerges. Vulnerability is fostered through self-compassion and sharing of feelings, thoughts, and experiences, which can lead the way for intimacy. Intimacy can be expressed through positive touch (i.e., a hand on a shoulder, hugs, and kisses), communication (both sharing and listening), and sex. Intimacy during infertility leads to additional challenges as intimacy becomes tied to sex for procreation and not a means of connecting for enjoyment or pleasure.

Providing a foundation for growth

Trauma recovery can become an opportunity for growth. The experience can allow for "positive reconfigurations of identity" by reworking previous ego weaknesses and solidifying them into a more committed and effective self (p. 91) [39]. Within the negative associations of trauma, resilience can exist and growth can occur. Resilience is considered "the capacity for individuals to recover functioning after exposure to stress-induced dysregulation" (p. 4) [23,40]. It is built out of previous models of coping and attachments. Research around stress and trauma supports the idea that finding meaning and purpose assist in creating and fostering resilience [41]. Realistic optimism, or belief in a brighter future with an assessment of reality, is also a common characteristic in resilience research.

Emerging literature suggests the idea of "posttraumatic growth," which proposes that growth can occur in five areas, including (1) a strengthening of self-perception; (2) increase in sense of new possibilities; (3) improvement in human relationships; (4) increase in appreciation of life; and (5) a renewed or strengthened spirituality [42]. Factors, such as early attachment foundations, affect regulation, biology, social supports, and culture, all influence resilience and growth.

Self-regulation, or the ability to control one's feelings, emotions, and behaviors, develops through early secure attachments to care providers. Trauma can cause an emotional dysregulation of the physical and psychological body responses. The reciprocal process between the care providers and children that promotes self-regulation is coregulation. Coregulation is established through (1) a positive, responsive relationship; (2) a structured environment that offers safety; and (3) teaching and modeling of self-regulation [43]. Coregulation, which helps to activate the social engagement nervous system, provides "reciprocal regulation of our autonomic states [so] that we feel safe to move into connection and create trusting relationships" (p. 4) [30]. Self-regulation in psychotherapy can be built through skill building and the use of a coregulation approach between the patient and the clinician as well as between a couple. Coregulation can be achieved through deep breathing exercises and positive touch or sensate focus exercises [44], as well as, calmly mirroring behaviors and feelings.

To provide trauma-informed care, the Substance Abuse and Mental Health Services Administration (SAMSHA) provides six guiding principles [1]:

- safety;
- trustworthiness and transparency;
- peer support;
- collaboration and mutuality;
- empowerment, voice, and choice; and
- cultural, historical, and gender issues.

These principles must be continually attended to throughout work with a survivor of trauma and may also be useful to those who have not experienced trauma. The principles suggest beginning by establishing a physically and psychologically safe environment where communication is clear and open, in an effort to build and maintain trust. A provider should share the power and decision making, being conscious not to model previous trauma relationships. A survivor's strengths and experiences are also used as a foundation for care. Trauma-informed care includes understanding, recognizing, and moving beyond cultural stereotypes and biases, taking into account different racial, ethnic, gender, and cultural considerations and needs in a sensitive manner. These principles will be referenced in considerations for the case example.

Assessment

To assess for the couple's needs and understand the nature of the histories they present, examine both the individuals and the couple. Assessment can be broken into four parts: (1) understanding the problem, (2 and 3) individual sessions to obtain histories, and (4) a feedback session. The following case example utilizes this format, elaborated further, to describe the issues to consider.

The first session should be used to gather information about the relationship history, fertility journey and coping, and to gain a better understanding of why the couple is coming in. Listen, reflect back, and clarify, as needed, to obtain a deeper understanding, avoiding any problem solving. The next sessions should address individual coping with infertility and fertility diagnosis, family history, medical history and medications, trauma history or other important turning points, sexual history, history of counseling (and feelings about it), social supports, and religious or cultural considerations. The final session should address feedback from the previous sessions that help to identify goals of counseling and the types of counseling that may be utilized to help achieve those goals. For the purposes of this chapter, the assessment will concentrate on trauma and infertility information gathering as a vehicle to address the couple's sexual relationship.

Table 11.1 provides suggested questions to ask and incorporate in the course of the assessment. These are important areas to address but should not necessarily be asked formulaically. While these topics bring up ideas and issues to cover and focus on, the questions provide a gateway to begin, continue, and guide discussion when a patient is unsure what to say.

Understanding the problem

Jillian, Caucasian cisgender female, age 36, walked into the door attentive to her husband, Mike, Caucasian cisgender male, age 37, making sure he was okay. Mike wheeled himself in wearing shorts and two prosthetic metal legs. When they sat down in my office, Jillian placed her face in her hands, and Mike placed his hand on her shoulder. She moved her body away from his touch. Mike began by sharing that they have been married 10 years and have struggled to grow their family for the last 3 years. He noted that they had planned to grow their family around 8 years ago, but while on deployment in Afghanistan, Mike was injured. He didn't share much about the injury but noted that his injury put growing their family on pause. Mike went through many extensive surgeries and spent about a year in and out of the military hospital. It took another few years for them to regain some normalcy, and after about 5 years, they decided they were ready to grow their family. They knew because of the injuries, as well as Jillian's history of polycystic ovarian syndrome, they would need to use fertility treatment. He shared this story with little emotion, just stating the facts. Jillian jumped in to correct his account of their fertility treatments. She wept as she shared their journey which included two failed in vitro fertilization (IVF) cycles, with one miscarriage. She noted that going through the IVF cycles brought up a lot of her own feelings of the many surgeries her husband underwent after he was injured.

TABLE 11.1 History gathering.

Medical history

- Could you tell me about your medical history?
- What are your ongoing medical needs?
- What medication are you on?
- Do your medical providers know you are trying to achieve a pregnancy?
- How do you feel about your body?

Trauma history

- What are the pertinent parts of your trauma, your experience, and life you think would be helpful for me to know about?
- In what ways have you dealt with [the trauma]? Are there ways you have not dealt with [the trauma]?
- Tell me about your recovery process. What has been the most challenging part of your recovery?
- How has [the trauma] impacted your relationship?
- What helped you in your recovery? Physically? Mentally? Socially?
- What does your family know? Have they been supportive?
- What has been your experience with counseling?

Partner's experience of trauma

- How did you find out about [the trauma]?
- What was the recovery like for you?
- Who was supportive and helpful during that time?
- What have been the most challenging parts for you?
- In what ways, has your relationship(s) changed since [the trauma]?
- What does your family know? Have they been supportive?

Sexual history (general)

- When has your sexual relationship together been the healthiest? What has it been the most disappointing?
- How do you hope for your sexual relationship to change? What would it look like?
- How interested have you been in sexual activity?
- How often have you felt like you wanted to have sex?
- Is anything being done at this time to address the sexual functioning issues you have?
- [For male] How difficult has it been for you to get an erection when you wanted to?
- When you have had sexual activity, how much have you enjoyed it?
- How would you rate your ability to have a satisfying orgasm/climax?
- Have you discussed any applicable sexual functioning issues you may have with your medical team?

Sexual history (in relation to trauma)

- How satisfying did you perceive sex life to be prior to [the trauma]? (0—not satisfying, 10—extremely satisfied)
- In what ways has your sex life changed since [the trauma]?
- To what degree does [the trauma] affect your ability to have a normal sexual relationship?
- On a scale of 1–10, where was your sexual functioning [pretrauma]? (1 being terrible and 10 being perfect) Where would you rate yourself now? Tell me why those numbers are different [or in what way has it stayed the same (if rating is the same)?]

Fertility and family building

- What is your relationship like to your family of origin?
- Have you always wanted to have children? Has this changed since [the trauma]?
- What are your worries/concerns, if any, with building a family outside of natural intercourse?
- What have you discussed about ways to grow your family with your partner?
- Has your journey to grow your family felt traumatic? If so, in what ways?
- How has your fertility treatment impacted your relationship?
- How does the infertility diagnosis impacted you individually? as a couple?
- How has your coping been? What are you observations about how your partner has been coping? How have you been coping as a couple?
- How has communication been about the infertility experience?
- What concerns do you have about fertility treatment moving forward?

Jillian described struggling to make challenging decisions about fertility treatment, and Mike was resistant to discuss other options. Jillian described how disengaged Mike had been throughout fertility treatment. They differed on how much to share with their friends and family. Since Mike hadn't wanted to talk about their treatment, she began using social media to find out about other's infertility experience, which provided both positive and negative experiences. Mike interjected that he was unsure how to support his wife, as no matter what he did she was always upset with him, and she constantly talked about their infertility. He whispered, "This is all my fault." Jillian was frustrated that Mike did not seem to be as invested as she was. Mike described that it is the only thing on her mind, and she only wants to have sex when she is ovulating. He has been having difficulties "performing on demand." Jillian added that having a baby felt like the last thing on their checklist to show that she and Mike had beaten the combat injury. Their infertility made the injury recovery feel ongoing.

This case example illustrates a couple with multiple traumas: deployments, injury, miscarriage, and infertility. While their histories will be important to gather, letting the patients guide the conversation at this point and providing empathy and reflective listening, will help to provide an initial foundation for safety. It is important initially to clearly lay out expectations for how the counseling will work and provide space to think about what they hope to get out of it.

The purpose of the initial session is to get to know the couple, hear their story, and what they bring into your office. This goal is achieved by engaging, listening, and asking questions pertinent to why they are coming in. The therapeutic relationship is a chance to model safety and affect regulation. This couple show dysregulation through the chronic stress of the aftermath of the injury and subsequent infertility. Particularly with a trauma history, the first goal of a clinician is to provide safety through a nonjudgmental and empathetic space. Trust can be established by communicating and maintaining clear boundaries and roles as a clinician, asking relevant questions, and providing autonomy and empowerment to the patient to provide information they feel comfortable sharing. Where appropriate, clinicians may ask permission to inquire about topics and give permission for them to decline sharing information. Even when consent about treatment seems like a given, asking the patient permission and approval can help to establish safety and model language to use within the relationship. This approach provides collaboration with the patient, leveling the power differential.

Relationship history gathering is an essential part of understanding sexual history, which Table 11.1 does not address. While providing a full couple's assessment is beyond the scope of this chapter, some information to gather from this couple would include:

- Their relationships with their families of origin;
- How/when they met and what initially attracted them to each other;
- How their relationship grew, over what period of time, and how they made the decision to commit to each other (and marry);
- How their families feel about their relationship; and
- What stands out as positives and negatives in their time together.

These concepts help to understand strengths that exist, as well as, understand whether the issues presented are newer to the relationship and related to the current crisis or preexisting areas of need.

As a couple, they have experienced the trauma of infertility and Mike's injury. Often men and women process and experience infertility in very different, unique ways. The gender differences of how Mike and Jillian experience their infertility are quite common [12]. Due to the nature of treatment and pregnancy, the woman is typically identified as the patient. This role reversal in fertility treatment may not be a role Jillian nor Mike are comfortable with or used to due to previous dynamics with Mike's recovery. As Jillian takes the more active role of treatment, Mike is more easily able to detach from feelings around the infertility. Understanding and discussing how gender, as well as cultural (i.e., military influence), differences may be playing out in the communication can be helpful. These variances also can take effect in how the trauma was processed within the relationship. Focusing on what the experience is like as a couple provides a way for the couple to grow together. Regardless of the cause, infertility is a couple's issue.

Partner 1 history gathering

When asked about where he would like to start, Mike jumped into describing his injury. He was age 29 and stationed in Afghanistan as a noncommissioned officer in the Marines. He quickly recounted details about being "blown up" after stepping on an improvised explosive device (IED). His injuries included bilateral leg amputations and a loss of one testicle (with atrophy to the remaining one). While people can see his leg amputation, Mike shared that very few people know about his genital injury. He is not sure how to tell people about the injury and unsure what they will think. Mike described a history of posttraumatic symptoms, including flashbacks, night terrors, and anger and guilt, related to his military deployments, not specific to the injury. He has received individual counseling and been on psychiatric medications, and he reports that his posttraumatic symptoms have been stable for about 3 years, when they started fertility treatment. He also plays on an adaptive ice hockey team, which has helped with his physical and mental health recovery. Mike acknowledged that he has talked a lot about his injury, but fertility considerations in relation to his genital injury had never really been discussed. He has begun to have feelings of anger around his injury and guilt that his wife has not been able to become pregnant. He worries that after the injury, the infertility will be too much for his wife and she will leave him. Mike discussed some ambivalence around the relationship and having children. While he very much loves Jillian and wants to start a family with her, he also reports that he would be fine if he never has children and if Jillian left him. Mike also described a paradoxical struggle with infertility, often fluctuating throughout the session between feeling that the infertility is a "real kick to his [psychological] balls" and the worst outcome of his injury to feeling that life would be okay without children and "it's not that bad." Mike discussed a decreased sex drive and difficulties with his testosterone levels. He noted that he has struggled to have the same sexual relationship with his wife, as he did preinjury, and this is even more complicated since beginning fertility treatment.

This case illustrates a complex trauma which has caused various changes to everyday life from the psychological aspects of recovery to the new physical limitations. The physical limitations can be a reminder of a vast change of identity. Due to his leg amputations, Mike has had to change the way he functions and needs to rely on others to help him with everyday tasks. Jillian has taken on the role of caregiver. For this couple, exploring each of their roles and expectations in the household is important to addressing their intimate relationship. These roles can have a direct shift for the sexual relationship. For example, if Jillian is the one helping Mike shower, the sexual nature of the relationship loses meaning, as caring for his naked body is now a task not an invitation to be intimate. Finding solutions and alternatives to separate these roles is important (e.g., hiring a care worker to help with some of those self-care tasks).

Mike also has experienced various psychological traumas and moral injury related to his deployments. His response to the infertility is a defense that has been referred to as "protective ambivalence" [45]. His ambivalence about having children helps him to cope and detach from the strong emotions he had associated with his injury. However, it is also preventing him from relating to his wife about infertility.

The protective ambivalence is not something to be addressed immediately due to the current state of crisis. As the therapeutic relationship develops, part of addressing and understanding ambivalence will create an environment of vulnerability with his wife, allowing Mike to acknowledge his conflicting feelings and explore his fears about himself and their relationship. Some of his loss of interest in sex is tied to ambivalence and trauma. Thus providing openness to explore his ambivalence helps to address some of the sexual issues that occur for him.

A key feature of this case example is that Mike is currently receiving counseling and psychological support to address his trauma. His involvement in adaptive sports is an example of social engagement to decrease his trauma response. If he is comfortable, it can also be helpful to collaborate with his other professional care providers. At the same time it is important to give him permission to decline, as a way of establishing safety and building trust. Individual problems should be dealt with in individual therapy, but those that impact the couple should be dealt with together as a couple. There are certainly aspects of the trauma that will be helpful to deal with on a more individual level, such as dealing with the daily aspects of deployment, while others should be examined on a couple level, where the trauma enters the relationship. While Mike was injured, the aftermath was experienced together as a couple, and the injury continues to impact and alter the functioning of their relationship.

Addressing medical history and understanding the ongoing physical needs of the recovery will help to understand the sexual dysfunction, distinguishing what is physiologically going on for him and what is psychologically occurring. The reproductive trauma, or the injury to his genitals, meaningfully impacts biology by changing testosterone levels that affect psychological wellbeing and the ability to engage in social and intimate relationships. In addressing the sexual issues, it is important to consider testosterone levels. While testosterone supplements can help with sex drive and energy, it can decrease sperm count [46]. Part of the work will be to help the patient to educate, advocate, and communicate needs effectively with healthcare providers about sexual function and intentions to procreate.

Partner 2 history gathering

Jillian came into the session ready to talk. She described feeling traumatized from the experience of being in the hospital with her husband and not being sure whether he would survive. Jillian worked hard to get Mike the care he needed and often went outside the military hospital system to get additional care, despite what others advised. Because of her efforts, they were able to get care for Mike that the military system did not have in place at the time of this injury.

Jillian initially went through fertility treatment at the local military hospital, where Mike was treated, but she noted that she didn't want to receive treatment there, due to the trauma association she experienced with her husband's recovery. However, due to healthcare system constraints, she had to receive care at the military hospital. Eventually she was referred out to a local fertility clinic for additional care. The fertility and medical procedures continue to cause her anxiety. The fertility medication caused her to gain 15 pounds, and she has felt angry with her body. Jillian described struggling to see other "wounded warrior" families grow their families and not have the same struggles she and Mike had with infertility. She described being left behind. She has wondered what life would be like if Mike had not been injured, and they had been able to start having children earlier.

Jillian also shared that she has a history of sexual abuse which occurred when she was about 8 years old, perpetrated by a neighbor. She had counseling for this in the past. However, due to the invasive nature of the fertility treatment, she acknowledged that recently, thoughts of that experience have been recurring. She noted she feels numb particularly when she has vaginal ultrasounds, making sex even less desirable. She is even beginning to worry about carrying a pregnancy. Mike is aware of her sexual abuse history and has always been supportive of her sexual boundaries.

Trauma does not solely affect the direct trauma recipient. It impacts those connected to that person as well. This case clearly shows how trauma can impact those close to the victim. Mike was not the only one who experienced a trauma. However, for Jillian, her experience can often be minimized compared to Mike's, causing her to feel disenfranchised, but she too experienced a trauma when she learned about her husband's injury. Understanding, acknowledging, allowing, and empowering Jillian to explore her experience with her husband's injury allows room to understand the impact on the relationship. It may even be helpful to reframe "Mike's injury" to something that identifies and incorporates the couple experience, such as "our recovery from injury."

There are three relationships to consider in trauma recovery: each partner's relationship with the self and the relationship between partners. Mike and Jillian should also explore the impact of the trauma as a couple. While the recovery is something Jillian and Mike experienced together, they have distinct experiences and varying emotional processes. Hearing about the other person's experiences can bring up anxiety and worry so it may be avoided. Many of the feelings are assumed and often not accurate, causing more friction in the relationship. Being able to discuss and understand how it is and has impacted them individually and as a couple allows for a more authentic, harmonious connection.

Infertility triggers previous trauma experience. Jillian notes that the infertility feels like the last item on the checklist to recovery. The infertility experience stunts her ability to address these previous conflicts or wounds, creating a sense of loss and being stuck [19]. In the course of treatment, the clinician can help Jillian to name and articulate her losses. These ambiguous losses can be harder to navigate, freezing the grief process. Recognize the grief and loss, naming the experience as ambiguous, and finding ways to memorialize can help in the mourning process. Yet, also acknowledge what remains, the positives coming from the experience, and help imagine a new hope for the future to facilitate in establishing resilience. Use of the reproductive story model can help Mike and Jillian to identify their previous assumptions and explore various new chapters for growing their family.

Body image issues are often a central theme with trauma, infertility, and sex [47]. We often hold trauma in various parts of our bodies, whether the brain or tension in the back or gastrointestinal issues. Because of trauma, body changes that can occur with fertility treatment and subsequent pregnancy can feel unsafe due of a lack of control related to what is happening within the body. Pregnancy is a body experience, and while pregnancy can be a very healing process, it can also be a trigger and cause distress, due to a lack of control and worry.

Jillian has experienced the trauma of her husband's injury and recovery, miscarriage, as well as, sexual abuse. Transvaginal ultrasounds and even ultrasound of the belly can feel like a crossing of personal boundaries and safety. Ideally, even though consent for these procedures is assumed, having the provider ask permission can help give the patient autonomy. This permission and consent is not always realistic so finding alternatives for the patient to gain empowerment and voice can be helpful.

Trauma can cause us to shut off parts of our body. Infertility, too, impacts the body, making it feel broken. Fertility treatment medications can cause weight gain and hormonal/emotional shifts. Identify triggers that are mobilizing the trauma response of fight-flight-freeze. Helping a client to understand how the trauma impacts the body and where it is being held can reconnect the body to the self, rather than staying in a state of fight-flight-freeze. It can be helpful to educate Jillian on the trauma response she is experiencing and help Mike and Jillian to begin to activate the social engagement nervous system through coregulation.

Feedback

Three topics to cover are areas of strengths (what each individual brings in and the couple brings in), areas that could be strengthened, and types of treatment to be utilized (as well as what adjunctly could be utilized, and how the work will be approached). For Mike and Jillian, there are several areas of strength to acknowledge.

First is that their relationship is resilient. Many couples do not make it as long as they have with all that has been put in front of them. They have continued to persevere and already have key elements for the foundation of resilience that have brought them this far. In the broader picture, Jillian chose to be actively involved in Mike's recovery and Mike allowed her to be a part of it. This approach is ultimately a protective factor in recovery. There may have been smaller areas where this is not happening or did not happen, but ultimately, they have chosen their love and commitment to one another. In the past the involvement in recovery may have been assumed. Moving forward it may be help for each to ask and give permission to be a part of their recovery, "Would you let me be a part of your past and future?." Addressing any areas of misunderstanding, fear, and hurt that happened after Mike's injury and during fertility treatment will help to open communication, increase connection, and strengthen the relationship.

Provide praise for coming to receive support and having a joint commitment to their relationship. There are many reasons why this may have been difficult. With both Mike and Jillian's trauma histories, putting trust in a provider takes vulnerability. The fact that they have even come in the door to receive support is another protective factor. Relationships can end when communication stops, a partner withdraws emotionally, and a person does not include their partner in healing or a partner refuses to cooperate in recovery [33]. Trauma can allow an opportunity to renew and strengthen a relationship. Adjustment and change is hard, but putting in the work to communicate and address trauma recovery can help to establish new, healthy, and mutually satisfying ways to relate physically, emotionally, and sexually.

While providing feedback to Mike and Jillian has therapeutic merit, it should be done with care, caution, and opportunity for their voices to be heard about next treatment steps. There should be a reciprocal process of exchange about moving forward in treatment. Begin by engaging the couple in the feedback by inquiring about what it has been like during the process and to understand their goals. It can be helpful to start by asking, something such as, "Is there anything new you have learned about yourself, partner, or marriage in what we have discussed over the last few session?" and then "What do you feel you need help with, and what would you like to get out of this work?" Once the couple has had a chance to answer, the clinician can ask something such as, "Over the course of the last few sessions, we have discussed many topics and areas that are currently difficult. Would you feel comfortable with me providing some of my insights and feedback of what I think would be helpful moving forward?" Although this is likely assumed, this permission and consent model is important therapist behavior in the work moving forward and provides a safer space for the patient to decide what to work on. Other permission questions may include:

- I believe it could be helpful if I provide some feedback of what I've noticed and observed over the last few sessions. Do you think it would be helpful if I provide some insight into what I think might be useful moving forward?
- If at any point, you are uncomfortable with what we are talking about or not ready to discuss the topic, please let me know. You can simply say, "Can we talk about this another time?" or "I am not ready to talk about this."

This session is about providing education on the therapeutic processes that may be utilized, continuing to establish and articulate boundaries of the relationship, and determining goals for counseling. The clinician may also contribute some suggested goals, but it is important to be clear that ultimately the patients should determine and decide what to work on. While sex is an important part of an intimate relationship, it should be something that the patients want to work on and discuss. For example, ask, "Would it be helpful to talk about sex and finding some ways for you to reengage pleasure and establish boundaries in your intimate relationship?"

Identifying family of origin issues and strengths can be a way to begin to identify attachment styles that may impact self-regulation. These attachment styles can help to understand what may or may not be working in the relationship. Helping them understand how their own actions are influencing the relationship can lead to changes and effective coregulation.

Provide psychoeducation and insight on how infertility and trauma may be impacting their physical and emotional intimacy: when is the right time to work on these sexual issues? Now! Rebuilding the sexual relationship can feel daunting, but the longer you wait, the harder it gets. The sexual relationship may decrease during fertility treatment, as sex feels like a job, rather than a joy. This cycle may then continue through a pregnancy, as anxieties can be high after going through fertility treatment. Both members of the couple might be worried that sex will cause harm to the pregnancy and baby. Once the baby has arrived there is a lack of sleep, tiredness and the sexual relationship again gets pushed off. Normalize the experience and help to provide understanding and decipher where the medication and health issues (with the help of referrals to appropriate medical care providers) versus psychological blocks, distress, and lifestyle issues might impact the sexual relationship.

A colleague once shared with me something a client of hers said, "Fighting the fear is often worse than fighting the fight." This saying is something I refer back to and acknowledge in my therapeutic work. It can feel scary to share emotions, feelings, and experiences about a trauma with someone else. How are they going to react? Will they still love me? Will they judge me? Our assumptions and fantasies are so often worse than the reality. Once we know what we are facing, we can figure out ways to address it, reframing this idea from a trauma response of "fighting the fight" to a relaxation response of "safely adjusting to reality."

Special considerations

This case example highlights a heteronormative, Caucasian relationship. Yet there are important consideration for this couple. As the trauma-informed guiding principles acknowledge, cultural, historical, and gender issues are a separate point and should be attended to in a conscious and caring way. Within these three issues exists marginalized groups (e.g., LGBTQ+, racial minorities, physically, mentally, or intellectually disabled persons, military combat veterans, etc.) who may experience traumas at an increased rate due to systemic oppressions that exist. There are two considerations for this couple: the military culture and experience with being physically disabled (Mike's amputations). Questions to consider for this case could include:

- Are you currently in the military or retired? What branch of the military did you serve? What was your rank? What was your job in the military? What was your length of time in the military? If retired: how did you exit the military? Are you enrolled in the VA (Veterans Affairs)?
- How did you decide to join the military? How would you describe your experience?
- How long after marriage was he deployed? Were there any previous deployments? How did they connect when they were away? What was reunification like for them as a couple?
- What has been your experience and observations in interacting with the world while utilizing a wheelchair and/or using prostheses?

Understanding these unique aspects of this case is important in providing competent care. Follow the clients lead to use appropriate language.

Clinical considerations

My area of work is reproductive health and fertility mental health counseling. I am not a certified sex therapist, but it is impossible and naïve to not include the topic of sex when working with couples, particularly in infertility treatment. I believe there is a professional obligation to address needs and not perpetuate shame, stigma, and silence, even if it is uncomfortable. Yet, we need words and education to begin to discuss these sensitive topics. As a provider, whether medical or mental health, it is important to be aware of our own feelings, biases, and experiences around sex and trauma. While our own experiences may help us to relate to a patient, our experiences are our own and do not equate to appropriate knowledge of the client's experience. Our experiences are shaped by our subjective values and prejudices and do not take into account varying cultural, historical, and gender issues. When talking about sex in the context of the therapeutic relationship, I find many are uncomfortable with the conversation. Thus, a good place to start is by acknowledging how uncomfortable it can be to talk about sex, especially with a stranger. Also, directly and confidently using accurate terminology (i.e., intercourse, erection, penis, and vagina) can be a model for the client to be more comfortable.

Sex may be innate, and sexual desire may be unconsciously, hormonally, and biologically based. However, love-making, or sex as a way to express love, commitment, and connection, is learned. Love-making comes though self-exploration, self-advocacy, and communication of sexual pleasures, desires, and turn-offs. The good news is that this can be learned, but it does take work. Goals of "love-making" are for it to feel good, comfortable, and a connection with your partner. This connection can occur through verbal communication of desires, letting go of expectations, and finding a variety of sexual expressions other than penetrative sex.

Baby-making is another concept to separate from love-making. When trying to grow a family, sex, and love-making turns into baby-making, becoming a task to do rather than something enjoyable. As many as four in five couples undergoing fertility treatment experience erectile dysfunction or inhibited sexual desires with the "on demand" protocols, as Mike and Jillian are experiencing [46]. This "baby-making" model sets up failure in sex by taking away the importance of pleasure in sex [48]. The many purposes of sex include reproduction, anxiety reduction, pleasure, self-esteem, and relationship closeness [48,49]. In working to establish boundaries and expectation, the clinician can help a couple to distinguish these concepts and find ways to discriminate the purpose and intention. For example, the couple may reserve "baby-making" for another area of the house than their bedroom or schedule sex outside of ovulation in an effort to focus on pleasure and connection in the relationship.

Communication is a key element to helping couples work through their trauma and sexual issues. There are various forms of communication, including verbal (spoken words) and nonverbal (facial expressions, body language, tone of voice, etc.). Sex is also a form of nonverbal communication with a partner and is an opportunity to convey love and commitment. Each partner should learn words and a confidence to convey what is wanted and not wanted sexually, while being able to say no and hold boundaries when it feels unsafe. Always ask and never assume feelings and expectations [33]. Mills and Turnbull [11] suggest that after a trauma, to have a reciprocal intimate relationship, each member of the couple must be a LOVER: Listen; Observe; Verify; Emphasize; Reassure/Rebuild/Repair.

Begin the work by building the relationship between the partners in the couple, as well as, the couple and the therapist. Establish helpful tools to open communication, through mirroring, validation, and empathy [50]. Provide safety and establish stability. One challenge with this is that although the trauma might be over, the couple infertility stressor and/or trauma is ongoing. There are ways to find stability outside of this ongoing stressor. For example, put limits on when and how long the couple can talk about the infertility (i.e., couple schedules a time to talk about the infertility and put a timer on for 20 minutes).

Next allow an opportunity to process the trauma(s) as a couple. Socratic dialog, which includes clarifying questions, examining assumption, evaluating objective evidence, and challenging unhelpful beliefs, provides useful techniques to help empower the survivor to process the trauma and experience [51]. Make sure there is enough time in the session to discuss the trauma, process, and wrap up to close up the discussion of the trauma. The goal of processing is not to get rid of the thoughts, but rather to make them a part of the normal memory so they do not activate the trauma response.

Through processing of the trauma, the clinician should also provide tools to elicit the parasympathetic nervous system and relaxation response, lowering heart rate, and slow breathing [52]. Primary techniques include mediation, mindfulness, and deep breathing. These help to connect the body response to the psychological response occurring during the processing. Physical activity and social supports can also be used to help with activating a relaxation response. The relaxation response can help in many areas of recovery, including as a foundation for sexual pleasure and function [48].

Rebuild and reframe for the "new normal." This process will involve establishing and reconceptualizing the sexual identity. In the case example, Mike is stuck in comparing his current sexual function with his sexual functioning prior to the injury, setting himself for unrealistic expectations. McCarthy and McCarthy [53] suggest creating positive, realistic expectations for the relationship; addressing sexual dysfunction as a couple's issue rather than an individual one; providing and establishing options to explore the sexual relationship beyond intercourse; and communicating desires. Help let go of expectations by setting up for a "good enough sex" model where the focus is on obtaining couple satisfaction through intimacy as a primary focus and pleasure as a function [48]. The clinician should help the couple to desire sex not only for the partner but also for each individual self, connecting three elements of sex: physical pleasure, emotional need, and passion.

Conclusion and takeaways

The body is physically and psychologically impacted by trauma and infertility, which can interrupt intimate relationships. The body also holds trauma in different locations. Sex can be used as tool to help a couple reconnect and rebuild from trauma and infertility. Learning empowerment to take control of the body, sex, and intimacy can be a healing experience if done with care, thought, and education. Clinicians should help couples create methods that establish a physically and psychologically safe environment for building vulnerability and trust. The following are takeaways from this chapter in providing trauma-informed care within infertility and sexual issues:

- Treat trauma, infertility, and sex as a couple's issues.
- Be aware of power differentials in providing care. Ask for permission and receive consent, even when it seems assumed.
- Help to provide empowerment and autonomy in decision making.

- With trauma comes dysregulation, of which infertility can be a trigger. It is important to establish safe "holding places" within the therapy to help patients gain control.
- The body can be physically and psychologically impacted by trauma and infertility which can interfere with the sexual relationship. "Immobilization without fear" can lead to a healthy sexual relationship [30].
- Social engagement is a strategy to establish a decreased trauma response of fight or flight and freeze or collapse. Coregulation and the use of deep breathing and mindfulness can also be used to activate the relaxation response.
- Address sexual issues early in treatment. Separate and provide psychoeducation around the ideas of sex, lovemaking, and baby-making.

References

[1] Substance Abuse and Mental Health Services Administration. SAMHSA's concept of trauma and guidance for a trauma-informed approach. Vol. HHS Publication No. (SMA) 14-4884. Rockville, MD: Substance Abuse and Mental Health Services Administration; 2014.
[2] American Psychiatric Association. Diagnostic and Statistical Manual of Mental Disorders (DSM-5 (R)). 5th ed. Arlington, TX: American Psychiatric Association Publishing; 2013.
[3] Boss P. Ambiguous loss: learning to live with unresolved grief. Cambridge, MA: Harvard University Press; 2009.
[4] Beck CT. Birth trauma: in the eye of the beholder. Nurs Res 2004;53(1):28—35.
[5] Boals A. Trauma in the eye of the beholder: objective and subjective definitions of trauma. J Psychother Integr 2018;28(1):77—89.
[6] Van der Kolk BA. The body keeps the score: mind, brain and body in the transformation of trauma. Harlow: Penguin Books; 2015.
[7] Jaffe J. Trauma and the reproductive story [Internet]. Psychotherapy.net. Available from: <https://www.psychotherapy.net/article/grief/trauma-and-the-reproductive-story>; 2019[cited September 11, 2020].
[8] Galst JP. The elusive connection between stress and infertility: a research review with clinical implications. J Psychother Integr 2018;28(1):1—13.
[9] Rooney KL, Domar AD. The relationship between stress and infertility. Dialogues Clin Neurosci 2018;20(1):41—7.
[10] De Silva P. Impact of trauma on sexual functioning and sexual relationships. Sex Relat Ther 2001;16(3):269—78.
[11] Mills B, Turnbull G. Broken hearts and mending bodies: the impact of trauma on intimacy. Sex Relat Ther 2004;19(3):265—89.
[12] Peterson B. Fertility counseling for couples. In: Covington SN, editor. Fertility counseling: clinical guide and case studies. Cambridge: Cambridge University Press; 2015.
[13] Burns LH, Covington SN. Psychology of infertility. In: Covington SN, Burns LH, editors. Infertility counseling: a comprehensive handbook for clinicians. New York: Cambridge University Press; 2006. p. 1—19.
[14] Mills B. Impact of trauma on sexuality and relationships. Sex Relat Ther 2001;16(3):197—205.
[15] Zisook S, Shear K. Grief and bereavement: what psychiatrists need to know. World Psychiatry 2009;8(2):67—74.
[16] Doka KJ, Martin TL. Grieving beyond gender, understanding the ways men and women mourn. New York: Routledge; 2010.
[17] Janoff-Bulman R. Shattered assumptions. New York: Free Press; 2010.
[18] Cann A, Calhoun LG, Tedeschi RG, Kilmer RP, Gil-Rivas V, Vishnevsky T, et al. The Core Beliefs Inventory: a brief measure of disruption in the assumptive world. Anxiety Stress Coping 2010;23(1):19—34.
[19] Jaffe J, Diamond MO. Reproductive trauma: psychotherapy with infertility and pregnancy loss clients. Washington, D.C.: American Psychological Association; 2010.
[20] Bretherton I. The origins of attachment theory: John Bowlby and Mary Ainsworth. Dev Psychol 1992;28(5):759—75.
[21] Bowlby J. Attachment and loss: attachment, vol. 1. Harlow: Penguin Books; 1969/1991.
[22] Main M, Solomon J. Discovery of an insecure-disorganized/disoriented attachment pattern. In: Brazelton TB, Yogman MW, editors. Affective development in infancy. Westport, CT: Ablex Publishing Corporation; 1986. p. 95—124.
[23] Hill D. Affect regulation theory: a clinical model. 1st ed. New York: WW Norton; 2015.
[24] Knapp DJ, Norton AM, Sandberg JG. Family-of-origin, relationship self-regulation, and attachment in marital relationships. Contemp Fam Ther 2015;37(2):130—41.
[25] Madison G, Dutton E. Sex differences in crying. Encyclopedia of evolutionary psychological science. Cham: Springer International Publishing; 2020. p. 1—4.
[26] Verma R, Balhara YPS, Gupta CS. Gender differences in stress response: role of developmental and biological determinants. Ind Psychiatry J 2011;20(1):4—10.
[27] Mather M, Lighthall NR, Nga L, Gorlick MA. Sex differences in how stress affects brain activity during face viewing. Neuroreport. 2010;21(14):933—7.
[28] Cannon WB. The wisdom of the body. Am J Med Sci 1932;184(6):864.
[29] Taylor SE, Klein LC, Lewis BP, Gruenewald TL, Gurung RAR, Updegraff JA. Biobehavioral responses to stress in females: tend-and-befriend, not fight-or-flight. Psychol Rev 2000;107(3):411—29.
[30] Dana DA. The polyvagal theory in therapy: engaging the rhythm of regulation. New York: WW Norton; 2018.
[31] Levine PA. In an unspoken voice: how the body releases trauma and restores goodness. New York: North Atlantic Books; 2012.
[32] Elliott R, Bohart AC, Watson JC, Greenberg LS. Empathy. Psychotherapy (Chic) 2011;48(1):43—9.
[33] Maltz W. The sexual healing journey: a guide for survivors of sexual abuse. 3rd ed. New York: William Morrow Paperbacks; 2012.
[34] Herman J. Trauma and recovery: the aftermath of violence — from domestic abuse to political terror. New York: Basic Books; 2015.
[35] Brown B. Power of vulnerability: teachings on authenticity, connection and courage. Louisville, CO: Sounds True; 2012.
[36] Aakvaag HF, Thoresen S, Wentzel-Larsen T, Dyb G, Røysamb E, Olff M. Broken and guilty since it happened: a population study of trauma-related shame and guilt after violence and sexual abuse. J Affect Disord 2016;204:16—23.

[37] Galhardo A, Cunha M, Pinto-Gouveia J. Psychological aspects in couples with infertility. Sexologies 2011;20(4):224–8.
[38] Øktedalen T, Hoffart A, Langkaas TF. Trauma-related shame and guilt as time-varying predictors of posttraumatic stress disorder symptoms during imagery exposure and imagery rescripting—a randomized controlled trial. Psychother Res 2015;25(5):518–32.
[39] Wilson JP. Trauma and the epigenesis of identity. In: Wilson JP, editor. The posttraumatic self: restoring meaning and wholeness to personality. New York: Routledge; 2006. p. 69–116.
[40] Cicchetti D. Resilience under conditions of extreme stress: a multilevel perspective. World Psychiatry 2010;9(3):145–54.
[41] Southwick SM, Charney DS. Resilience: the science of mastering life's greatest challenges. Cambridge: Cambridge University Press; 2012.
[42] Levers LL, editor. Trauma counseling: theories and interventions. New York: Springer Publishing; 2012.
[43] Rosanbalm KD, Murray DW. Caregiver co-regulation across development: a practice brief. OPRE Brief #2017-80. Washington, D.C.: Office of Planning, Research and Evaluation, Administration for Children and Families; 2017. Available from: https://fpg.unc.edu/sites/fpg.unc.edu/files/resources/reports-and-policy-briefs/Co-RegulationFromBirthThroughYoungAdulthood.pdf.
[44] Masters WH, Johnson VE. Human sexual inadequacy. Philadelphia, PA: Lippincott Williams and Wilkins; 1970.
[45] Covington LS. Combat-related reproductive trauma: implications for quality of life and the reproductive narrative. Bryn Mawr, PA: Graduate School of Social Work and Social Research of Bryn Mawr College; 2018.
[46] American Society for Reproductive Medicine. Testosterone use and male infertility. Reproductivefacts.org. Available from: <https://www.reproductivefacts.org/news-and-publications/patient-fact-sheets-and-booklets/documents/fact-sheets-and-info-booklets/testosterone-use-and-male-infertility/> [cited September 11, 2020].
[47] Gillen MM, Markey CH. A review of research linking body image and sexual well-being. Body Image 2019;31:294–301.
[48] Metz ME, McCarthy BW. The "Good-Enough Sex" model for couple sexual satisfaction. Sex Relat Ther 2007;22(3):351–62.
[49] Mezzich JE, Hernandez-Serrano R. Psychiatry and sexual health: an integrative approach. New York: Jason Aronson; 2006.
[50] Hendrix H, Hunt HL. Getting the love you want: a guide for couples. New York: Simon & Schuster; 2005.
[51] Resick PA, Monson CM, Chard KM. Cognitive processing therapy for PTSD: a comprehensive manual. New York: Guilford Publications; 2017.
[52] Benson H, Klipper MZ. The relaxation response. London: Fount; 1984.
[53] McCarthy B, McCarthy E. Enhancing couple sexuality: creating an intimate and erotic bond. New York: Routledge; 2019.

CHAPTER 12

How the medicalization of reproduction takes the fun out of the process

Alice D. Domar[1], Alison J. Meyers[1] and Elizabeth A. Grill[2]

[1]Domar Centers for Mind/Body Health, Waltham, MA, United States [2]Center for Reproductive Medicine, Weill Cornell Medical College, New York, NY, United States

Highlights

Purpose of chapter:
The objective of this chapter was to analyze the recent research on the bidirectional relationship between infertility-related stress and sexual dysfunction in men, women, and the couple.

Importance:
The psychological and sexual implications of infertility-related stress can have long-term effects even after withdrawal or completion of fertility treatment. Addressing these issues early may eliminate long-term consequences.

Main ideas:
Women and men with infertility often report increased rates of sexual challenges and changes in sexuality; however, these consequences of infertility often go ignored. Sexual challenges can often manifest into changes in interpersonal relationships, sexual satisfaction, and can negatively affect fertility treatment outcomes. There are numerous marital, sexual, psychosocial, and clinical interventions which may be efficacious in decreasing the impact of infertility on sexuality.

Summary:
Infertility-related stress as a result or cause of sexual dysfunction is an important factor to consider when addressing the symptoms of an infertility diagnosis. Decreasing sexual dysfunction may lead to significant changes in psychological and physical well-being in affected patients, and therefore should not be overlooked.

Introduction

Stress can have positive purposes in terms of productivity, motivation, and cognitive function. However, when stress becomes too extreme, negative consequences may arise [1]. Particularly, severe or chronic life stress leads to increased release of glucocorticoid stress hormones, and can significantly negatively impact an individual's biological and emotional well-being, affecting almost all realms of their life [2]. Stressful experiences can severely impact sexual function, desire, and satisfaction in the man, woman, and couple as a unit; and the degree of the stressful experience may be correlated with higher rates of sexual dysfunction. While it is critical that sexual dysfunction be addressed in affected individuals, optimal dyadic sexual function is crucial for a *couple's* relationship success, in addition to preserving the patients' emotional well-being and self-perception [3].

While there are many causes of significant stress resulting in sexual dysfunction and changes in one, or both, partner's sexuality, this chapter will focus on the psychosocial and clinical effects of infertility-related stress on sexual dysfunction in the man, woman, and couple. Infertility patients often characterize their diagnosis as their most stressful life experience, comparable to cancer, human immunodeficiency virus (HIV), and other serious medical manifestations, validating that the psychological effects of the diagnosis must not be neglected [3]. Infertility-related stress is multifaceted. The diagnosis of infertility and the subsequent treatment process may lead to psychological consequences ranging from depression, to anxiety, to general distress [4]. Sexual dysfunction and changes in intimacy between a couple are another element constituting the numerous emotional and clinical consequences of the infertility diagnosis. Additionally, the physical stress of infertility treatments is yet another important component. In this chapter, the effects of general stress on sexuality will be outlined. Subsequently, the psychological effects of infertility-related stress will be discussed with specific attention paid to changes in sexuality and intimacy in the man, woman, and couple. Furthermore, the dyadic effects of sexual dysfunction within a couple necessitate the discussion of potential treatment interventions for sexual dysfunction specifically related to infertility.

Case study

Katelyn (37) and Steve (39) had been together for 4 years before marrying 2 years ago. One of the reasons they had waited to marry and start their family were their mutual career goals. Katelyn is in finance, had rapidly climbed the promotion ladder, and is now finally in a position of security, power, and an extremely high earning potential. However, she works 60–80 hours/week routinely and often goes into the office on weekends. Steve has been equally successful in the academic world and is currently a tenured Professor at an Ivy league institution. However, his workload has lessened with his seniority and he finds himself with a lot of time at home while Katelyn is still at the office. The couple have been trying to have a baby on their own since they married. Although Katelyn is thin, with a body mass index of 19 kg/m^2, she does have fairly regular menstrual cycles. Steve was tested and found to have a significant male factor, so they were advised to go straight to in vitro fertilization (IVF) with intracytoplasmic sperm injection (ICSI) in which a single sperm is injected directly into an egg to induce embryo formation. Both members of the couple reported that prior to their infertility, their sex life had been satisfying and somewhat adventurous. But once the workup was completed, according to Steve their sex life basically disappeared.

Upon sitting down with their clinic's Mental Health Professional (MHP), both members of the couple expressed sadness and disappointment with their physical relationship. But they were not previously aware of what their partner had been thinking about

Katelyn explained that she had always been an intense person, and in fact thrived on living a bit on the edge. But she had come to realize that the stress of her job, which was increasing substantially with her increasing job responsibilities, was beginning to overwhelm her. She felt inadequate and underprepared. She began to experience a variety of stress-related symptoms, including insomnia, tearfulness, headaches, and anxiety. She was devastated by their infertility and as her friends and family members became pregnant easily, she pulled away and lost her sources of social support. Her libido vanished. And there did not seem to be any point to making love if Steve's sperm count was too low to allow conception to occur on its own.

At the same time, Steve was reeling from the male factor diagnosis. He needed reassurance from Katelyn that she still felt that he was a man in her eyes, and began to push for more frequent episodes of love making. Katelyn was feeling anxious, sad, and overwhelmed and the last thing she wanted was to feel pressure to have sex.

The two of them were able to communicate effectively and to even see where their partner was coming from. Steve had not realized how awful others' pregnancies were for Katelyn and Katelyn had not realized that Steve's diagnosis made him feel guilty and less virile.

Katelyn was encouraged to learn a variety of stress management and relaxation strategies that led to a decrease in her psychological symptoms. Steve was reassured that a sperm count has nothing to do with manhood. As Katelyn calmed down and began to feel more in control of her feelings, her desire for Steve increased. And as Steve came to accept that sperm count and virility are in no way connected, he began to feel less insecure and pressured Katelyn less. At their final session, they held hands and felt grateful that they were able to happily connect physically again.

Background

General stress and sexual dysfunction in men and women

Sexual dysfunction is common, with 40%–45% of adult women and 20%–30% of adult men reporting one or more manifestations of sexual dysfunction [5]. Life stress is a major contributor to sexual dysfunction in both males and females, and can have serious implications on the physiological, psychological, and relationship well-being of affected individuals. In this section, the physiological and psychological impact of excess stress in men, women, and the couple regarding sexual function will be addressed.

In males, chronic stress can affect testosterone production due to interference in the hypothalamic–pituitary–gonadal (HPG) axis as a result of stress hormone release, leading to a decline in sexual desire and libido [2]. Additionally, stress over an extended period of time can cause erectile dysfunction (ED) or impotence [6]. Researchers have shown that chronic stress can result in diminished sperm production and maturation, causing difficulties for reproduction for couples who are trying to conceive [6]. Further, researchers report that men who have experienced two or more particularly stressful life events in the past year had a lower percentage of sperm motility and a lower percentage of sperm with normal morphologies in comparison to men who did not experience particularly stressful events [6]. Chronic stress in men can impact both the biological ability to engage in sexual activity as well as the psychological connotations around sex and their own self-image.

Unmistakably, sexual dysfunction caused by stress in men can have psychological implications. The inability to be sexually active due to a clinical complication or psychological manifestation can affect a man's sexual identity, self-perception, and may increase feelings of failure, worthlessness, and shame [3]. Barlow [7] suggests that sexual dysfunction due to psychological manifestation is based on cognitive interference and anxiety. This model concludes that sexual dysfunction is attributed to an inappropriate attentional focus that tends to the negative outcomes of sex such as performance anxiety. Further, neutral distracting stimuli may inhibit arousal and sexual function [7]. Thus severe stress can have significant consequences on not only sexual identity and emotional well-being but also the organic ability to reproduce.

In females, excessive stress can have deleterious effects on menstruation leading to more aberrant or irregular cycles, in addition to an increase in pain or duration of the cycle. Stress may also worsen premenstrual symptoms creating reproductive and sexual difficulties [6]. Additionally, changes in hormone production as a result of stress can substantially negatively impact sexual function. Higher levels of glucocorticoids in women released from the adrenal gland in response to extreme stress can inhibit the HPG axis, which is critical for control of reproduction and sexual responses. Glucocorticoids can interfere with the successful release of gonadotropin releasing hormone, luteinizing hormone, and follicle stimulating hormone. Accordingly, a reduction in gonadotropin release can result in decreased production of gonadal steroids such as estradiol and testosterone, both of which have mediating effects on female genital arousal [2].

Excess stress greatly increases the likelihood of developing psychological symptoms such as anxiety and depression. In fact, depression caused by excess stress is one of the leading complications in pregnancy and postpartum adjustment [6]. Psychologically, stress can interfere with sexual function due to both emotional and cognitive changes, distracting the individual from sexual cues toward negative outcomes [2]. Hamilton et al. [2] investigated the effects of chronic stress on female sexual arousal. Fifteen women with high chronic stress and 15 women with average stress were measured in genital and psychological arousal after watching an erotic film. Results revealed that women in the high-stress groups had lower levels of genital arousal and higher levels of cortisol, a hormone produced by excess stress. Interestingly, psychological arousal was not significantly different between the group with high-stress and the control group [2]. In a 2004 study examining the effects of prolonged stress on female rat sexual function, results showed that the high-stress experimental group experienced reduced receptivity to males. Additionally, the high-stress group experienced changes in sex hormones, endocrine factors, and neurotransmitters, likely signifying the mechanisms of how chronic stress modifies sexual behavior [8]. In summary, severe stress can significantly impact the physiological and psychological aspects of female sexual function.

Sexual dysfunction can have significant implications for personal well-being and relationship satisfaction [9]. Sexuality between a couple is a bidirectional relationship. The desire, arousal, and sexual identity of one partner affects that of the other. For example, researchers from one study [10] reported that the sexual function and satisfaction of women with partners with ED was significantly lower than women with partners without ED. A total of 632 sexually active couples were analyzed using the Female Sexual Function Index (FSFI) and the International Index of Erectile Function. Almost half (42.9%) of female participants reported sexual difficulty, and 15.0% of men reported mild-to-moderate (ED). From this, the female partners of men with ED revealed significantly lower scores on the FSFI than those with male partners without ED [10]. Moreover, sexual dysfunction of one partner heavily influences the sexual function of the other. Thus treating stress-related sexual dysfunction is vital to optimal sexual function and intimacy within a relationship. Modern population-based studies evaluating the incidence of sexual dysfunction in the United States are scarcely available. Nevertheless, data from the National Health and Social Life Survey observed sexual dysfunction in 43% of women and 31% of men [11]. Likewise, a review of domestic and international studies observed similar percentages of the prevalence of sexual dysfunction in men and women [5]. Stress in general has many psychosocial and clinical consequences when it comes to sexuality and intimacy in a relationship. The etiology of sexual dysfunction is multidimensional; however, research has shown that significant stress can result in loss of sexual desire, function, and satisfaction. For instance, in men and women, researchers have shown that higher-self reported stress in daily life, such as before a job interview or big exam, is associated with lower levels of sexual activity and individual satisfaction within a relationship [9]. Sexual dysfunction as a result of stress can have severe implications on various factors of life, and as stress is exacerbated by additional factors such as infertility, the impact on sexual function is also intensified. In subsequent sections, the effects of specifically infertility-related stress on sexuality will be addressed.

Infertility—prevalence, etiology, and diagnosis

Infertility is defined as the "failure to establish a clinical pregnancy after 12 months of regular and unprotected sexual intercourse" [12]. It is estimated that one in eight couples have difficulty conceiving and sustaining a pregnancy [13]. Research on the specific prevalence varies, but studies have reported that the diagnosis affects approximately 12%—18% of women aged 15—44, and roughly 7% of men [12,14]. Researchers from one study assessed the global infertility rates between 1990 and 2010 in 190 countries, revealing 48.5 million couples, 19.2 million suffering from primary infertility, while 29.3 were diagnosed with secondary infertility [15].

The reasons for infertility can include both female and male factors. In females, reproduction can be impaired by altered function of the reproductive organs, illnesses, or by psychological factors. In men, Starc [15] lists three potential categories for infertility etiology: unobstructive etiology (production of sperm problem), obstructive etiology (transportation of sperm problem), and coital infertility (problems with ejaculation or impotence) [15]. Diagnosing infertility is a multifaceted processes. Women may receive a gynecologic examination from their obstetrician/gynecologist (OB/GYN), and may be asked to generate detailed reports on their menstrual and gynecological history [16]. Both partners may be asked about medications, risk factors such as smoking and chemotherapy, family history of infertility-causing diseases, and previous or existing sexually transmitted infections (STIs). The male partner may be asked to give a sperm sample to assess semen quality and sperm function. If no obvious etiologies are observed, the female partner will likely receive blood work, a physical examination of the thyroid gland, breasts, pelvis, and may be asked to complete cervical cultures and/or a transvaginal sonogram. Anatomic abnormalities can also be evaluated using a hysterosalpingogram [16]. Summarily, testing for infertility causes for males and females falls into three categories: hormonal, anatomic, and female egg factors [16].

Evidently, an infertility workup, including the extensive process to which one can obtain an accurate diagnosis, tends to be not only physically but also psychologically exhausting and distressing for all individuals involved. Unfortunately, the diagnosis can lead to an extensive procedure of medical attention and treatment, resulting in more arduous psychological and physical experiences.

Psychological impact of infertility

The inability to conceive naturally often results in feelings of low self-esteem, distress, guilt, and shame. And despite the high prevalence of infertility, the majority of infertile couples do not share their story with friends and family, thereby increasing their vulnerability to debilitating psychological disorders [17]. Individuals and couples that undergo assisted reproductive technology (ART) treatment with hopes of having a biological child are at increased risk of experiencing psychological troubles. In fact, researchers from one study found that 40.8% of infertile women assessed suffer from clinical depression, in addition to 86.8% women reporting symptoms of anxiety [17].

In another study, 352 women and 274 men receiving infertility treatment were evaluated for depression and anxiety. A total of 56% of the women and 32% of the men reported clinical levels of depressive symptoms. Additionally, 76% of the women and 61% of the men reported clinical levels of anxiety [18]. A study in Denmark consisting of 42,000 women who underwent ART treatment evaluated women for depression, reporting 35% of positive cases;[19] another study found 15% of women and 6% of men reported severe depression after 1 year of unsuccessful infertility treatment [20]. In a recent study, 60 married women, 30 fertile and 30 infertile, were evaluated for depression, anxiety, and stress. The results of the study indicate significantly higher rates of depression (10.83 + 8.37 vs 4.17 + 3.21; $P<.000$), anxiety (11.60 + 8.48 vs 5.50 + 4.24 $P<0001$), and stress (19.67 + 8.40 vs 12.10 + 6.76 $P<.000$) in infertile women compared to fertile controls [21].

Maroufizadeh et al. [22] performed a cross-sectional study evaluating 330 infertility patients (122 men, 208 women) on the Hospital Anxiety and Depression Scale (HADS). The results showed that infertile couples were very likely to have psychological symptoms such as anxiety (49.6%) and depression (33%). Additionally, individuals with at least one fertility treatment failure had significantly higher rates of anxiety and depression than those who have not yet had a treatment failure [22]. Bakhtiyar et al. [23] assessed 180 infertile and 540 fertile women in a matched case-control study using the WHOQOL-BREF (WHO Quality of Life-BREF instrument) to evaluate physical, social, environmental, and mental dimensions constituting one's quality of life. The results indicate significant effects of infertility on physical, social, and mental health ($P<.001$) compared to controls. Environmental health was statistically unaffected by infertility [23].

In one study, only 21% of women and 11.3% of men undergoing infertility treatment reported receiving mental health services [18]. Because psychological symptoms have shown be correlated to in negative pregnancy outcomes and discontinuation rates of fertility treatment, these data emphasize the need for the promotion of mental healthcare [18,24].

Women with infertility frequently characterize their diagnosis as their most stressful life experience [16,25]. Studies have shown that infertility is a stressor comparable to devastating manifestations such as cancer, AIDS, and loss of a loved one. Domar et al. [3] evaluated 149 women with infertility, 136 with chronic pain, 22 in the process of cardiac rehabilitation, 93 with cancer, 77 with hypertension, and 11 with HIV. The results of this study show that women with infertility had scores assessing psychological well-being comparable to cancer, cardiac rehabilitation, and hypertension patients, and had lower scores than the HIV-positive and chronic patient participants; the anxiety and depression scores of women with infertility were not significantly differently from all other groups excluding the chronic pain patients. From this, infertility can be classified as equally distressing as other serious medical conditions such as cancer [3]. Additionally, Vaughan et al. [26] reported that infertility-related stress was still paramount in the midst of the global COVID-19 pandemic amongst patients in Boston. A questionnaire assessing the top three stressors was collected and analyzed from 2202 nonpregnant women with infertility over three separate time courses between 1 January 2019 and 1 April 2020. Even during the surge in the Boston area, infertility was the most frequent top stressor reported by the participants [26].

For many, infertility diagnoses result in significant psychological and clinical manifestations spanning their emotional, physical, mental, and sexual health. Sexual function and successful conception are imperative aspects of most marital relationships, and have significant impacts on marital success and the quality of life of both partners. Unfortunately, the diagnosis of infertility not only presents marital challenges but also forces those facing infertility to confront familial and societal pressures, financial burdens for ART treatments, and physical and psychological drains [3]. Sexual dysfunction and changes in an individual's sexuality are significant consequences of infertility, and must be medically and/or psychologically addressed.

The impacts of infertility-related stress on sexuality

As the psychological and physical burdens of infertility treatment increase, couples often experience changes in their sexuality. They no longer see sex as an activity of enjoyment, love, romance, and intimacy. Rather, sex becomes an instrument for the sole purpose to conceive a child. Sexual intercourse becomes a scheduled chore around ovulation and the "fertile window," accompanied by feelings of distress, despair, and worry about failure [3,16,27]. Unsuccessful family planning can result in negative self-image, altered self-respect, changes in sexuality, and may impact marital and interpersonal satisfaction [15]. Additionally, as an infertility diagnosis persists, and the years of childlessness increase, the effects on sexual function manifest and consequently worsen [16]. Infertile couples have reported psychosexual problems ranging from loss in libido, changes in sexual desire, spontaneity, and ability to orgasm [28]. The interplay between infertility and sexuality can largely impact one's reproductive potential, interpersonal relationships, martial relationship, and self-image. Studies have associated the psychological, physical, clinical, and financial burdens of ART treatment with increased marital conflict, changes in marital intimacy, decreased sexual self-esteem, feelings of shame and guilt, and changes in the frequency of sexual activity [16]. Thus sexual dysfunction and infertility can significantly impact an individual's physical and psychological well-being.

Sexual dysfunction may have an etiological role in infertility, or it may be a result of the disorder secondary to psychological stress in one or both partners. Whether sexual dysfunction is a preexisting condition, or a side effect of the stress of infertility and accompanying treatment, it can feel devastating, compounding the existing disappointment of childlessness, distress of medical treatment, and feelings of guilt and shame [16]. Statistically, preexisting sexual dysfunctions have only a minor etiological role in infertility, impacting approximately 5% of infertility cases. In these cases, male ED and anejaculation, in addition to female vaginismus, are the only clinical sexual dysfunctions inhibiting natural conception [3]. Psychological factors such as severe stress have been shown to contribute to male fertility by mechanisms such as interfering with spermatogenesis. Additionally, extreme physical stress can alter testosterone levels also negatively affecting sperm production [29]. Most commonly, the stresses of infertility and psychological effects such as anxiety and depression are the leading causes of changes in sexual function within a couple [3].

As the psychological effects of infertility manifest, individuals may consider the use of antidepressant medications such as selective-serotonin reuptake inhibitors (SSRIs) to mediate such emotional distresses. SSRIs are used for a wide range of psychological disorders, including major depressive disorder, general anxiety, posttraumatic stress disorder, eating disorders, panic disorder, and more. While these medications may work to compound the negative psychological effects of infertility often contributing to comorbid sexual dysfunction, these prescriptions can also have a biological impact on sexual ability, including changes in libido and desire. Unfortunately, the common side effects on sexuality due to the use of antidepressant drugs often leads to changes in patient's compliance with the treatment medication and ultimately complete cessation of the treatment resulting in increased negative psychological symptoms [30].

Infertility and sexuality in men—clinical implications

Preexisting clinical factors and psychological stressors impacting male fertility can hamper sexual function. The most common male sexual dysfunctions likely to affect male fertility include those that cause ED, and impact sexual desire, arousal, and ejaculation abilities. The etiology of ED comprises a mix of different clinical and psychogenic factors. Particularly, men with chronic conditions such as hypertension, heart disease, and diabetes have an increased risk of developing ED. Certain lifestyles also impact the risk of ED, including obesity, cigarette smoking, and a sedentary lifestyle. Depression and other psychological dysfunctions have also been linked to ED development, and these dysfunctions are linked to changes in sexual confidence and performance anxiety as well. Certain medications are also linked to male sexual dysfunction, including diuretics, beta-blockers, and various antidepressants. Six percent of men evaluated for infertility have concomitant pathologies, including malignancies, genetic abnormalities, and endocrinopathy. Summarily, whether the cause is vascular, hormonal, pathological, drug-induced, anatomic, neurogenic, or psychological, the effects are the same. Decreased sexuality and desire in addition to clinical sexual dysfunctions not only limit a man's fertility and ability to reproduce but also can have significant negative impacts on marital success, quality of life, and self-image [3,30,31]. Further, male sexual function tends to decrease with a male factor cause for infertility. For example, men with reduced sperm counts experienced a parallel decrease in sexual function, impacting a couple's sex life and associated intimacy [32].

An additional complication of male infertility is the increase in the rate of sexual dysfunction within couples. Clinical manifestations in men not only impact the ability to naturally conceive a child but also affect the other partner's sexual function, marital satisfaction, and intimacy [32]. As previously mentioned, sexual function is a dyadic process impacting both partners in a sexual relationship; therefore the psychological and physiological factors in men must also be addressed in women.

Infertility and sexuality in men—psychosocial implications

Sexual disinterest and loss of satisfaction are frequently observed in both men and women experiencing infertility. The monthly on-demand intercourse, or in men, ejaculation for infertility treatment collections, often makes sexual activity outside of these times "purposeless" for both the man and woman [29]. Frequently, men experiencing infertility develop performance anxiety, sexual avoidance, and even sexual aversion as opposed to enjoyment and satisfaction. Schedules and unspontaneous intercourse can decrease libido in 10% of patients, and

ED may occur in 20% of men [3,33]. Men experiencing infertility, whether personally or with their partner, are linked with higher rates of ED, depressive symptoms, lower self-esteem, higher anxiety, increased somatic symptoms, and greater sexual dysfunction in their relationship [32].

Some studies report that men experience less distress and sexual effects than women in an infertile relationship. Nevertheless, the dyadic essence of a sexual relationship eventually leads to significant changes in male sexual function, desire, and satisfaction. Researchers assessing the sexual function of 308 infertile women found that the rate of women who presented a sexual problem in their male partner had significantly higher incidences of sexual dysfunction in themselves than in the fertile control group consisting of 308 healthy women ($P > .05$) [34]. Male infertility has emotional ramifications ranging from higher incidences of depression, decreased relationship stability, higher anxiety, lower self-esteem, and an increase in dysfunctional sexual relationships. Additionally, men report a decreased ability to control ejaculation and a decrease in personal performance satisfaction [3]. In one study by Ozkan et al., 56 infertile men and 28 fertile men were evaluated based on sexual function and rates of depression. The results showed that infertile men had significantly higher impaired sexual function and higher rates of depressive symptoms than healthy male controls. In fact, 85.9% of infertile patients had diagnosable mild-to-moderate ED [35].

One of the most common psychosexual manifestations of infertility includes hypoactive sexual desire disorder, now known as female sexual interest/arousal disorder [Diagnostic and Statistical Manual of Mental Disorders (DSM)-V] involving episodic or contextual responses to emotional or physical strains of infertility, affecting one's sexual desire [36]. Sexual aversion disorder, which existed in the DSM-IV and is no longer recognized as an "official" sexual dysfunction is also a consequence of infertility consisting of anxiety, fear, and/or disgust when they are in a sexual context or even think about sex [36]. Hence the psychological implications of infertility must be addressed as it may result in sexual dysfunction in the male partner.

Infertility and sexuality in women—clinical implications

The emotional, physical, and financial stress of an infertility evaluation, diagnosis, and treatment are exacerbated by regimented intercourse. The interference in the spontaneity of a couple's sexual relationship interferes in marital intimacy and sexual function. Importantly, these effects seem to manifest more frequently in the female partner [3,37,38].

Common types of sexual disorders, as described by Tayebi et al., in women include sexual desire disorders, sexual arousal disorders, orgasmic disorders, and sexual pain disorders (vaginismus, dyspareunia) [39]. Vaginismus, now known as genitopelvic pain/penetration disorder (DSM-V), is the only clinical manifestation in women that can directly inhibit pregnancy. Nevertheless, sexual dysfunction in women and couples tends to be a product of infertility rather than a direct cause [3]. Vaginismus affects approximately 1% of the population and is a condition in which vaginal spasms occur and prevent penetration during intercourse. Vaginismus may influence a woman's ability to conceive and impact her sexual identity and femininity. Interestingly, the disease used to be attributed to a somatic manifestation of an underlying psychological problem, but it is frequently the result of gynecological disorders, including endometriosis, pelvic pain, or vestibulitis. In one study examining pregnant women with vaginismus, 100% of the participants described feelings of anxiety and anger immediately before sexual intercourse, validating the damaging effect vaginismus has on not only the ability to procreate but also on the psychological conception of sex [40].

Multiple studies have evaluated the effects of infertility on sexual function in women. In one study of 121 women with infertility, 26% of the participants reported sexual dysfunctions. In a subsequent study, 61.7% of infertile female participants were identified to have a high risk of sexual dysfunction [34,38]. In an additional study, 236 infertile women were examined for sexual dysfunction. Slightly more than half (55.5%) of the infertile women reported some form of impaired sexual function [41]. In another study, the prevalence of sexual dysfunction between 50 infertile women and 50 fertile women was compared. The vast majority of infertile women (90%) suffered from some form of sexual dysfunction, while only 26% of fertile women did [42]. Notably, some studies did not find significant differences in the sexual function between fertile and infertile women [43,44].

As the years of childlessness increase, particularly in secondary infertility patients, the psychological and emotional effects of infertility-related stress worsens [3]. Tanha et al. [45] evaluated 191 primary and 129 secondary infertility female patients compared with 87 fertile controls. The results showed that sexual function was negatively impacted in all infertile women, and importantly, secondary infertility was linked to more severe results [45].

Additional factors may exacerbate women's reported stress levels. One study examined the difference in reported stress and sexual function of women with infertility with and without polycystic ovary syndrome (PCOS). The results showed that women with infertility in addition to PCOS had significantly higher reports of stress than women without PCOS. There was no difference in the reports of sexual dysfunction between the two groups [46]. Thus it is important to address comorbid manifestations in infertility patients that may impact patient's psychological health and sexual function.

Infertility and sexuality in women—psychosocial implications

Infertility-related stress has important psychological and sexual implications in female patients [47]. Researchers from one study reported that compared to fertile controls, women undergoing infertility treatment were significantly more depressed and anxious. Additionally, infertile women showed lower self-esteem, sexual satisfaction, and sexual self-esteem than fertile women [48]. A study assessing the emotional and sexual state of 50 women with infertility reported 33% of the participants to be clinically depressed, 59% with high distress, and a mean FSFI score indicating sexual dysfunction [49]. Pakpour et al. [50] examined 410 women with primary infertility and 194 women with secondary infertility in comparison to healthy controls based on sexual satisfaction. Results showed that infertile women reported significantly lower sexual satisfaction than fertile controls, with individuals with secondary infertility having the worst scores [50]. Finally, in one study assessing sexual function in women with primary and secondary infertility compared to healthy controls using the FSFI survey, researchers found that the total scores measuring sexual function in all domains (arousal, desire, and satisfaction) were significantly lower in all infertile women [45]. Oskay et al. [34] evaluated 308 infertile and 308 fertile women using the FSFI. The total mean FSFI score for infertile women was 24.58 and 26.55 for the fertile control group, indicating a significant difference. Additionally, 61.7% of the infertile women had scores accepted as high risk for female sexual dysfunction [34].

Researchers have determined that female distress levels are higher than their male spouses with respect to "grief, guilt, denial, anxiety, cognitive disturbance, and hostility" [16]. Reasons for this include that women report feeling social responsibility for conceiving and sustaining a pregnancy, and experience feelings of failure with reproductive and sexual functions exacerbated by existing medical terminology such as "premature ovarian failure" and "incompetent cervix" [16]. Additionally, women view the role of mother as a key piece of their femininity, gender identity, and sexuality. Further, fertility treatment is more invasive and intrusive for women than men, potentially distorting a sexual relationship. Finally, coping strategies are different between men and women. For instance, women cannot imagine life without children and may subsequently develop depressive symptoms, while men tend to deny the diagnosis and implications and remain active going about their daily lives [16]. Overall, research has shown that women experience greater psychological distress than men in response to infertility and often assume more personal responsibility for failed conception, in addition to enduring the majority of invasive medical treatment [16]. Nevertheless, addressing both partners' challenges is imperative to successful treatment.

Infertility and sexuality in the couple—marital implications

It is estimated that 10%−60% of couples have sexual problems related to infertility, affecting intimacy, couple sexual function, marital well-being, and sexual satisfaction [51,52]. Couples experiencing infertility often have increased rates of sexual dysfunction and decreased sexual satisfaction, and the results of various studies emphasize the dyadic effects of infertility within a couple. In one study, 88 women and 45 couples receiving fertility treatments completed measures of adult attachment and sexual functioning. Results showed that the frequency and type of sexual dysfunction varied: 14.8% pain and 58% decreased desire in women, and 6.7% dissatisfaction with orgasm and 28.9% decrease in desire in men. Additionally, attachment avoidance predicted lower levels of sexual satisfaction. Finally, this study emphasized the partner effect. Specifically, men's sexual avoidance was related to their partner's difficultly achieving orgasms [53]. In an additional study, when 200 women with infertility and their husbands were evaluated on sexual function using the FSFI and Sexual Health Inventory for Men, both the male and female partner scores in the group experiencing infertility had significantly lower scores in sexual function and satisfaction. Further, husbands of women with infertility experienced significantly higher rates of ED. These results emphasize the dyadic quality of infertility-related stress, both from a clinical and psychosocial perspective [31]. Yangin et al. recruited 102 infertile couples who were examined based on sexual satisfaction, reporting that 37.3% of women and 33.3% of men were sexually unsatisfied in their relationship [54].

The results from studies pertaining to intimacy and well-being in couples experiencing infertility vary, with some suggesting that infertility is actually associated with increases in marital satisfaction. For instance, researchers from one study revealed that infertility subjects presented higher scores on marital intimacy than couples not experiencing infertility. This interesting study suggests that infertility may function as a couple's cohesion factor during medical treatment [55]. This phenomenon is also seen in one study comprised of 125 couples with infertility and 125 fertile couples, who completed various questionnaires assessing martial and sexual satisfaction. The mean scores for sexual satisfaction for the infertile group was 63.67, and was 46.37 for the fertile group. Further, the mean scores for marital satisfaction were 44.03 for the infertile and 36.20 for the fertile group, indicating that infertile couples may have higher marital and sexual satisfaction than fertile controls [56]. Finally, one study examining 221 women with infertility revealed that 88.5% of the participants had good marital intimacy in emotional, psychological, intellectual, sexual, physical, spiritual, esthetic, and social domains [57].

Researchers in Rwanda recruited 312 infertility patients who were evaluated on marital well-being, specifically regarding domestic violence, sexual dysfunction, and divorce rates. Results showed that infertility patients reported more domestic violence, union dissolutions, and sexual dysfunctions than healthy control couples [58]. This study necessitates the need for psychological intervention in infertility patients experiencing distress, as this presents a higher likelihood of developing challenging and even dangerous circumstances.

In conclusion, studies reveal interesting results that marital intimacy may not be affected, or may even be enhanced with infertility-related stress, suggesting that the significant togetherness of such a major stressor may act as a cohesion factor for couples [55]. Other speculations for this increase in marital satisfaction include the exclusion of the financial and social burden of having children [56]. However, most research which assessed the sexual function and sexual satisfaction of married couples experiencing infertility revealed significant decreases in both areas. Thus it is imperative that the psychological and sexual effects of an infertility diagnosis are appropriately addressed so that couples may maintain sexual satisfaction and function.

Infertility-related stress on sexuality and pregnancy—treatment outcomes

A frequently disputed area in reproductive medicine is the potential influence of psychological factors such as stress, depression, anxiety, and so on, on pregnancy rates. Dozens of studies have examined the interplay between pregnancy rates and psychological symptoms prior to and during ART cycles. Some have shown no relationship; however, many have revealed that higher rates of distress before and during treatment correlate with lower pregnancy rates [46]. Ostensibly, there are many explanations for these varying results; nonetheless, the relationship between stress and sexual function in infertility patients likely has a significant role.

As previously mentioned, general stress and psychological symptoms can have negative impacts on sexual function and human sexuality. Hence the high prevalence rates of psychological distress in infertility patients, exacerbated by the notion that sex is no longer for enjoyment but for conception alone, substantially increases the need for psychological and sexual intervention. Importantly, the psychological and sexual effects of infertility may have a significant impact on fertility treatment outcomes. Researchers in one study found that the more distressed a patient is prior to starting IVF treatment, the less likely it is that she will conceive. Researchers from this study showed that stress level was correlated to number of retrieved oocytes, number fertilized, pregnancy success rates, live birth rates, and birth weight [59,60]. Frederiksen et al. [61] evaluated 39 studies assessing the effects of psychological intervention on pregnancy rates and psychological outcome. The results of the study demonstrate statistically significant effects of psychosocial intervention on clinical pregnancy [risk ratio = 2.01; confidence interval (CI) 1.48–2.73; $P < .001$] and combined psychological outcomes (Hedges $g = 0.59$; CI 0.38–0.80; $P = .001$). Additionally, meta-regression showed that larger decreases in anxiety were associated with improvement in pregnancy rates [61]. Domar et al. [62] conducted a study of 143 women less than 40 years of age who were about to start their first IVF cycle. Participants were randomly assigned to complete a 10-session Mind/Body Program (MB) consisting of psychological intervention and education on relevant coping skills for infertility, or assigned to a control group. The participants were followed for two IVF cycles. The researchers found that at cycle 1, pregnancy rates for all subjects was 43%. The majority of the mind/body patients had not attended the program, however, prior to undergoing their cycle. At cycle 2, pregnancy rates for the MB group was 52% and only 20% for the controls [62]. Thus an intervention tending to the psychological effects of infertility was correlated to higher pregnancy rates in infertile patients, emphasizing the need to address nonclinical manifestations of the diagnosis.

Reducing psychological distress and cognitively restructuring the connotation of the "task" of sex may not only improve affect and psychosocial functioning but also improve sexual function and intimacy between couples. While there are no definitive studies confirming the positive linear relationship between psychological improvement and pregnancy rates, one can speculate that improved sexual function and psychological function is certainly a beneficial result of clinical and psychological intervention. Further, increased sexual activity may result in an increase likelihood of naturally conceiving [4].

Consultation, referral, and treatment options

All too often, the psychological and sexual problems of infertile couples go ignored. The medicalization of the diagnosis eliminates the humanity and accompanying emotional devastation of infertility [63]. Action to address the sexual implications of infertility-related stress should be taken when sexual dysfunction impacts medical intervention and infertility treatments, poses problems for the couple's marital relationship, and/or if sexuality and sexual health are highly important to the couple.

Assessment should evaluate whether the sexual impacts is: "(1) preexisting or secondary to infertility; (2) generalized or situation specific (e.g., problems more likely to occur when collecting a sperm sample, when the woman is ovulating); and (3) related to medical conditions or medications associated with infertility (e.g., endometriosis, prostatitis, and medications such as clomiphene or gonadotropins)" [56]. Management of the effects of infertility-related stressors on sexual dysfunction is best provided by a combination approach that effectively addresses the interplay between clinical and psychosocial factors. Having a consultation with an experienced sex therapist is the best way to start and sexual pharmaceuticals can be discussed if counseling is not quickly effective [3,64]. Depending on the rapport, relationship, comfort level, preference, and resource availability, a physician or infertility specialist may choose to personally treat a couple or refer them to a sex therapist, infertility, or marital counselor [3,65]. Subsequent sections will address the various treatment options for infertility-related sexual dysfunction, including marital intervention, sex therapy, psychosocial intervention, and clinical and pharmaceutical intervention.

Marital intervention—the couple

Couples tend to be reluctant to discuss sexual aspects of their relationship, especially when sexual functioning may be problematic, embarrassing, or atypical. Infertile couples are even more resistant to discussing sexual dysfunction for fear of disrupting or jeopardizing medical fertility treatments [36]. Nevertheless, addressing the sexual aspects of their relationship is imperative to marital satisfaction, psychological well-being, and successful fertility treatments. Further, martial intervention has been proven effective in reducing sexual dissatisfaction in couples, strengthening couples' marital health. For instance, couples with infertility completed surveys pertaining to their marital and sexual satisfaction before and after their participation in an enrichment program involving marriage and sex counseling. Results showed a significant increase in martial and sexual satisfaction scores among couples following the program ($P < .001$) [66]. In a randomized controlled trial of 100 couples with infertility, those who received three couple's therapy sessions consisting of marital counseling had higher sexual and marital satisfaction 3 months later in comparison to the control group who did not receive couples therapy [56,67]. In an additional study with 60 females undergoing IVF, those who received collaborative counseling on marital satisfaction reported higher levels of martial satisfaction than the control group [68]. Thus the effectiveness of martial intervention should be emphasized when discussing treatment options of sexual dysfunction.

In many couples, infertility and accompanying sexual dysfunction lead to feelings of guilt, shame, and loss of self-esteem. Oftentimes, in couples, one partner blames themselves or the other for the inability to naturally conceive. In this case, psychological and marital intervention is critical in addressing sexual and emotional health before the infertility diagnosis, and what the patient's view of causation is. Importantly, findings may reveal that the sexual problems are not a result of infertility, rather reflect a more fundamental relationship problem, necessitating marital intervention [52]. If sexual problems seem to reflect more fundamental relationship programs, it may be true that those issues take precedence over further infertility treatment [16].

Notably, issues of gender and culture are paramount: threats to femininity and masculinity, comfort when discussing sexuality, and the importance of parenthood must be addressed. Also, it is necessary to validate the experience of affected couple's feelings of shame, guilt, and inadequacy to enhance the therapeutic bond [52]. Overall, collaborative and open dialog is a necessity in marital intervention regarding sexual dysfunction.

Sex therapy

Sex therapy can be highly beneficial for individuals experiencing the sexual consequences of infertility. Sex therapists can use the "sexual status exam," and act essentially as detectives whose detailed accounts and inquiries help unveil the causes of sexual dysfunction and associated emotional symptoms [36]. Importantly, the management and treatment of sexual dysfunction is best provided by an approach combining the physical and psychosocial factors.

Research has shown that sex therapy and cognitive-behavioral approaches to treat ED, a common sexual manifestation as a result of psychological distress or other pathological factors, can be effective in reducing many of the sexual symptoms of the ED diagnosis. Commonly, this type of treatment revolves around providing psychoeducation about healthy erectile function, promoting mindfulness during sex, reducing performance anxiety, increasing communication between couples about sexual techniques, promoting the use of appropriate sexual stimulation, and encouraging a more flexible sexual life which is paramount when tending to infertility patients. Regular masturbation exercises are recommended emphasizing self-stimulation exercises in low-stress contexts with the goal to eventually pair relaxation with sexual arousal and reduce sexual stress [69]. Sex therapy for sexual dysfunctions in infertility patients must carefully educate patients to restructure intrusive, negative thoughts relating to infertility and sexual function. Additionally, sex therapists must work to reveal possible underlying psychological issues that could affect their mental and physical health in the future [69].

Psychosocial intervention

The medicalization of infertility, while critical for certain ARTs and medical procedures, has inadvertently resulted in an increase in the neglect of the emotional and psychological aspects of an infertility diagnosis, including changes in sexuality. Fortunately, various psychological interventions addressing such problems have been efficacious in eliminating some of these deterring effects [63]. Psychological interventions emphasizing stress management and coping skills have been associated with decreasing some of the most deleterious emotional effects accompanying infertility [63].

Numerous studies have evaluated the efficacy of psychosocial interventions to mediate the psychological effects of infertility. Boivin performed a review of some of the psychosocial interventions for infertility, considering the results of 380 studies. The results showed three main themes: psychosocial interventions were most effective in reducing negative affect than changing interpersonal functioning such as marital and social functioning; pregnancy rates were high unaffected by psychosocial interventions; group programs emphasizing education and skills training were substantially more effective than counseling interventions emphasizing emotional expression, thoughts, and feeling related to infertility; finally, the study revealed that men and women equally benefitted from psychosocial interventions [70]. Frederiksen et al. reviewed 39 studies assessing psychological intervention effects on pregnancy rates and psychological outcomes (depression, anxiety, stress, and marital function). The results showed that there were statistically significant effects on pregnancy rates and a variety of psychological symptoms from psychosocial interventions [61].

However, research on the impact of psychological interventions in the infertility arena are sparse. In one study on 70 women with infertility, those who received two psychoeducational sexual counseling sessions had higher sexual function and satisfaction 4 months later in comparison to the control group [52,71].

Unfortunately, there have been limited empirical studies available on the effectiveness of psychosocial interventions for infertile individuals on sexual dysfunctions. Nevertheless, the effectiveness of psychosocial interventions of the general emotional implications of infertility present promising results for their use for sexual dysfunctions.

Psychoeducation to aid in appreciating the impact depression, anxiety, stress, and marital conflicts may have on the manifestation of ED is imperative for a successful treatment solution. In fact, referral of ED patients to a mental health specialist is recommended by the Canadian, American, and European Urological Associations [69].

Clinical intervention

Depending on the etiology of one's sexual dysfunction, certain medications may be suited to treat the symptomology. For instance, if psychological distress seems to be the main contributor to sexual dysfunction, antidepressants may be prescribed to the affected individual. In fact, 9.2% of reproductive-age women report using antidepressants [72].

If the sexual dysfunction is a result of an underlying clinical condition, pharmaceutical or invasive sexual dysfunction treatment may be recommended [73]. For example, phosphodiesterase-5-inhibitors (PDE5I)such as sildenafil, vardenafil, avanafil, and tadalafil may be prescribed to ED patients. Men and women preferred tadalafil for clinical symptoms as well as self-esteem, confidence, and sexual satisfaction [69]. Other medical interventions for ED include vacuum constriction devices, transurethral suppositories (MUSE), and intracavernosal injection therapy (IT). Surgical interventions include penile implants, arterial revascularization, and venous surgery [69]. Unfortunately, the rate of discontinuation of pharmacological treatment for disorders such as ED is very high (30%—80%) most commonly due to comorbid conditions in addition to marital problems, cost, lack of effectiveness, and ED recovery. This high dropout rate validates the need for a combinations approach—psychological, marital, and/or clinical [69].

It is crucial that clinical examinations must focus on addressing the underlying medical conditions. A diagnosis of infertility and associated sexual dysfunction may be the result of a clinical manifestation, thus addressing the clinical manifestation may be efficacious in eliminating psychological and sexual effects. Additionally, removal of medications and/or cessation of alcohol, tobacco, and recreational drugs may be necessary for successful treatment [36].

Prevention of sexual dysfunction in infertile couples

To prevent sexual dysfunction manifestation in infertile couples, it is necessary to address the importance of their sexual relationship and educate them on common sexual problems related to the infertility experience. Additionally, assessing the pros and cons of treatment procedure in terms of sexual consequences is imperative to being honest and open with the couple. In a treatment setting, professionals should give the couple permission to discuss these problems and establish a safe, comfortable environment—normalizing these sexual effects of infertility and minimizing the commonly accompanied guilt and stigma. If necessary, physicians and psychologists should accommodate treatment approaches to religious or culture proscriptions. Further, efforts should be made to emphasize the ways a couple can keep their sexual relationships rewarding, erotic, interesting, and enlivened by, for example, exploring different forms of sexual expression [36].

Conclusion

Summarily, general life stress is a noteworthy source of the manifestation of sexual challenges and changes in intimacy between partners. Furthermore, when additional sources of stress are added, the prospect of developing sexual issues increases. An infertility diagnosis can result in substantial psychological consequences such as anxiety, depression, and general distress in the man, woman, and couple as a unit often contributing to changes in sexuality within a couple. Infertility can have an etiological role in or be a result of sexual dysfunction; nevertheless, the medicalization of an infertility diagnosis can be said to "take the fun out of the process." Coexisting clinical and psychosocial factors of infertility can contribute to sexual challenges. Infertility-related sexual dysfunction can have implications in personal and marital well-being, in addition to sexual health and fertility treatment outcomes, however, the sexual effects of infertility are often neglected. Sexual dysfunction associated with infertility cannot be ignored, and appropriate treatments targeting the biological and psychological issues must be enacted. Depending on the underlying etiology of the sexual challenges and psychological manifestations related to infertility, treatments may include marital intervention, sex therapy, psychosocial intervention, involving group therapy, mindfulness training, and cognitive-behavioral techniques, and pharmacologic interventions. Understanding the effects of infertility-related stress on sexuality is essential to the efficacious treatment of these patients. An emphasis on the couple as a dyadic unit must be made, and an integration of various treatment approaches, including sex, marital, and psychosocial therapy in addition to clinical treatments to target all possible causes and manifestations should be encouraged [3]. In this chapter, the psychosocial and clinical implications of infertility-related stress on the sexuality and intimacy of the man, woman, and couple was discussed. Treatment outcomes related to neglect of these psychological and sexual manifestations were addressed. Additionally, the potential treatment interventions for the individual and couple was outlined.

Key points

- **Stress on sexuality:** Chronic stress can negatively implicate male and female sexual and reproductive potential. In males, chronic stress can affect testosterone production due to interference in the HPG axis as a result of stress hormone release, leading to a decline in sexual desire and libido [2]. In females, excessive stress can have negative effects on menstruation leading to more aberrant or irregular cycles, in addition to an increase in pain or duration of the cycle. Stress may also worsen premenstrual symptoms creating reproductive and sexual difficulties [6].
- **Infertility-related stress:** Infertility is defined as the "failure to establish a clinical pregnancy after 12 months of regular and unprotected sexual intercourse" [12]. Studies have reported that the diagnosis affects approximately 12%–18% of women aged 15–44, and roughly 7% of men [12,14]. Infertility is often accompanied by psychological distress. About 352 women and 274 men receiving infertility treatment were evaluated for depression and anxiety. A total of 56% of the women and 32% of the men reported clinical levels of depressive symptoms. Additionally, 76% of the women and 61% of the men reported clinical levels of anxiety [18]. Only 21% of women and 11.3% of men undergoing infertility treatment reported receiving mental health services [18]. Studies have shown that infertility-related stress is comparable to the stress experienced by cancer, cardiac rehabilitation, and hypertension patients [3]. Additionally, studies have shown that infertility remains the top stressor for affected patients even during the COVID-19 pandemic [26].
- **Infertility—Taking the fun out of the process:** As the psychological and physical burdens of infertility treatment increase, couples often experience sexual challenges. They no longer see sex as an activity of enjoyment, love, romance, and intimacy. Rather, sexual intercourse becomes a scheduled chore around ovulation and the "fertile window," accompanied by feelings of distress, despair, and worry about failure [3,16,27]. Schedules and unspontaneous intercourse can decrease libido in 10% of patients, and ED may occur in 20% of men [3,33]. It is estimated that 10%–60% of couples have sexual problems related to infertility, affecting intimacy, couple sexual function, marital well-being, and sexual satisfaction [51,52].
  - **Clinical factors:** Preexisting clinical factors impacting fertility and sexual function may include vaginismus in women and ED in men. Sexual challenges may also manifest as a result of infertility-related psychological distress, or may be a cause of distress.
  - **Psychological factors:** Frequently, men experiencing infertility develop performance anxiety, sexual avoidance, and even sexual aversion as opposed to enjoyment and satisfaction. Studies assessing the emotional and sexual states of five women with infertility reported high levels of clinical depression, distress, and sexual dysfunction [49].
- **Treatment outcomes—Pregnancy:** Frederiksen et al. [61] evaluated 39 studies assessing the effects of psychological intervention on pregnancy rates and psychological outcome. The results of the study demonstrate statistically significant effects of psychosocial intervention on clinical pregnancy (risk ratio = 2.01; CI 1.48–2.73; $P < .001$) and combined psychological outcomes (Hedges $g = 0.59$; CI 0.38–0.80; $P = .001$). Additionally, meta-regression showed that larger decreases in anxiety were associated with improvement in pregnancy rates [61].
- **Treatment options for infertility-related sexual challenges:** Treatment options for infertility-related stress and sexual challenges include psychosocial intervention, marital intervention, sex therapy, and pharmacologic methods.
  - **Marital intervention:** In a randomized controlled trial of 100 couples with infertility, those who received three couple's therapy sessions consisting of marital counseling had higher sexual and marital satisfaction 3 months later in comparison to the control group who did not receive couples therapy [56,67].
  - **Sex therapy:** Sex therapy for sexual dysfunctions in infertility patients must carefully educate patients to restructure intrusive, negative thoughts relating to infertility and sexual function. Additionally, sex therapists must work to reveal possible underlying psychological issues that could affect their mental and physical health in the future [69].
  - **Psychosocial intervention:** Psychological interventions emphasizing stress management and coping skills have been associated with decreasing some of the most deleterious emotional effects accompanying infertility [63]. Boivin performed a review of some of the psychosocial interventions for infertility, considering the results of 380 studies. The results showed three main themes: psychosocial interventions were most effective in reducing negative affect than changing interpersonal functioning such as marital and social functioning; pregnancy rates were high unaffected by psychosocial interventions; group programs emphasizing education and skills training were substantially more effective than counseling interventions emphasizing emotional expression, thoughts, and feeling related to infertility; finally, the study revealed

that men and women equally benefitted from psychosocial interventions [70]. Other components of psychosocial intervention may include cognitive-behavioral therapies and mindfulness trainings.
- **Clinical intervention:** Depending on the etiology of one's sexual dysfunction, certain medications may be suited to treat the symptomology. For instance, if psychological distress seems to be the main contributor to sexual dysfunction, antidepressants may be prescribed to the affected individual. If the sexual dysfunction is a result of an underlying clinical condition, pharmaceutical or invasive sexual dysfunction treatment may be recommended [73]. PDE5Is such as sildenafil, vardenafil, avanafil, and tadalafil may be prescribed to ED patients, and medications treating vaginismus or other clinical manifestations in the female partner may be administered.
- **Prevention:** To prevent sexual dysfunction manifestation in infertile couples, it is necessary to address the importance of their sexual relationship and educate them on common sexual problems related to the infertility experience.

References

[1] Yaribeygi H, Panahi Y, Sahraei H, Johnston TP, Sahebkar A. The impact of stress on body function: a review. EXCLI J 2017;16:1057—72. Available from: https://doi.org/10.17179/EXCLI2017-480.

[2] Hamilton LD, Meston CM. Chronic stress and sexual function in women. J Sex Med 2013;10(10):2443—54. Available from: https://doi.org/10.1111/jsm.12249.

[3] Grill E, Khavari R, Zurawin J, Flores Gonzales JR, Pastuszak AW. Infertility and sexual dysfunction (SD) in the couple. In: Lipshultz LI, Pastuszak AW, Goldstein A, Giraldi A, Perelman MA, editors. Management of sexual dysfunction in men and women: an interdisciplinary approach. New York: Springer; 2016.

[4] Rooney KL, Domar AD. The relationship between stress and infertility. Dialogues Clin Neurosci 2018;20(1):41—7.

[5] McCabe MP, Sharlip ID, Lewis R, et al. Incidence and prevalence of sexual dysfunction in women and men: a consensus statement from the Fourth International Consultation on Sexual Medicine 2015. J Sex Med 2016;13(2):144—52. Available from: https://doi.org/10.1016/j.jsxm.2015.12.034.

[6] American Psychological Association. Stress effects on the body. Published online 2020. https://www.apa.org/helpcenter/stress/effects-male-reproductive.

[7] Barlow DH. Causes of sexual dysfunction: the role of anxiety and cognitive interference. J Consult Clin Psychol 1986;54(2):140—8. Available from: https://doi.org/10.1037/0022-006X.54.2.140.

[8] Yoon H, Chung WS, Park YY, Cho IH. Effects of stress on female rat sexual function. Int J Impot Res 2005;17(1):33—8. Available from: https://doi.org/10.1038/sj.ijir.3901223.

[9] Bodenmann G, Atkins DC, Schär M, Poffet V. The association between daily stress and sexual activity. J Fam Psychol 2010;24(3):271—9. Available from: https://doi.org/10.1037/a0019365.

[10] Jiann B, Su C, Tsai J. Is female sexual function related to the male partners' erectile function? J Sex Med 2013;10(2):420—9. Available from: https://doi.org/10.1111/j.1743-6109.2012.03007.x.

[11] Laumann EO, Paik A, Rosen RC. Sexual dysfunction in the United States: prevalence and predictors. JAMA 1999;281(6):537. Available from: https://doi.org/10.1001/jama.281.6.537.

[12] Vander Borght M, Wyns C. Fertility and infertility: definition and epidemiology. Clin Biochem 2018;62:2—10. Available from: https://doi.org/10.1016/j.clinbiochem.2018.03.012.

[13] Domar AD, Zuttermeister PC, Friedman R. The psychological impact of infertility: a comparison with patients with other medical conditions. J Psychosom Obstet Gynaecol 1993;14(Suppl):45—52.

[14] Lotti F, Maggi M. Ultrasound of the male genital tract in relation to male reproductive health. Hum Reprod Update 2015;21(1):56—83. Available from: https://doi.org/10.1093/humupd/dmu042.

[15] Starc A. Infertility and sexual dysfunctions: a systematic literature review. Acta Clin Croat 2019;58(3):508—15. Available from: https://doi.org/10.20471/acc.2019.58.03.15.

[16] Grill E, Schattman GL. Female sexual dysfunction and infertility. In: Lipshultz LI, Pastuszak AW, Goldstein AT, Giraldi A, Perelman MA, editors. Management of sexual dysfunction in men and women. New York: Springer; 2016. p. 337—42. Available from: http://doi.org/10.1007/978-1-4939-3100-2_29.

[17] Ramezanzadeh F, Aghssa MM, Abedinia N, et al. A survey of relationship between anxiety, depression and duration of infertility. BMC Womens Health 2004;4(1):9. Available from: https://doi.org/10.1186/1472-6874-4-9.

[18] Pasch LA, Holley SR, Bleil ME, Shehab D, Katz PP, Adler NE. Addressing the needs of fertility treatment patients and their partners: are they informed of and do they receive mental health services? Fertil Steril 2016;106(1):209—215.e2. Available from: https://doi.org/10.1016/j.fertnstert.2016.03.006.

[19] Sejbaek CS, Hageman I, Pinborg A, Hougaard CO, Schmidt L. Incidence of depression and influence of depression on the number of treatment cycles and births in a national cohort of 42,880 women treated with ART. Hum Reprod 2013;28(4):1100—9. Available from: https://doi.org/10.1093/humrep/des442.

[20] Lund R, Sejbaek CS, Christensen U, Schmidt L. The impact of social relations on the incidence of severe depressive symptoms among infertile women and men. Hum Reprod 2009;24(11):2810—20. Available from: https://doi.org/10.1093/humrep/dep257.

[21] Khan AR, Iqbal N, Afzal A. Impact of infertility on mental health of women. Int J Indian Psychol 2019;7(1):804—9. Available from: https://doi.org/10.25215/0701.089.

References

[22] Maroufizadeh S, Karimi E, Vesali S, Omani, Samani R. Anxiety and depression after failure of assisted reproductive treatment among patients experiencing infertility. Int J Gynecol Obstet 2015;130(3):253—6. Available from: https://doi.org/10.1016/j.ijgo.2015.03.044.

[23] Bakhtiyar K, Beiranvand R, Ardalan A, et al. An investigation of the effects of infertility on Women's quality of life: a case-control study. BMC Womens Health 2019;19(1):114. Available from: https://doi.org/10.1186/s12905-019-0805-3.

[24] Shreffler K, Gallus K, Peterson B, Greil AL. Couples and infertility. 1st ed. The handbook of systemic family therapy, 3. New York: John Wiley & Sons Ltd; 2020. p. 385—405.

[25] Freeman EW, Boxer AS, Rickels K, Tureck R, Mastroianni L. Psychological evaluation and support in a program of in vitro fertilization and embryo transfer**Supported in part from the Mudd Expense Fund. Fertil Steril 1985;43(1):48—53. Available from: https://doi.org/10.1016/S0015-0282(16)48316-0.

[26] Vaughan DA, Shah JS, Penzias AS, Domar AD, Toth TL. Infertility remains a top stressor despite the COVID-19 pandemic. Reprod Biomed Online 2020;41(3):425—7. Available from: https://doi.org/10.1016/j.rbmo.2020.05.015.

[27] Luk BHK, Loke AY. Sexual satisfaction, intimacy and relationship of couples undergoing infertility treatment. J Reprod Infant Psychol 2019;37(2):108—22. Available from: https://doi.org/10.1080/02646838.2018.1529407.

[28] Elstein M. Effect of infertility on psychosexual function. BMJ 1975;3(5978):296—9. Available from: https://doi.org/10.1136/bmj.3.5978.296.

[29] Elliott S. The relationship between fertility issues and sexual problems in men. Can J Hum Sex 1998;7(3):295—303.

[30] Atmaca M. Selective serotonin reuptake inhibitor-induced sexual dysfunction: current management perspectives. Neuropsychiatr Dis Treat 2020;16:1043—51.

[31] Gabr AA, Omran EF, Abdallah AA, et al. Prevalence of sexual dysfunction in infertile vs fertile couples. Eur J Obstet Gynecol Reprod Biol 2017;217:38—43. Available from: https://doi.org/10.1016/j.ejogrb.2017.08.025.

[32] Kizilay F, Sahin M, Altay B. Do sperm parameters and infertility affect sexuality of couples? Andrologia 2018;50(2):e12879. Available from: https://doi.org/10.1111/and.12879.

[33] Sigg C. [Sexuality and sterility]. Ther Umsch Rev Ther 1994;51(2):115—19.

[34] Oskay UY, Beji NK, Serdaroglu H. The issue of infertility and sexual function in Turkish women. Sex Disabil 2010;28(2):71—9. Available from: https://doi.org/10.1007/s11195-010-9158-4.

[35] Ozkan B, Orhan E, Aktas N, Coskuner ER. Depression and sexual dysfunction in Turkish men diagnosed with infertility. Urology 2015;85(6):1389—93. Available from: https://doi.org/10.1016/j.urology.2015.03.005.

[36] Grill EA, Perelman MA. The role of sex therapy for male infertility. In: Goldstein M, Schlegel PN, editors. Surgical and medical management of male infertility. Cambridge: Cambridge University Press; 2013. p. 2014—8.

[37] Moro M, Rossi R, Borioni S, Pala A, Simonelli C. T05-O-14 sexual desire in infertile patients. Sexologies 2008;17(1):S8V6. Available from: https://doi.org/10.1016/S1158-1360(08)72750-6.

[38] Nelson CJ, Shindel AW, Naughton CK, Ohebshalom M, Mulhall JP. Prevalence and predictors of sexual problems, relationship stress, and depression in female partners of infertile couples. J Sex Med 2008;5(8):1907—14. Available from: https://doi.org/10.1111/j.1743-6109.2008.00880.x.

[39] Tayebi N, Mojtaba S, Ardakani Y. Incidence and prevalence of the sexual dysfunctions in infertile women. Eur J Gen Med 2009;6(2):74—7. Available from: https://doi.org/10.29333/ejgm/82644.

[40] Achour R, Koch M, Zgueb Y, Ouali U, Rim BH. Vaginismus and pregnancy: epidemiological profile and management difficulties. Psychol Res Behav Manag 2019;12:137—43. Available from: https://doi.org/10.2147/PRBM.S186950.

[41] Bakhtiari A, Basirat Z, Aghajani, Mir M-R. Sexual dysfunction in men seeking infertility treatment: the prevalence and associations. Casp J Reprod Med 2015;1(3):2—6.

[42] Czyżkowska A, Awruk K, Janowski K. Sexual satisfaction and sexual reactivity in infertile women: the contribution of the dyadic functioning and clinical variables. Int J Fertil Steril 2016;9(4):465—76. Available from: https://doi.org/10.22074/ijfs.2015.4604.

[43] Alihocagil Emec Z, Ejder Apay S, Ozorhan EY. Determination and comparison of sexual dysfunctions of women with and without infertility problems. Sex Disabil 2017;35(1):59—72. Available from: https://doi.org/10.1007/s11195-016-9471-7.

[44] Jamali S, Rasekh J, Javadpour S. Sexual function in fertile and infertile women referring to the Jahrom Infertility in 2011. Jundishapur J Chronic Dis Care 2014;3(1):11—20.

[45] Tanha FD, Mohseni M, Ghajarzadeh M. Sexual function in women with primary and secondary infertility in comparison with controls. Int J Impot Res 2014;26(4):132—4. Available from: https://doi.org/10.1038/ijir.2013.51.

[46] Basirat Z, Faramarzi M, Esmaelzadeh S, Abedi Firoozjai S, Mahouti T, Geraili Z. Stress, depression, sexual function, and alexithymia in infertile females with and without polycystic ovary syndrome: a case-control study. Int J Fertil Steril 2019;13(3):203—8. Available from: https://doi.org/10.22074/ijfs.2019.5703.

[47] Kucur Suna K, Ilay G, Aysenur A, et al. Effects of infertility etiology and depression on female sexual function. J Sex Marital Ther 2016;42(1):27—35. Available from: https://doi.org/10.1080/0092623X.2015.1010673.

[48] Zayed A, Adel, El-Hadidy M. Sexual satisfaction and self-esteem in women with primary infertility. Middle East Fertil Soc J 2020;25(1):1—5. Available from: https://doi.org/10.1186/s43043-020-00024-5.

[49] Carter J, Applegarth L, Josephs L, Grill E, Baser R, Rosenwaks Z. A cross-sectional cohort study of infertile women awaiting oocyte donation: the emotional, sexual, and quality-of-life impact. Fertil Steril 2011;95(2):711—16. Available from: https://doi.org/10.1016/j.fertnstert.2010.10.004.

[50] Pakpour AH, Yekaninejad MS, Zeidi IM, Burri A. Prevalence and risk factors of the female sexual dysfunction in a sample of infertile Iranian women. Arch Gynecol Obstet 2012;286(6):1589—96. Available from: https://doi.org/10.1007/s00404-012-2489-x.

[51] Wischmann TH. Sexual disorders in infertile couples. J Sex Med 2010;7(5):1868—76. Available from: https://doi.org/10.1111/j.1743-6109.2010.01717.x.

[52] Sexuality in the transition to parenthood. In: Hall KSK, Binik YM, Rosen NO, Byers S, editors. Principles and practice of sex therapy. 6th ed. New York: The Guilford Press; 2020.

[53] Purcell-Lévesque C, Brassard A, Carranza-Mamane B, Péloquin K. Attachment and sexual functioning in women and men seeking fertility treatment. J Psychosom Obstet Gynecol 2019;40(3):202—10. Available from: https://doi.org/10.1080/0167482X.2018.1471462.

[54] Yangin H, Kukulu K, Gulşen S, Aktaş M, Sever B. A survey on the correlation between sexual satisfaction and depressive symptoms during infertility. Health Care Women Int 2016;37(10):1082–95. Available from: https://doi.org/10.1080/07399332.2015.1107067.

[55] Galhardo A, Cunha M, Pinto-Gouveia J. Psychological aspects in couples with infertility. Sexologies 2011;20(4):224–8. Available from: https://doi.org/10.1016/j.sexol.2011.08.005.

[56] Masoumi S, Garousian M, Khani S, Oliaei SR, Shayan A. Comparison of quality of life, sexual satisfaction and marital satisfaction between fertile and infertile couples. Int J Fertil Steril 2016;10(3):290–6.

[57] Pasha H. Marital intimacy and predictive factors among infertile women in Northern Iran. J Clin Diagn Res 2017;11(5):13–17. Available from: https://doi.org/10.7860/JCDR/2017/24972.9935.

[58] Dhont N, van de Wijgert J, Coene G, Gasarabwe A, Temmerman M. "Mama and papa nothing": living with infertility among an urban population in Kigali, Rwanda. Hum Reprod 2011;26(3):623–9. Available from: https://doi.org/10.1093/humrep/deq373.

[59] Rooney K, Domar AD. Emotional and social aspects of infertility treatment. In: Dubey AK, editor. Infertility: Management and Treatment. New Delhi, India: Jaypee Brothers Medical Publishers; 2012.

[60] Klonoff-Cohen H, Chu E, Natarajan L, Sieber W. A prospective study of stress among women undergoing in vitro fertilization or gamete intrafallopian transfer. Fertil Steril 2001;76(4):675–87. Available from: https://doi.org/10.1016/S0015-0282(01)02008-8.

[61] Frederiksen Y, Farver-Vestergaard I, Skovgard NG, Ingerslev HJ, Zachariae R. Efficacy of psychosocial interventions for psychological and pregnancy outcomes in infertile women and men: a systematic review and meta-analysis. BMJ Open 2015;5(1):e006592. Available from: https://doi.org/10.1136/bmjopen-2014-006592.

[62] Domar AD, Rooney KL, Wiegand B, et al. Impact of a group mind/body intervention on pregnancy rates in IVF patients. Fertil Steril 2011;95(7):2269–73. Available from: https://doi.org/10.1016/j.fertnstert.2011.03.046.

[63] Cousineau TM, Domar AD. Psychological impact of infertility. Best Pract Res Clin Obstet Gynaecol 2007;21(2):293–308. Available from: https://doi.org/10.1016/j.bpobgyn.2006.12.003.

[64] Boivin J, Gameiro S. Evolution of psychology and counseling in infertility. Fertil Steril 2015;104(2):251–9. Available from: https://doi.org/10.1016/j.fertnstert.2015.05.035.

[65] Perelman MA. Sex coaching for physicians: combination treatment for patient and partner. Int J Impot Res 2003;15(S5):S67–74. Available from: https://doi.org/10.1038/sj.ijir.3901075.

[66] Masoumi S, Khani S, Kalhori F, Ebrahimi R, Roshanaei G. Effect of marital relationship enrichment program on marital satisfaction, marital intimacy, and sexual satisfaction on infertile couples. Int J Fertil Steril 2017;11(3):197–204. Available from: https://doi.org/10.22074/ijfs.2017.4885.

[67] Vizneh M, Pakgohar M, Babaei G, Ramezanzadeh F. Effect of counseling on quality of marital relationship of infertile couples: a randomized, controlled trial (RCT) study. Arch Gynecol Obstet 2013;287:583–9.

[68] Latifnejad Roudsari R, Rasoulzadeh, Bidgoli M. The effect of collaborative infertility counseling on marital satisfaction in infertile women undergoing in vitro fertilization: a randomized controlled trial. Nurs Midwifery Stud 2017;6(2):e36723. Available from: https://doi.org/10.5812/nmsjournal.36723.

[69] Kalogeropoulos D, Larouche J. An integrative biopsychosocial approach to the conceptualization and treatment of erectile disorder. In: Hall KSK, Binik YM, editors. Principles and practice of sex therapy. 6th ed. New York: The Guilford Press; 2020.

[70] Boivin J. A review of psychosocial interventions in infertility. Soc Sci Med 2003;57(12):2325–41. Available from: https://doi.org/10.1016/S0277-9536(03)00138-2.

[71] Karakas S, Aslan E. Sexual counseling in women with primary infertility and sexual dysfunction: use of the BETTER model. J Sex Marital Ther 2019;45(1):21–30. Available from: https://doi.org/10.1080/0092623X.2018.1474407.

[72] Evans-Hoeker EA, Eisenberg E, Diamond MP, et al. Major depression, antidepressant use, and male and female fertility. Fertil Steril 2018;109(5):879–87. Available from: https://doi.org/10.1016/j.fertnstert.2018.01.029.

[73] Reddy M, Ms V. Pharmacological advances in the management of sexual dysfunction. Indian J Psychol Med 2017;39(3):219. Available from: https://doi.org/10.4103/0253-7176.207318.

CHAPTER

13

Unintended infertility: labor markets, software workers, and fertility decision-making

Sharmila Rudrappa

Department of Sociology, University of Texas at Austin, Austin, TX, United States

Introduction

Madan is a 45-year-old Indian immigrant software engineer working for a multinational company in Austin, Texas. His wife Menaka, a year older than him, is also a software engineer in the same company. They first met when they were employed in a smaller firm in Bangalore, South India, in the late 1990s. They fell in love and were married by 2001. The following year, Menaka became pregnant but opted for an abortion. Madan said: "we wanted to have a married life together. And plus, we were young, and we wanted to focus on our careers." Menaka found herself pregnant again in 2004, however this turned out to be an ectopic pregnancy that resulted in a miscarriage. Her right fallopian tube was destroyed. In 2006, already married for 5 years and worried that Menaka was now 33 years old, they began trying for a pregnancy in earnest. However, her cycles were uneven, and Madan traveled extensively for work. Madan explained that they had no time for sex. In order to achieve a pregnancy they opted for an intrauterine insemination twice, in 2008 and 2009, both of which failed.

By 2011, Madan had been promoted at work and was asked to move to Texas. In a few months, Menaka followed him. They were both on L-1 visas, which allow a company to transfer employees from its offshore offices, such as in India, into the United States.[1] Madan and Menaka's lives got more complicated. While they were happy to be together, their work pressures coupled with anxieties around their nonpermanent status in the United States exacerbated stress levels in their personal lives. Together they decided that they wanted to obtain permanent residency in the United States before attempting to have a baby. This meant they would need to work harder in order to prove their value as workers so their company would sponsor their permanent residency.

Madan explained that they hardly had the energy for sexual intimacy. "Plus," he added, "when you've been married for that long it's hard to sustain desire. And having sex just to get pregnant felt like a duty rather than fun." They opted for their first in vitro fertilization (IVF) in 2013, which failed. Madan and Menaka were depressed. They loved each other deeply, and had managed their careers so they could be together across India and the United States. They had been married for 12 years, but they felt there was no spark in their marriage. Their marriage was unfulfilling, and sex unproductive in terms of achieving pregnancy, but their work was rewarding. They were achieving success in their professional lives. Their company finally sponsored their permanent residency in 2013, and reluctantly, in 2014, because Menaka was turning 41, they had their second IVF attempt. To their delight, they were successful. Menaka had a difficult pregnancy but gave birth to a healthy boy in October 2014. Madan stated "I have my 4-year-old son. I love being a dad, but I don't want another child.

---

[1] L-1A and L-1B visas are temporary work permits for foreign workers in the United States, which allow companies to make intracompany transfers of employees in managerial positions, or transfer of employees who have specialized knowledge. The L-1 visa is a nonimmigrant category and is valid for a relatively short period of time of between 3 months and 5 years. See https://www.uscis.gov/forms/explore-my-options/l-visas-l-1a-and-l-1b-for-temporary-workers.

I used to give more than 100% to my job. I went that extra mile for work. Not anymore. Now I put in exactly what I need to put in. Nothing more. Nothing less."

At the end of our conversation, when we spoke in October 2018, I asked Madan if he wanted to add anything. "Just this," he said, "we should never have had that first abortion, but that's all in the past now. If I were to do it again, I would do it completely differently. When we were first married, we had no problems with fertility, but we messed it up. My only advice to young couples is don't wait. Have a child as soon as you can. Soon work takes over, and there is so little time for anything else. Don't put it off."

I start this chapter with this vignette to underscore key aspects to my research on infertility among high-wage information technology workers in India. First, the obvious; infertility is not a given, but emerges over the life course of a heterosexual couple. They may start their lives together resisting fertility, but over time they might come to a point in their lives when they seek fertility assistance. Second, workplaces, especially high-wage employment, entails huge amounts of intellectual/emotional/physical labor and significant time commitments from both men and women, which shapes their fertility decisions. And third, it is not just the actions of women, who are almost always blamed for delaying fertility, but those of men too, as they work incredibly hard to build their professional careers, which shapes couples' fertility decision-making.

Defining unintended infertility

There is much research on unintended fertility that is understood as women having unplanned pregnancies [1,2]. Worldwide, an estimated 44% of pregnancies were unintended in 2010−14. In developed regions of the world, unintended pregnancies fell from 64 per 1000 in 1990−94 to 45 per 1000 in 2010−14 among women aged 15−44 years. In the same time interval, in the same age cohort, unintended pregnancy rates fell from 77 to 65 per 1000 women in the developing world [3]. Unintended fertility accounts for more than 40% of all births in the United States [4]. Data from 2015 in India show a rate of 70.1 unintended pregnancies per 1000 women aged 15−49 years [5].

However, there is very little research on *unintended infertility*. By unintended infertility I am referring to individuals and couples who initially do not face fertility challenges, but, over their life course, find themselves in situations that lead them into making decisions that lead to subsequent medically indicated infertility. In this new research I examine how labor markets and fertility decision-making are intertwined.

Research into labor markets and infertility is not new. There is a whole body of research that attributes decreased female fertility to women's labor market participation [6−9]. In the developing world, the negative correlation of fertility with women's formal employment is seen as an unmitigated positive. Women's empowerment is positively associated with education, formal labor market participation, and increased gender rights, which are all seen as having a depressing effect on birth rates [10,11]. While this is a desired outcome in the developing world, the very opposite is true in the developed world which faces falling birth rates. Women's labor force participation, increased age of women who are first-time mothers, and the accompanying decreased female fertility have become a problem in these countries [12,13].

Much of the early infertility literature too, often shaded in moralistic terms, blamed women for the growth of the infertility industry. The reasoning was that if career-minded women did not delay their fertility, there would be no need to exploit younger women for their ova or other infertility services. Moreover, individual women's delayed childbearing was seen as having a public health outcome, because advanced maternal age was associated with common fetal and obstetric complications. Also, children born to older women were more likely to have cerebral palsy, and neurocognitive and psychiatric disorders [14].

Rather than blaming women for focusing on their careers, my aim here is to show that fertility decision-making by both men and women under growing socioeconomic precarity is fraught with risk. New research in the United States focuses on high-wage women who freeze their eggs to optimize career goals without compromising fertility [15,16]. However, large numbers of people in the global south also navigate the competing demands of the workplace and fertility decision-making. Many workers, especially in migrant-sending countries like India, have attempted to balance labor market trends with fertility decision-making for decades in what can be best described as the complex choreography between workplace demands and fertility aspirations. Moreover, while fertility decisions have been singularly attentive to women and their career trajectories, my current investigations lead me to examine how the working lives of *men* affect their female partners' fertility trajectories. The focus, then, is on men and sperm [17−19]. Through examining the reproductive lives of information technology (IT) personnel in Bangalore, I suggest that there is an emergent mode of reproduction intimately tied to labor market pressures and precarious high-wage work which shape intimacy, and ultimately, fertility seeking among men and women.

Meeting with couples undergoing fertility assistance

When I first began research into surrogacy in Bangalore, south India, in 2008−12, I spent a considerable amount of time in infertility clinics. A large percentage of the clientele in these clinics was information technology workers who were trying to get pregnant. Various infertility doctors in Bangalore also remarked on the over-representation of IT workers among their patients. The preponderance of these workers is not a statistical anomaly, because Bangalore is a global site for a plethora of firms engaging in various facets of the IT industry, from research and development, to backroom business processing firms, and call centers. Beginning with Texas Instruments, which established offices in the city in 1985, various other IT firms moved to Bangalore during the 1990s and 2000s, making it India's largest IT hub. Today, the city contributes over 30% of India's IT exports, with India-based global companies such as Infosys, Wipro, and Mindtree housed in the city and the International Tech Park in the satellite town of Whitefield. Many of my interviewees, if they were Bangalore based, lived in and around Whitefield; I write more on that subsequently.

Paralleling the growth of IT firms were medical firms providing assisted reproductive technologies. In 2013, there were just over 20 assisted reproductive technology clinics in Bangalore, including Cambridge Infertility Clinic, Bangalore Assisted Conception Center, Ankur Fertility Clinic, Gunasheela IVF Center, and Fertility Clinic at the Apollo Hospitals. Many of these emerged from the mid-2000s onwards. Close to a decade later, there are many more.

In 1950, Bangalore's population was 745,999; today, 70 years later, it stands close to 12.5 million. In 2001 there were 2985 people per km^2; by 2011 there were 4378 people per square kilometer in the city.[2] Various other Indian cities are now equally important for global IT firms, but Bangalore is irrevocably shaped by its global importance for information technology production and outsourcing. The city contributes more than 87% of the state of Karnataka's economy, and accounts for 98% of the state's software exports.[3] That more IT workers are represented among those who seek fertility assistance in Bangalore is not surprising, because the city has a larger percentage of these workers. Madan and Menaka's struggles with infertility were part of a larger pattern of what many IT workers were going through.

When we first met in 2011, I had been somewhat dismissive when Dr. Viji, an infertility specialist in Bangalore, told me that, "most of the IT couples don't have medically indicated infertility. Instead, they simply don't have time for sex. It's easier for them to come to us to get pregnant than to make time for each other. Ninety percent of them, I tell you, this is what is happening." The problem according to her, then, was not a standard medical diagnosis of infertility; instead, the diagnosis of infertility was interwoven with sexual intimacy. Given the pervasiveness of this "problem" in Bangalore, I thought I could easily recruit interviewees; yet that turned out not to be the case. The problem, in large part, had to do with the fact that I did not want to recruit interviewees through Bangalore's infertility clinics because I felt such a practice was invasive. Instead, I recruited interviewees through Fertility Dost, which is an online support group for women undergoing fertility assistance, I conducted eight in-person, telephone, and Skype interviews with men and women in Austin, TX, and the Indian cities of Jaipur, Kolkota, Gurgaon, Mumbai, and Bangalore. I was also a silent participant on WhatsApp discussions among Fertility Dost members for 11 months (2019−20).

To make up for the low numbers of interviews, I conducted "expert interviews" with infertility specialists and marriage counselors who work with IT couples in Bangalore. As a methodological tool, expert interviews are useful when access to interview subjects is limited. In my case, there were few people who wanted to be as candid as Madan was in admitting to the relative sexlessness of their marriages. Experts, such as marriage counselors and assisted reproductive technology (ART) specialists, meet with a large number of people who are of interest in my study. These experts, then, provide me with generalizations about their clientele, which gives me a sense of broad patterns. My data presented here, based on interviews with eight people using ARTs, four marriage counselors, and four infertility doctors, point to the broad trends among IT workers in Bangalore that shape their fertility decision-making.

I want to note that this is an ongoing study, and the findings presented here are preliminary, but indicative of larger patterns. All of my interviewees indicated that workplace demands compromised marital relationships. In the subsequent sections I analyze the information my interviewees shared with me.

---

[2] https://worldpopulationreview.com/world-cities/bangalore-population.

[3] https://www.karnataka.com/profile/bangalore-main-revenue-generator-karnataka/.

Workplace demands and relationship needs

The eight women and men I interviewed who were undergoing fertility assistance all elaborated on work-related reasons, but all also had medical conditions, that affected fertility, the primary one being polycystic ovarian syndrome (PCOS).[4] Many of the women on the Fertility Dost WhatsApp discussion group also indicated that PCOS was the most common reason for female infertility. PCOS is a hormonal disorder that leads to irregular menstrual cycles and ovarian cysts that make pregnancy challenging. Though the causes of polycystic ovarian syndrome are unknown, there is general agreement that it runs in families. Insulin resistance and type II diabetes, and PCOS are correlated.[5] Stress, poor dietary choices, and lack of exercise exacerbate the symptoms. Nonpharmacological approaches to ameliorating symptoms include reducing stress, weight loss, exercise, and low-carbohydrate diets rich in fruits, vegetables, and whole grains that are effective in lowering insulin levels.

All of these nonpharmacological approaches to tackling PCOS need dedicated time, yet the one thing all of my interlocutors lacked was time. Time, for the individuals undergoing infertiltiy assistance, was absolutely critical. Their lives were ruled by anxieties around time. Infertility as a "disorder" is defined as the inability to achieve pregnancy after 12 months of regular unprotected sex. Time, again, becomes imperative as women chart uneven menustral cycles. And again, time matters for women and men as they wait anxiously for egg maturation after ovarian hyperstimulation, and the anguishing waiting period between embryo transfer and a successful pregnancy. However, time took on a particular resonance for my interviewees. In addition to the notion of time so acutely felt by individuals undergoing fertility assistance, my interlocutors said they lacked time to exercise; they lacked time to cook for themselves; and mostly, they lacked time for their relationships. Work left them exhausted, with little time for social or sexual intimacy.

Chitra and Chetan are in their mid-30s and live in Gurgaon and London, separated from one another. Chitra explained that when the couple lived together in Gurgaon, before her husband's transfer, it was normal for her to work 12–13 hours per day. Sometimes she clocked in 15–16-hour workdays to return home around 2:00–3:00 a.m. She also traveled frequently, with 1–2-week trips every month. Chetan also traveled often, but to make matters worse, he had been transferred to London 9 months before our interview. Chitra got her company to send her to their London office so she could be with her husband. In the 4 months they were together they attempted to have unprotected sex four to five times, she said. However, each time Chitra got a urinary tract infection. They therefore tried their first IVF in March 2019, which failed. When we spoke, Chitra had requested a transfer back to Gurgaon where she was gearing up for her second IVF. She had her sister and mother nearby in Delhi for support. Her husband provided long-distance emotional support and sperm from London.

Initiating sexual activity was far more challenging for individuals in arranged marriages, which are prevalent among Indian couples. Tanuja, who lives in Gurgaon, explained that her husband regularly put in 11–12-hour workdays, which was very challenging in the early days of their marriage because theirs "was an arranged marriage and we were just figuring out to be intimate." Because she knew no one in Gurgaon and her husband was always at work, Tanjua found a job with a firm that worked off-site with companies in Singapore. Because Singapore is 2.5 hours ahead in time, Tanuja had to be at work by 6:00 a.m. and returned home by 7:00 p.m. After her husband returned around 10:00 p.m. they ate dinner together at close to 11:00 p.m. every night. She was eventually diagnosed with polycystic ovarian syndrome and used IVF to get pregnant.

Like the two couples I discuss here, my five other interviewees also shared that couple time was a scarce resource. However, not all these individuals were IT workers. One was a journalist in a major newspaper who had male indicated infertility, and another was a woman who worked for a pharmacy company, coordinating clinical trials for the company. Professionals in these highly demanding jobs, like the IT couples I had interviewed, also faced infertility, indicating that, perhaps, demands on time and workplace stress are not isolated to IT workers, but are more widespread.

Based on the interviews, I could see that individuals' time was taken up by what I saw as four work demands. These are:

1. The long hours put into everyday work;
2. The extra effort and time put into work simply to keep their jobs;
3. Long commute times in cities like Bangalore or Gurgaon; and finally,

---

[4] Four of the women had PCOS; two women had endometriosis; one woman had irregular periods, and a ruptured fallopian tube; and one man suffered unexplained male infertility.

[5] Indians have very high rates of type II diabetes.

4. The frequent out-of-town or overseas travel for work.

Time demands of work: Indian IT workers shared that work schedules are far more demanding in Indian cities like Gurgaon, Noida, and Bangalore than in American cities like San Jose, Phoenix, or Austin.[6] The work culture in India is that everyone starts their day late, around 10:00 a.m. and stays at work often past 8:00 p.m. Though they could telecommute from home, the unwritten expectation was that they would show up at the office and clock in long hours. Clocking longer hours did not make these workers more productive according to them, but demonstrated to colleagues that they were reliable, steadfast workers.

Others like Tanuja did not adhere to the Indian work culture (that is, starting the workday at 10:00 a.m.). Instead, they dialed into Sydney, Stockholm, or San Jose. Tanuja's day started when her compatriots in Singapore clocked in, 2.5 hours earlier than her fellow Indian workers. But her day ended at the same time as the Indian workers' workdays, around 7:00 or 8:00 p.m. Many IT workers were like Tanuja; they plugged into schedules set by US Pacific Standard Time, or Singapore Standard Time. The everyday routines of life—of going to sleep, eating regular meals— that are embedded in the time zones of their specific geographic locations are now disembedded, as their workdays are shaped according to time zones halfway across the world. As a result, my interviewees were expected to be on call, especially when working on projects with tight deadlines. Weekends could be spent on the telephone; or, they had to be available during vacations. While some individuals expressed that this was good because work proceeded at a faster pace, being on call regularly also compromised the quality of the time they spent together as a couple. Work-related demands were almost constantly on their minds. They had no "down time."

Job security anxieties: Not only was work more demanding, but the IT workers also felt they had to prove to their companies that they were deeply committed to their workplace. As Madan, whose words I open with, said to me "I used to give more than one hundred percent to my job. I went that extra mile for work." Though he was not told to do so, he felt he needed to show his allegiance to his firm, and a commitment to building his career. In other words, he had to be an entrepreneur who, by investing in himself as a worker, showed his sense of responsibility to his firm. As an L-1 visa holder, he worried that he would lose his job, and along with that, his home in the United States because he would *have* to return to Bangalore. Finally, after his company in Austin, TX, sponsored his permanent residency, he expressed that he "put into work exactly what I need to put in. Nothing more. Nothing less."

Unlike Madan who now has job security, workers in India faced deep precarity, and so they worked long hours. One could imagine that as older workers they had spent more time at the firm and had greater security because they had workplace seniority. Instead, they felt their positions were far more precarious as they aged. They could always be replaced by younger, cheaper workers. They expressed that it would be next to impossible to find employment as older workers who had been laid off. Therefore they put in tremendous amounts of effort simply to show their commitment to their careers, and hold onto their jobs.

Commuting to work: All eight interviewees indicated that one factor that has to be considered in contributing to stress is their commutes to work. One interviewee, a newspaper employee who worked in Gurgaon, said that he spent 3 hours commuting to work every day. He said that he arrived at work exhausted, and when he reached home in the evenings he was enervated. In a city like Bangalore, with intense population densities and poor urban planning and a confounding city design, a drive of 7–10 kms can easily take 45 minutes to an hour. Some of my interviewees, especially the women, preferred not to drive and instead used Uber to commute to work because they found it very stressful to negotiate noisy, disorderly traffic. They also said that they could attend meetings and other work-related matters on the telephone as they commuted to work.

Travel for work: In addition, almost all the individuals I spoke with worked in jobs that required frequent travel within India and abroad. Chitra, for example, traveled for up to 2 weeks for work off-site. Many declared that they enjoyed such travel, but it also meant that they were apart from their partners for significant parts of the month, including during the women's fertility windows. Some couples were separated for much longer, because, like Chetan, spouses were posted overseas.

---

[6] This is from my previous research conducted in the mid-2000s with IT workers whose H-1B visas in the United States had expired, or were downsized, and could no longer be legally employed there. Many had returned from California, Arizona, and Texas to Bangalore, to staff the explosion of IT-related development that changed the city's physical and economic landscape fundamentally. See Rudrappa S. Cybercoolies and techno-braceros: race and commodification of Indian information technology guest workers in the United States. University of San Francisco Law Review 2009; 44(2):353–72.

High-wage couples in IT work—whether both, or one spouse in such employment—seemed to experience time in unusual ways. Their work time stretched into much of the day, and the time they spent with each other shrank. As a result, emotional and physical intimacy was compromised. However, their biological clocks ticked on. The only way out, then, was to use ARTs to meet their fertility aspirations. Charis Thompson [20] uses the term ontological choreography to describe medical, social, emotional, legal, and financial matters that are coordinated to achieve pregnancy in ART clinics. I like the term choreography because it fundamentally describes the coordination and organization of bodies and motion, and different systems—the ART clinic, the IT firm, and the finances—across physical space and time. Achieving pregnancy, when heterosexual couples are coordinating work demands and relationship needs, requires a sequencing of events in time and space in order to be sexually intimate at the right time in order to have a successful pregnancy. Often, my preliminary research indicates that such sequencing is challenging for men and women given the demands of high-wage work. Finding time for each other, it seems, is increasingly challenging for heterosexual couples caught up in global labor markets.

Marriage counselors who work with IT couples in Bangalore

While the eight individuals spoke extensively about the individual challenges they faced in making time for their spouses, the four marriage counselors I met with in Bangalore spoke extensively, but in broad generalizations, about the IT couples they worked with.[7] They all were unsurprised that IT couples tended to be overrepresented among ART users in the city. Almost all the couples they worked with who had problems with marital intimacy, IT couples faced unique challenges. Because work was demanding, and social (class) pressures were intense to earn large paychecks, IT workers were highly stressed, which then affected their libidos, they said. The general anxieties they experienced at work transferred to their marriages.

The second issue that the marriage counselors emphasized was that many IT professionals came from all over India to Bangalore only because of work. As a result, they were unfamiliar with the city, and had no friends because much of the socializing in the city is centered around extended family and childhood friendship networks. Newcomers, then, become socially isolated. IT workers were geographically isolated from the rest of Bangalore also, because they tended to live near or in the satellite town of Whitefield, which is perceived as an IT professional worker enclave. To avoid long commutes, workers prefer to stay close to their workplaces, but this creates its own issues. Because they spent so much time at work, and because they knew no one outside of work, they formed tight friendship bonds with coworkers, and not anyone else. Their social networks in the larger city were very limited. The four marriage counselors I spoke with said that extramarital sexual encounters were rampant among IT workers because they shared far more time with coworkers who felt more real than their spouses at home.

Moreover, all four counselors noted that a larger number of IT men among their clientele were addicted to pornography. They noted that this was in large part because of the rhythm of work in an IT firm. IT workers labored intensely on one aspect of the project and sent it over to other teammates or another team who then worked on different aspects that project. During these down times, the IT protagonists hit a lull period during the workday, and sat idle. It was during these times that they turned to porn on their smart phones. Radha, a marriage counselor in Bangalore who works almost exclusively with IT couples, noted that pornography was far more preferable to some of her clients than sex with real people, including their spouses. Almost all porn users among her clientele were men.

Emergent modes of reproduction

Tracing the human embryo in assisted fertility interventions, Charis Thompson says that the biomedical mode of reproduction is characterized by its own systems of exchange and value, notions of the life course, epistemic norms, hegemonic political forms, security, hierarchies, and definitions of commodities and personhood [20]. She then elucidates that this mode of reproduction does not stand in isolation, but is intimately tied to the economy, notions of science, and identity and kinship. An economic characteristic of capitalist modes of production, explains Charis Thompson, is that workers risked being alienated from their labor; in the biomedical mode of reproduction, individual patients risk being alienated from their bodies and body parts [20]. I use Charis

---

[7] I deliberately selected marriage counselors who worked mostly with IT couples.

Thompson's formulations to visualize new modes of reproduction in the forms of sexual inactivity and concomitant biomedicalization of reproduction that I have witnessed among Indian IT workers.

The IT workers in this preliminary study seem to experience a profound alienation, yet simultaneously encounter new genres of relationships. While the home is experienced as an alienated and isolating space and the spouse as an inscrutable being who has become a stranger, the workplace becomes deeply meaningful as high-wage workers spend increasing amounts of time with coworkers. Social conventions, however, dictate that procreation is a necessary means to attain proper upper-middle class masculinity and femininity; and that such procreation is tolerable only within marriage. Accordingly, couples endure marriages that often seem sexless, and therefore, unconventional (or perhaps the marriage = sex assumption as the norm itself needs to be reexamined). As sexual intimacy with spouses become unmanageable, aspirations to fertility are achieved mainly through medically assisted means.

The second point I want to make is that work is immaterial for IT workers. That is, they are not dealing with tangible products that have volume, weight, and other such characteristics of materiality. Instead, the products of information technology work are intangible; lines of code that manipulate data into web pages and content, app developers, systems analysts, programmers, cloud architects, and network engineers. Caught up in cycles of production of immaterial commodities, might their sexual orientations also be stimulated by the immaterial, that dealing with the materiality of a partner's body and bodily desires is far more alienating than images of extraordinary sexual acts that flicker on their phone screens?

Conclusions

My early research on purely Indian IT workers points to compelling directions which need further exploration. How does one understand their aspirational fertility and heterosexual family-making given the emotional and sexual alienation heterosexual couples in my study feel for each other? Maybe some individuals and couples prefer biomedical modes of reproduction versus achieving fertility through more conventional means, namely sex? What does it mean to have children? What efforts do individuals make in order to reach heteronormative reproductive desires, and what does it mean to be successful in achieving such desires? And finally, how might we theorize IT workers and their spouses as not aberrant asexual or overly sexed beings, but as pioneers in emerging forms of intimacy and family-making?

When I presented these research findings in a workshop organized in Taiwan in summer 2019, I had interesting conversations with my Japanese, Taiwanese, and South Korean colleagues: might the low fertility rates among East Asian couples, especially among highly educated professionals, be attributable to similar processes as I have observed in India? Might similar processes of fertility decision-making be occurring among highly educated couples in the United States and Europe as well, where both partners are embedded in high-wage labor markets that demand substantial time and effort from employees? The purpose of this research is *not* to minimize medically indicated infertility. Instead, I hope to understand the ways by which professionals in high-wage jobs organize their homes and personal lives to accommodate the demands of the globally networked workplace, which can lead to the onset of medically indicated infertility. Rather than blaming individual men and women for focusing solely on careers, my hope is to make interventions toward more humane workspaces that allow for fuller social, family, and intimate lives.

References

[1] Wildsmith E, Guzzo EB, Hayford SR. Repeat unintended, unwanted and seriously mistimed childbearing in the United States. Perspect Sex Reprod Health 2010;42(1):14–22.
[2] Finer LB, Zolna MR. Declines in unintended pregnancy in the United States, 2008–2011. Engl J Med 2016;374:843–52.
[3] Bearak J, Popinchalk A, Alkema L, Sedgh G. Global, regional, and subregional trends in unintended pregnancy and its outcomes from 1990 to 2014: Estimates from a Bayesian hierarchical model. Lancet Glob Health 2018;6(4):e380–9.
[4] Rajan S, Morgan SP, Harris KM, Guilkey D, Hayford S, Guzzo K. Trajectories of unintended fertility. Popul Res Policy Rev 2017;36(6):903–28.
[5] Singh S, Shekhar C, Acharya R, Moore AM, Stillman M, Pradhan MR, et al. The incidence of abortion and unintended pregnancy in India. Lancet Glob Health 2018;6(1):e111–20.
[6] Butz WP, Ward MP. The emergence of countercyclical U.S. fertility. Am Econ Rev 1979;69(3):318–28.
[7] Becker G. A treatise on the family. Cambridge, MA: Harvard University Press; 1981.
[8] Brewster K, Rindfuss RR. Fertility and women's employment in industrialized nations. Annu Rev Sociol 2002;26(1):271–96.

[9] Thevenon O. Increased women's labour force participation in Europe: progress in the work-life balance or polarization of behaviours? Population 2009;64(2):235–72.

[10] Phan L. Measuring women's empowerment at household level using DHS data of four Southeast Asian countries. Soc Indic Res 2016;126(1):359–78.

[11] Upadaya UD, Gison JD, Withers M, Lewis S, Ciaraldi EJ, Fraser A, et al. Women's empowerment and fertility: a review of the literature. Soc Sci Med 2014;111–20 (0).

[12] Billari F, Kohler H-P. Patterns of low and lowest-low fertility in Europe. Popul Stud 2004;58(2):161–76.

[13] Frejka T, Sardon J-P. First birth trends in developed countries: persisting parenthood postponement. Demogr Res 2006;15:147–80.

[14] Balasch J, Gratacós E. Delayed childbearing: effects on fertility and the outcome of pregnancy. Curr Opin Obstet Gynecol 2012;24(3):187–93.

[15] Goold I, Savulescu J. In favour of freezing eggs for non-medical reasons. Bioethics 2009;23(1):47–58.

[16] Mertes H. Does company-sponsored egg freezing promote or confine women's autonomy? J Assist Reprod Genet 2015;32(8):1205–9.

[17] Inhorn M. The New Arab man: emergent masculinities, technologies, and Islam in the Middle East. Princeton (NJ): Princeton University Press; 2012.

[18] Almeling R, Waggoner M. More and less than equal: how men factor in the reproductive equation. Gend Soc 2013;27(6):821–42 2013.

[19] Culley L, Hudson N, Lohan M. Where are all the men? The marginalization of men in social scientific research on infertility. Reprod Biomed Online 2013;27(3):225–35.

[20] Thompson C. Making parents: the ontological choreography of reproductive technologies. Cambridge, MA: The MIT Press; 2007.

CHAPTER

14

Traditional Chinese Medicine, infertility, and sexuality dysfunction

Denise Wiesner

Yo San University of Traditional Chinese Medicine, Los Angeles, CA, United States

Love is of all passions the strongest, for it attacks simultaneously the head, the heart and the senses. Lao Tzu

Chinese Medicine has been around for over 3000 years with its basis coming from thousands of documents written between 500 BCE and the 1930s. Included in these texts are information about Taoist philosophy, for example; herbal medicine, the philosophy of Chinese Medicine based on Taoist thinking, and the approach to treating diseases. As Chinese Medicine was disseminated to other countries there also became differences in approach. Today, there exists Korean style acupuncture, Japanese style acupuncture, ear microsystem acupuncture, traditional acupuncture, classical five-element style, and Traditional Chinese Medicine (TCM). TCM is a standardization of a long history of information in an effective model that is primarily taught in Europe and the West. There are, however, scholars of classical Chinese Medicine who seek to educate that TCM is a diluted form of the medicine. Nonetheless, this chapter will primarily refer to TCM and it's principles.

To understand the rich history of Chinese Medicine and its views on sexuality and fertility would be a scholarly endeavor so I will leave it to the translators of the classics. For our purpose in this chapter, I hope to impart a basic understanding of the principles of TCM and how it is used in modern times so we can integrate this knowledge into a Western framework. The World Health Organization's (WHO) "…latest version, ICD-11, is the first to include a chapter on TCM—part of a warming to the practice under former director-general Margaret Chan, who led the WHO from 2006 to 2017." [1] There is amazing and practical information on TCM that could help Western medicine practitioners form a different perspective on standardized care and treatment of fertility and sexual dysfunction. Let's start by looking at concepts in TCM to form a basic understanding of its principles and then apply TCM to gynecology, fertility, and andrology specifically sexual dysfunction and fertility care.

Chinese Medicine uses concepts that are different from Western medicine but correlate to Western medicine diagnosis. To understand this language takes years of study. Ted Kaptchuck in his famous book, *The Web That Has No Weaver* tells us that Chinese Medicine is interested in, "the relationship between X and Y" while Western medicine is asking "what X is causing Y." Both are valid treatment strategies. And the goal of the Chinese Medicine practitioner is to bring the configurations into balance, to restore harmony to the individual [2].

The first important concept to understand that many would call the basis of TCM is that of YIN and YANG as stated in the *Yellow Emperor's Classic of Internal Medicine* (Neijing) which is composed of two books the Ling Shu and the Su Wen. Compiled during the 1st-century CE, the Neijing provides a framework for Chinese Medicine based on Taoist philosophy. It offers practical advice on how-to live-in balance with nature. In a translation by Ilsa Veith, it is stated, "The principle of Yin and Yang is the basis of the entire universe. It is the principle of everything in creation. It brings about the transformation to parenthood; it is the root and source of life and death" [3].

To further elaborate, yin energy is feminine in nature. It is lunar energy containing the qualities of cool, moist, nourishing; and rest, stillness, and receptivity. Yang energy is masculine in nature. It is the sun energy containing the qualities of warm, transformative, generative, active, and initiating. These two energies are trying to achieve balance in nature and in our bodies. When we are dealing with sperm and eggs, we can see yin and yang at play. The eggs (yin in nature) receive the eager sperm (yang in nature) that swim to find the egg in the fallopian tube and life is made.

Chinese Medicine also uses concepts such as dampness, wind, heat, cold, repletion, and vacuity to diagnose and describe patterns. TCM asks if the condition is internal or external, meaning is the imbalance caused by something outside the body such as a pathogen or is the problem an internal one like an imbalance in the microbiome or gut flora? Jill Blakeway, in her book, *Making Babies, a Proven 3-Month Program for Maximum Fertility*, uses different language to describe the Chinese patterns of imbalance. She uses the concepts of tired, dry, stuck, pale, and waterlogged to describe fertility types perhaps to make the concepts that are taught easier for the Western mind to grasp [4]. To fully understand Chinese Medicine and therefore the treatment principles that are used, we must understand TCM diagnosis.

However, it is impossible to enumerate the complexities afforded by a TCM diagnosis because there are many techniques used. Patient profiles are somewhat explained by an eight-parameter pattern diagnosis (yin/yang, hot/cold, internal/external, and vacuity/repletion) but there are other ways to diagnose including the five-element wheel which contains: earth, metal, water, wood, and fire. In this system, all the five elements engender each other such that if there is an imbalance in one it causes an imbalance in another. This idea of cause and effect and a circular pattern is different from a linear model. As it relates to infertility and sexuality, TCM practitioners seek to balance the whole system and look at all areas of a person's life and health. Unlike Western medicine that looks at specific areas of the body with blood tests, ultrasounds, x-rays, and MRIs, the ancient Chinese did not have these tools and so relied on clues the body would give about its status. They looked at the tongue, felt the pulse, looked at the complexion, smelled the patient, and asked questions. However, in the 18th century, male doctors were not allowed to examine female patients and so the women, behind a screen, used jade dolls to point out their ailments [5]. Luckily, that practice is not done today. A modern TCM practitioner looks for patterns and uses all the patient's signs like Sherlock Holmes to come up with a treatment strategy.

To illustrate, an intake at a TCM clinic involves asking about all body systems including respiration, elimination, sleep, diet, and emotions even if someone is only coming in for infertility. Furthermore, practitioners are trained to ask women about the quality and quantity of their menstrual blood as it helps to establish a diagnosis. For example, a woman with a lot of purple painful clots during her menses could be diagnosed with Qi and blood stagnation. We might find that this woman also has a dusky color tongue and a wiry pulse and pain on intercourse. The Western medicine equivalent diagnosis could be endometriosis. In a review of evidence for TCM and sexual dysfunction, the authors say,

> Compared with Western biomedicine, TCM offers a more interdisciplinary and individualized approach to disease and its treatment. This embrace of individual idiosyncrasy in diagnosis and treatment presents a challenge to Western biomedical research norms that rely almost exclusively on quantitative methods that compare large and homogeneous groups with a fixed diagnosis and treatment regimen. [6]

The individualized approach makes TCM hard to study.

For Chinese Medicine practitioners the goal of treatment is about "nourishing life" (yang-sheng) meaning to nurture the body, mind, and spirit in harmony with the natural rhythms of life and thereby foster health. According to Sandra Hill in an article she wrote for Monkey Press, "specific *yang-sheng* texts have been found which date back to the 3rd and 2nd centuries BCE. Some of these texts specify stress, diet, exercise, and sexual practices which are considered to enhance the vitality and possibly even lengthen life" [7]. This is well suited with fertility and sexuality because both people need to nourish their bodies and take care of their three treasures: Jing, Qi, and Shen.

The Three Treasures: Jing, Qi, and Shen

Jing

Jing is the first concept of the three treasures in Chinese Medicine. Jing presides over growth, maturation, and aging in TCM. It is about our genetic inheritance. Prenatal Jing or innate Jing is a fixed amount that we get from our parents like a savings account and that is why it is of the utmost importance to have two healthy people when procreating. Postnatal Jing or acquired Jing is based on our lifestyle. We can think of it as the environment that turns the genes on like epigenetics. Factors such as toxins, emotions, drugs, exercise, psychological state, illness, and certain herbs and supplements influence our epigenetics and therefore our Jing.

Jing also refers to the quality of the sperm and egg says Jane Lyttleton in her book, *Treatment of Infertility with Chinese Medicine* [8]. In Chinese Medicine there are many herbs that are called Jing tonics. They work on the level of the sperm and egg.

To enhance fertility, we must work on the Jing. A crazy lifestyle ages us prematurely and therefore does not create good quality Jing. We all know of people that age faster than others. It's as though they dip into their savings account and withdraw all their money. Some are already born with a deficiency in their Jing. We see this in women who have very small uteruses, women who have primary ovarian insufficiency, or men that age rapidly or have azoospermia from an unknown cause. It is interpretation that correlates the Chinese concept of Jing with the Western concepts I have mentioned before. Practitioners of Chinese Medicine believe they can influence postnatal Jing (aka. quality of sperm and eggs) by helping patients with diet, lifestyle, and giving acupuncture and herbs. In the Su Wen, one of the classic books in the *Yellow Emperor's Classic of Internal Medicine*, Qi Bo, the mythological Chinese doctor, employed by the Yellow Emperor (Huangdi) as his minister explains that, "The people of today … through their lust they exhaust their essence, through their wastefulness they dissipate their true *qi*" [9].

Many of the texts on sexuality for males talk about conserving Jing. "Nothing is more important for the Qi of the man than the Jing of the penis" [10]. As Chinese Medicine students we are taught that men should not ejaculate too much as to not waste their precious Jing. Men can learn techniques to refrain from always ejaculating. Mantak Chia talks about them in his books on Taoist cultivation. He says, "For 8000 years of Chinese history, the sexual Kung Fu Method of retaining the seminal fluid during the act of love remained a deep secret" [11]. It was said that emperors had high demands for sexuality from their wives and concubines and needed to have a way to not exhaust themselves. For the principles of fertility, not ejaculating is not applicable. However, if a man is exhausted after ejaculating, we can use herbal medicine to help his energy and guide him to limit his ejaculations outside of the fertile window. There are specific qi-gong exercises to help men strengthen their sexual energy and will be looked at in the section on male sexual dysfunction. As far as Jing and sexuality goes for women, we do not lose sperm but instead lose blood every month, therefore sex is not limited.

Qi

The second concept to understand is Qi or vital energy. This is an elusive concept for Westerners. It is about our overall energy that we get from digesting and processing foods and the air we breathe. Not only do we need to eat well but we must be able to break the food down. Chinese Medicine talks about this as having good Spleen/Stomach Qi as part of the earth element. However, the energy of the Chinese "Spleen" is not only about digestion but related to an emotional state. The emotion of an out of balanced spleen energy is over worrying and overthinking which can activate the sympathetic nervous system. In Western society, many people suffer from digestion problems; irritable bowel, constipation, colitis, SIBO, and diarrhea to name a few. These issues can wreak havoc on the body and lead to low energy. How does this affect fertility and sexuality? Inflammation is not good for fertility and bad digestive symptoms such as abdominal pain and bloating are not conducive to love making. If women and men do not feel good in their bodies, they might not desire to have sex.

According to a cross-sectional design study of 151 Dutch heterosexual couples that completed an online survey measuring body image, sexual satisfaction, and perceived relationship quality, "within individuals, a more positive body image was linked to higher perceived romantic relationship quality through greater sexual satisfaction. No gender differences were found" [12].

How does Chinese Medicine help a patient feel good in their body and have more vital energy? We start at the center. We make sure that digestion is strong. According to Li Dong-Yuan's *Treatise on the Spleen and Stomach: A Translation of the Pi Wei Lun* it is said that the spleen and stomach give rise to original Qi. He also underscores the importance of diet and emotional factors as causes of disease [13].

Having a healthy sex drive while trying to conceive demands healthy vital energy. Individuals that are tired and have inflammatory chronic health conditions might not have a strong libido.

Jenny, a patient of mine, complained she was always exhausted and did not have a sex drive. Her diet consisted of sandwiches and snack foods like potato chips, and candy. She drank a lot of coffee during the day. She also complained of bloating and gas. When I examined her tongue and pulse, I noticed her tongue was flabby with a thick white coat indicating that she had spleen Qi deficiency with dampness. We needed to work on her diet and lifestyle. I palpated her abdomen which felt like play-doh—an indication of Qi deficiency. When we press on the belly of patients, we want to feel good muscle tone. I gave her herbs to help digestion and recommended she eat warming foods like cooked vegetables, salmon, and rice. Cold foods in Chinese Medicine are bad for digestion and for fertility. In 3 months working with me, Jenny had more Qi and an improved sex drive and in three more months she conceived.

Western medicine treatments like hormone injections can make a woman feel bloated, fat, and unattractive. When we approach patients, we evaluate the quality of their Qi. Do they have enough to nourish a fetus? Do they have enough Qi to make a baby?

Do you know women and men that are always tired? Maybe they do not nourish themselves well. TCM believes that if you have little energy you will have a hard time making blood and blood is important for women because it is what nourishes a fetus (more on that later).

Shen

The third of the three treasures is Shen or translated as spirit, god, and consciousness. Shen resides in the upper part of the body in a person's heart. It is the spark of life that inhabits one's eyes. This is our true essence. When we love it is with our heart. It is the infinite and invisible energy of love that brings couples together and it is what consciously creates a child. For true intimacy couples can practice eye gazing because it helps them to connect. David Schnarch, author of *Passionate Marriage*, recommends couples eye gaze when making love [14]. Results of a study that looked at a functional MRI showed that mutual gaze provides a communicative link between humans by sharing the message of "I am attending to you" [15].

Fertility comes with many challenges and it can disconnect couples and lead to sexual dysfunction or can exacerbate a preexisting condition. Helen and Larry came to see me because they had been trying to conceive for a year but were having difficulty. As it turned out, 36-year-old Larry thought he needed to take Viagra to have an erection. Helen would send him texts when she was ovulating that said, "sexy time" to give him a heads up about her fertile window. Larry did not like these texts because they made him feel pressured. In fact, when they both came to see me, sex was not happening during her fertile window. Together we came up with a different solution to let Larry know Helen was ovulating. I suggested putting a calendar in their closet and having Helen mark the days she was ovulating so that Larry could know. I also suggested they have a date night once a week to spend more intimate time together that did not revolve around baby making. They agreed. I saw each of them individually for acupuncture and herbs. Larry was working and getting his master's degree. He was stressed. He told me he had been using Viagra since his twenties. His diagnosis using Chinese Medicine, was stuck Liver Qi and excessive anxiety damaging the Heart and Spleen. He had energy but it was not moving down to his penis. Instead he was in his head worrying about whether he would get an erection for baby-making sex. When they were not trying to conceive, he had no issues. I used acupuncture to settle his nervous system and move energy. I also wrote him a herbal formula to address his circulation. I treated Helen as well. She was worried that she could not get pregnant because she had polycystic ovary syndrome (PCOS). She did get pregnant in our first week together but then had an early miscarriage. Two months later, they fell pregnant again and told me their relationship and sex life had improved.

TCM texts on gynecology, sexuality, and fertility

One of the famous texts, Fu Xing Zhu's Gynecology, was written in the early Qing dynasty and has information on gynecological conditions such as vaginal bleeding, menstrual irregularity, and conditions of pregnancy and postpartum. Not much was written about women's sexual dysfunction in this text albeit a mention of genital pain as it relates to postpartum is included. Sun Simiao also wrote an enormous and comprehensive encyclopedia titled, *Essential Prescriptions for Every Emergency worth a Thousand in Gold (Bei Ji Qian Jin Yao Fang)* around CE 652 which contains three scrolls on gynecology. According to Lorraine Wilcox, an acupuncturist who interprets the classic texts in Chinese Medicine, "The old books did not discuss women's sexuality much. They were interested in her ability to procreate. Beyond that, doctors were not interested in her level of sexual desire or sexual satisfaction. At least, if that concerned them, they did not write about it" [16]. It might have been because Confucianism was the dominant school of ethical and moral thought for more than 2000 years (551~479 BCE). In a study called, "How does traditional Confucian culture influence adolescents' sexual behavior in three Asian cities?" it was stated, that "Confucianism sees sexuality as taboo and forbids discussion about sex," as well as talking about the subordinate role of women as compared to men in a culture that valued the birth of male children [17]. Happily, this is changing culturally in modern Asia. The only sexual reference that I found was by Giovani Maciocia, who said,

> With regard to sexual frustration, Qing dynasty's Chen Jia Yuan wrote very perceptively about some women's emotional longing and loneliness. Among the emotional causes of disease, he distinguishes "worry and pensiveness" from "depression." He basically considers depression, with its ensuing stagnation, due to emotional and sexual frustration and loneliness. [18]

Another ancient Chinese medical text, *The Yellow Emperor's Classic of Internal Medicine (Neijing)* provides a framework for procreation by explaining a 7-year trajectory for women and an 8-year trajectory for men. For example, it is said, every 7 years a woman goes through a change; at age 14 conception is possible and by 49 a woman is all dried up. As for the 8-year cycles for men it is said at age 16, kidney energy is ample and men can procreate, and by age 40 kidney energy begins its decline. We understand the Taoist philosophy of cultivation of Qi when The Yellow Emperor asked his advisor Qi Bo how men in their later years produce offspring. Qi Bo answers, "those who follow the Tao, the Right Way can escape old age and keep their body in perfect condition. Although they are old in years, they are still able to produce offspring" [2]. The Yellow Emperor, who reigned in China from 2697 to 2598 BCE, had three female sexual advisors whose names are The Plain Girl, The Harvest Girl, and The Mystery Girl, and one male doctor. He asks questions on sexuality in The Plain Girl's Classic (Su-Nu Ching) recorded between the 3rd and 4th century BCE. In his book, *The Chinese Sexual Yoga Classics Including Women's Solo Meditation Text*, Douglas Wile translates the Art of the Bedchamber [10].

Diagnosing according to Traditional Chinese Medicine

When TCM doctors look at the signs and symptoms, feel the pulse, look at the tongue, and observe their patients, they can diagnose their issues. I will never forget when one of my colleagues told me a story of a famous Chinese Medicine practitioner who treated a woman with bad eye problems. She had been to many doctors and no one could figure out what was the cause, so she flew out to see him. He asked her many questions, felt her pulses and spent time. In the end, he told her to stop using the mascara she was using. As it turns out, she was using a new brand of mascara and when she stopped using it her eye problems disappeared. Good practitioners of Chinese Medicine use their intuition, look at the person, and see what is going on. It is not just a linear medicine.

TCM practitioners first develop a conceptual framework to understand and diagnose the body/mind/spirit of those trying to become pregnant and those with sexual dysfunction. We look through the lens of the five elements, the eight principles (eight principles are yin/yang, interior/exterior, hot/cold, and excess/deficient), and the eight extraordinary channels, to come up with a treatment plan using acupuncture, herbs, and lifestyle suggestions. Below are two of these paradigms: the five elements and the eight extraordinary channels.

The five elements, fertility, and sexuality

The five elements: earth, metal, water, wood, and fire are a complex system for the diagnosis and treatment in Chinese Medicine. According to Lonnie Jarret, in his book, *The Clinical Practice of Chinese Medicine*, "As an environmentally based paradigm, the five-element system holds the potential for healing nature as it lies broken both within and around us" [19]. This is just a brief look into the organ systems in Chinese Medicine as they relate to fertility and sexuality.

Reproduction and sex drive fall into the energy of the Kidneys (water element) which also contain the 7- and 8-year cycles for both women and men that were mentioned earlier. When kidney energy is robust, individuals age gracefully, have good reproductive energy and a strong will. When the kidney energy is out of balance, symptoms can include low back pain, knee pain, tinnitus, and fear. Fear, in its positive side can help us learn to keep safe. However, women who fear their biological clocks are running out disconnect from their fertile nature. The antidote is to connect with love, compassion, and gratitude and live in the present moment. The kidney energy also has a direct effect on the urogenital function as it controls the opening and closing of the anus and vagina in women and anus and urethral meatus in men. Chinese Medicine also differentiates between people with more cold symptoms such as feeling cold, cold hands and feet (yang deficiency) to people that run hot, have night sweats, or flush easily (yin deficiency). This is a complex pattern diagnosis.

The liver energy (wood element) is about free moving energy in our bodies. Liver also governs the sinews and tendons. When there is disharmony in this element, people can be frustrated and angry. They will frequently sigh. This can also occur when one party is sexually frustrated. The Liver meridian also encircles the genitals and is often treated for sexual problems.

The heart energy (fire element) governs blood. It is also connected to the kidney energy. Some of the signs and symptoms of issues in the heart energies are insomnia, palpitations, and sadness—many of the symptoms that women going through fertility treatments have. There is a special channel that connects the heart energies to the kidney energies called the Chong vessel or Penetrating vessel (see below). If a woman has shock or trauma it can interrupt her ovulation, it also can lead to sexual dysfunction. This is because the heart disconnects from the kidney energy. Heart energies govern the spirit and for a man, if there is sudden shock, the heart energy will also disconnect to the kidney energy and by extension to the penis, possibly leading to impotence.

The spleen energy (earth element) as we saw earlier, has to do with digestion and absorption. It also is how we extract the nutrients from food to make blood. If we eat greasy and processed foods, we will have poor digestion. Blood is also important in Chinese Medicine because it nourishes our bodies and is especially important for women as we lose blood every month. Women and men who do not have enough Qi and blood (they do not have to be anemic) will have a pale complexion and have low energy. It is said that Qi and blood work together. The earth's emotion when out of balance is worrying. For love making to occur, couples must be in the moment. For example, if a man is worried about getting an erection, he usually will not. If the spleen energy is not functioning dampness can occur, which might look like frequent yeast infections, allergies, and a feeling of heaviness—not conducive to baby making.

The lung energy (metal element) is about the breath. Although it is not given that much importance in TCM gynecology, in most all other traditions, the breath is the gateway to calm the body. Lung energy is about letting go, grief and moving the energy down. It is said that sadness and sorrow that is prolonged can scatter the Qi which can lead to a decreased sexual drive. Lungs also govern the Qi of the entire body and are linked with the spleen energy. Breathing helps increase the parasympathetic response: rest and digest. Breathing practices can help increase sexual fire by relaxing the body. When we treat women postmiscarriage, we inevitably treat the lungs.

Using these five elements as a framework is one way to diagnose a condition in TCM. Frequently there is pathology in more than one organ system because when one element is out of balance it can affect the others. This model is circular with no ending and no beginning—just like the circle of life.

The Eight Extraordinary vessels, fertility, and sexuality

When TCM practitioners want to help a patient express their authentic self, they can treat the eight extra energy pathways in the body because they supply all the meridians of the body with life force and blood. Who we are is formed from what we have inherited physically as well as emotionally. If we have experienced past trauma or unresolved emotions, it can be held in the eight extraordinary channels of the body. These vessels are also likened to our epigenetic inheritance. When we work with fertility and sexuality it is important to treat the eight extras. My understanding of them is from Jeffrey Yuen, an 88th generational Taoist priest of the jade purity school. Here is a tiny glimpse into the eight extras. They are complex in character and require a greater depth of understanding then is presented here.

Chong Mai (Penetrating vessel)—This is thought of as the vessel that contains the genetic material passed on from past generations. It is the vessel that connects the heart energy to the reproductive organs. This pathway needs to be cleared of trauma, sorrows, and unprocessed emotions so we do not pass them on to future generations. It is also the vessel that is associated with gynecological problems. Shock and trauma can disrupt a woman's menstrual cycle because it scatters the heart energy making it unavailable to connect to the reproductive organs. We can see this in Western medicine as the disconnection between the hypothalamic/pituitary and ovaries.

Ren channel (Conception vessel)—As its name implies, this vessel connects to all aspects of a woman's natural cycle including fertility, conception, pregnancy, labor, birth, and menopause. This vessel asks the question, who am I and how was I nurtured by my primary caretaker? It's about self-love. Located from the middle of the perineum (Ren 1) all the way up the front center of the body, this channel's acupuncture points are most always treated for sexual or gynecological conditions.

Du channel (Governing vessel)—It is called the vessel of individuality and presides over the yang aspect of the body (the spine) and the process of becoming self-aware or self-actualized. When there is disruption in this vessel, women and men with this pathology might have a difficult time going forward with their life when it comes to fertility. The lack of motivation can also exist in a pattern of coldness and lack of libido.

Dai channel (Belt vessel)—This channel is wrapped around the torso like a belt and is where trauma can be stored if it is not released. Dai imbalances could be represented by gynecological and infertility conditions associated with damp conditions like too much vaginal discharge and pain that wraps around from back to front. People with issues in their Dai Mai often carry excess weight around their middle.

Yin Wei and Yang Wei (linking vessels)—Asks the question, what is my life's purpose? When these vessels are in balance, we meet life's challenges with grace. A strong Yang Wei protects us from the outside and a strong Yin Wei nourishes us from the inside. Mental emotional problems like depression and anxiety, a common plight of infertility patients, are represented by the Yin Wei Mai. Back, shoulder, and hip pain along the lateral aspect of the body are represented by the Yang Wei Mai.

Yin and Yang Qiao vessels (vessels of one's stance)—Asks the question, am I comfortable in my body? Do I know who I am even in the darkest aspects of myself? When the Yin Qiao is not in balance all we want is to close out the world and go inside because of feelings of inadequacy, common when women and men have fertility challenges. Women who have genital pain and fibroids because of past trauma can have an imbalance in the Yin Qiao Mai. The Yang Qiao is about how we hold tension in our bodies that can result in pain in the body, headaches, agitation, and insomnia. This is equated with the frenetic journey to do repeated western fertility attempts without taking a break.

The eight extra vessels are complex channels used for complex problems. The Chinese Medicine practitioner will go to these after attempts have been made using the 12 regular channels and the patient has not improved.

Modalities used in Traditional Chinese Medicine

Acupuncture

Acupuncture is the use of stainless-steel needles inserted into over 365 acupuncture points on the body. These points are on special energy pathways called meridians and there are 12 main meridian channels. Their names are: Liver (Liv), Spleen (Sp), Stomach (St), Gallbladder (GB), Small Intestine (SI), Pericardium (P), Triple Burner (SJ), Heart (HT), Kidney (Kid), Large Intestine (LI), Lung (Lu), and Bladder (UB). There are also eight extraordinary meridians aforementioned. Special microsystems exist on the ear, hand, and scalp. In a review study, it was said, "acupuncture needles, either manipulated manually or stimulated using a low current and frequency, have been documented to be a neurophysiological basis for modulating the activity of peripheral and central neural pathways" [20]. Research also exists on acupuncture and its effects on fertility. It is well known that it is challenging to study acupuncture in randomized control trials. For example, in a review study on acupuncture and fertility the researchers stated, "Acupuncture has the highest level of evidence for its use in improving male and female fertility outcomes although this evidence is inconclusive" [21]. One reason is because of the use of a sham acupuncture needle. Any pushing of an acupuncture point will affect an outcome on a body. Furthermore, protocols in many studies are different and sample sizes are usually small. That does not mean, however, that acupuncture for fertility and sexual pain is not effective. More research needs to be done.

It is important to remember that TCM uses a whole systems approach. We diagnose based on an individual's signs and symptoms and treat not only with acupuncture but also with herbs, diet, and lifestyle. Standardized acupuncture point and herbal protocols, while used in randomized controlled trial (RCT) studies, are not the way TCM doctors practice. In a metaanalysis looking at acupuncture and its effects on infertile women that were not using assisted reproductive techniques, the researchers concluded, "Acupuncture and its combined therapy may be effective for treating female infertility. However, the included studies are not robust enough to draw a firm conclusion due to the not robustly sampled quality of the included studies. Future high-quality RCTs are needed to confirm our findings" [22].

Electroacupuncture

Electroacupuncture (EA), where electrodes are attached to needles, is used for pain but also for fertility. In a study it was shown that, "EA can enhance oocyte maturation and fertilization rate, and reduce the granulosa-cell apoptosis index in an IVF program" [23].

Cupping

Cups are put on the skin to create suction and help with pain, inflammation, and blood flow. There are many theories of how cupping works. Immunomodulation theory suggests that "changing the microenvironment by skin stimulation could transform into biological signals and activate the neuroendocrine immune system" [24].

Moxabustion

Moxabustion is the burning of mugwort herb over acupuncture points. It is used in Chinese Medicine to warm areas of the body with the intention of stimulating circulation and lymphatic flow. It is used to turn breech babies and, in some studies has been found to help with fertility [25].

Herbal medicine

In the TCM gynecology clinics in China, herbal medicine is the preferred treatment modality. Anywhere from 6 to 12 single herbs are blended together to make herbal formulas that are used orally as well as vaginally and rectally. Each herb has a taste, temperature, and organ system that it goes to. Herbs are used to treat many conditions based on Chinese diagnosis. Herbal medicine for conditions such as PCOS, endometriosis, low sex drive, dysmenorrhea, impotence, and low egg quality, are now being researched. According to a study, "As well as with IVF, Chinese Integrative Medicine is believed to improve outcomes when used in relation to unexplained infertility, early ovarian failure, PCOS, and amenorrhoea ... ovarian problems or where the patient wants to conceive quickly, such as with advancing age (35 years plus) or for other personal reasons" [26].

In a review study the researchers said, "In modern China, TCM is used to treat infertility in both men and women. Although no individual Chinese herb is considered especially useful for promoting fertility, more than 100 different herbs, usually given in complex formulas comprising of 12 or more ingredients, are used in the treatment of infertility with the purpose of correcting a functional or organic problem that caused infertility" [27].

We will explore herbs used to treat infertility and sexual disorders in this chapter. I have presented the names of the herbs in Pin Yin which is the official romanization system for Standard Chinese in mainland China. See addendum for Latin names.

Eastern medicine: an alternative perspective on sexual dysfunction and fertility care

By the time a patient goes into a Western clinic for fertility treatments my experience is that many Western doctors that I have interviewed do not ask about sexual problems. One of the reproductive medicine doctors I interviewed told me that a couple came to see him for fertility treatments because they never had intercourse.

What is sexual dysfunction as it pertains to fertility? Persistent, recurrent difficulty with sexual response, arousal, desire, orgasm, or pain. Causes include stress, fatigue, medication/drug use, environment, trauma, health issues, pain, hormonal issues, and relationship issues.

With all the pressure of trying to conceive on schedule, many patients throw in the towel and just look to Western reproductive medicine for help. Situations like the inability to get an erection when under stress, low sex drive, vaginismus, vulvodynia, and inability to ejaculate limit a couple from trying to conceive naturally. However, many couples carry a great deal of shame around sexuality and often do not share with their doctor the reason for seeking Western medicine. Let's take a look at what they are and how Chinese Medicine treats these conditions.

Sex drive and reproduction in Traditional Chinese Medicine

Sex drive is complex. For a woman there are many factors that dictate her sex drive. In Rosemary Basson's sexual response model that differs from Masters and Johnson linear model, she suggests that female sexual response is more cyclical in nature. Sometimes for women, desire can follow arousal [28] Men, studies show, are more visual than women and the Taoist say are quick to boil whereas women are slow to boil. Issues around sex drive seem to surface when couples are trying to conceive. From mismatched lovers, timing, lack of foreplay to pressure to perform, sex drive can become a complex issue to tackle. I often see diminished sex drive in couples trying to conceive as a response to how mechanical sex has become. In addition, old traumas can also resurface at this time. If that is the case, we can treat the eight extra channels which are energy pathways on the body (see The Eight Extraordinary vessels, fertility and sexuality section). Sometimes it takes relaxing the individual and treating the liver energy that gets stuck or working on calming fear and treating the kidney and heart energies. The sad truth is that women and men do not talk about their libidos. Surveys of women who self-reported low sexual desire and associated distress showed that up to 80% had not mentioned the issue to a health care provider, with at least 50% reporting that discomfort or embarrassment contributed to their unwillingness to seek treatment [29]. Sometimes, TCM practitioners are the first to ask about a fertility patient's sex drive.

In Chinese Medicine we look at the whole person to assess sex drive. Following are factors that can contribute to a low libido from a TCM perspective.

1. Too much dampness in the body can decrease libido. This can be caused from a diet of greasy, fatty food which can lead to obesity. We know that body image plays a role in sex drive. If trauma is at play, acupuncture points and herbs would be chosen that get rid of dampness. Patients also need counseling to cut out alcohol, refined foods, sugar, and strengthen their digestive function (Spleen Qi).
2. Low kidney energy is the first organ system we look at. As mentioned earlier, kidney energy governs reproduction and sexuality. We must have good kidney energy to make a baby and we can boost the kidney energy through herbs, acupuncture, and lifestyle.
3. Heart and Kidney not communicating can also wreak havoc on sex drive. Although not much is written about this as it pertains to Chinese Medicine, TCM practitioners can help patients by instructing one partner to attune to their partner's energy first by connecting the heart energy and then moving it down to the loins. In the book, *Taoist Sexual Meditation*, there is a sexual qi-gong practice for women to help link a man's heart center to his eyes. It is about hovering the woman's hands over the heart space of her partner and moving the hands toward his eyes while the man is laying down. When stimulating a woman's sexual energy, a partner can try to move energy downward to the lower legs with the same hovering hands [30].
4. The diagnosis of Liver Qi stagnation or bottled up energy does not lead to a healthy sex drive. When we repress our emotions both good and bad it leads to stagnation. Some people feel they do not deserve pleasure. Others, because of trauma, block pleasure, and do not feel anything. Wherever there is stuck energy, we must treat the liver, especially because the channel encircles the genitals.

Acupuncture can be beneficial in helping libido. In a very small study, *Acupuncture in Premenopausal Women With Hypoactive Sexual Desire Disorder: A Prospective Cohort Pilot Study*, it was found that 5 weeks of acupuncture therapy was associated with significant improvements in sexual function, particularly desire. This supports a role for acupuncture as a therapeutic option for women with low desire and for more studies to be done [31]. In another study on *Efficacy of Acupuncture Treatment of Sexual Dysfunction Secondary to Antidepressants Design*, participants received a TCM assessment and followed an acupuncture protocol for 12 consecutive weeks. The acupuncture points used were Kidney 3, Governing Vessel 4, Urinary Bladder 23, with Heart 7, and Pericardium 6. Participants also completed a questionnaire package on a weekly basis. The results were, "Significant improvement among male participants was noted in all areas of sexual functioning, as well as in both anxiety and depressive symptoms. Female participants reported a significant improvement in libido and lubrication and a nonsignificant trend toward improvement in several other areas of function" [32].

Herbal medicine is used frequently with low sex drive. Herbs are mixed together based on a patient's pattern of imbalance. Rarely are the herbs given individually. Following is a list of five of the individual herbs that have been researched for libido although there are many others.

1. Horny Goat Weed (Epimedium yin yang huo)—This herb increases libido, improves erectile dysfunction (ED), and regulates hormones in both sexes. It contains the flavonoid: icariin. Dosage is 500 mg 2—3 times a day. Not good for people with low blood pressure.
2. *Cynomorium songaricum (Suo yang)*—In a study, it was found that there were dose-dependent effects on sexual function. Promotes male fertility by strengthening the spermatogenesis in the golden hamsters [33]. This herb can adjust hypothalamic-pituitary-gonadal axis by increasing E2 and make related biomedical indexes and hormone receptors normal. It can relieve perimenopausal syndrome and perimenopausal syndrome with depression.
3. Cordyceps (Dong Chong Xia Cao) enhances cellular energy, normalizes immune function, enhances athletic performance, restores normal energy stores, and increases sexual function. It is good for sperm health and restores libido in men and women. Dosage is about 500—1000 mg once a day. Both serum testosterone and 17-estradiol

were increased in a study published in the *American Journal of Chinese Medicine* in rats after 5 weeks of taking the herb cordyceps. In human females enhances estradiol production 17-estradiol in biology of reproduction [34].

4. Herba Cistanche (Rou Cong-Rong)—One of the best pharmaceutical gifts of TCM it is said. The chemical constituents: volatile oils, nonvolatile phenylethanoid glycosides, iridoids, lignans, alditols, oligosaccharides, and polysaccharides. Studies show antioxidant, neuroprotection, and antiaging effect. Applied in formulas for chronic renal disease, impotence, female infertility, morbid leucorrhea, profuse metrorrhagia, and senile constipation. It can improve mitochondrial function, is good for increasing sex hormones, and also used for brain function [35].

5. Ashwagandha (*Withania somnifera*): Protects the body and brain from stress-related elevations in cortisol, corrects low testosterone, supports antioxidant levels, boosts the immune system, improves energy levels, and alleviates symptoms of anxiety and depression [36].

Case study: low sex drive and trauma

Alice, a 33-year-old woman came to see me because she had hypothalamic amenorrhea and wanted to conceive. She had a history of sexual abuse and was very sensitive to her surroundings. Alice was an exercise trainer and I educated her about not working out so much and eating a higher calorie and fat diet. She also complained that her sex drive was low but when I asked about it further, she said her husband also had a low sex drive and they barely had intercourse. It turned out he was also molested when he was young. The first task was getting her to ovulate again. I diagnosed her with Kidney and Heart not communicating and imbalance in the Chong, Ren, and Du channels. She had done therapy but was not convinced it did anything. Over 9 months I worked with her giving her herbs and acupuncture. I specifically did EA on points in her lower abdomen and added acupuncture points to stimulate her hypothalamus-pituitary-ovarian axis like Yintang (between the eyebrows) and Du 20 (on the top of the head). I told her to drink goat milk. She finally got her period back. I gave them exercises to do together to build intimacy: microcosmic order breathing (see below) hugging and eye gazing. She told me that they finally had intercourse and 3 months later she conceived.

Microcosmic orbit breathing

Sit in a comfortable position in a chair or on the floor. Touch the tongue to the roof of the mouth, just behind the teeth to activate the channels. Begin to use abdominal breathing, inhaling and exhaling nine times. Breathe gently, so there is no sense of urgency or forcefulness. Feel the energy in the perineum (Ren 1) and engage the **pubococcygeus muscle (PC)** muscle and inhale it up the spine to the top of the head (Du 20). Then exhale down the front of the body down to the genitals gently releasing the PC muscle. The motion is circular. Once you get the hang of it, you can go from nine times to 36, and eventually 72 times, until you experience a sense of warmth in the genitals.

Stress, fertility, sexuality, and Traditional Chinese Medicine

Over the years Western medical doctors have referred me their infertility patients so that I can help them with "stress." We can all agree that Western medicine treatments add strain to the already emotionally loaded journey that individuals and couples go through when they have difficulty conceiving. Stress is a Western concept and Taoism has many effective coping strategies to manage it. As we have seen, the yin/yang theory is a key principle in TCM. We must balance doing (yang) with receiving (yin). I explain to my female fertility patients that women receive the sperm/embryo even if they use Western reproductive medicine. So as much as they want to make it happen it is equally important to for them to let go of control. Another concept in Taoism is called "wuwei." This means do nothing and everything gets done. It's not to say that individuals should not take action but part of the frustration and stress around infertility is the lack of control many individuals and couples feel. The pressure around trying to conceive can also create problems in a couple's intimacy. Taoism, based on the cycles and rhythms of nature, can help couples understand there is a time and place for storms, blossoming, growth, and death. It's the stress of a grain of sand in an oyster that makes a pearl.

When individuals come to my office for treatment it might be the only time in their day (besides sleeping) that they get to unplug. They are literally pinned down and finally can drop into the parasympathetic nervous system. Even acupuncture points in the ear can activate the vagus nerve such as the point "Shen men" located in the ear's triangular fossa.

As practitioners we look to the stress that individuals feel and break it down into TCM patterns. We determine what is the root cause of the stress and how it manifests in a person's body. Some individuals have "heart energy" issues with symptoms such as palpitations and insomnia while others have stuck Liver Qi and experience frustration and anger. Many have multiple patterns. The idea in all treatments is to bring the body/mind/spirit back into balance. We might give individuals meditations or qi-gong exercises to do as homework as well as herbs to calm the nervous system. It's no wonder that the classic formula Xiao Yao Wan translated as free and easy wanderer is coveted by my patients who have anxiety.

Case: stress, infertility, and sexuality

My patient Alexis came to me to help her conceive her first child naturally. She was diagnosed with uterus didelphis and also had two cervixes. No one knew how long it would take her to conceive but she did within 6 months and birthed a healthy baby girl. A few years later they were ready to try again, and within months she conceived. Everything was going along smoothly until with genetic tests it was confirmed that this baby boy had a genetic disorder that would severely affect its quality of life and that Alexis was a carrier for. Then came the agonizing decision about what to do about this baby. She went to many doctors only to find out that this disease would cripple her child and lead to severe pain. They made the decision to terminate, a decision that she never felt good about. For their next child (1 year later), they decided to do in vitro fertilization (IVF) and genetically test the embryos for this genetic mutation. When she came to see me, she had high levels of stress. She was not having any sexual relations with her husband, and the doctor told her she had few follicles.

Alexis decided to take every supplement for fertility in hope that it would improve her body. It did not and in fact, her estrogen dropped to 4 pg/mL. Her fertility doctor called me. When I worked with Alexis I told her to stop all supplements (I rarely say that). I had her listen to guided meditations, come in for acupuncture and try to reconnect to her husband. She had already seen a grief therapist. Within 2 months of following my plan, her estrogen went to 23 pg/mL. The lesson of this story is when the body is in "stress" it is not fertile and TCM can help bring the person back to health.

Male sexual problems and Traditional Chinese Medicine

Erectile dysfunction

ED is a condition in which one is unable to get or keep an erection firm enough for satisfactory sexual intercourse. ED can be a short-term or long-term problem. There are many causes of ED such as cardiovascular disease, high blood pressure, other medical conditions, certain medications, smoking, low testosterone, relationship issues, stress, trauma, and depression (see Chapter 4 for a detailed discussion from a Western medicine perspective).

Diagnosis of erectile dysfunction in Traditional Chinese Medicine

In the book, *The Principles of Chinese Medical Andrology, an integrated Approach to Male Reproductive and Urological Health*, Bob Damone states that the ancestors called ED "Yang wilt" [37]. ED can happen with fertility challenges. The mind overtakes the body and it becomes psychogenic in nature. The diagnosis according to Chinese Medicine is different depending on signs and symptoms. For example, excessive anxiety can damage the Heart or Spleen with signs of over worry and over concern. This also may be due to working too much. I receive many questions from women who want to know how to help their partners who are focused on their professional life and not focused on baby making. If men think that baby making is another job, it can cause inability to perform. Furthermore, the worry about not performing can also lead to ED.

Another TCM diagnosis is depression of Liver Qi which would look more like anger and frustration that is repressed. Men confide in me that they get irritated because their partners only want to have sex during the fertile window.

A third TCM pattern causing ED is fear and fright damaging the Heart and Kidney. This might be due to a traumatic event and can show up in men who have PTSD, including those in the military.

On the physical side, causes of low libido and therefore ED are Kidney essence, Kidney yang, or Kidney yin deficiency. We can see these patterns in older men. The Kidneys are the root of sexuality and the fire of desire needs to be stirred in order for an erection to happen. If there is Kidney yang deficiency a man could be suffering from a chronic condition with symptoms such as coldness, tiredness, and low libido. In a Kidney yin deficiency situation, a man would have more heat signs such as night sweats, constipation, and a parched throat. He may be working long hours with little rest.

ED can also be caused by outside forces like damp heat pouring downward from too much alcohol and greasy food which can lead to obesity. Cold-evil, a product of men who work in damp and cold conditions can also obstruct the Liver channel. I liken this to men who work on fishing boats in the Bering sea. Chronic diseases can also lead to ED as well as physical trauma from surgeries. Blood flow is essential for an erection to transpire. The TCM diagnosis in these situations is phlegm and/or blood stasis in the ancestral sinew (fancy word for penis). A varicocele is an example of blood stasis.

Traditional Chinese Medicine treatment of erectile dysfunction

Chinese Medicine deals with all of these issues differently. We diagnose with patterns and then use herbal medicine, acupuncture, and lifestyle management to treat the condition. From the view of modern medicine, acupuncture treatment can regulate nerve sensitivity and improve the blood supply of peripheral blood vessels, which achieves the efficacy. In a systematic review to assess the effectiveness and safety of acupuncture for ED researchers looked at 22 randomized studies, 14 looked at psychogenic ED, those with a psychological origin instead of a physical one. The researchers found no difference between EA and sham acupuncture. Acupuncture combined with drug therapy was said to have a better cure effect. The review also found that acupuncture combined with herbal medicine had better improvements in ED than acupuncture alone. There was also a high or unclear risk of bias due to insufficient or inadequate reporting of the information. The controls included no treatment, sham acupuncture, herbal medicine, or conventional medicine [38].

Studying acupuncture is fraught with difficulties, but the takeaway is that acupuncture and herbs can be effective in providing care for men with ED. It is especially useful when combined with other treatment modalities such as psychotherapy, and Western medicine or when men do not like to take phophodiesterase-5 (PDE5) inhibitors and want an alternative.

In clinical practice we choose acupuncture points and herbal formulas based on the pattern of diagnosis for individuals. Acupuncture treatment frequency is twice a week for 12 treatments. Some use low-frequency electrostimulation for ED (5 Hz and up to 10 mA). There are many possible herbal and acupuncture point combinations.

Main acupuncture points: Ren 4, Ren 3, Bl 23, BL 32, Sp 6, Kid 3, St 36, Ren 1, and Du 1.

Excessive anxiety damaging the Heart or Spleen (ED). Treatment Principle: supplement Spleen Qi, nourish the heart, calm the spirit and raise the wilted sinew. Acupuncture: P6, Sp 6, Ren 4, St 36, Yintang, Bl 23, Bl 15 Herbal formula: Modified Gui Pi Tang—add shan zha for food stagnation, chai hu, sheng ma for hemorrhoids, add Ba ji tian, and Bu gu zhi.for sp/kid yang deficiency.

Fear fright damaging Heart and Kidney (ED). Treatment Principle: supplement the Kidney, nourish the Heart, calm the spirit and regulate the Chong Mai. Acupuncture points: Ren 4, Ren 3, Bl 23, Bl 32, Sp 6, Kid 3, St 36, Ren 1, Du 1, Herbal Formula: Modified Xuan Zhi Tang and Yuan Zhi Wan adding chai hu, shi chang pu, suan zao ren from Bob Damone's Principles of Chinese Medical Andrology [37].

Treatment of Liver Qi stagnation (ED). Treatment principle: Course the Liver, resolve depression. The Formula is Modified Chai Hu Shu Gan Wan or Yue Ju wan—add he huan pi, shi chang pu, wu gong (two pieces), dan shen, hong hua, chi shao for blood stasis and bai ji tian, rou cong rong and tu si zi, yin yang huo for kidney yang, if too much heat remove sheng ma and add zhi zi and mu dan pi, add yu jin, and Xiang Fu, for Kidney. Acupuncture: Ren 3, Ren 4, Liver 3, LI4, Liver 5, GB 34, Sp 6, Ren 1, Du 1, Kid 3, and St 36.

Decline of the fire of the Kidneys (not enough energy to raise the penis). Points include: Ren 4, Du 4, Ub 23, Kid 3, and add moxa. If Heart and Spleen are involved: Bl 15, Ht 7, and Sp 6. Herbal formulas include: You Gui

Wan or modified Jin Gui Shen Qi Wa add du zhong, wu wei zi, ba ji tian, lu jiao jiao, yin yang huo, xian mao, and he shou wu.

Damp heat pouring downward. In this condition it is best to have a physician diagnose the patient. This condition can be from infections and other outside forces. We can treat them with Chinese Medicine. Acupuncture points: Liver 5, liver 8, Sp 9, St 40, Bl 19, and Bl 28. Herbal formula: Long Dan Xie Gan Tang.

Blood stasis obstruction. Erections are about blood flow. We see this in varicocele, tobacco use, heart disease, and diabetes. Acupuncture points: main ones plus: Sp 6, Bl 17, Sp10, St 37, and St 39. Herbal formula: modified Xue Zhu Yu Tang.

Case Study 1—erectile dysfunction

Eddie was a 42-year-old divorced man with two children. He complained of ED. He would drink alcohol 5–6 days a week and would have more when he was dating. Eddie did not smoke but chewed Nicorette gum for more than 20 years. He took Viagra to achieve an erection. He showed me pictures of him cooking in his house and I noticed how spotless everything was. He was athletic and ran the hills in addition to his physical job where he was always on his feet. When we started talking about his divorce his face turned red and he got agitated. In fact, he told me he "hated" his ex-wife. He had just met someone that he really liked, and she wanted to have a baby. He was anxious about this new relationship. He did not want to have to depend on Viagra. His pulses had a choppy and wiry quality and his tongue was a dusky purple color. We equate these findings with Liver Qi stagnation turning into fire and blood stagnation. I had to first have him stop chewing Nicorette gum then gave him herbs and acupuncture. After a few months, he noticed that he was more relaxed. He started to communicate more with his partner and was using less Viagra and told me his erections had improved.

Case Study 2— erectile dysfunction

A 34-year-old man, Eric, came to see me on the advice of his wife because he had very low sperm count, and they were trying to conceive. He said when he was in his twenties, he felt like he would have a hard time making a baby. He was right. During the process of trying to conceive, his wife also came in for treatment and complained that she had to work hard to get Eric to get an erection and it was exhausting. My advice to both of them was to go away for the weekend, and not "try" to baby make. To help him break the cycle of worrying that he would not be able to get an erection I had him take Viagra and practice the deer exercise (see below). Meanwhile, I put him on a Chinese herbal tonic to nourish the Kidney energy and also to nourish the Heart and Spleen. To their doctor's surprise, his sperm count increased and he was able to provide a sample instead of having a testicular aspiration. They succeeded on their first IVF.

The male deer exercise

Strengthens the males kidney Jing. Chinese doctors use this exercise to help with impotence and premature ejaculation (PE). This is practiced every day in the morning possibly with a morning erection.

1. Sit on a chair or cross legged on a pillow naked below the waste.
2. Take a few deep breaths to get centered and relaxed in your body.
3. Cup the right hand around the testicles gently and rest the right thumb on the base of the shaft of the penis.
4. Massage the area between the navel and pubic bone, called the dan tian clockwise 81 times in a circular motion with the left hand.
5. Repeat numbers 3 and 4 but change hands.
6. Rest hands on lap in the position where the hands are made into fists and the thumb is enclosed.
7. Then, contract the perineum muscles (the pelvic floor) while maintaining regular breathing for about 1 minute if you can. Relax this for another minute. Repeat nine times.

Herbal medicine and erectile dysfunction

Herbs are powerful tools to help support not only fertility but also sexual response. In a review study, the following herbs were shown to have properties that helped with sexual function when tested on laboratory animals. The researchers said,

It was revealed that the mechanisms of Chinese herbs for treating ED might involve changes in nitric oxide synthase (NOS)-NO-cyclic guanosine monophosphate (cGMP) pathway, cyclic adenosine monophosphate (cAMP), testosterone level, transforming growth factor β1 (TGFβ1)/Smad2 pathway, oxidative stress as well as intracellular Ca^{2+} concentration. Some Chinese herbs ameliorate ED through one pathway, others involve several pathways." [39]

This is consistent with the traditional use of the herbs. Some of those included:

1. Rhizoma Ligustici Chuanxiong (Chuan xiong)—an extract Ligustrazine is a vasoactive component shown to relax rabbit cavernosal smooth muscle.
2. Extract of *Ginkgo biloba* was shown to enhance noncontact erection by increasing dopamine contents in some parts of the brain of male rats.
3. *Tribulus* (Ba ji li)—has aphrodisiac properties but mechanism is unknown.
4. *Morinda officinalis* (Ba Ji tian)—improved sexual response in rats, but the mechanism is unknown.
5. Herba *Cistanche* (Rou cong rong)—increases sex hormones in rats.
6. Semen cuscutae (Tu si zi)—restores the testosterone level and androgen receptor expression in the kidney and testicle.
7. Ginseng—Korean red ginseng extracts could enhance erectile function in patients.
8. *Lycium barbarum* (goji berry)—the administration of *L. barbarum* polysaccharides could promote nerve regeneration and erectile function recovery in rats suffering from cavernous nerve injury.
9. Berberine (extract from huang lian) could induce relaxation of corpus cavernosum by enhancing eNOS mRNA expression.
10. Icariin extract from epimedium (yin yang huo) was reported to increase the circulating testosterone level in rats with damaged reproductive systems.

There are other researched formulas like Shugan Yiyang (SGYY) capsules that in a study improved ED of rats by regulating mediators of NOS-cyclic guanosine monophosphate pathway. It also significantly upregulated vascular endothelial growth factor, insulin-like growth factor, protein kinase B, and improved vascular endothelial function thereby improving erectile function of rats [40]. This formula contains herbs like leech, earthworm, and centipede which contain thrombin inhibitors and some traditional Chinese herbs to fortify the yang energy. Mixed in are other herbs. One herb, chai hu, is said to regulate the Liver, improve frustration, and also researched for its functions: immunomodulatory antipyretic hepatoprotective choleretic, autophagy-inducing sedative and analgesic antihyperlipidemic antiviral and anticancer function [41].

There are many other herbal formulas for ED but this is just a snapshot to help you understand how TCM works.

Ejaculatory dysfunction

Besides ED, there are other conditions that affect men who are wishing to make a baby. In a review in Reproductive Medical Biology, researchers said, "Our new classification categorizes men into two groups as follows: (1) men with inability to ejaculate (retrograde ejaculation, anejaculation, intravaginal ejaculatory dysfunction) and (2) men requiring an abnormal time for ejaculation (DE, delayed ejaculation)" [42]. The latter two depending on the cause can be cotreated with TCM because they have an impact on fertility.

According to a study published in the journal, *Translational Andrology and Urology*, there's not "a single pathogenetic pathway ... for sexual disorders generally and that is also true for Delayed Ejaculation (DE) specifically." In fact, a variety of biological, psychosocial, behavioral, and cultural factors contribute to "trigger, reinforce, or worsen the probability of DE occurring." They include high blood pressure, antidepressants [especially selective serotonin reuptake inhibitors (SSRIs)], intimacy issues, and performance anxiety (both common during fertility challenges), ambivalence about having a baby, and anger or resentment toward a partner [43].

As an adjunct treatment to masturbation training, there are also cases of effective treatment with oral administration of yohimbine (a sympathetic α-2 receptor antagonist) 1 hour before sexual intercourse. In some animal models, it is used for delayed ejaculation [44].

A case on intravaginal ejaculatory dysfunction

Les came to see me because his wife wanted him to improve his sperm. They were planning for a second IVF cycle and wanted to do everything possible so it would be successful. When I worked with Les individually, I found out that he could not ejaculate inside his wife, Julie. In fact, his first wife divorced him because of it. There was so much difficulty around baby making that sex with his wife became strained. They forgot to enjoy it.

I worked on his liver energy and his Ren channel (Conception Vessel). Acupuncture was the vehicle to connect his mind and body. Les was able to release stuck energy and feelings. He was able to talk about the shame he felt and literally get it off his chest. When I explained to him some causes: a psychogenic one and also a masturbatory style that does not translate to vaginal stimulation, he took a deep breath and the strained look he had on his face melted away. I gave them homework to enjoy and practice touch exercises to regain intimacy. They both came back to me and told me that sex had significantly improved; however, they were still on for the IVF the next month. I did recommend Les talk to a therapist to look at healing underlying issues that were preventing him from ejaculating in his partner. As it turned out the IVF was a success.

Premature ejaculation and Traditional Chinese Medicine

PE for some men trying to conceive can be acquired meaning it has not happened before and for others it can be lifelong. The definition of PE is ejaculation that always or nearly always occurs prior to or within *about 1 minute* of vaginal penetration from the first sexual experience (LPE), or a clinically significant reduction in latency time, often to about 3 minutes or less (acquired PE). We know that it can have negative personal consequences for some men and others avoid sexual intimacy altogether. TCM offers solutions for PE with acupuncture and herbs. As always, it's important to diagnose the underlying pattern. In one study it was concluded, "Our results confirm previous reports on the efficacy and safety of dapoxetine. Although less effective than dapoxetine (an SSRI for PE) acupuncture had a significant ejaculation-delaying effect." In this study the following points were used: BL 30, Bl 52, ST 26, LI4, LIV3, Ren 3, and Yintang—twice a week for 20 minutes and the patients were followed up in a month [45]. Although SSRIs are used for PE, they are not recommended for fertility, says Dr. Philip Werthman, a Reproductive Urologist in Los Angeles. An option is to use herbs and acupuncture.

In another study the researchers showed that acupuncture can extend the ejaculation latency to a certain extent. On the basis of TCM theory, acupuncture can regulate the balance of Qi and blood by stimulating acupuncture points to improve human body function. Studies have shown that acupuncture points: tianshu (ST25), zusanli (ST36), and taichong (LIV3) can adjust neurotransmitter 5-HT levels and reduce nerve sensitivity [46].

When it comes to PE (I like to call it early ejaculation) and fertility, chances are the limiting factor is the amount of pleasure with each experience. Some couples shy away from engaging in sex because of shame around this issue. For some men early masturbation style can lead to PE and the edging practice below can help to retrain them.

Edging practice for early ejaculators

When self-pleasuring, men should notice the point of no return when ejaculation is inevitable. They should stop all self-touching and practice slow breathing until the urge to ejaculate has passed. Instructions are to tighten the PC muscle and press Ren 1 located on the perineum and maybe squeeze the base of the penis with a hand. Then when the urge has passed, continue with stimulation. (For a detailed discussion of Western approaches to ejaculatory problems see Chapter 5).

Female sexual issues

Females are complex beings. Every month women get their menstrual bleed called Tian gui in Chinese Medicine. Some women have issues such as irregular cycles, PCOS, endometriosis, and amenorrhea; and these can affect not only their ability to procreate but also their sexuality. There are many causes of female sexual issues (Fig. 14.1).

Traditional Chinese Medicine for sexual dysfunctions; dyspareunia, vulvodynia, vaginismus

In my clinic, I treat women with gynecological conditions and women who are trying to conceive. I often see women who have pain in their genitals and pain with intercourse. They do not readily volunteer this information until asked and then they want to know if Chinese Medicine can help them.

There are many words defining women's genital pain. Dyspareunia is one and is often defined as, "a persistent or recurrent genital pain that occurs just before, during or after intercourse" [47].

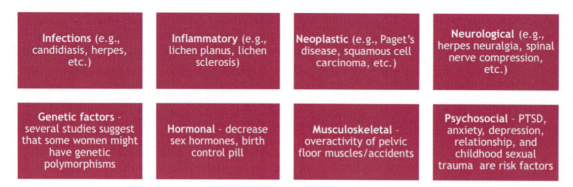

FIGURE 14.1 Causes of female sexual issues.

Many causes of dyspareunia exist. Sometimes it is from scant lubrication possibly caused from not enough sexual arousal or medications such as antihistamines, antidepressants, and some birth control pills. Other causes can be injury or local trauma to the vulva and vagina, infections, inflammations (skin disorders), cancers, and neurologic disorders such as postherpetic neuralgia, hormonal and postoperative/chemotherapy, and musculoskeletal problems [48]. A referral to a physician for diagnosis is essential.

Some women's pain is due to vaginismus. According to the International Society for the Study of Vulvovaginal Disease (ISSVD), "Vaginismus occurs when the muscles around the vagina tighten when something enters the vagina (penis, tampon, menstrual cups, getting a pelvic examination, etc.)" [48]. When the muscles in the vagina tighten and cause pain, women become fearful that this will happen again and fear can perpetuate this condition. We address fear in TCM by looking at the kidney energy.

Another type of pain is vulvodynia. According to the National Vulvodynia Association, "Vulvodynia, simply put, is chronic vulvar pain without an identifiable cause. The location, constancy and severity of the pain vary among sufferers. Some women experience pain in only one area of the vulva, while others experience pain in multiple areas. The most commonly reported symptom is burning, but women's descriptions of the pain vary" [48].

According to the fact sheet from the American College of Obstetricians and Gynecologists, "vulvodynia is pain that lasts 3 months or longer" [49]. Some women have pain on one site of the vulva and others have pain on the vestibule (around the opening of the vagina) called vestibulodynia. There are two types of vulvodynia provoked and unprovoked. Provoked is when pressure is applied to the vestibule with such things as tampon insertion, intercourse, a gynecological examination, prolonged sitting, and/or wearing tight-fitting pants. Medical doctors use a moist cotton swab to touch the vulva and have the patient report their localized pain, known as the "Q-tip test." Primary vulvodynia, which occurs on the first attempt at vaginal penetration and secondary vulvodynia when the first attempt was fine but later attempts caused pain. Unprovoked or generalized vulvodynia occurs when a woman has pain without touch. However, many can have a mix of provoked and unprovoked. The symptoms include stinging, burning pain, and hypersensitivity of the external genital area. In addition, pain can occur on the clitoris called clitorodynia. Women with this condition are in so much pain that they rarely want to be touched in that area let alone have intercourse.

The current treatment for these conditions is multifaceted. According to UCLA's Gail and Gerald Oppenheimer Family Center for Neurobiology of Stress and Resilience, "No one therapy has been proven successful and up to 50% of women, even after treatment of vulvodynia, continue to experience pain that interferes with general functioning and can prevent sexual intercourse" [50].

Research on Traditional Chinese Medicine and female sexual pain

As we have seen, research on TCM at this point in time, is fraught with difficulty. Although we will review the studies here, in my clinical experience I have seen great results with my patients. Below is a review of studies on female sexual pain and acupuncture.

In a 1999 study published in the *Journal of the Royal Society of Medicine*, the researchers gave weekly acupuncture on four points known for external genital pain: Sp 6, Sp 9, Liv3, and LI4. Patients reported feeling better and also liked time spent with the practitioner. The researchers think that the release of beta endorphins can change an overactive pain response [51].

In one pilot Scandinavian study in 2001, a small number of women had acupuncture one to two times per week for 10 sessions. They reported less pain and better quality of life. Measurements were all significantly higher after both the last acupuncture treatment and at 3 months follow-up, compared to before treatment was started [52].

According to a 2014 review study in *Chinese Medicine*, American guidelines for treatment of vulvodynia do not support usage of acupuncture whereas the British guidelines support usage of acupuncture. The researchers concluded that "there is insufficient data to argue for the efficacy of acupuncture for treatment of unprovoked vulvodynia, and no data on the efficacy of acupuncture for treatment of provoked vulvodynia." They called for well-designed and performed trials of acupuncture for treatment of vulvodynia [53], finding describing much of current acupuncture research.

In a 2015 pilot study published in the *Journal of Sexual Medicine*, researchers found that when patients received acupuncture two times per week for 5 weeks for a total of 10 sessions the reports of vulvar pain and dyspareunia were significantly reduced [54].

In a 2017 study published in the *Journal of Complementary and Alternative Medicine*, the researchers broke vulvodynia into two different TCM patterns; one heat and one cold and found that there might be a difference in how the women in the study experienced pain but further studies with a larger number of people need to be done [55].

The National Institute of Health (NIH) is supporting a study on acupuncture and vulvodynia at the NIH McLean Center for Complementary and Alternative Medicine, due to the significant number of women affected (16%). This study protocol for a pilot pragmatic controlled trial will compare two groups of acupuncture treatments with the standard of care of physical therapy, pain medications, and nerve blocking [56].

In another study, *Acupuncture Augmentation of Lidocaine Therapy for Provoked, Localized Vulvodynia: A Protocol for Feasibility and Acceptability Study*, the researchers broke the patients into different TCM diagnosis groups and then applied different treatments. The TCM diagnosis pertaining to the affected acupuncture channels were: Qi and blood stagnation in the Liver channel, fire in the Liver channel, and cold in the Liver channel engendering fire. The secondary TCM diagnosis were: Liver Qi stagnation; Liver/Spleen disharmony, damp-heat accumulation in the lower burner; phlegm/damp accumulation, Spleen Qi deficiency, Heart blood deficiency, and Heart blood deficiency. The conclusion was, "In this early-phase research, acupuncture augmentation of lidocaine was acceptable. The study procedures, with modifications, may be feasible for future investigation. Both acupuncture techniques showed a favorable effect; however, the contribution to pain relief is undetermined" [57]. One of the pluses in this study was that it was more in alignment with TCM theory. Clearly more research needs to be done.

Chinese medical theory and female sexual pain

According to *Concise Traditional Chinese Gynecology*, the external genitalia of women are closely related to the Liver (Liv), Kidney (Kid), Chong, and Ren channels [58]. Also, the *Handbook of Obstetrics and Gynecology in Chinese Medicine, an Integrated Approach* [59] contains a chapter on disorders of the vulva. Some are caused by chronic infections leaving lesions or thickening of the skin on the vulva possibly leading to pain. Also noted are atrophic changes from lack of estrogen leading to dyspareunia or vulvar deficiency. This would be synonymous with Kidney, Liver yin deficiency, or in Western terms an imbalance in the endocrine and/or immune systems. We see Kidney yin deficiency (possibly associated with lack of estrogen) most prevalent in older women although some women in their thirties have low estrogen and vaginal dryness. In making a differential diagnosis, a TCM practitioner must be clear about the causes of vaginal dryness. Our Chinese diagnosis has to determine whether the patient has other Kidney yin deficiency signs such as night sweats, red tongue, rapid pulse, low back pain, dry mouth, and scanty urination. The emotion of the kidney energy is also fear. This can be a factor in vaginismus. Since kidney energy is first and foremost of our reproductive energy, we must assess its function or determine if the vaginal dryness is because of lack of foreplay. It is important to inquire about a patient's sexuality or any related trauma. When treating vaginismus, in the five-element model, we can also treat the Pericardium channel which is called the heart protector to help with past wounding. According to Lonnie Jarret in *The Clinical Practice of Chinese Medicine*, the acupuncture points on the Pericardium channel empower the heart to be nourished by intimacy and also help let go of past pain or heartbreak [18]. In the world of fertility, miscarriages or failed IVFs can be a cause of pain for many individuals.

Because the Liver channel runs through the genitals, many women who experience pain in the vulva have a diagnosis of Liver Qi stagnation. This can be diagnosed by other signs and symptoms such as anxiety, frustration, and a feeling of being stuck in situations. The patient may sigh frequently, complain of difficulty in taking a full breath and have hypochondriac pain. The patient can also complain of vaginismus as the constrained Liver Qi does not allow the muscles to relax. In many blog posts women call their pain their "angry vag" and since the Liver's emotion is anger, Liver Qi stagnation would be a fitting Chinese diagnosis. Liver Qi stagnation can also lead to Liver fire. The patient would have more fire signs such as headaches, dizziness, a bitter taste, thirst, and red tongue with a wiry rapid pulse.

Another treatment strategy used in Chinese Medicine for chronic conditions is the diagnosis of blood stasis. One of my professors at Emperor's college used to say that if a patient has had a chronic condition then treat blood stasis. This would be analogous to improving blood flow and microcirculation to the vulva, allowing nutrients and oxygen to get to the area. We might also find signs and symptoms that would confirm this diagnosis such as a dusky purple tongue and a sharp stabbing pain. In an article, "Investigations from a TCM perspective," the author talks about other signs to look for with blood stasis including trauma, surgery, dark menstrual blood with clots, fibroids, endometriosis, and a choppy pulse, with a dark red or purple tongue [60]. We can use both herbs and acupuncture to treat this pattern.

In TCM there is limited information on the specific conditions of vulvodynia or dyspareunia as TCM primarily focuses on patterns of imbalance and menstrual conditions. Many books such as Giovanni Maciocia's book, *Obstetrics and Gynecology* [61] talk about pain as it relates to conditions such as endometriosis and addresses the vulva with the concept of vulvar itching which can stem from infections such as candida, genital eczema, herpes, and bacterial vaginosis (dampness in the lower burner). Vulvar pain on its own is not spoken about directly. In fact, there is limited reference to sexual dysfunctions for women. So, Chinese differential diagnosis for vulvar problems is extrapolated from research and clinical experience.

TCM practitioners can derive a treatment strategy based on diagnosis signs such as tongue, pulse, and the quality of pain. Some women talk about a burning sensation and this would be synonymous with heat. Obviously, if the pain is due to an infection there would be a purulent discharge.

For vulvodynia and dyspareunia, we would want to know if there has been any history of sexual abuse. Putting all the factors together a practitioner can come up with an effective treatment plan.

Lichen sclerosus and Traditional Chinese Medicine

Lichen sclerosus is a common chronic skin disorder that most often affects genital and perianal areas sometimes seen in young women that want to conceive. It is a condition that is not commonly understood and creates a lot of shame in women who have it. Lichen sclerosus presents as white crinkled or thickened patches of skin that tend to scar and often will cause adhesions. It primarily involves the nonhair bearing, inner areas of the vulva and can result in a buried clitoris (phimosis) and a labia minora that will resorb/shrink. Sexual intercourse can be very uncomfortable. Many treatments in Western medicine exist with the most common being topical steroids. In Chinese Medicine, the diagnosis can be any combination of these: damp heat in lower burner, Kidney and Liver yin deficiency, blood deficiency creating dryness and wind, fire accumulating in Liver, and Heart blood stasis. Our treatment principle is activating blood, eliminating stasis, promoting tissue regeneration, clearing heat, detoxifying, removing dampness, and relieving itching. To treat lichen sclerosus, patients drink special herbal combinations and receive acupuncture based on their pattern diagnosis. A patient of mine, in her thirties with lichen sclerosus felt like she was not normal "down there." She did not want to have intercourse with her husband not only because of pain but also because of her eroded labia that made her feel bad about herself. With months of work, her symptoms of itching and burning abated and she accepted her condition. Her medical doctor was surprised.

Traditional Chinese Medicine treatment plans for female problems

Acupuncture treatment is based on pattern diagnosis. For vulvodynia some common points are Liver 5, Ren 3, St 30, and back points, including BL-32–BL-34 with continuous milliamp. Other acupuncture points that can be added include: Sp 6, LV 3, GB 34, Sp9, and BL43. To get the best results all treatments are given twice a week for 6 weeks for a total of 12 treatments and then we reevaluate.

Herbal medicine is also based on pattern identification and is not as forgiving as acupuncture. Obviously, we would modify these formulas based on the need of the individual but here are some examples of traditional uses for herbal formulas. If there is a Kid/Liv Yin def—herbal formulas include: Zuo Gui Wan and Liu Wei Di Huang Wan. For a diagnosis of Liver Qi stagnation the formulas used can be: Si Ni San and Xiao Yao San. If damp heat is involved the formula Long Dan Xie Gan Tang is a good fit. We can also modify formulas with nourishing yin herbs that include: sheng di, mu dan pi, mai men dong, xuan, shen, zhi mu, di gu pi, han lian cao, nu zhen zi lian zi, and shi hu. If we want to clear more heat we can add huang bai. For pronounced Qi stagnation we can add: xiang Fu, qing pi, yu jin, and chuan lian zi. For blood stasis herbs are used such as: dan shen, ji xue teng, chi shao, yan hu suo, niu xi, pu huang, and yu jin. For calming, herbs used are: suan zao ren, yuan zhi, hu po, and he huan pi (uterine stimulant). Lastly for Qi and blood deficiency added herbs include: huang qi, dang shen, dang gui, and e jiao.

Most patients that come for female conditions have already been checked out by an Ob-Gyn. They are more than willing to do what is suggested to make their pain go away. Some are also given topical estrogen or testosterone to put on their vulvas. It is essential to work with a medical doctor because it is not in the scope of a Chinese Medicine practitioner to examine the vulva.

Because we cannot do the Q-tip test on the vulva to assess vulvodynia pain, we need to have the patient rate their pain on the Visual Analog Scale for the following: intercourse, insertion of a toy, finger, or just with touching themselves with a Q-tip. Patients can also keep a pain journal. If they are experiencing vaginal dryness causing discomfort, we evaluate improvement of dryness and other symptoms.

Vaginal steaming

Patients ask me about vaginal steaming as they have read that it can help them get pregnant. Internet searches reveal, significant controversy over "V-steam." One PubMed article referred to it as sorcery. Insignificant research exists to tout the benefits of this ancient modality. However, it may be effective for treating infections, soothing tissues, and promoting fertility. Let's work backwards. To get pregnant, a woman needs good fertile cervical mucous. During the fertile window, this cervical mucous needs to be more alkaline to allow the sperm to live in it and make its way to the uterus. Proper pH can be impacted by infections such as yeast overgrowth, urea plasm, mycoplasm, and other problems in the vaginal microbiome or a more alkaline pH can then lead to infections. While some claim a "V-steam" cleans out the uterus, that would be inaccurate. The vagina is self-cleaning so I do not recommend regular steams. The Chinese do use vaginal and rectal delivery of herbs for infections. Mugwort is the traditional herb that is used for a "V-steam." Videos touting the benefits of vaginal pearls at "cleaning out" the vagina are widely disrtibuted. Care should be taken when discussing this with patients. Not everyone's vagina needs to be cleaned! However, if a woman is suffering from frequent bacteria vaginosis and other problems, it might be that her flora and fauna are not healthy. Taking herbs orally, using probiotics, eating a healthy diet with no sugar or refined products, and possibly vaginal steaming can be helpful.

Case study: vaginismus

A patient of mine, who was trying to conceive suffered from vaginismus and low back pain. The causative factor of the dyspareunia was the frequent painful bladder infections she would regularly get after having intercourse with her husband. After a while she feared having sexual relations and just the slightest touch inside her vagina caused her pain. Her Ob-Gyn diagnosed her with vaginismus and sent her to a pelvic floor physical therapist (PT). She and the PT worked on using small dilators to expand her vagina. She was instructed not to have intercourse with her husband which further exacerbated her anxiety about conceiving. She also started seeing a therapist. When she came to see me for treatment of low back pain which she said was caused by exercise and as an afterthought she revealed she had vaginismus. Over time, I saw that her diagnosis was clearly a combination of Kidney def and Liver Qi stagnation with disruption of the Chong Mai and Yin Qiao Mai. She also experienced difficulty falling asleep and had hot feet at night. I gave her acupuncture, including the points: Kid 6, Lu 7, Liver 2, UB 23, 24, 25, Ub 32, ear shen men, and Du 20. I alternated this treatment with working on the Chong and Yin Qiao meridians with the points: Sp 4, P6, Kid 6, Lu 7 Liv 8, Kid 11, Ren 17, Kid 27, and Ren 1. She worked on releasing fear that was held in the muscles of her vagina. In a few sessions she said not only was her back pain better, but her vaginismus was improving, and she was able to use a bigger dilator. She was only able to come to the clinic once a week and sometimes missed sessions. Given enough time and with a combination of treatment modalities her pain started to subside and she was able to try to conceive.

Conclusion

TCM can offer a great deal when it comes to sexual dysfunction in the infertility setting. As practitioners, we can evaluate the body, mind, and spirit and address each of these as one system. Although limited quality studies examine whole systems, Chinese Medicine, including acupuncture, herbs, lifestyle, and dietary therapy together can be employed in the clinic setting. A few small studies have examined these modalities individually. Their results are limited in their generalizability. However, anecdotal reports of successful outcomes are abundant. Helping women and men conceive is one of the goals of Chinese Medicine as it is about living in harmony with nature and finding the middle path. When we are out of balance, our planet and those that inhabit it suffer. We are forced to reevaluate what "fertility" means. Although Western intervention has a significant ability to help, we cannot turn a blind eye to the causes of imbalance in our society and planet that contribute to infertility. The best approach is an integrative one where collectively we work with all modalities to ensure the conception of the next generation.

References

[1] Nature.com. The World Health Organization's decision about traditional Chinese Medicine could backfire. Nature 2019;570(7759):5. Available from: https://www.nature.com/articles/d41586-019-01726-1 [accessed 13.07.20].
[2] Kaptchuk T. The web that has no weaver. Cork: BookBaby; 2014.
[3] Veith I. Huang ti nei ching su wen: The yellow emperor's classic of internal medicine. Baltimore: Williams & Wilkins; 1949.
[4] Blakeway J, David SS. The fertility plan: a proven three-month programme to help you conceive naturally. New York: Little, Brown; 2009.
[5] Imbler S. Chinese women once had to point out their medical troubles on ivory dolls. Atlas Obscura. Available from: <https://www.atlasobscura.com/articles/chinese-medical-doll>; 2019 [cited July 13, 2020].
[6] Chubak B, Doctor A. Traditional Chinese Medicine for sexual dysfunction: review of the evidence. Sex Med Rev 2018;6(3):410–18.
[7] Hill S. Yang sheng 養生 nourishing life. Monkey Press. Available from: <https://www.monkeypress.net/blog/yang-sheng-%E9%A4%8A-%E7%94%9F-nourishing-life>; 2018 [cited 14 July 2020].
[8] Lyttleton J. Treatment of infertility with Chinese Medicine. Edinburgh: Churchill Livingstone; 2013.
[9] Maxwell D. The clinical utility of the concept of Jing in Chinese reproductive medicine. Asian Med 2012;7(2):421–54.
[10] Wile D. Art of the bedchamber. Albany: State University of New York Press; 1992.
[11] Chia M, Winn M. Taoist secrets of love. Santa Fe: Aurora Press;; 1999.
[12] Van den Brink F, Vollmann M, Smeets M, Hessen D, Woertman L. Relationships between body image, sexual satisfaction, and relationship quality in romantic couples. J Fam Psychol 2018;32(4):466–74.
[13] Li G, Flaws B. Li Dong-yuan's treatise on the spleen & stomach. Boulder, CO: Blue Poppy Press; 2004.
[14] Schnarch D. Passionate marriage, keeping love and intimacy alive in committed relaitonships. New York: Norton & Company; 2009.
[15] Koike T, Sumiya M, Nakagawa E, Okazaki S, Sadato N. What makes eye contact special? Neural substrates of on-line mutual eye-gaze: a hyperscanning fMRI study. eNeuro. 2019;6(1).
[16] Wilcox L. In an e-mail interview about female sex in the classics (zhenjiu@gmail.com); March 2020.
[17] Gao E, Zuo X, Wang L, Lou C, Cheng Y, Zabin L. How does traditional Confucian culture influence adolescents' sexual behavior in three Asian cities? J Adolesc Health 2012;50(3):S12–17.
[18] Maciocia G. Sexual life in Chinese Medicine. Available from: <https://giovanni-maciocia.com/sexual-life-in-chinese-medicine/>; 2020 [cited July 17, 2020].
[19] Jarrett L. The clinical practice of Chinese Medicine. 1st ed. Stockbridge, MA: Spirit Path Press; 2006. p. 189.
[20] Zhou W, Benharash P. Effects and mechanisms of acupuncture based on the principle of meridians. J Acupunct Meridian Stud 2014;7(4):190–3.
[21] Miner S, Robins S, Zhu Y, Keeren K, Gu V, Read S, et al. Evidence for the use of complementary and alternative medicines during fertility treatment: a scoping review. BMC Complement Altern Med 2018;18(1):158.
[22] Yun L, Liqun W, Shuqi Y, Chunxiao W, Liming L, Wei Y. Acupuncture for infertile women without undergoing assisted reproductive techniques (ART). Medicine 2019;98(29):e16463.
[23] Kusuma A, Oktari N, Mihardja H, Srilestari A, Simadibrata C, Hestiantoro A, et al. Electroacupuncture enhances number of mature oocytes and fertility rates for in vitro fertilization. Med Acupunct 2019;31(5):289–97.
[24] Aboushanab T, AlSanad S. Cupping therapy: an overview from a modern medicine perspective. J Acupunct Meridian Stud 2018;11(3):83–7.
[25] Zhaofeng L, Hui i, Hao M, Wang X, Yu Y, Ma Y. Herb-partitioned moxibustion on navel for anovulatory infertility: a randomized controlled trial. Zhongguo Zhen Jiu 2017;37(8):819–23. Available from: https://pubmed.ncbi.nlm.nih.gov/29231340/ [cited July 18, 2020].
[26] Qu F, Wang F, Robinson N, Hardiman P. Women's health and Chinese integrative medicine. J Zhejiang Univ Sci B 2017;18(3):183–5.

[27] Zhou J, Qu F. Treating gynaecological disorders with traditional Chinese Medicine: a review. Afr J Tradit Complement Altern Med 2009;6(4):494–517.
[28] Basson R. Rethinking low sexual desire in women. BJOG 2002;109(4):357–63.
[29] Clayton A, Kingsberg S, Goldstein I. Evaluation and management of hypoactive sexual desire disorder. Sex Med 2018;6(2):59–74.
[30] Frantzis B. Taoist sexual meditation. Berkeley, CA: North Atlantic Books; 2012.
[31] Oakley S, Walther-Liu J, Crisp C, Pauls R. Acupuncture in premenopausal women with hypoactive sexual desire disorder: a prospective cohort pilot study. Sex Med 2016;4(3):e176–81.
[32] Khamba B, Aucoin M, Lytle M, Vermani M, Maldonado A, Iorio C, et al. Efficacy of acupuncture treatment of sexual dysfunction secondary to antidepressants. J Altern Complement Med 2013;19(11):862–9.
[33] Lee J, Oh H, Kwon J, Jeong M, Lee J, Kang D, et al. The effects of *Cynomorium songaricum* on the reproductive activity in male golden hamsters. Dev Reprod 2013;17(1):37–43.
[34] Chang Y, Jeng K, Huang K, Lee Y, Hou C, Chen K, et al. Effect of *Cordyceps militaris* supplementation on sperm production, sperm motility and hormones in Sprague-Dawley rats. Am J Chin Med 2008;36(05):849–59.
[35] Li Z, Lin H, Gu L, Gao J, Tzeng C. Herba Cistanche (Rou Cong-Rong): one of the best pharmaceutical gifts of traditional Chinese Medicine. Front Pharmacol 2016;7:41.
[36] Nasimi Doost Azgomi R, Zomorrodi A, Nazemyieh H, Fazljou S, Sadeghi Bazargani H, Nejatbakhsh F, et al. Effects of *Withania somnifera* on reproductive system: a systematic review of the available evidence. Biomed Res Int 2018;2018:1–17.
[37] Damone B. Principles of Chinese medical andrology. Boulder, CO: Blue Poppy Press; 2008. p. 235–6.
[38] Lai B, Cao H, Yang G, Jia L, Grant S, Fei Y, et al. Acupuncture for treatment of erectile dysfunction: a systematic review and meta-analysis. World J Mens Health 2019;37(3):322.
[39] Li H, Jiang H, Liu J. Traditional Chinese medical therapy for erectile dysfunction. Transl Androl Urol 2017;6(2):192–8.
[40] Yan X, Li J, Yang F, Huang X, Tan K, Dong L, et al. Shugan Yiyang capsule for the treatment of erectile dysfunction. Medicine. 2019;98(44):e17646.
[41] Law B, Mo J, Wong V. Autophagic effects of Chaihu (dried roots of Bupleurum Chinense DC or Bupleurum scorzoneraefolium WILD). Chin Med 2014;9(1):21.
[42] Otani T. Clinical review of ejaculatory dysfunction. Reprod Med Biol 2019;18(4):331–43.
[43] Perelman M. Psychosexual therapy for delayed ejaculation based on the Sexual Tipping Point model. Transl Androl Urol 2016;5(4):563–75.
[44] Abdel-Hamid I, Elsaied M, Mostafa T. The drug treatment of delayed ejaculation. Transl Androl Urol 2016;5(4):576–91.
[45] Sahin S, Bicer M, Yenice M, Seker K, Yavuzsan A, Tugcu V. A prospective randomized controlled study to compare acupuncture and dapoxetine for the treatment of premature ejaculation. Urol Int 2016;97(1):104–11.
[46] Zhao Q, Dai H, Gong X, Wang L, Cao M, Li H, et al. Acupuncture for premature ejaculation. Medicine 2018;97(35):e11980.
[47] Mayo Clinic Staff. Painful intercourse (dyspareunia)—symptoms and causes. Mayo Clinic. Available from: <https://www.mayoclinic.org/diseases-conditions/painful-intercourse/symptoms-causes/syc-20375967>; 2020 [cited 24 July 2020].
[48] Bornstein J, Goldstein A, Stockdale C, Bergeron S, Pukall C, Zolnoun D, et al. 2015 ISSVD, ISSWSH and IPPS consensus terminology and classification of persistent vulvar pain and vulvodynia. Obstet Gynecol 2016;127(4):745–51.
[49] American College of Obstetricians and Gynecologists. Retrieved from: <https://www.acog.org/-/media/For-Patients/faq127.pdf?dmc=1&ts=20181026T1753255104>; n.d.
[50] <http://uclacns.org/about-cnsr>.
[51] Powell J, Wojnarowska F. Acupuncture for vulvodynia. JRSM 1999;92(11):579–81.
[52] Danielsson I, Sjoberg I, Ostman C. Acupuncture for the treatment of vulvar vestibulitis: a pilot study. Acta Obstet Gynecol Scand 2001;80(5):437–41.
[53] Nwanodi O, Tidman M. Vulvodynia treated with acupuncture or electromyographic biofeedback. Chin Med 2014;05(02):61–70.
[54] Schlaeger J, Xu N, Mejta C, Park C, Wilkie D. Acupuncture for the treatment of vulvodynia: a randomized wait-list controlled pilot study. Sex Med 2015;12(4):1019–27.
[55] Schlaeger J, Cai H, Nenggui X, Steffens A, Lin W, Wilkie D, et al. Patterns differ by pain types? Beginning evidence supporting the concept. J Altern Complement Med 2017;23(5):380–4.
[56] Fan A, Alemi S, Zhu Y, Rahimi S, Wei H, Tian H, et al. Effectiveness of two different acupuncture strategies in patients with vulvodynia: study protocol for a pilot pragmatic controlled trial. J Integr Med 2018;16(6):384–9.
[57] Hullender Rubin L, Mist S, Schnyer R, Rowe R, Wimberly A, Leclair C. Acupuncture augmentation of lidocaine therapy for provoked, localized vulvodynia: a protocol for a feasibility and acceptability study. Meridians JAOM 2018;5(4).
[58] Nanjing College of Traditional Medicine. Concise traditional Chinese gynecology. Nanjing, Jiangsu: Jiangsu Science and Technology Publishing House; 1987.
[59] Chin Y, Hakim C. Handbook of obstetrics & gynecology in Chinese Medicine. Seattle, WA: Eastland Press; 1998.
[60] Szmelskyj I, Aquilina L, Szmelskyj A. Acupuncture for IVF and assisted reproduction. Edinburgh: Elsevier; 2015.
[61] Maciocia G. Obstetrics and gynecology in Chinese Medicine. London: Elsevier Health Sciences UK; 2014.

Addendum

Herbal medicine

Herbal formulas: Pin Yin/Western name

1. Gui Pi Tang—Restore the spleen decoction, ginseng and longan combination

2. Xuan Zhi Tang plus Yuan Zhi wan (modified)—Mind diffusing decoction plus Yuan Zhi
3. Chai Hu Shu Gan Wan—Bupleurum to dredge the liver
4. Yue Ju Wan—Escape restraint pill
5. Jin Gui Shen Qi Wan—Kidney Qi pill from the golden cabinet
6. Long Dan Xie Gan Tang—Gentian decoction to drain the liver
7. Xue Fu Zhu Yu Tang—Drive out stasis from the mansion of blood decoction
8. Zou Gui Wan—Restore the left decoction
9. Liu Wei Di Huang Wan—Six-ingredient pill with Rehmannia
10. Si Ni San—Frigid extremities powder
11. Xiao Yao San—Rambling powder, free and easy wanderer
12. You Gui Wan—Restore the right decoction

Individual herbs: Pin Yin/Latin

1. Shan Zha—Fructus Crataegi, hawthorne berry
2. Chai Hu—Rx Buplerum, thororax root
3. Sheng Ma—Cimicifugae Rhizoma, black cohosh
4. Ba Ji Tian—Radix Morindae, Indian mulberry
5. Bu Gu Zhi—Rx Psoralea Frui
6. Yuan Zhi—Radix Polygalae
7. Shi Chang Pu—Rhizoma Acori Tatarinowii, Sweetflag rhizone
8. Suan Zao Ren—Semen Zizyphi Spinosae—sour jujube seeds
9. He Huan Pi—Albizia Bark, Cortex Albiziae
10. Wu Gong—Scolopendra subspinipes—cenitpede
11. Dan Shen—Salvia miltiorrhiza—Chinese sage
12. Hong Hua—Rx Carthamus, safflower
13. Chi Shao—Red Peony Root—Paeoniae radix rubra
14. Zhi zi—Fructus Gardenia
15. Mu Dan Pi—Moutan cortex, tree peony bark
16. Yu Jin—Curcumae root, turmeric tuber
17. Xiang Fu—Rhizoma Cyperi, nutgrass
18. Du Zhong—Eucommia bark
19. Wu Wei Zi—Fructus Schizandrae, magnolia berry
20. Lu Jiao Jiao—Cervi Conus Colla, deer antler glue
21. Yin Yang Huo—Herba Epimedii, horny goat weed
22. Xian Mao—Curculigo Rhizome, Rhizoma Curculiginis
23. He Shou Wu—Polygonum multiflorum, Fo-ti
24. Chuan Xiong—Ligusticum chuanxiong, Szechuan lovage root
25. Ginkgo Biloba—Maidenhair
26. Ba Ji Li—Tribulus, Caltrop fruit
27. Korean Ginseng
28. Gou Qi Zi—Lycium fruit, Gou ji berry
29. Huang Lian—Rhizoma Coptidis
30. Sheng Di Huang—Chinese foxglove root, Radix Rehmannia
31. Mai Men Dong—Ophiopogon tuber
32. Xuan Shen—Radix Scrophularia
33. Zhi Mu—Rhizome Anemarrhena
34. Di Gu PI—Cortex Lycii, Chinese wolfberry
35. Han Lian Cao—Herba Ecliptae
36. Nu Zhen zi—Fructus Ligustri Lucidi, Privet fruit
37. Lian Zi—Semen Nelumbinis, lotus seed
38. Shi Hu—Herba Dendrobii, stem of orchid of Southeast Asia
39. Huang Bai—Cortex Phellondendri, Amur cork tree bark
40. Qing Pi—Green tangerine peel
41. Chuan Lian Zi—Fructus Tossendan, Sichuan Pogoda tree fruit
42. Dan Shen—Salvia miltiorrhiza

43. Ji Xue Tang—Spatholobus stem
44. Yan Hu Cao—Rhizoma Corydalis
45. Niu XI—Radix Achyranthis Bidentatae
46. Pu Huang—Pollen Typhae, Cattail pollen
47. Hu Po—Succinum, Amber
48. Huang Qi—Radix Astragalus
49. Dang Shen—Radix Codonopsis
50. Dang Gui—Radix Angelicae Sinensis
51. E Jiao—Donkey Hide Gelatin, Colla Corii Asini

CHAPTER 15

Sex, religion, and infertility: the complications of G-d in the bedroom

Julie Bindeman
Integrative Therapy of Greater Washington, Rockville, MD, United States

Historical overview of sex, religion, and assisted reproductive technology

Sex

Examining the history of sex is akin to the retelling of human history. Without sex, as pertains to reproduction, *Homo sapiens* would be unable to continue as a species. Throughout history sex has been, and continues to be, interwoven into the systems that human beings created. Thus, it is of no surprise that religions have significant rules and mandates regarding sex: who can have it, its purpose, what it can look like, and more. Religions are not static edifices though: they change and adapt as they grow and recede in popularity. As the religions controlling sex and sexuality evolved, the dovetailing between sex and religion, by its nature, drove continuous evolution in the rules, restrictions, and expectations regarding sex.

In early humankind, people and societies were primarily nomadic. This meant that their religious preferences needed to be nomadic as well so that they could be continued and literally carried. As religions became prominent, so did the necessity for formal places to worship, such as churches or temples. Humanity's movement away from hunter gatherers to a more agrarian society was a driving force leading to formal places of worship [1].

An examination of the Medieval period provides a good example of the evolution of sex within a religious framework. While not often discussed, the early Middle Ages are actually considered to be a significant period of sexual abandon [2]. While the Christian Church proselytized and enforced total abstinence within its clerical ranks it was unable to instill this belief in society as a whole. To combat this, the Church began to create a belief system where chastity was perceived as a value and virtue and overt sexuality or sexual interest was associated with sin and damnation. This push and pull around how sex and sexuality are seen and accepted is repeated time and again throughout history. Religion and religious organizations are often the predominant forces behind efforts to define acceptable sexual standards. This dichotomy stands out strongly during the Victorian age as well during which the religious pull toward chastity was strong. The eminent neurologist, Dr. Sigmund Freud, using the culture of chastity around him, codified a theory of mind that included sexual impulses and desires as both normal and as a key motivating force within human beings [3]. Another key time in human history when sexuality and religion became at odds with one another was the 1960s and began with the "free love" movement. This was a time when religious morays around sex were seemingly abandoned by many youth of the generation. The catalysts for this about-face in terms of sexuality were manifold: a war in Vietnam, the invention of the birth control pill, and Betty Friedan's revolutionary tome, *The Feminine Mystique*, to list several [4]. To the current day, the reverberations of this time period continue to be sorted out. For instance, the invention of the birth control pill shifted, and continues to shift, the dynamics between men and women, as women have more control than solely abstinence around their reproductive choices [5]. Religious institutions had many differing responses to this seismic shift. The more "liberal" leaning institutions were able to find ways to adapt their teachings on sex and sexuality, whereas more "conservative" institutions employed previously successful tactics such as shame, guilt, and godliness as their response [2,6].

The creation of birth control proved to be the first modern building block in the evolution of assisted reproductive technologies (ARTs). If people could now control when *not* to get pregnant, surely technology could be applied to assist the one in eight couples who were unable to become pregnant [7,8]. The advent of new technology required religions to come up with guidance to share with followers that might need to engage in using medical advances as the manner in which to grow their families. Religions turned to their ancient sources and texts to find new interpretations that justified their new stances. In order to understand how Judaism, Christianity, and Islam perceive ART, it is important to first get a sense of each religion's origins.

Origin of Judaism

Of the three religions under discussion, Judaism is the oldest. According to the Jewish calendar, the religion is over 5780 years old, though historical documentation suggests that Judaism is closer to 4000 years old. Judaism's oldest prophet and seeming "founder" is Abraham; the first human that G-d[1] revealed themself to. G-d and Abraham made a special covenant wherein G-d promised to Abraham that his descendants would be the "chosen people" in exchange for evidence of belief in G-d's singularity. This evidence was to be provided in the form of circumcision of every Jewish male [9]. The story of Abraham contains the first of many instances of infertility spoken about within the Hebrew Bible, also known as the Old Testament, the first five books, which are known as the Torah. In addition to the Torah, Judaism has several other sacred texts that inform understanding of the original Torah. These texts include the Mishnah, the Talmud, and the Midrash. Each of these texts represents recordings of oral history, commentary by religious leaders, or expansion on concepts within the Torah or other texts [10]. There are also more modern commentaries, and all continue the conversation between generations and authors about interpretations of Torah and managing the laws and traditions in modern, at the time the texts were written, life.

The texts of Judaism incorporate stories as well as rules or commandments, 613 of which are contained in the entire Torah, by which Jews are to live their lives by. These laws or Halacha provide great detail for the manner in which they must be carried out, by whom, and how. Included in them are the manner in which food is killed and prepared, known as the laws of kashrut (kosher), as well as laws pertaining to sex and cleanliness or ritual purity, which are called the laws of niddah [11]. There are three major denominations of Judaism: Orthodox, Conservative, and Reform. Each denomination varies in how adherent it is to the text of Torah and its interpretation by commentators writing after the Torah was completed. Formal worship leaders of each denomination are rabbis, translated from the Hebrew as "my teacher" [12].

Origin of Christianity

Chronologically, the next of the three religions to emerge was Christianity. The age of the Christian faith matches the year of the Gregorian calendar and thus is over 2020 years old. Christianity's sacred text centers on two main volumes: The Old Testament and the New Testament, which, between the two, constitutes a total of 66 books. The key distinguishing feature between Judaism and Christianity is the belief in Jesus Christ. Christians believe that Jesus was the direct son of G-d, born through a virgin mother, who died for his love of humanity. In his death he is believed to have absolved humanity of their sins by taking them upon himself. Several days after Jesus' death, it is believed that he was resurrected, which is seen as the first Christian-based miracle.

The New Testament includes many subsidiary writings including: the Gospels which are named for the prophets who wrote them, letters that speak to how the Church should operate known as the Epistles, Acts of the Apostles that represent a "part two" of the Gospels that speaks to what happened after Jesus' death and resurrection, and the final book Revelation which speaks to the end of days [13]. Christianity takes on many forms and is considered to be the most practiced religion around the world [13]. The three most common denominations include Catholic, Protestant, and Eastern Orthodox. Within the Protestant denomination there exist multiple sects that include, among others, Baptists, Lutherans, Evangelicals, Methodists, and Seventh Day Adventists. Generally speaking, those that practice within the framework of Catholicism or Orthodoxy are considered to maintain more literal views of the sacred texts, though certainly Evangelical churches and Seventh Day

---

[1] G-d will denote how the name of the monotheistic deity is represented in this chapter. Within a Jewish framework, withholding a letter in text is seen as a way of separating humans from the divine.

Adventists take on a similar view and variety exists within each church as well as within practitioners. Worship leaders of a church are called ministers or priests.

Origin of Islam

The youngest of the monotheistic religions is considered to be Islam, which is believed to have been founded by the prophet Muhammad 613 years after Christianity was founded. Those that follow the religion are called Muslims. Islam grew due to a caliphate system, or a system of succession based upon designated rulers, which enabled there not to be a gap in leadership should a leader die or be killed [14]. After Muhammad's death, there was a split in Islam, creating two main sects that exist today: Sunni and Shi'a. Adherents to Islam consider their sacred text as the Qur'an, originally given to Muhammad, through the prophet Gabriel [14]. Additional principles and understanding of the laws come from: the *Sunnah* which are traditions, or "common laws"; *ijma* a consensus, or a standardization of legal theories; and *ijtihad* individual thoughts, which for Shi'a Muslims continue to evolve, whereas for Sunni Muslims, remain static. Muslims view both Jews and Christians as other "people of the book" with the idea that their prophets were also divine messengers from G-d, with Muhammad being the last in that line [15].

The Islamic legal system is called *Sharia* law, which guides adherents in their daily behaviors. There is no hierarchy in Islam: thus, clerics aren't seen as direct links to Allah, rather, each individual has their own relationship with the divine. Those that guide the prayers in their houses of worship (mosques) are called imams [16]. In the United States, imams often function similarly to their priest or rabbinical counterparts. Ulema is the term for an Islamic scholar, though no one such scholar is thought to have more authority than others [17].

Assisted reproductive technology

Before commencing the core examination of religion and sex, one additional overview is necessary: the context for ART. Within the various concepts about sex and religion, ART is by far the newest. Originating in 1978 with the birth of the first "test tube" baby, Louise Brown, ART has only been around for a short time. This historic event occurred when Robert Edwards, an embryologist, and Patrick Steptoe, an obstetrician-gynecologist, joined together to create the first human embryo outside of the body (in vitro), transfer it back to the uterus, resulting in a live birth. Though the procedure had been tried before, none of the attempts resulted in a living baby. In the 1940s, two earlier researchers, John Rock, MD and Miriam Menkin, MA, were able to prove that embryos could be created in vitro [18]. This new technology enabled those that were unable to conceive an option for parenthood.

Over the next 42 years, the technologies and processes within ART have continued to advance, presenting more feasible options for those diagnosed with infertility or socially infertile.[2] ART positively affects many different reproductive issues, such as: people with low ovarian reserve, or who don't produce ova, may use donor eggs; people with low, impaired, or no sperm may use donor sperm; embryos may be created by intended parents and implanted within a surrogate's uterus; test blastocysts may be used to determine chromosomal anomalies within a cell line; gametes may be retrieved and preserved for future use; and mitochondria from a donor may be used to eradicate disease within an egg from an intended mother. These advancements, and more, continue to push the envelope in terms of what is seen as ethical and moral within a society as well as within religious groups [19,20].

Judeo-Christian views on sexuality and sex

Before looking at Judeo-Christian perspectives on ART, it is imperative to first understand how each religion views sex and procreation. All three religious perspectives include prohibitions regarding premarital sex as well as the assumption that sex is between a man and a woman. In the Old Testament, sex is not referred to overtly, but rather obliquely as "to lie with," "to sleep with," or "knowing" (hence the colloquialism of "know them in the Biblical sense"). The ancient text was first translated into Greek and eventually English. Through the various

---

[2] Social infertility refers to circumstances such as being a single parent by choice or someone that identifies as LGBTQ+ and might not have within a partnership all of the components necessary for spontaneous reproduction.

iterations the original meaning can be modified or even lost, and so euphemisms emerged instead. One can surmise that the original authors were also uncomfortable using plain language to describe anatomy or acts [21].

An additional context to consider is that most religions are patriarchal in nature and have a vested interest in matters of kinship as well as inheritance or property. This lens complicates the perspective of sex as most instances are spoken from a male point of view or how the female is seen *in relation* to the male, just as humans are viewed as subservient to G-d. For example, Genesis 2:18–2:25 recounts the process in which Adam was given a companion by G-d,

> **18** The Lord God said, "It is not good for the man to be alone. I will make a helper suitable for him." **19** Now the Lord God had formed out of the ground all the wild animals and all the birds in the sky. He brought them to the man to see what he would name them; and whatever the man called each living creature, that was its name. **20** So the man gave names to all the livestock, the birds in the sky and all the wild animals. But for Adam[3] no suitable helper was found. **21** So the Lord God caused the man to fall into a deep sleep; and while he was sleeping, he took one of the man's ribs[4] and then closed up the place with flesh. **22** Then the Lord God made a woman from the rib[5] he had taken out of the man, and he brought her to the man. **23** The man said, "This is now bone of my bones and flesh of my flesh; she shall be called 'woman,' for she was taken out of man." **24** That is why a man leaves his father and mother and is united to his wife, and they become one flesh. **25** Adam and his wife were both naked, and they felt no shame [22].

From a literalist perspective, woman is made from man and the last sentence makes the point that the human body, stripped of adornments, was not something about which to feel shame. Shame was felt only after eating from the tree of knowledge in the next chapter, which also set up the hierarchy (see below) of:

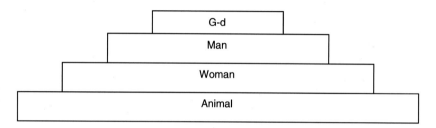

As Judaism served as the outline for Christianity and Islam, the internalization of nakedness and shame growing into sex being shameful can be seen as a natural extension. While the Old Testament doesn't speak about sex directly, much of the beginnings of Genesis speak to parentage, which is, until the time of Abram, spoken as those who fathered children rather than as pairs of people. This clearly emphasized the importance of patrilineal descent. The Old Testament spells out the importance specifically of a woman's virginity, which can be tied to ensuring that only a man's actual children (i.e., sons) will stand to inherit both his name and his riches, and that bastard children will be separated out [21]. Thus virgin girls are considered more of a "prize" than their nonvirgin counterparts. This is a perspective that continues to the current day and is found across many faiths. Within the more adherent factions of all three religious' groups, virginity at marriage, for both sexes, continues to be both an expectation and a virtue as it demonstrates a strong faith in G-d and one's commitment to following the faith's traditions and teachings with regard to sexual intercourse.

The Old Testament specifies what sexual relationships are considered godly versus those that are considered forbidden. The sexual sins of adultery and desiring a woman who belongs to another man, take prominence within the Ten Commandments (Commandments 7 and 10, respectively: "Thou shalt not commit adultery" and "Thou shalt not covet".) [21].

There are standing arguments pointing to biblical text citations condemning same-sex attraction. Initial citations include Leviticus Chapter 18 verse 22 ("You shall not lie with a male as with a woman; it is an abomination.") [22] and Chapter 20 verse 13 ("If a man lies with a male as with a woman, both of them have committed an abomination; they shall be put to death; their blood is upon them.") [22]. One nonliteral interpretation offers that this was important due to cleanliness and hygiene practices in ancient times, whereas another suggests that this was the role for Jews, who adhere to the Old Testament, but not for Christians who adhere to the New Testament, which sets aside a New Kingdom [23,24]. It should be noted that within the texts, homosexuality is

---

[3] Or *the man*.

[4] Or *part of the man's sides*.

[5] Or *part*.

described solely within the framework of gay relationships and is silent in terms of lesbian relationships. Interpretations relate to the patriarchal system established within the Bible and Torah. In addition, this interpretation of Leviticus separated Judaism from other religions that were focused on more of a cult basis or the worship of many gods and embraced homosexual activity. Islam has a formal term for illicit sexual acts: zina. Included as zina is anything outside of heterosexual sex within a marriage as well as adultery. Unlike both Judaism and Christianity, in Islam, there is no confessional model, thus no place to unburden oneself of such a secret [25].

It is in service and advantageous to all religions to promote heterosexual relationships. Without them, faith groups fail to gain adherents. Catholicism sets forth three guidelines for sex, that it is: unitive, procreative, and voluntary. According to Reverend Schaefer, "Therefore, sex that is casual and doesn't create a bond is not unitive, nor is any sex that happens outside the marital bond, because marriage is how two become 'one flesh.' Sex that uses birth control is not procreative (which is understood as being open to procreation, not requiring that every act of intercourse result in a pregnancy). In the same way, homosexual sex was often rejected because it could not be procreative. And finally, rape, abuse, etc. are not appropriate expressions of sexuality because they are not voluntary" [26].

As more progressive arms of each religion have adapted to the cultural and societal changes that modernity offers, the view on sex has become somewhat more flexible. Developing a religious context for sexual pleasure is based upon embracing sexual pleasure, looking at sex as part of the larger religious context, and creating rules within religious observance that sanction sex [27]. While even the most progressive sects wouldn't encourage unsafe sexual practices outright or condone casual sex, they might be more likely to refrain from passing judgment. This extends to views on same-sex relationships, though in this instance, the progressive wings of religions are explicit in their support of same-sex relationships. Another relationship in which religions are less vocal about is solo relationships (which would incorporate masturbation), looking at them as a way for people to experience the pleasure that their own body is capable of feeling.

Orthodox Judaism prepares new brides by teaching them about sex and sexuality. The specific teacher will have oversight on the curriculum in which she[6] uses, and whether or not she explicates beyond sex for procreative purposes, or if she teaches about how a woman's own body can be a source of pleasure. Orthodox men receive premarital counseling as well that focuses on the halachic matters related to marriage, typically contained in the Talmud. Some teachers also discuss female anatomy and sexual response but there is no standardized curriculum, leading to uneven outcomes. In Orthodoxy, there is a paradox between sexual urges, which are not seen as permissible versus sex within a marriage, which is considered to be a mitzvah or commandment [28]. The Talmud has sections that are evocative in terms of citing what sexual positions are permissible between a married couple, though their interpretations are anything but explicit. Typically, the understanding is that the husband is the one who controls these interactions. In Orthodox Judaism, masturbation is prohibited by the Torah, as it results in "wasting seed" or semen unable to be given the opportunity to be procreative, which was taken from Genesis 38:8–10, the story of Onan [22]. Different Talmudic rabbis have varying interpretations about what is considered to be a waste of seed, and interestingly, as long as masturbation is not being practiced, all types of penetrative sex are permitted, which seems to be in direct conflict with the words of the Torah, but perhaps accounts for attempts over the centuries to modernize [29]. In fact, the ketubah (the legal marriage contract within Judaism) explicitly repeats Talmudic law in which the husband must sleep with his wife "regularly for her pleasure and benefit" [29].

Surveys of Evangelical Christian practitioners also view most sex acts as permissible, with the caveat that each member of the couple consents, thus ensuring that both spouses have a voice as to what is explored sexually. There is a shift from the viewpoint that sex is a means to an end (thus procreative) to the sense that in and of itself can be seen as almost a spiritual journey. Thus, there can be a wide berth of acceptability of what can happen within the sanctity of a union of marriage. However, most people have been taught within their religious contexts that sex is "sinful," which can be a difficult framework to extricate oneself from to the more open framework of sexual enjoyment [27]. This is considered to be the "inhibition paradox" in which sex is tied to negative messages from religious authorities and practitioners are then expected to fully embrace sex once part of a marital union [27].

The United Methodist Church (UMC) is an example of how Christianity has evolved thinking and continues to balance values and morals found within sacred texts. The UMC's Revised Social Principles (2020) speak to

---

[6] Such teachers are called kallah teachers, as "kallah" is Hebrew for "bride," and take classes themselves to conduct the training. Many are married to rabbis, and all are cisgender women.

human sexuality as a gift and values intimacy as equal to celibacy as both are valid choices. The Principles further promote marriage, but also recognize the necessity of divorce, and view all forms of gender and sexual expression as meaningful ones. In such ways, the UMC seems to be threading the needle of working to keep consistency in their practices while also adapting to a changing culture [30].

Pre-Cana (Cana meaning marriage) is the formalized process of premarital counseling within the Catholic Church that began in the 1970s as a way to combat climbing divorce rates. Though a couple does not need to seek out Pre-Cana specifically, it is recommended that some kind of premarital counseling occurs. Within Pre-Cana, US bishops require education around family planning [31].

Within the world of Islam, sex can be a sign of religious commitment. Often, there is a Western perpetuated myth through the media that, within Islam, women are seen as subservient (sexually and otherwise) to men, yet within the actually practicing culture, sexuality is seen as part and parcel of being human [32]. The definition provided by Hiber and Colombini sums up an important way to consider sexuality:

> Sexuality is a central aspect of being human throughout life and encompasses sex, gender identities and roles, sexual orientation, eroticism, pleasure, intimacy and reproduction. Sexuality is experienced and expressed in thoughts, fantasies, desires, beliefs, attitudes, values, behaviors, practices, roles and relationships. While sexuality can include all of these dimensions, not all of them are always experienced or expressed. Sexuality is influenced by the interaction of biological, psychological, social, economic, political, cultural, ethical, legal, historical and religious and spiritual factors [33].

The practice of Islam is not only that of a religion with specific theology, but also as a means in which to live one's everyday life. A Muslim marriage contains the concept of *Nikah*, a marriage contract in which is explicated the ways that sexuality is expected to be expressed within the framework of the marriage. The contract can contain parts that are legally sanctioned as well as morally so and tends to contain two additional concepts: *Tamk'n* (the wife's submission) and *Nafaqa* (maintenance) [32].

More seems to be written within the Sunni perspective about sexuality than from the Shi'a point of view. There is a framework within Muslim texts that speaks to the importance of sexual drives or instincts in particular, managing these aspects of being human. One Imam (Ghazali) believes that sexual instinct should only be used to perpetuate the social order and for social health. Additionally, sexual instinct is thus used as a way to serve Allah as its main goal is not pleasure, but reproduction [34]. *Tamk'n*, though considered to be the wife's submission, might also be thought of as a pathway of worshiping Allah, and to do so, the act must be given of one's own volition, as to not be consensual would be a rebuke to Allah rather than a way of showing praise [35]. Research continues to positively support the connection between marital commitment and satisfaction with religiosity [36,37]. Inherent to *Nafaqa* appears to be this principle. Being a more legalistic religion, rather than guided by complex theology, Islam seems to be a religion of being and doing [38].

For many Muslims, there is no formal counseling or meetings to discuss expectations for a marriage outside of the *Nikah*. In some cases (seen to be the exception, rather than the rule), couples will meet with an imam, and these meetings reportedly consist of looking at what living a faith-based life will look like for the couple [39]. Unlike within Orthodox Judaism or Catholicism, there is no Islamic curriculum to pull from, so whatever teachings are based upon the Qur'an are not necessarily consistent outside of that text.

Judeo-Christian views of homosexuality and status

There is a group of practitioners from various religious homes that, up until recently, have been absent in the conversation about reproduction: LGBTQ+ individuals and couples. Herein lies a challenge when two parts of an individual's identity are not able to work in concert with one another: their faith and their sexuality. Inherent to faith-based members who also identify as gay or lesbian is the challenge to reconcile these two parts, which can be complicated by not only the messages within their religious texts, but also how the community internalizes these messages. As previously mentioned, most religions offer biblical citation of Genesis and Leviticus as a way to justify homophobic viewpoints or condemning this identity as being "against G-d." However, there are people who consider themselves to have both a strong faith and belong to the LGBTQ+ community.

The 21st century has brought about unprecedented legal protections and validation for Lesbian and Gay people, including in 2015, the monumental American Supreme Court decision in Obergefell v. Hodges declaring equality in marriage [40]. This case demonstrated how public sentiment and opinion towards LGBTQ+ -identified people has dramatically changed, which was also helped by progressive religions willing to condone and celebrate LGBTQ+ unions. There continues to be pushback from more conservative religious points of view, as evidenced by the delicate balance between religious rights and LGBTQ+ rights, such as Masterpiece Cakeshop v. Colorado Civil Right Commission, where the American Supreme Court ruled narrowly for the petitioner saying they could refuse service to those that strayed from their religious viewpoints [41,42]. Even within religious persuasions, viewpoints on LGBTQ+ can be nuanced.

Judaism, as previously discussed, has several denominations within it and, unsurprisingly, each sees homosexuality through a different lens. The Reconstructionist, Reform, and even Conservative movements all express a welcoming posture towards LGBTQ+ individuals and, as a formal position, are affirming. This affirmation includes marriage equality [43–45]. The formal positions have evolved within each grouping at different points in time, with the Reform and Reconstructionist groups having a longer history of inclusivity [46]. Within the Orthodox community however, LGBTQ+ inclusion can be a vastly different picture.

Typically, Orthodox Judaism is thought of and viewed as a singular grouping of people. However, there are at least two separate groupings that are worth discussing separately: the Ultra-Orthodox and the Modern Orthodox. Modern Orthodoxy works to maintain traditional Jewish practices while also embracing living amidst a modern cultural context and is considered to be a minority within a minority. Both communities signed onto a joint statement affirming that those that identify as LGBTQ+ should be treated with respect as a fellow human being, though were unable to condone sexual practices or unions for those that identify as nonheterosexual, coming back to the text of the Torah [47]. However, some of the Hassidic (a branch of Ultra-Orthodox practice) rabbis chose to abstain from signing at all [48]. There is a line that is towed: certain sexual acts are seen as forbidden, however as the idea of an "orientation" is outside of the Torah's purview, one is able to confer that identity upon oneself [49].

Though homosexuality is not condoned, within the Modern Orthodox context, individuals who come out as homosexual are more likely to be accepted and included by their immediate families. That being said, the communal view might not match the family's view, and the heteronormative expectation around procreation makes continuing to live as a Modern Orthodox Jewish individual extremely difficult. In the Ultra-Orthodox community, gay men (especially) either try to "pass" as heterosexual including potentially getting married to a member of the opposite sex and keep their homosexual identity a secret or choose to leave the community [48]. The latter is seen as a tremendous loss as most of one's support and livelihood is self-contained within the Ultra-Orthodox community. It also might mean the loss of family, as Ultra-Orthodox parents of an "out" child have difficulty understanding this concept of sexuality, as within Orthodoxy, there is an expectation and norm of heterosexuality. If one is not heterosexual, then they are unable to follow the provisions of the Torah [50].

Coming from a framework that the Bible is the literal word of G-d makes condoning sexual orientations and nonconforming behavior outside of heterosexuality a near impossibility. The tendency, from religiously conservative communities, is to use the original words of G-d and attempt to adapt to a modern context around these scriptures [49]. The United Nations General Assembly put forth a statement that condemned all forms of violence taken against those within the LGBTQ+ community [51]. As a response, the Catholic Church, under Pope Francis, worked to toe the line between decrying violence and the subjugation of people as well as defining what can be condoned within the faith. This balance essentially affirmed that Catholics were able to self-identify as lesbian or gay, but sexual actions along these identities would not be accepted. Thus, LGBTQ+ people, in order to preserve their Catholic faith and their sexual identity, would need to live a life of celibacy [52]. This statement was not without reverberations: applauded by other sects of Christianity with an originalist text focus and decried by those that adhere to a more contemporary focus. While attitudes, even within more conservative communities, have trended positively in views of LGBTQ+ individuals, religious institutions walk a precarious balance [53].

Similar to its more textualist cousins, Islam gives "hegemonic status to heterosexuality" as all of its sources for religious thought and dialogue are explicit in their disapproval of homosexuality [54,55]. It cites similar passages in the Old Testament, particularly the story of Lut (Lot) and his experiences as G-d was about to destroy the City of Sodom, as told in Genesis, 19:1–8. Lot has a conversation with the townsmen who noticed he took in two angels of G-d. Lot tries to discourage the townspeople from having sexual relations with the angels, offering up his daughters instead [22,56].

This singular story has permeated not only within Islam, but within the culture of Muslim-majority countries as the principle of heterosexism remains the unassailable norm, and intolerant views of homosexuality are seen to be valid based upon the religious view, as it is spoken in both the Qur'an and the Hadith [57]. Additionally, Sharia defines homosexuality as a crime where the punishment can range depending upon the disruption to the social order (i.e., if the perpetrator was married, this is seen as worse than if both were single) [57]. Similar to

Christianity and Orthodox Judaism, the overarching view around homosexuality in Islam is that it is "unnatural" and goes against "the natural order" G-d prescribed of one man and one woman [58].

It would make sense to address the potential psychological harm that can come from disparities in one's sexual identity and one's religious identity. This kind of cognitive dissonance has a particular name: spiritual cognitive dissonance (SCD), coined in 1957 by Leon Festinger [59]. As in all types of cognitive dissonance, there is a sense of inner disharmony between two thoughts or experiences or especially between two closely held beliefs. SCD has been shown to contribute to depression, anxiety, suicidal ideation, self-loathing, feelings of social exclusion, or posttraumatic stress disorder: all of which cause significant suffering for an individual [60,61]. It makes sense that an individual might go to great lengths in which to eradicate this dissonance, the process of which can be painful. Examples of problem solving, or minimizing the felt cognitive dissonance include: mixed orientation marriages [50]; conversion therapy [58,62]; refusal to self-identify as gay [61]; self-isolation [55]; rejection of religious identity [48,49]; or the adherence to a new religious identity that doesn't come into conflict with the person's sexual orientation [63]. It is possible that LGBTQ+ people that also identify as a religious minority (such as Orthodox Jews) must also manage the mantle of being a double minority.

The Minority Stress Model[7] conceptualizes that those individuals that are part of "stigmatized social categories are exposed as a result of their social, often a minority, position" [64] and are thus more apt to suffer due to the reactions to their minority qualities from others (often nonminority members) in their environment. When using this framework of minority stress, it identifies a potentially exacerbated cause of stress: the actual interactions a person might have with heterosexism, prejudice, or stigmatization as well as the perceived and feared potential reactions that a person might encounter [64]. Again, these aspects can set up a person of minority status to have mental health and physical issues as a result of their social stressors. Interestingly, cognitive dissonance might also impact family members upon a person's "coming out." They too, might need to figure out how, if at all, to reconcile the perception of their kin going against the family's faith. This can cause families to react in several distinct ways: they might shun their family member in order to keep ties with scripture or religious doctrine; they might see the text as not applicable to their particular family member or situation; or they attempt to question the family member to assist in relieving the dissonance by "mending" the gayness [49]. In this context, "mending" can be seen as cognitively (or in practice) figuring out a way to remove their family member's sexual identity as if it were a spot on a garment.

From all three of these major religious perspectives, the primary argument (outside of citing scripture or religious sources) against homosexuality is that it fails to continue to perpetuate the species. From a religious point of view, it also then fails to add more future adherents to the faith. Prior to the advancement and discovery of ARTs, this could be seen as a somewhat valid argument. Yet, even for heterosexual couples that struggle to conceive, religion proves to be mixed on how it interprets the storied line in Genesis (9:1) "G-d blessed Noah and his sons, and said to them, 'Be fruitful and increase, and fill the earth.'" [56].

Judeo-Christian perspectives on infertility and assisted reproduction

Infertility in the Old Testament

The Old Testament is filled with stories of both fertility and infertility, and the ancient solutions proposed, in many ways, mirror some of today's options. Yet religious responses to infertility vary greatly, and as technology continues to advance, the questions around ethics, suitability, and textual basis continue to swirl. Many cite the shorthand of the famous quote from Genesis, "Be fruitful and multiply" as the mandate that speaks to G-d's will in terms of procreating. Certainly, there are many questions that can be asked if difficulty should occur in the attempts at procreation vis-a-vis one's relationship with G-d, for if conception and family building are G-d's will, then why do some people struggle with infertility?

To attempt to answer this question, it is useful to look at the Old Testament and what it might say about family building. Much of the beginning of Genesis serves as a genogram before the reader is ever even introduced to Abram (the birth name that the nation building patriarch was given, prior to his circumcision, thus conversion to Judaism where he was conferred the name Abraham). In the background of Genesis, readers learn of G-d's great power and will: from the destruction of Sodom to both fertility and infertility on G-d's whim, as "G-d healed

---

[7] The Minority Stress Model, as it was proposed by Richard Lazarus and Susan Folkman, speaks to race as the stressor and has since been expanded to include other minority groups.

Abimelech and his wife and his slave girls, so that they bore children; for the LORD had closed fast every womb of the household of Abimelech because of Sarah, the wife of Abraham" (Genesis 21:17–18) [56]. In the next verse, we learn of Sarah's advanced maternal age (thus the cause of her infertility) and yet, because of G-d's will, she is able to bear Abraham a son, Isaac. While Abraham's age is noted as 100, the Old Testament seems to infer that the cause of childlessness rested with Sarah. The miracle to be known was that Sarah was able to create life from her body to fulfill G-d's promise that Abraham would be the father of a great nation, and thus, trusting in G-d enables dreams to come true. Previously, Abraham had impregnated a servant, Hagar (the first documented surrogate), in order to continue his line. It seems that the first infertile couple had come to this decision (at G-d's suggestion) together, but once Sarah bore Isaac, the extended family arrangement became tenuous, and Sarah wanted Hagar and her son Ishmael to leave their house. Abraham manages this moral conflict (having to choose between his sons) with another promise of G-d: his son Ishmael will lead a separate nation, as he was from Abraham's "seed" [56].

Infertility seems to have a generational component when it comes to Abraham's lineage: as Isaac and his wife Rebekah also struggled to conceive. The Old Testament specifically elucidates that Rebekah was barren until G-d intervened after Isaac's prayer, enabling her to conceive twins. One of these twins, Jacob, has an arranged marriage with two sisters: Rachel and Leah. As Leah was the elder daughter, she was given first to Jacob, though he had assumed that his work for her father, Laban, would be to betroth Rachel. After seven more years of labor, Jacob was awarded Rachel as a second wife. Genesis states (29:31–35) that Leah was "unloved and he [G-d] opened her womb; but Rachel was barren" and continues to outline her conceiving four sons for Jacob. Rachel understandably felt jealous of her sister's fertility and begged her husband to impregnate her. Jacob, perhaps from family lore, knew the answer to Rachel's infertility would be in G-d's hands, not his. The couple agreed on a traditional surrogacy[8] arrangement with one of Rachel's maids, and in this arrangement, she bore two sons for Jacob and Rachel. As this worked, Rachel then engaged for a second traditional surrogacy relationship to unfold, from which two more sons were born. This relationship seemed to be different than that of Abraham and Hagar, as Rachel raised these boys as her own, whereas Hagar, rather than Sarah, raised Ishmael. Though Leah had appeared to be barren after conceiving four sons, she later gave birth to three more children: two more sons and a daughter. At this point, Genesis speaks to (30:22–24) G-d "remember[ing] Rachel; G-d heeded her and opened her womb. She conceived and bore a son, and said, 'G-d has taken away my disgrace.'" [56]. For Rachel, the ability to bear her own child that came from her genetic line, rather than the experience of raising children, was the validation she needed of her own worth.

The themes of infertility and jealousy are repeated and go hand in hand within the Old Testament. Another often cited story is the one of Hannah, one of the wives of Elkanah (his second wife being Peninnah). Biblical code for infertility is a "closed womb," which was the plight of Hannah, whereas Peninnah had children. Hannah's jealous feelings were exacerbated by the taunting she endured by Peninnah, who is framed to be Hannah's rival. Hannah weeps to the priest, Eli, who understands her grief as drunkenness and confronts her. Upon returning home, Hannah is said to have conceived Samuel, who she will later offer up to G-d as thanks (I Samuel, 1; 1–28) [56]. The story of Hannah is the most elucidated story of infertility as it includes the multitude of emotions and remedies to try to cure the ailment [65]. The Old Testament seems to assume that difficulties with conception are universally female factor issues. The one exception to this is spoken as a law within the section of Deuteronomy 25:5–10 that speaks to what shall happen to a widow upon her husband's death prior to the couple bearing a son, is that she shall marry the brother of her husband [56]. This section infers the potential cause of infertility as being male-factor, and the pull to have a child (and one who maintains the genetic and inheritance line) is strong enough to suggest that the woman remarry her brother-in-law. This harkens back to the story of Onan and in addition to the spilling of seed, speaks to inheritance [65].

These are the more storied depictions of fertility within the Old Testament and they amount to the following proclamations around infertility that reverberate within the present-day landscape and the availability of ART. It is notable that G-d makes the promise of fertility to the Jews seven separate times in Genesis [65]. This general command ("Be fruitful and multiply") has also been etched into the ethos of both Christianity and Islam, and has been expanded not only from a commandment, but also framed as a blessing. Thus, doing G-d's will means to procreate, and a failure to do so, intimates that one is cursed, or willingly choosing to not walk the path of G-d. With this as a background, it might make more sense to look at the biblical roadblocks that an Orthodox Jewish couple might conceptualize or perceive when facing the inability to conceive on their own.

---

[8] Traditional surrogacy refers to the practice of the oocyte and surrogate being the same person, thus the genetic connection is between the surrogate and the man who has impregnated her.

Navigating Jewish infertility

When a Jewish Orthodox couple passes the threshold of a reproductive endocrinologist's office, in many ways, they carry what other patients that might be in the waiting room also hold: fear, nervousness, and hope. However, in addition to these emotional areas, Orthodox Jews are also carrying with them the laws of Torah and the spirit of Niddah (family purity laws), that might directly come into opposition with advice they might be given about the life they are trying to create. In terms of the physician's role within Orthodox Judaism, doctors are seen primarily as healers, and their duty is to preserve life. However, infertility is seen as a medical ailment in need of healing, so treatment can be permissible [66]. It is important to note is that there is no universal teaching or prescription when it comes to various aspects of infertility treatment from a definitive source. Rather, individual rabbis take into consideration various factors and will provide advice based upon the data that they have collected (usually from the religious texts, the individual couple's circumstance, Halacha, and other rabbinical opinions on the topic). Therefore, on how close a couple's treatment might match a clinic's typical standard protocols will also depend on the specific rabbi [67].

Some overall nuances that a physician might experience with Orthodox couples relate to when they are available for treatment. Shabbat (sunset on Friday night into sunset on Saturday evening) is a literal time of rest, as it is stated within the creation story in the Torah. Orthodox Jews will refrain from using electronics, cars, transportation (other than walking), the exchange of money, and many other practices that are seen as commonplace on other days of the week. Rather, they spend that time with family and at a synagogue, in prayer. Thus, Shabbat will be a time when, even if treatment necessitates, an Orthodox couple will likely be unable to comply. This would extend to monitoring basal body temperature, the use of ovulation testing kits, as both were seen to disobey the prohibition against work on the Sabbath [68]. These prohibitions will be the same for other Jewish holidays and celebrations, which might (especially in the Fall, which has a cycle of several Holy Days and festivals) mean that treatment must be postponed. Another timing issue that Orthodox Jews will be aware of is when they might be within the menstrual cycle.

Separate from the yearly calendar, there is a part of Halacha that includes monthly visits to the Mikveh (ritual bath) at the end of the menstrual cycle. Preparation includes checking oneself for blood once menstruation has ceased and looking for the cloth to be unstained for a consecutive week. During this time (called Niddah), the couple goes to great lengths to avoid all touching one another, including separating their beds as well as with the passing of food. Touch (including sexual relations) can resume once the woman has immersed herself at the Mikveh and is considered to be "clean." At this point, it is a mitzvah (or "good deed") for the couple to have sexual relations [69]. Another potential complication is if a woman bleeds after a self-examination for cleanliness, the "clock" resets for the full 7-day consecutive cycle of no blood in the cloth [68]. If peak fertility occurs during niddah, a rabbi would have to grant permission for treatments to proceed, as all sexual contact is to be ceased [66,68,69]. A couple might need a rabbi to weigh in if any kinds of testing or treatment during niddah might cause bleeding (an event that is exceedingly rare, but not impossible) in terms of what the path forward would look like while retaining ritual purity [70].

The physical examination process by a physician might proceed a bit differently than it could with other couples. First, the woman will be examined, though oftentimes for nonobservant Jews or those of other faiths, the recommendation might be to have a semen analysis prior to initiating invasive testing on the female. An Orthodox couple will want to abstain from any semen collection as it is seen as forbidden under the rules of Halacha for a man to "waste seed" [66,68]. (This is based upon the story of Onan in Genesis 38.7–10, as he refused to impregnate the widow of his brother, who was childless, and from here, it was extrapolated that "spilling seed" or masturbating was unconscionable [56,68].) Obtaining a sperm sample (without rabbinic approval) can be done through post-coital testing, whereas the sperm is collected within a nonspermicidal condom, as the sex act (versus masturbation) is in line with adherence to the teachings of the Torah and Talmud [68]. A second workaround can be found in using a specific condom that has a hole at the base, so that while it is possible for sperm to potentially reach an egg, the condom can also secure a sample while the couple is able to engage within the spirit and letter of the religious laws [66].

A second aspect to consider when evaluating an Orthodox man who might potentially be suffering from male factor infertility is how to conduct a testicular biopsy, should that be necessary. The conflict comes from a passage in Deuteronomy (23.2) that renders both a castrated man or a eunuch as unable to enter the synagogue, or "congregation of G-d" [56,70]. Scholars have debated whether an incision, such as what might be necessary for testicular sperm extraction (TESE), would technically render a man as castrated. Continued debate looks at whether a healed incision would be seen as restoring the sense of fertility, thus the technique of micro-TESE may be considered to be halachically acceptable [70].

An issue that can frequently occur is when two (or more) of the commandments are in conflict with one another, such as "be fruitful and multiply" and "thou shalt not murder" (Exodus 20.13) [56]. This would be the case (in theory) for disposition of unused embryos. In this instance, Jews believe that life doesn't begin (meaning that a person isn't ensouled) until 40 days after conception (prior to that, it is considered to be water) [71]. Thus, at this point, discarding unused embryos would not constitute murder, as an embryo is not yet a person [71]. For less stark commandments (such as not being able to observe Sabbath or denying treatment), "be fruitful and multiply" is often cited as the commandment that trumps others, and so there is a possibility that a rabbi might give his proverbial blessing to allow treatment to continue. That being said, modifying the protocol and cycle using birth control to ensure Halachic purity is another medical option [72].

To ensure that embryos, which are created using a couple's own gametes, stay safe, a variety of steps are suggested so that the containment of the embryos follows a strict chain of possession and can be proven to be that of the couple, as not to confuse potential inheritance concerns that might arise. Such steps might be having a mashgiach (halachic or spiritual supervisor) oversee all laboratory procedures and ensure that the lab itself is kept within halachic standards [73]. Ensuring that embryologists, lab technicians, and others that might be handling gametes are labeling samples correctly and placing them within the correct cryopreservation containers would be another way of overseeing the process to protect against an error which would result in a nonbiological child to one of the parents, which would be the religious equivalent to adultery [73].

Navigating a path forward can become more complicated if the need for donor gametes presents itself, and here again there might be conflict within two pieces of Jewish law: the strong tenet to procreate which comes against the idea of inheritance. Prior to the availability of ART, couples would be allowed to divorce if a child was unable to be conceived within a decade of the marriage. This is one of the rare occurrences where Jewish law allows for something typically forbidden, in order to fulfill a commandment, showing the importance of procreation to the religion [71]. Indeed, as an alternative to using donor gametes, a couple would be allowed to divorce to attempt procreation with a new partner.

Using donated sperm is the perceived equivalent to adultery—an expressed prohibition within the Torah—as it is seen as a child born out of wedlock, even if socially being raised by the married couple. There are future oriented concerns for the marital relationship in raising a child that does not bear a genetic relationship to both parents. A second potential problem with donor eggs or sperm is of genetic lineage: children would not know fully their own genetic information and history, which is seen as a potential issue around identity for that child. An additional issue is that according to Talmudic law, the sperm donor, and not the intended father, would be considered the father of the offspring, raising concern about inheritance [11,66]. This is especially problematic if the surname of a couple is either Cohen or Levi, as those surnames are derived from the priestly class of biblical times [66].

Judaism is a rare religion where matrilineal descent is considered important. This goes back to the Torah, and the story of Rachel and Leah, where Rachel was carrying a girl while Leah was carrying a boy, and these fetuses were exchanged so that Rachel mothered Joseph, while Leah mothered Dinah. The concern about a sexual relationship outside of marriage is also eradicated with ovum donation, as no extramarital "sex" can occur, converse to donor insemination [66]. The Mishnah is clear that a person who begins an action, must complete it, so from this teaching, rabbis will confer that a Jewish woman who bears a child (thus both beginning and completing an action) is seen as the mother, regardless of the genetic origins of the ova that was used to create that child [11]. According to Jewish law and tradition, that child would be born as a Jew, based upon matrilineal descent. In order to ensure that marriages remain intact, it would be essential for the donor to be unmarried [11].

As with all donor scenarios, the idea of consanguinity bears importance, and perhaps more so, given that Orthodox Jews tend to be a more insular community that marries within itself. However, using donor gametes might also be seen as a way to solidify the love and respect that a couple holds for one another given the lengths they would go to in order to fulfill the commandment of procreation [74]. Once again, for a couple to use donor gametes, it would be important to have the blessing of a rabbi, who can understand that this route is one of a last resort, rather than one entered into initially [11,74].

Despite the halachic and marital factors in using donor gametes, it is widely suggested that couples using donor gametes *do not* keep this genetic secret from their children or from other family members [11]. Additionally, prior to taking this step, couples might want to talk through how they will manage the potential stress on their marriage as time goes by as well as to ascertain that both parties are truly consenting to going forward with using donor gametes [11]. Given the precedent set in the Old Testament, it would be assumed that

Judaism would give couples who needed to use a surrogate its blessing, but the reality takes some of the principles that have been discussed into consideration, making surrogacy a more complex process.

This chapter has already spoken of several biblical instances where a traditional surrogate arrangement was sanctioned so that a patriarch would be able to continue his lineage. Surprisingly, surrogate arrangements have several concerns that rabbis postulate and consider, making outright condoning of surrogacy not possible. As discussed, Judaism is a religion of matriarchal descent, which would thus (in the eyes of the religion) make the surrogate deemed the mother of the child she was carrying, even in the common cases where the surrogate has no genetic connection to the child. If the surrogate was married, the child born could be seen as the result of an adulterous relationship, which would give the child the distinction of being *mamzer* (illegitimate) [11,66]. Ways of overcoming such obstacles are to ensure that the embryo created is of the genetics from the intended parents. If there is a concern about the Jewish status of the child, they can be formally converted (a girl in the mikvah and for a boy, circumcision, just as would be done in an adoption context). A conversion would also sever genetic links [66]. Additionally, the surrogate should be single, divorced, or widowed to ensure that adultery is not a circumstance or context that can be perceived as the child being born into [11]. Finally, the surrogate should be Jewish, to ensure (without conversion) that the child is also Jewish [11].

Orthodox Judaism has some opinions around other aspects of reproductive technologies, such as preimplantation genetic testing for aneuploidy (PGT-A), cryopreservation, sex selection, embryo donation, and multiple pregnancy reduction and abortion. Beginning with PGT-A, an embryo that has yet to be implanted hasn't been conferred legal status as a person, as until the 41st day of gestation, an embryo is still considered to be "water" [11,66,74]. This enables embryos to be tested, cryopreserved, and would allow for an early abortion (though this becomes more complex as gestational age increases) [11,66,74]. PGT-A and genetic testing are widely encouraged within all of the Jewish community as there are specific genetic conditions that are prevalent, such as Tay-Sachs. In fact, many people undergo carrier screenings prior to marriage to ensure that the match is also genetically a good one [75].

One element to preimplantation genetic testing is the ability to test for sex. Sex selection is considered to be sanctioned by religious authorities within Judaism, as the Talmud seems to have its own instructions for conceiving a child of a particular sex [66]. There is a "requirement" for a Jewish man to have two children, one of each sex, but to fulfill the commandment of procreation, at least one son is needed [11]. In this instance (for family balancing), sex selection would not be considered out of bounds and in fact is condoned [66].

Embryo donation (as well as gamete donation) is considered to be a sacred responsibility, as a person is partnering not only with an intended family, but also with G-d [74]. Yet it can be seen as dichotomous: using donated gametes assists Jews in the commandment of procreation, yet donating one's own genetic material to others, isn't always seen as an in-kind arrangement. One argument for this uneven approach is that some tasks, particularly those that are ritual-bound, are a responsibility solely for Jews to partake in, whereas others are only appropriate for non-Jews to partake in [74]. Once again, to donate an embryo (as to receive a donated embryo), a couple would need to consult with their rabbi for specific guidance. Judaism doesn't necessitate the permanent freezing of embryos, but opinions are mixed within the Orthodox responsa (a written response from a religious authority, such as a rabbi, in order to answer a question or problem) when it comes to discarding embryos: some rabbis believe that cryopreservation for potential future children is important, others believe that embryos can be discarded if they will be unused, and donating unused embryos for scientific endeavors also yields mixed opinions [11,66,74]. However, with cryopreservation, the onus is on protecting the identity of the father for lineage and inheritance cohesion [11].

Finally, it is important to consider the stances of Judaism in issues of selective reduction of a multifetal pregnancy and abortion. Once again, discrepancies tend to follow within the political divisions that each sect of Judaism belies. Inside of Orthodoxy, there is a distinction as to when selective reduction or abortion can be practiced. Abortion on demand is never deemed to be a sanctioned action, and for multifetal reduction or a termination for medical reasons to ensue, specific principles must be evidenced, such as the life or health of the mother [11,66]. There have been instances when abortion has been mandated by a rabbi in order to save the life of a mother [66]. Additionally, abortion may be condoned if the health risk to the mother was one of mental health [66]. In a multifetal situation, both fetuses are seen to have equal rights, and only if one is considered to be a *rodef* (or aggressor) that threatens the growth of another, is this seen as ample justification to reduce the number [11,66]. Reduction is then decided based upon medical necessity, as the maximum number of fetuses should be left implanted [66]. As with so many other aspects of reproductive technology, specific decisions for a couple are often necessary to be made in consultation with their rabbi and, depending upon his points of view and the responsa he credits, will inform the path of treatment that a couple can continue upon. This being said, it is also not uncommon for couples to speak with several rabbis as a way to resolve tension between interpretations of the halachic value of certain procedures and their desire to be parents. This tactic of searching for a sympathetic spiritual advisor is a common thread through multiple religious perspectives as couples navigate a permission structure in which to build their families.

Infertility in the New Testament

In addition to the Old Testament, modern-day Christians also adhere to the stories and advice garnered from the New Testament, which has its own understanding about fertility. The backbone of Catholic theology lies within the structure of the nuclear family, seen as "domestic churches" within the larger body of the Church [70]. Within that structure, children are the "supreme gift of marriage" according to the Catechism of 2002 [76]. Marriage, in and of itself, is seen as an arrangement of G-d, thus a holy and sacred endeavor [70]. The Book of Matthew (19.6) regards marriage as "They are no longer two therefore, but one flesh" [77]. While procreation is the ultimate expression of a marriage, it is not the sole purpose for marriage. Couples should be able to give of themselves fully to their partner, thus there should not be any type of encumbrance within the sex act, which can yield difficulties when it comes to fertility testing of individuals [70,76].

References to infertility are not as frequent within the New Testament. There are only five explicit references that relate to infertility and potential ways of solving the problem of childlessness, two of which are stories of the New Testament's storied women. The first is found in Luke, Chapter 1:1–25, which tells the story of a priest named Zachariah and his wife Elizabeth, who were childless. Upon praying, Zachariah was visited by the angel Gabriel, who alerted him that his prayer had been heard and would be answered: G-d would grant the couple a son for them to call John [77]. However, Zachariah didn't believe this news, and as a result, was rendered mute [77]. Part of this story breaks with what had previously been instructive of what one might do should they experience infertility within the Old Testament, which followed the path of: infertility (in the form of being barren); acknowledgment of the pain this causes; taking action; meeting or communicating with G-d; conception; birth; and naming [78]. However, the New Testament, in this story, doesn't follow the previously laid out plans set up within the Old Testament. Rather, Elizabeth and Zachariah accepted their childlessness—it's not seen as a crisis—and looked at their age as the cause [79]. Additionally, the couple does not protest or acknowledge the pain that childlessness might have upon them. The couple did not seek out G-d's intervention, rather G-d, in the form of an angel, came to them. Another striking difference is that the infertility narratives within the Old Testament are centered around the women expressing their grief for not having a child, whereas in this story, Elizabeth plays a supporting role. However, the end of the path is similar: Elizabeth and Zachariah conceive, give birth, and name their child as a homage to G-d in gratitude [79].

Immediately following this story, comes the story of Mary, the mother of Jesus and the cousin of Elizabeth (Luke 1:26–80). The nuance of Mary is her conception absent sexual intercourse, and the subsequent virgin birth. Both Elizabeth (in her older age) and Mary (a virgin) were shown the power of G-d in their stories of conception, and reiterate that those who are faithful and believe will yield the rewards of G-d [79]. Interestingly, Mary was not seeking pregnancy. There is nothing in the passage that references her hopes for a child, and yet given the timeframe in which she lived, it is a safe expectation that this was a path she would go down. G-d's plan for Mary differed from that offered to the Hebrew Patriarchs, which was about nation building and lineage [79]. This story starts to lay groundwork on birth being the work of three: the father, mother, and G-d.

The next several references to barrenness (which continues to be the coded term for infertility) relate to Jesus' direct teachings. Later in Luke (23:26–31), while Jesus was on the cross, he spoke directly to the women: those with children and those that were childless.

> (28) Daughters of Jerusalem do not weep for me, but weep for yourselves and for your children. (29) For the days are surely coming when they will say, "Blessed are the barren, and the wombs that never bore, and the breasts that never nursed." (30) Then they will begin to say to the mountains, "Fall on us"; and to the hills, "Cover us." (31) For if they do this when the wood is green, what will happen when it is dry? [77].

This can be understood to highlight and show importance to those that typically aren't seen (both by society and perhaps within a religious organization): those without children. Perhaps it also serves as a contrast between the fertile and the infertile, whereas both have a place within heaven and within Christianity [79]. Additionally, Jesus *does not* make a promise to infertile women about future fertility, as previous stories within the Old Testament and the few in the New Testament demonstrate [80]. This might lay groundwork in the idea that one can be whole and be childless, and thus counter the notion that infertility is a result of G-d's disfavor [80].

Infertility is mentioned overtly in two other places within the New Testament: first in Hebrews 11:8—12, which seems to recapitulate Sarah's barrenness, and Abraham and Sarah's reward (the great nation born to them) as G-d promised in their son Isaac [77]. This section reiterates the importance of the belief in G-d, with the parallel that believers are the ones to whom G-d will deliver. The final place where infertility is overtly mentioned is in Galatians 4:27:

Rejoice, you childless one, you who bear no children,
burst into song and shout, you who endure no birth pangs;
for the children of the desolate woman are more numerous
than the children of the one who is married [77].

Galatians, in the same chapter, mentions the progeny of Abraham where one was born to a slave and the other to his legitimate wife. This chapter speaks in a dichotomy where both those that have children and those that don't (or can't) are seen to have a place before G-d. Directly after the quoted passage, Galatians goes on to talk about the importance of inheritance within the confines of marriage, which might be a holdover from ideas within the Old Testament, and sets up more evidence in how families should be formed: within marriage between a man and woman [77].

Where Christians and Catholics seem to struggle to navigate infertility and its treatment lies less within the New Testament, but instead within the Old Testament. Typically, the difficulties with treatments such as in vitro processes lie within ideas of the womb and the sacredness of that space. Two passages speak to the nature of the womb, Job 31:15, "Did not he who made me in the womb make them? And did not one fashion us in the womb?" and Psalm 139:13, "For it was you who formed my inward parts; you knit me together in my mother's womb." This is reiterated in Isaiah 44:2; 44:24; 46:3; 49:1; and 49:5. It tends to be sealed within Jeremiah 1:5 "Before I formed you in the womb I knew you, and before you were born I consecrated you; I appointed you a prophet to the nations." This passage in particular (as well as in combination with the aforementioned) solidifies the notion that the process of conception needs to occur in utero.

Navigating Christian infertility

A Catholic[9] couple embarking on a fertility journey may take some time before heading to see a reproductive endocrinology and infertility specialist (REI), first trying to resolve their infertility through the guidance of their OB/GYN and priest. Family building is seen as the "ultimate expression of G-d's love and grace" [81] and is especially painful for those with a strong faith background, as it can initially feel like a rebuke from the Almighty. In several devout Christian subgroups, life begins at the moment of conception (following the guidance within the passage above from Jeremiah), and conception needs the three parts of man, woman, and G-d. With this as a background, stepping into an REI's office, that might offer options outside of the realm of the expected "conception trinity," is extremely difficult. Churches include a heavy family focus, so seeking out support within that community can also be fraught [82].

Catholicism, in its system of beliefs set out by the *Donum Vitae* in 1987 (Respect for Human Life in Its Origin and on the Dignity of Procreation) and reaffirmed in 2008 in *Dignitas Personae* (The Dignity of a Person) articulates an opposition to IVF, as the procedure occurs outside of the sacrament of procreation as a marital act [83,84]. To take conception into a laboratory is seen as a rupture of the very nature of reproduction, as G-d is no longer that third party, but rather other humans are [83]. Remember, sex is seen by the Church as serving two functions: it is unitive and procreative; thus, methods of reproduction must meet both these standards [85].

Despite this, there are aspects of ART that are sanctioned by the Church, as long as the act can be considered unitive and procreative. Morally and religiously acceptable methods to assist with conception are: any medications that could enhance ovulation or other types of hormonal techniques, use of NaPro, natural procreative technology (which speaks to monitoring women's reproductive health), surgical interventions that will enhance opportunities for procreation, and perforated "collection" condoms that can collect semen during intercourse that can later be used for IUI [82,83]. Without the use of the specialty condoms, the Church prohibits IUI, as it takes the unitive piece away from procreation [86]. GIFT (gamete intrafallopian transfer) is also seen as a technology

---

[9] Catholicism will be used here as its writings on the topic of ART are the most extensive and can be seen as the most restrictive. Additionally, Catholicism is the most popular denomination amongst the Christian subsets, encompassing 50% of those that identify as Christian, according to the Pew Report in 2011.

that can be in line with the Church's teachings, as long as the sperm is transferred back within the woman's fallopian tube [87].

It is no surprise that the Catholic Church prohibits the use of donated eggs, sperm, or embryos. All of the above do not occur within the marriage (thus aren't unitive) and are outside of the marriage directly being procreative. Given that the Church believes that life begins at the moment of conception, and that the Church has an obligation to preserve the dignity of all people, such practices do not align with the dictums set forth in *Dignitas Persone* [84]. Accordingly, the Catholic Church opposes selective reduction and abortion [86]. Interestingly, abortion is not spoken about within the Bible, but the decision is based on these later decrees and statements [88].

Surrogacy within the views of the Catholic Church is black and white: it is a practice that is prohibited as it takes procreation away from the couple and G-d, it occurs outside of the marital relationship (with the introduction of a gestational carrier), and it is seen as doing harm to the eventual child that will be born [89]. While those that enter an altruistic surrogacy arrangement might mean no harm (for example, a woman undergoing chemotherapy, and her sister carrying the pregnancy on her behalf), there is a view that the child might suffer emotional harm in the form of confusion about their origin story [90]. Additionally, children might be worried about why their "birth mothers" gave them away [90]. Finally, surrogacy within the form of a commercial arrangement is also seen as exploitative as it is seen as akin to selling children [90].

The Catholic Church differs from Judaism, in that kinship is not such a strong value, that infertility would be acceptable grounds for divorce [83]. This paves the way for adoption as an acceptable form (as well as an encouraged route) for family building. Typically, couples prefer to adopt an infant that is similar to their own ethnicity and race, in order to approximate a sense of family blending and belonging [91]. However, it is not always possible to find a child that matches a couple's ethnicity or racial identity. Therefore some couples might need to reconsider what attributes are important for their future child. These children might differ from the fantasized version of what that child might look like. Some couples have an "ah-ha" moment when they learn that the path to adopting a child with special needs might yield quicker results to parenting [91].

For devout couples that choose not to adopt, utilizing more invasive technologies can contradict their belief system. There can be solace within the concept of "moral femininity" [83], which aligns an individual's gender and spiritual identity. This can empower a woman to feel solidified within her morality, as she has not only "talked the talk" but also "walked the walk." While this shift doesn't take away the pain that infertility can engender, it allows for a perspective that might assist in healing [83].

One final notable aspect is the Church's reaction to those that have children using any of the various ART methods. The Church adheres to ethics within science and, to that end, affirms its positions on ART [87]. However, the Church also acknowledges the imperfections that exist as a part of being human, and the power to be forgiven, especially within the Church setting. The Church would be able to forgive couples that use donors and ART outside of the condoned methodologies and would welcome the resulting children with open arms [87].

In many ways, Protestants straddle the middle when it comes to ART. There are no singular directives or specific ethical guidelines that inform the practice of assisted reproduction. Members of the Protestant designation can both participate with IVF practices or choose not to. Generally speaking, ART should be considered by married couples within the faith. Cryopreservation is not encouraged and selective reduction is not a condoned practice [86].

Infertility in the Qur'an

Islam, as previously mentioned, is guided by the Old and New Testaments in addition to the Qur'an. The Qur'an itself contains a few infertility stories. The first (which is also seen in the New Testament) is about the prophet Zachariah and his wife's inability to bear a child, which G-d intervenes in after Zachariah prays, and corrects the course, enabling them to become pregnant [92]. The Qur'an cites the tale of Abraham (as seen in the Old Testament), who also is granted parenthood after prayer to G-d. The Qur'an sees children as blessings from Allah, and childlessness underscores Allah's power and dominion, explicitly (42:49–50) "He bestows offspring to whom He wills and makes some individuals barren" [92]. Children are desirable, but not a human need. The choice to use medical systems to remedy infertility is something that is acceptable but not obligatory [92]. Additionally, parents that are childless are not viewed as wanting or lacking, in contrast to other perspectives [92]. Another important dictum of the Qur'an is: "The Holy Qur'an also says: And one of [Allah's] signs is, that

He has created for you mates from yourselves, that you may dwell in tranquility with them, and has ordained between you Love and Mercy" (Al-Roum: 21) [93].

Specifically, the Qur'an doesn't offer much more than the Old and New Testaments do in terms of examples of infertility. Rather, it reiterates these stories that reverberate within the earlier religions and offers additional guidance through fatwas (a ruling on a point of Islamic law given by a recognized authority) to think through modern technological advances. The Qur'an also highlights that marriage (and thus children) are between a husband and his wife. It should be noted that Islam is a religion where kinship (which determines paternity and property arrangements) is extremely important, and this can factor in decision-making for couples struggling with infertility [94]. The Qur'an affirms the importance of marriage (13:38), family formation (16:27, 42), and procreation (16:49—50) [86]. A further philosophical difference that Islam has, making it more similar to Judaism than Christianity, is its view about when life begins. In Islam, a developing fetus is not thought to be "ensouled" until the 120th day of gestation [86].

Fatwas that speak to a variety of points within the assisted reproductive continuum also vary between the Sunni and Shi'a traditions. Women who are infertile might be concerned about the trajectory of their marriage, as they might be seen as "damaged goods," which could justify a divorce [95]. This viewpoint is less religion-focused, but culturally dependent within countries with a Muslim majority. Fatwas (because of the variance between the subsects of Islam) can provide immense relief for couples struggling with infertility, or a clarity in the choice to stop treatments and become child free.

Navigating Muslim infertility (Sunni Muslims)

Sunni Muslims make up about 90% of all people that identify with Islam [86]. Two fatwas issued on assisted reproductive care are: Al-Azhar Religious Institution in Cairo, Egypt (1980) and that by the Islamic Fikh Council (based in Mecca, Saudi Arabia) in 1984 [86]. In addition to these fatwas, two guidelines have also been issued: one from the Organization of Islamic Medicine based in Kuwait in 1991 and the other from the Islamic Educational, Scientific and Cultural Organization in Rabat, Morocco in 2002 [86]. These four documents or decrees allow for all types of ARTs to be used as long as the couple is using their own gametes and the wife's body to implant an embryo that is created from those gametes [86]. Specifically, permitted is [94]:

- Interuterine insemination (with the husband's sperm);
- In vitro fertilization (as long as the egg is from the wife, and the sperm from the husband);
- Intracytoplasmic sperm injection (as long as the egg is from the wife, and the sperm from the husband);
- Cryopreservation of any excess embryos, eggs, or sperm (as long as the egg and sperm are from a married couple with the designation to be used later by that couple);
- Postmenopausal women can use their own cryopreserved embryo or oocytes (in combination with her husband's sperm);
- Preimplantation genetic testing of aneuploidy for couples that might be high risk for genetic anomalies within their potential offspring;
- Multifetal pregnancy reduction, since life does not begin at conception;
- Embryo research on excess embryos donated by a couple;
- Uterine transplantation (an emerging technique).

This list provides a wide berth of options for Sunni couples struggling with infertility. However, if couples try using their own gametes without success, they are considered at the end of their options for family building. All forms of third-party donation (sperm, egg, and embryo donation) are taboo, as sperm donation specifically is viewed akin to *zina* or adultery [92—94]. Any form of surrogacy would match this same conclusion, that it was *zina* [92,94]. Resulting children from a surrogacy arrangement would be viewed as illegitimate, and unable to inherit from either parent [96]. Adoption is also considered to be an illicit practice, as it goes outside of the laws of inheritance, and thus a child conceived using donor gametes cannot even be adopted in order to gain legitimacy within a family [92,94,97]. Other forbidden practices include [94]:

- Posthumous reproduction;
- The use of an ex's gametes;
- Donor gametes (sperm or egg);

- Sperm banks for the purpose of selling donor sperm (one can cryopreserve sperm before a treatment such as chemotherapy);
- PGT-A to determine sex selection;
- Cloning;
- Genetic alteration of embryos (such as three-party IVF).

Some Sunni men have been sensitive to their wives' plight of being infertile and have created a kind of workaround. They will participate in egg donation by engaging in a *mut'a* (temporary marriage, typically seen within the Shi'a sect) which then would allow for an egg retrieval cycle to commence, and the resulting embryo created would be transferred to his wife [94]. This specific kind of polygynous situation is sanctioned within Islam.

While formal adoption, in the way that it is practiced throughout much of the world is prohibited within the Sunni world, Muslims are encouraged to take in abandoned children as a type of social adoption. These children are unable to take on the name of their adoptive families and are also unable to inherit [97]. While cared for by the families that take these children in, they aren't considered to be children of the adults that care for them, though there are families that shroud the genetics in secrecy to raise a child seemingly of their own [97].

The Sunni fatwas dictating the use of reproductive technology speak in tones of certainty around what is permissible and what is not and clearly stipulate that only a couple's own gametes and body must be used. However, the Shi'a perspective has layers of nuance in comparison, and has certainly been an influence in pushing Sunni couples to explore IVF in Shi'a-dominant regions [94].

Navigating Muslim infertility (Shi'a Muslims)

Whereas Sunni Muslims are the outright majority, Shi'a Muslims are the minority and tend to be concentrated geographically in Pakistan, Iran, Lebanon, Iraq, and Bahrain, although Shi'a Muslims have emigrated throughout the world [86,94]. Reproductive assistance follows the fatwa authored by Ayatollah Ali Hussein Khamenei in Iran (1999) [86], and is similar to the Sunni fatwas, with a glaring addition: for Shi'a Muslims, gamete donation is considered allowable [86,94]. The justification for this difference is that the Ayatollah wanted to ensure that the psychological toll of infertility (and its potential impact on the couple) was considered and called this allowance a "marriage savior" [94].

In practical terms, balancing the importance of inheritance and marriage with the introduction of donor gametes requires some complex explanation. Ayatollah Khamenei argued that egg donation wasn't inherently forbidden in a legal sense, as long as the infertile mother and the egg donor both abide by the religious parenting codes, thus the infertile mother in many ways is seen as an adoptive mother, and the resulting child would be able to inherit from the egg donor as that is the biological tie [94]. A child that is conceived using donor sperm is able to inherit from the sperm donor—the person that the child has the genetic and biological connection to [94]. However, the infertile father is seen as an adoptive father, so that the child can take his name, but is not expected to inherit [94]. The overarching argument that could be made to support the use of donor gametes is that the act of adultery is not occurring for procreation to occur [86].

Shi'a men will also engage in obtaining a *mut'a* in order to ease the way for egg donation, as the practice originates within this sect of the religion. This process entails the temporary union to occur between a man who is already married with an unmarried woman, with the arrangement being specified for its amount of time. The parties agree to a sum of money also. Next, the couple need to present in front of a religious court to ascertain if the donation is necessary or not. Witnesses must be present when a decision is made, in addition to the REI, as well as the agreement of both parties (including the infertile wife) [86,94].

Adding to the menu of what is permissible is gestational surrogacy. Surrogacy is permissible as long as care is taken so that no physical contact occurs during the procedures between unmarried couples [96]. Such a stark difference of opinion between the Sunni's and Shi'ites seem to exist due to the way each promulgates their laws, as Shi'a Muslims give more weight to individual fatwas rendered by individual jurists, versus a more collective jurisprudence within the Sunni community [96]. While the case around surrogacy seems to be fairly black and white between both sects, as most things, it's not always that clear. There are Sunni scholars who argue that surrogacy should be permitted as long as the intended parents' gametes are being used. While some Shi'a scholars argue that surrogacy should not be permissible under any circumstances [96]. As reproductive technologies continue to improve and completely new ones are created, both sects of Islam continue to grapple with the inherent bioethical concerns that emerge. A clear division has emerged in terms of where the proliferation of clinics geographically occurs in the Middle East, with Shi'a majority countries creating options that neighboring Sunni majority countries lack. This has led to reproductive tourism within the region itself [94].

A point to consider, pertinent across both sects of Islam, is the role of masturbation in order to provide a semen sample for any kind of assisted reproductive intervention. As in Christianity, masturbation has a connotation of sin and guilt, as well as illicit pleasure, as the pleasure of any type of sexual act ideally occurs within the sexual context of a man and his wife. Masturbation is not completely condoned, as it is thought to be a preventative step from *zina* [98]. For some men, the act of masturbating connotes homosexuality, also considered impermissible and forbidden. An additional potential conflict of semen is its dual purposes: it is both a cellular instrument to give life and a contaminant (for the reasons stated previously) [98]. Given this duality, many men perform ablutions (ritual washings) before prayer, which indicates their ambivalence about semen and providing a sample. Such a conflict can cause iatrogenic infertility vis-a-vis male orgasmic dysfunction, or the failure to ejaculate, in a way that is experienced as sex "on demand" [98].

Implications and recommendations

The intersection of religious belief, sex, and reproductive challenges presents unique circumstances for adherents as individuals navigate what is considered "permissible" according to their faith. The influence of religious belief can have an impact on sexual function. Placing infertility into the mix adds to the complexity. It is easy to see how concerns about masturbation to produce a semen sample for IUI could cause anxiety-related erectile dysfunction for observant Jews, Catholics, or Muslims. Such situations will present unique challenges for both the patient and the treating professional.

The majority of this chapter speaks to the three Judeo-Christian based religions and the potential faith-based impact on treatment for couples who experience infertility. Treating physicians or mental health providers who are missing the necessary religio-cultural knowledge might experience frustration with what can seem a limitation on potential options for a particular couple. However, religion can also provide a boon for treatment, as faith and its corollary, hope, can keep a couple engaged in treatment. There is a wide range of literature that supports spiritual involvement yielding better coping outcomes in the wake of medical diagnosis and techniques [99]. Specifically regarding ART, treatment positively correlates with an increased level of stress experienced by patients [100]. While the mechanism is not completely understood, some studies suggest that religion and spirituality, in the form of prayer as well as belief, can impact treatment outcomes for the better [99].

A more recent study looked at specific aspects of Jewish culture that might assist in managing the stress of infertility, narrowing them down to three coping strategies: seeking the support of G-d; seeking the support of rabbis; and seeking the support of the community [101]. Derived from work that looked at a wider range of religions and religious experiences, a tool, the RCOPE (an assessment measure that looks at the religious aspects of one's ability to cope with adverse experiences), was created. The RCOPE assesses how religion impacts a particular individual's coping experience [102]. A study of religious Jews found that seeking the support of a rabbi and seeking the support of G-d helped to reduce psychological distress but did not enhance a state of better psychological well-being [101]. Seeking recognition from the community, however, did enhance psychological well-being [101]. Knowing community clergy and religious-specific support options can assist patients in boosting their well-being and lowering their distress during treatment.

A common belief is that the more religious a person is, the more those coping styles interplay when problems arise in life. This belief was confirmed by a study of coping styles and religious beliefs as well as observance [103]. As infertility is a medical issue where people commonly feel a lack of control, being able to take back a semblance of control in the form of religious belief might be of benefit. To date, research doesn't clearly bear this out [103]. Another known factor is that those who are more religious tend to seek out more health-related help and interventions [104]. However, for reasons that this chapter has discussed, help seeking does not correlate in the same way when it comes to reproductive interventions [105]. Breaking down this disparity suggests that the pro-natalist nature of most major religions doesn't outweigh the moral and ethical concerns those religions speak to regarding the use of certain aspects of reproductive technologies [105].

Oftentimes, religion is seen as an anathema or an antagonist to beliefs based in science or social science. Religion, fundamentally, can be instrumental in one's search for significance (i.e., "Who am I?") [106]. The role of parenthood as an answer to generativity versus stagnation (the resolution of which is a major task in midlife according to Erik Erikson) can also be felt with the experience of infertility [107]. This kind of unexpected interruption of life's plans can aide in the questioning of one's significance. Religion, in times of strife, tends to be where people turn to answer questions about significance [106]. Additionally, religion can offer protectiveness in the following ways: prevention (preventing events that might pose a threat to religion, an example might be to not embark upon a visit with an REI); support (whether it be from G-d or community); purification (the religious mechanisms in place that assist a person to get back on track with piety—this might be confession, atonement, or prayer); and reframing (which can be for a situation, an individual, or even what is considered to be sacred) [106].

Religious coping can be broken down into three common approaches: self-directing, deferring, or collaborative [108]. Self-directing refers to people relying on their own attributes in order to cope; deferring relates to allowing G-d, rather than themself, to solve a particular problem; and in the collaborative approach, individuals work in concert with G-d to solve a problem. The same author found that a further breakdown could occur where traits were either classified as positive religious coping or negative religious coping. Positive religious coping methods come from the central idea that life has meaning and a secure relationship with G-d and include finding a positive appraisal in a negative situation; collaborative religious coping; seeking spiritual support from G-d, seeking support from clergy or other congregants, the helping of others, and forgiveness [108]. Negative religious coping methods come from a more tenuous relationship with G-d during times of trouble, a more pessimistic view of the world, and struggling to find a sense of significance [108]. Such methods might include questioning G-d's powers, anger toward G-d, discontent with clergy and/or congregation, and punitive religious appraisals of negative situations [108].

With the challenge of infertility, ensuring that patients have social involvement or religious fellowship have both been shown to have positive effects on mental health. The act of boosting mental health during fertility interventions is of utmost importance [109]. Another way in which religion can boost mental health is through meditation, or in religious terms, prayer [109]. One study showed an inverse correlation between depressive symptoms within fertility distress and spiritual well-being [109,110]. Another study showed that an individual's involvement within their faith as well as their relationship with G-d (including their idea of G-d) can impact treatment [109,111].

Religion can also be a benefit to treatment as those that adhere to a specific religious creed in their daily life show that they are more likely to follow a treatment plan closely [109]. Religious beliefs might also impact the lifestyle choices in eating that a person may make, which can also lead to better health as a starting point [109]. With these points being made, it should be noted that the study is equivocal in its findings [109].

Religious rituals can provide comfort for those undergoing treatment. For example, in Judaism, the use of the mikveh a ritual for niddah (purity), receives growing popularity to mark reproductive challenges [112]. There are few available Jewish prayers for infertility and pregnancy loss. However, there is an effort within the Reform, Reconstructionist, and Conservative communities to adapt or even create liturgy specific to these common situations [113,114]. In Christianity, there is also a growing movement to be inclusive of infertility as part of normative experiences that congregants might face, and the ability to support existing scripture while also adding acknowledgment during services that might be especially painful for those going through infertility (such as Mother's Day and Father's Day) [115]. In Islam, as in its religious cousins, there is a larger body for ritual and prayer upon the birth of a baby than for the death of one, or even for the continued struggle to conceive a baby. Some people will engage in prayer at *pirs* (saints or holy men), which is a tradition used widely to cure a variety of medical ailments [116]. Protective herbs or talismans created from *pirs* in one's homeland can be a substitute for actual travel [116]. The ability to address these ideas with patients demonstrates cultural understanding and can garner a deeper sense of trust within a process that might be filled with suspicion.

A significant difficulty of the infertility experience is the multisystemic nature of the disease. Among the domains impacted, in addition to the medical conditions that treatment addresses, are the individual's sense of self and personal psychology; religious or spiritual beliefs (the sense of why?); mental health; status in society; and the changes to a relationship as a result of infertility's fallout [117]. These domains overlap, as having children is the typical expectation of the individual, couple, religion, and society. In fact, childbearing has been described as an apex for women in terms of their sense of spiritual fulfillment, given that the process itself is miraculous [117–119]. Additionally, infertility removes a sense of connectedness to other women who are mothers [117]. Oftentimes, infertility is the first crisis that a couple experiences together. They can be ill-equipped both individually and collectively to understand that within the crises, each might have differing needs from the other. Religion can provide a guide to help shepherd both partners through [117]. A useful overview of each of the monotheistic religions and their views on various ART procedures can be found here Table 15.1.

TABLE 15.1 Religion and ART practices at a glance.

	Reform	Conservative	Orthodox	Sunni	Shia	Protestant	Catholic	Methodist
Premarital Sex	&							
Sex for pleasure**								
Sex for procreation								
Consent needed for sex								
Homosexuality								
IUI			*				*	**
IVF			**	**				**
GIFT				**	**			
Surrogacy			**					
Sperm Donation								
Egg Donation			***		^^			
Embryo Donation								
Embryo Cryopreservation						^		
Multifetal Reduction								
Adoption								

Columns grouped: Reform, Conservative, Orthodox = Judaism; Sunni, Shia = Islam; Protestant, Catholic, Methodist = Christian.

Table Notes:
& Teachings show sex to be a normative process, so there is no shame given with premarital sex
*With special condom used for collection and only with married partner
**Only with husband and wife's gametes/within a marriage
***Only with a Jewish Egg Donor
^Without wastage of embryos
^^Husband will need to have a temporary marriage (muta) with the donor so that she is his wife at the time.
Green--permissible (specifics noted by above chart)
Yellow--sometimes permissible (specifics noted by above chart)
Red--rarely permissible (specifics noted by above chart)

Toward the collaboration of religion with treatment

Physicians are experts in their studied specialty area and are loath to cross over into other areas of study. While this makes sense overall and is considered to be good practice (to not operate outside of one's scope of practice), opportunities for discussion and conversation tend to lessen as a result. Additionally, when operating within the confines of a busy schedule, the allotment of additional time to manage patient care can be strained, so the idea of adding more content and discussion points with a patient might feel onerous [120]. Patients will not expect their physician to be an expert in all things and going the extra mile to show compassion toward factors such as religious constraints within treatment will positively impact rapport [117]. Extending this to all potential people that might interact with a couple is also important. The ability to see that infertility is not only biological but impacts the wholeness of a person and their relationship is a key factor for patients feeling more connected and trusting toward their care providers [117]. Ensuring that religious practices and beliefs are part of any standard intake paperwork can assist in learning how patients orient themselves toward religion prior to a first appointment. Periodic assessments of physical, emotional, psychological, cultural, social, and spiritual needs enable patients to feel they are wholly cared for [103,109,117]. Including a place on intake forms to identify religious affiliation can go a long way to that end [120].

To reach this seemingly lofty goal, it would behoove clinics to offer all staff continued training in religious competencies [109]. This goes beyond the simplified explanation of what the basics of each religion encompasses and enables clinics to engage in nuanced conversations about common practices that might be misunderstood by certain religious populations. For example, the idea of modesty is strong within Judaism as well as Islam. Knowing how to manage modesty when treatment can feel intrusive and exposing is key. Oftentimes, clinics put the responsibility of the social sciences upon the nursing staff, with the expectation that they will balance patient's emotional needs, and potentially their spiritual ones as well. Clinics can rather offer a standard along the entire continuum of care within the clinic setting: ranging from reception, nurses, embryologists, and physicians.

Clinics often assign aspects of care to professionals within other disciplines, such as psychologists or other mental health professionals, as frequently, these professionals are not already embedded within the clinic setting. Ensuring that clinics have a good relationship with these off-site (as well as any on-site) professionals is important, to insure continuity of care. A similar model for religious issues makes sense. Working relationships with a variety of clergy promotes trust within religious communities that the beliefs of congregants will be understood. Conversely, many religious leaders have little idea of what occurs within a reproductive clinic, thus facilitating that conversation goes both ways in terms of education and understanding [120]. An additional benefit of maintaining faith relationships is to avoid the common experience of physicians not understanding, or even having a bias against, faith-based rationales [121]. Being able to have common parlance with various faith practices and an openness to discussing faith as part of the treatment plan would be felt as invaluable, as the converse feels demoralizing [121].

As these relationships are being built, simpler changes that can be made within the clinical setting can include familiarizing and creating religious-based resource lists (both local as well as national resources) [67]. There are several websites and even a call line to a rabbi for concerns about adherence to Orthodox Jewish laws around assisted reproduction[10] [122]. For Jewish patients, being knowledgeable about niddah as it can relate to oocyte retrieval is key, as well as having flexibility to modify an antagonist cycle in order to accommodate purity observances [72,122]. Additionally, having supplies to assist with sperm collection (such as specialty condoms, e.g., the "Kosher condom") or using a post-coital test as methods to rule out male factor concerns [122,123]. Using an organization, like Puah, that can ascertain the "kosherness" of a facility as well as provide specific supervisors that will maintain security of reproductive material from observant Jewish patients is another step to take [124,125]. While seemingly dramatic, this will ensure the genetics of the potential child and can avoid lab mix-ups, which would be especially difficult for certain families within the Orthodox community (such as a Cohen or Levi descendant) [124].

These relationships are partnerships. A rabbi or Halachic supervisor might also serve as a type of translator, between the medical professional and the patient, while occurring in real time [125]. By shifting perspective, these kinds of collaborations can yield a synthesis of information for all involved, rather than barriers to competent and holistic care [125]. This type of arrangement might be less relevant in both Christianity and Islam, as reproductive prohibitions are far more set than in Judaism, where there can be some flexibility depending upon which authority is queried. Regardless, knowledge of religious proscriptions makes sense so that patients are not inadvertently asked to do something they might consider sacrilegious.

In relation to male religious patients, sensitivity around semen collection is an aspect that can be modified in the clinical setting. It is important that any rooms used to collect semen are private and separate from other spaces within the clinic [98]. While common practice is for pornographic materials to be provided in collection rooms, this can also be uncomfortable for devout men, and so it should be ensured that there are spaces for these assistive tools to be placed that are out of sight for some men. Another idea might be to allow his wife to be with him to assist with masturbation [98].

While many people would benefit and appreciate spiritual care, it is also important to note that not every patient requires it [109]. Being able to apply a spiritual lens can add to a patient's experience, when that is a lens that they already use. The conversation between clinic and clergy is an important and ongoing one that can benefit both parties when applied. Clergy has much to learn from practitioners of reproductive medicine. Who is better positioned than those that see the pain of infertility each day to teach others what that looks like [82]?

---

[10] https://www.puahonline.org and https://www.boneiolam.org.

Though the field is often called ART, practitioners know that science plays a part. And yet these two pieces do not create babies in all cases: There is an ingredient that is missing from the overly simplistic equation of ART + science = a child. Those with a strong faith ethos believe that a divine spark or presence is necessary to ensure that a child can be created, even with the best science at humanity's disposal [67]. No matter what one's faith perspective (or lack thereof) might be, there is something magical about bringing a child into the world, given all of the pieces that need to align with precision. Perhaps it is important to remember that for some the treatment room contains four entities: the physician, man, woman, and G-d [126].

Summary

The desire to procreate is strong, often based upon internalized religious beliefs to "go forth and multiply." Much of American culture and religious institutions are built on the assumption that families are the foundation, and activities revolve around this premise. For religiously oriented couples, religion can potentially limit options that can be chosen when reproduction is not occurring spontaneously. Infertility, therefore, can cause a crisis of faith, or can cause people to become more aligned with their faith. Competent reproductive care must incorporate a knowledge of a patient's religion and the beliefs that they hold so that recommendations for treatment can be in accordance with these principles. Relationships with clergy can assist in managing a deference to individual beliefs and create an ongoing dialogue as well as provide resources for patients. Creating clinics that incorporate faith as part of the process can potentially help with outcomes, as it aligns the physician with the patient's beliefs for the outcome that all are striving toward.

References

[1] Aslan R. God: a human history. New York: Random House; 2018.
[2] Taylor GR. Sex in history. New York: Vanguard Press; 1954.
[3] Freud S. Three contributions to the theory of sex. Washington, DC: Nervous and Mental Disease Publishing; 1930.
[4] https://www.pbs.org/wgbh/americanexperience/features/pill-and-sexual-revolution/.
[5] Hills R. Sexual revolution then and now: hook-ups from 1964 to today. Retrieved August 12, 2020, from https://time.com/3611781/sexual-revolution-revisited/; December 2, 2014.
[6] Taylor C. Sex & christianity. Commonweal 2007;134(16):12−18.
[7] Inhorn MC, Patrizio P. Infertility around the globe: new thinking on gender, reproductive technologies and global movements in the 21st century. Hum Reprod Update 2015;21(4):411−26.
[8] Boivin J, Bunting L, Collins JA, Nygren KG. International estimates of infertility prevalence and treatment-seeking: potential need and demand for infertility medical care. Hum Reprod 2007;22(6):1506−12.
[9] https://www.history.com/topics/religion/judaism.
[10] https://www.britannica.com/topic/Judaism/Basic-beliefs-and-doctrines.
[11] Schenker JG. Assisted reproductive technology: perspectives in Halakha (Jewish religious law). Ethics Biosci Life 2008;3(3):17−24.
[12] https://www.britannica.com/topic/rabbi.
[13] https://www.history.com/topics/religion/history-of-christianity.
[14] https://www.history.com/topics/religion/islam#:~:text=Although%20its%20roots%20go%20back,of%20the%20prophet%20Muhammad%20life.
[15] https://www.britannica.com/topic/Islam.
[16] https://www.britannica.com/topic/imam.
[17] https://www.pbs.org/wgbh/pages/frontline/teach/muslims/beliefs.html.
[18] Marsh M, Ronner W. The pursuit of parenthood: reproductive technology from test-tube babies to uterus transplants. Johns Hopkins University Press; 2019.
[19] Klitzman R. Designing babies: how technology is changing the ways we create children. Oxford University Press; 2020.
[20] Klitzman R. Unconventional combinations of prospective parents: ethical challenges faced by IVF providers. BMC Med Ethics 2017;18(1). Available from: https://doi.org/10.1186/s12910-017-0177-x.
[21] Coogan MD. God and sex: what the Bible really says. New York: Twelve; 2011.
[22] Coogan M. The new Oxford annotated Bible: New Revised Standard Version: with the Apocrypha: an ecumenical study Bible. 4th ed Oxford University Press; 2010. Fully revised.
[23] https://www.hrc.org/resources/what-does-the-bible-say-about-homosexuality?utm_source = GS&utm_medium = AD&utm_campaign = BPI-HRC-Grant&utm_content = 456227624868&utm_term = gay%20in%20the%20bible&gclid = Cj0KCQjw7Nj5BRCZARIsABwxDKLmn5THzhegHec6FnqztP6KXRUNmua3ZoYy7YUP_cb2La1imglyHpAaAlGgEALw_wcB.
[24] https://www.nytimes.com/interactive/2015/06/05/us/samesex-scriptures.html.
[25] Inhorn MC. Islam, sex, and sin: IVF Ethnography as Muslim men's confessional. Anthropological Q 2018;91(1):25−51. Available from: https://doi.org/10.1353/anq.2018.0001.
[26] Schaefer M. First question [e-mail to the author]; July 4, 2020.
[27] Avishai O, Burke K. God's case for sex. Context 2016;15(4):30−5. Available from: https://doi.org/10.1177/1536504216684819.

References

[28] Rosenfeld J, Ribner DS. The newlywed's guide to physical intimacy. Jerusalem, Israel: Gefen Pub; 2011.

[29] Boyarin D. Carnal Israel: reading sex in Talmudic culture. Berkeley, CA: University of California Press; 1993.

[30] United methodist revised social principles. Nashville: The Publishing House of The United Methodist Church; 2020.

[31] Steinke AF. Does pre-cana need an overhaul? US Catholic 2016;81:27−30 Retrieved from: http://proxygw.wrlc.org/login?url = https://search-proquest-com.proxygw.wrlc.org/docview/1807075291?accountid = 11243.

[32] Khoei EM, Whelan A, Cohen J. Sharing beliefs: what sexuality means to Muslim Iranian women living in Australia. Cult Health Sex 2008;10(3):237−48. Available from: https://doi.org/10.1080/13691050701740039.

[33] Hilber AM, Colombini M. Promoting sexual health means promoting healthy approaches to sexuality. Sex Health Exch 2002;4:1−3.

[34] Mernissi F. The Muslim concept of active female sexuality. Women Sexuality Muslim Soc. 2000;19−35.

[35] Ahmad K. Islam: its meaning and message. 2nd ed. Islamic Council of Europe: distributed by News and Media; 1976.

[36] Mahoney A, Pargament KI, Tarakeshwar N, Swank AB. Religion in the home in the 1980s and 1990s: a meta-analytic review and conceptual analysis of links between religion, marriage, and parenting. J Fam Psychol 2001;15(4):559−96. Available from: https://doi.org/10.1037/0893-3200.15.4.559.

[37] Burdette AM, Ellison CG, Sherkat DE, Gore KA. Are there religious variations in marital infidelity? J Family Issues 2007;28(12):1553−81. Available from: https://doi.org/10.1177/0192513x07304269.

[38] Alghafli Z, Hatch T, Marks L. Religion and relationships in Muslim families: a qualitative examination of devout married Muslim couples. Religions 2014;5(3):814−33. Available from: https://doi.org/10.3390/rel5030814.

[39] Killawi A, Fathi E, Dadras I, Daneshpour M, Elmi A, Altalib H. Perceptions and experiences of marriage preparation among U.S. Muslims: multiple voices from the community. J Marital Family Ther 2017;44(1):90−106. Available from: https://doi.org/10.1111/jmft.12233.

[40] Obergefell, et al. v. Hodges, Director, Ohio Department of Health, et al., 576 U.S.; 2015.

[41] Craig v. Masterpiece Cakeshop, Inc. 370 P.3d 272 (Colo. App. 2015), cert. granted, 137 S. Ct. 2290; 2017.

[42] Velte KC. Why the religious right can't have its (straight wedding) cake and eat it too: breaking the preservation-through-transformation dynamic in masterpiece Cakeshop v. Colorado Civil Rights Commission. SSRN Electron J 2017. Available from: https://doi.org/10.2139/ssrn.3041332.

[43] Stance of faiths on LGBTQ issues: reform judaism. Retrieved August 30, 2020, from https://www.hrc.org/resources/stances-of-faiths-on-lgbt-issues-reform-judaism; n.d.

[44] Stance of faiths on LGBTQ issues: reconstructionist judaism. Retrieved August 30, 2020, from https://www.hrc.org/resources/stances-of-faiths-on-lgbt-issues-reconstructionist-judaism; n.d.

[45] Stance of faiths on LGBTQ issues: conservative judaism. Retrieved August 30, 2020, from https://www.hrc.org/resources/stances-of-faiths-on-lgbt-issues-conservative-judaism; n.d.

[46] Kaplan DE. The acceptance of gays and lesbians. American reform Judaism an introduction. New Brunswick, NJ: Rutgers Univ. Press; 2005, p. 209−32. Available from: http://www.jstor.com/stable/j.ctt5hj6xp.15.

[47] Helfgot N. Statement of principles nya. Retrieved August 30, 2020, from https://statementofprinciplesnya.blogspot.com/; July 28, 2010.

[48] Allen SH, Golojuch LA. "She Still Doesn't Want Me to Tell My Next-Door Neighbor:" the familial experiences of modern orthodox Jewish gay men. J GLBT Fam Stud 2018;15(4):373−94. Available from: https://doi.org/10.1080/1550428x.2018.1487811.

[49] Etengoff C, Rodriguez E. Gay men's and their religiously conservative family allies' scriptural engagement. Psychol Relig Spirit 2017;9(4):423−36. Available from: https://doi.org/10.1037/rel0000087.

[50] Zack E, Ben-Ari A. "Men are for Sex and Women are for Marriage": on the duality in the lives of jewish religious gay men married to women. J GLBT Fam Stud 2019;15(4):395−413. Available from: https://doi.org/10.1080/1550428X.2018.150637.

[51] Discriminatory laws and practices and acts of violence against individuals based upon their sexual orientation or gender identity. Retrieved August 30, 2020, from https://www.ohchr.org/Documents/Issues/Discrimination/A.HRC.19.41_English.pdf; November 17, 2011.

[52] Declaration on human rights, sexual orientation and gender identity. Retrieved August 30, 2020, from https://w2.vatican.va/roman_curia/secretariat_state/2008/documents/rc_seg-st_20081218_statement-sexual-orientation_en.html; December 18, 2008.

[53] Perry S, Whitehead A. Religion and public opinion toward same-sex relations, marriage, and adoption: does the type of practice matter? J Sci Study Relig 2016;55(3):637−51. Available from: https://doi.org/10.1111/jssr.12215.

[54] Yip AK. Embracing Allah and sexuality? South-Asian non-heterosexual Muslims in Britain. South Asians Diaspora 2004;294−310. Available from: https://doi.org/10.1163/9789047401407_016.

[55] Jaspal R, Cinnirella M. Identity processes, threat, and interpersonal relations: accounts from British Muslim gay men. J Homosex 2012;59(2):215−40. Available from: https://doi-org.proxygw.wrlc.org/10.1080/00918369.2012.638551.

[56] Tanakh The Holy Scriptures. Philadelphia, PA: The Jewish Publication Society; 1985.

[57] Siraj A. The construction of the homosexual "other" by British Muslim heterosexuals. Contemp Islam 2009;3(1):41−57. Available from: https://doi.org/10.1007/s11562-008-0076-5.

[58] Subhi N, Geelan D. When Christianity and homosexuality collide: understanding the potential intrapersonal conflict. J Homosex 2012;59(10):1382−402. Available from: https://doi.org/10.1080/00918369.2012.724638.

[59] Festinger L. A theory of cognitive dissonance. Stanford University Press; 1957.

[60] O'Flynne T. Spiritual cognitive dissonance in LGBTQQ people (Order No. 27544489). Available from ProQuest Dissertations & Theses Global. (2313355219). http://proxygw.wrlc.org/login?url = https://www-proquest-com.proxygw.wrlc.org/docview/2313355219?accountid = 11243; 2019.

[61] Pietkiewicz I, Kołodziejczyk-Skrzypek M. Living in sin? How gay catholics manage their conflicting sexual and religious identities. Arch Sex Behav 2016;45(6):1573−85. Available from: https://doi.org/10.1007/s10508-016-0752-0.

[62] Slomowitz A, Feit A. Does god make referrals? Orthodox Judaism and homosexuality. J Gay Lesbian Ment Health 2015;19(1):100−11. Available from: https://doi.org/10.1080/19359705.2014.975583.

[63] Anderton C, Pender D, Asner-Self K. A review of the religious identity/sexual orientation identity conflict literature: revisiting festinger's cognitive dissonance theory. J LGBT Issues Couns 2011;5(3-4):259−81. Available from: https://doi.org/10.1080/15538605.2011.632745.

[64] Meyer I. Prejudice, social stress, and mental health in lesbian, gay, and bisexual populations: conceptual issues and research evidence. Psychol Bull 2003;129(5):674—97. Available from: https://doi.org/10.1037/0033-2909.129.5.674.
[65] Moss CR, Baden JS. Reconceiving infertility: Biblical perspectives on procreation and childlessness. Princeton, NJ: Princeton University Press; 2015.
[66] Hirsh A. Infertility in Jewish couples, biblical and rabbinic law. Hum Fertil 1998;1(1):14—19. Available from: https://doi.org/10.1080/14647279820001989041.
[67] Kahn SM. Making technology familiar: orthodox jews and infertility support, advice, and inspiration. Cult Med Psychiatry 2006;30(4):468—80. Available from: https://doi.org/10.1007/s11013-006-9029-8.
[68] Kohane I. Empty cribs: infertility challenges for orthodox Jewish couples. ProQuest Dissertations Publishing; 2020.
[69] Knohl E. The marriage covenant: a guide to Jewish marriage. Ein Tzurim, Israel: Erscheinungsort nicht ermittelbar; 2008.
[70] Blyth E, Landau R. Faith and fertility: attitudes towards reproductive practices in different religions from ancient to modern times. London: Jessica Kingsley; 2009.
[71] Silber SJ. Judaism and reproductive technology. In: Woodruff T, Zoloth L, Campo-Engelstein L, Rodriguez S, editors. Oncofertility. Cancer treatment and research, 156. Boston, MA: Springer; 2010. Available from: https://doi.org/10.1007/978-1-4419-6518-9_38.
[72] Reichman D, Brauer A, Goldschlag D, Schattman G, Rosenwaks Z. In vitro fertilization for Orthodox Jewish couples: antagonist cycle modifications allowing for mikveh attendance before oocyte retrieval. Fertil Steril 2013;99(5):1408—12. Available from: https://doi.org/10.1016/j.fertnstert.2012.11.050.
[73] Shalev C. Seminar reasoning ultra-orthodoxy and the biopolitics of medically assisted reproduction in Israel. In 948201698 739798178 U. Auga, 948201699 739798178 C. V. Braun, 948201700 739798178 C. Bruns, & 948201701 739798178 J. Husmann (Authors), fundamentalism and gender: Scripture--body--community. Eugene, OR: Pickwick Publications; 2013, p. 220—43.
[74] Mackler AL. An expanded partnership with god? In vitro fertilization in Jewish ethics. J Religious Ethics 1997;25(2):277—304.
[75] Rose E, Schreiber-Agus N, Bajaj K, Klugman S, Goldwaser T. Challenges of pre- and post-test counseling for orthodox Jewish individuals in the premarital phase. J Genet Couns 2016;25(1):18—24. Available from: https://doi.org/10.1007/s10897-015-9880-2.
[76] Catechism of the Catholic Church. London: Burns Oates; 2002.
[77] Catholic Online. New Testament—Bible. Retrieved September 28, 2020, from https://www.catholic.org/bible/new_testament.php; n.d.
[78] Havrelock R. The myth of birthing the hero: Heroic Barrenness in the Hebrew Bible. Biblical Interpretation 2008;16(2):154—78. Available from: https://doi.org/10.1163/156851508X262948.
[79] Morris M. Rejoice, o barren woman? Infertility in the New Testament. ProQuest Dissertations Publishing; 2014.
[80] Pitre B. Blessing the barren and warning the fecund: Jesus' message for women concerning pregnancy and childbirth. J Study N Testam 2001;23(81):59—80. Available from: https://doi.org/10.1177/0142064X0102308103.
[81] Caler M. In God's hands: evangelical talk about infertility, God's will and family building. ProQuest Dissertations Publishing; 2012.
[82] Feske M. Rachel's Lament: the impact of infertility and pregnancy loss upon the religious faith of ordinary Christians. J Pastor Theology 2012;22(1):3—1—3—17. Available from: https://doi.org/10.1179/jpt.2012.22.1.003.
[83] Czarnecki D. Moral women, immoral technologies: how devout women negotiate gender, religion, and assisted reproductive technologies. Gend Soc 2015;29(5):716—42. Available from: https://doi.org/10.1177/0891243215591504.
[84] Murphy T. Dignity, marriage and embryo adoption: a look at Dignitas Personae. Reprod BioMed Online 2011;23(7):860—8. Available from: https://doi.org/10.1016/j.rbmo.2011.06.001.
[85] Kieser D. The female body in catholic theology: menstruation. Reprod Autonomy Horiz (Villanova) 2017;44(1):1—27. Available from: https://doi.org/10.1017/hor.2017.51.
[86] Sallam H, Sallam N. Religious aspects of assisted reproduction. Facts Views Vis ObGyn 2016;8(1):33—48.
[87] Metz L. Life-love, insight, fertility, experiences a podcast [Audio podcast]. https://lorimetz.net/2020/05/15/the-church-philosophy-on-conception/; May 15, 2020.
[88] Picardi P. Unholier Than Thou [Audio podcast]. https://crooked.com/podcast/the-sanctity-of-abortion/; September 4, 2020.
[89] Deonandan R. Thoughts on the ethics of gestational surrogacy: perspectives from religions, Western liberalism, and comparisons with adoption. J Assist Reprod Genet 2020;37(2):269—79. Available from: https://doi.org/10.1007/s10815-019-01647-y.
[90] Ford N. Catholicism and human reproduction: an historical overview. Australas Cathol Rec 2012;89(1):49—62.
[91] Jennings P. "God Had Something Else in Mind": family, religion, and infertility. J Contemp Ethnogr 2010;39(2):215—37. Available from: https://doi.org/10.1177/0891241609342432.
[92] Padela A, Klima K, Duivenbode R. Producing parenthood: Islamic bioethical perspectives & normative implications. N Bioeth 2020;26(1):17—37. Available from: https://doi.org/10.1080/20502877.2020.1729575.
[93] Serour G. Ethical issues in human reproduction: Islamic perspectives. Gynecol Endocrinol 2013;29(11):949—52. Available from: https://doi.org/10.3109/09513590.2013.825714.
[94] Inhorn M, Tremayne S. Islam, assisted reproduction, and the bioethical aftermath. J Relig Health 2016;55(2):422—30. Available from: https://doi.org/10.1007/s10943-015-0151-1.
[95] Höbek Akarsu R, Kızılkaya Beji N. Spiritual and religious issues of stigmatization women with infertility: a qualitative study: spiritual and religious issues of stigmatization. J Relig Health 2019;. Available from: https://doi.org/10.1007/s10943-019-00884-w.
[96] Shabana A. Foundations of the consensus against surrogacy arrangements in Islamic Law. Islamic Law Soc 2015;22(1/2):82—113. Available from: https://doi.org/10.1163/15685195-02212p03.
[97] Inhorn MC. "He Won't Be My Son": Middle Eastern Muslim men's discourses of adoption and gamete donation. Med Anthropol Q 2006;20(1):94—120.
[98] Inhorn M. Masturbation, semen collection and Men's IVF experiences: anxieties in the Muslim world. Bod Soc 2007;13(3):37—53. Available from: https://doi.org/10.1177/1357034X07082251.
[99] Braga D, Melamed R, Setti A, Zanetti B, Figueira R, Iaconelli A, et al. Role of religion, spirituality, and faith in assisted reproduction. J Psychosom Obstet Gynaecol 2019;40(3):195—201. Available from: https://doi.org/10.1080/0167482X.2018.1470163.

References

[100] Boivin J, Schmidt L. Infertility-related stress in men and women predicts treatment outcome 1 year later. Fertil Sterili 2005;83(6):1745–52. Available from: https://doi.org/10.1016/j.fertnstert.2004.12.039.

[101] Nouman H, Benyamini Y. Religious women's coping with infertility: do culturally adapted religious coping strategies contribute to well-being and health? Int J Behav Med 2018;26(2):154–64. Available from: https://doi.org/10.1007/s12529-018-9757-5.

[102] Pargament K, Koenig H, Perez L. The many methods of religious coping: development and initial validation of the RCOPE. J Clin Psych 2000;56(4):519–43. Available from: https://doi.org/10.1002/(SICI)1097-4679(200004)56:43.0.CO;2-1.

[103] Grinstein-Cohen O, Grinstein-Cohen O, Katz A, Katz A, Sarid O, Sarid O. Religiosity: its impact on coping styles among women undergoing fertility treatment. J Relig Health 2017;56(3):1032–41. Available from: https://doi.org/10.1007/s10943-016-0344-2.

[104] Schiller P, Levin J. Is there a religious factor in health care utilization?: a review. Soc Sci Med 1988;27(12):1369–79. Available from: https://doi.org/10.1016/0277-9536(88)90202-X (1982).

[105] Greil A, McQuillan J, Benjamins M, Johnson D, Johnson K, Heinz C. Specifying the effects of religion on medical helpseeking: the case of infertility. Soc Sci Med 2010;71(4):734–42. Available from: https://doi.org/10.1016/j.socscimed.2010.04.033 (1982).

[106] Pargament KI. Religious methods of coping: resources for the conservation and transformation of significance. In: 990858690 765921488 E. P. Shafranske (Author), Religion and the clinical practice of psychology. Washington, DC: American Psychological Association; 1996, p. 215–239.

[107] Snarey J, Son L, Kuehne V, Hauser S, Vaillant G. The role of parenting in men's psychosocial development: a longitudinal study of early adulthood infertility and midlife generativity. Dev Psychol 1987;23(4):593–603. Available from: https://doi.org/10.1037/0012-1649.23.4.593.

[108] Pargament KI. The bitter and the sweet: an evaluation of the costs and benefits of religiousness. Psychol Inq 2002;13(3):168–81. Available from: https://doi.org/10.1207/S15327965PLI1303_02.

[109] Roudsari R, Allan H, Smith P. Looking at infertility through the lens of religion and spirituality: a review of the literature. Hum Fertil 2007;10(3):141–9. Available from: https://doi.org/10.1080/14647270601182677.

[110] Domar A, Penzias A, Dusek J, Magna A, Merarim D, Nielsen B, et al. The stress and distress of infertility: does religion help women cope? Sex Reprod Menopause 2005;3(2):45–51. Available from: https://doi.org/10.1016/j.sram.2005.09.007.

[111] Sewpaul V. Culture religion and infertility: a South African perspective. Br J Soc Work 1999;29(5):741–54. Available from: https://doi.org/10.1093/bjsw/29.5.741.

[112] Searle S. Living water, sacred space: an outsider's look at contemporary mikveh practice (Order No. MR45327). Available from ProQuest Dissertations & Theses Global (304489588). Retrieved from http://proxygw.wrlc.org/login?url=https://www-proquest-com.proxygw.wrlc.org/docview/304489588?accountid=11243; 2008.

[113] Burton G. Finding liturgy for infertility and pregnancy loss. Eur Jud 2017;50(1):123. Available from: https://doi.org/10.3167/ej.2017.500116.

[114] Cardin NB. Tears of sorrow, seeds of hope: a Jewish spiritual companion for infertility and pregnancy loss. Woodstock, VT: Jewish Lights Pub; 2007.

[115] Gruner MH. A proposal for a local church infertility ministry (Order No. 3718898). Available from ProQuest Dissertations & Theses Global. (1713693639); 2015.

[116] Shaw A. Rituals of infant death: defining life and islamic personhood. Bioethics 2014;28(2):84–95. Available from: https://doi.org/10.1111/bioe.12047.

[117] Romeiro J, Caldeira S, Brady V, Hall J, Timmins F. The spiritual journey of infertile couples: discussing the opportunity for spiritual care. Religions (Basel, Switz) 2017;8(4):76. Available from: https://doi.org/10.3390/rel8040076.

[118] Prinds C, Hvidt N, Mogensen O, Buus N. Making existential meaning in transition to motherhood—a scoping review. Midwifery 2014;30(6):733–41. Available from: https://doi.org/10.1016/j.midw.2013.06.021.

[119] Callister L, Khalaf I. Spirituality in childbearing women. J Perinat Educ 2010;19(2):16–24. Available from: https://doi.org/10.1624/105812410X495514.

[120] Braddock III C, Snyder L. The doctor will see you shortly: the ethical significance of time for the patient-physician relationship. J Gen Intern Med 2005;20(11):1057–62. Available from: https://doi.org/10.1111/j.1525-1497.2005.00217.x.

[121] Scully J, Banks S, Song R, Haq J. Experiences of faith group members using new reproductive and genetic technologies: a qualitative interview study. Hum Fertil (Cambridge, Engl) 2016;20(1):22–9. Available from: https://doi.org/10.1080/14647273.2016.1243816.

[122] Kol S. Ultra-Orthodox Jews and infertility diagnosis and treatment. Andrology (Oxf) 2018;6(5):662–4. Available from: https://doi.org/10.1111/andr.12533.

[123] Haimov-Kochman R, Adler C, Ein-Mor E, Rosenak D, Hurwitz A. Infertility associated with precoital ovulation in observant Jewish couples; prevalence, treatment, efficacy and side effects. Isr Med Assoc J 2012;14(2):100–3.

[124] Carlson K. How to make a Kosher baby. Natl Post (Tor) 2009;11(172):A1.

[125] Ivry T. Kosher medicine and medicalized halacha: an exploration of triadic relations among Israeli rabbis, doctors, and infertility patients. Am Ethnol 2010;37(4):662–80. Available from: https://doi.org/10.1111/j.1548-1425.2010.01277.x.

[126] Dutney A. Religion, infertility and assisted reproductive technology. Best Pract Res: Clin Obstet Gynecol 2006;21(1):169–80. Available from: https://doi.org/10.1016/j.bpobgyn.2006.09.007.

PART IV

Looking forward

CHAPTER

16

Thoughts on education, reproduction, and sexual function. Futures directions and obstacles

Angela K. Lawson
Northwestern University, Evanston, IL, United States

A brief history of reproductive education

The example of the US education system

Sex education in schools (the first exposure to reproductive education albeit education about how not to conceive) was introduced in the United States in 1914 with the formation of the American Social Hygiene Association. Even more of a taboo in the early 1900s than today, discussions of sex and sex education were largely unheard of. It was not until 1936 that the first newspaper articles on sexually transmitted infections (STIs) were published. Early education focused on STI prevention and the "menace" of prostitution among soldiers in World Wars I and II. College and University professors, youth leaders, and parents (deemed the child's first sex educator) were also recipients of these early educational efforts [1]. Public efforts to provide school-based sex education were largely resisted at the time (e.g., the "Chicago Experiment"); however, a limited form of improvised sex education (e.g., discussion of reproduction in animals, insects, and plants), often unbeknownst to parents, was offered in as many as 45% of schools in 1927 [2,3].

Public school sex education transitioned in the 1940s and 1950s to focus on "family life education," which included more benign topics such as marriage, relationships, finances, and childbearing. This change in focus of sex education made such education more palatable to parents. The sexual revolution of the 1960s and 1970s, the introduction of birth control pills, legalization of abortion, and publication of the Kinsey Reports on human sexuality in 1948 and 1953 all challenged established social norms about sex and sex education and ushered in a call for morally neutral comprehensive school-based sex education (CSE), which included information about how to engage in safe sex [2].

US Federal government involvement in family planning and sex education began in 1964, when President Lyndon Johnson dedicated federal funding to family planning services and in 1970 President Nixon continued this funding through Title X of the Public Health Service Act. The Act was amended in 1978 by President Carter and mandated that sex education be created to target a teenage audience in an effort to reduce teen pregnancies [2,4]. Backlash toward CSE was increasingly evident in the 1980s and in 1981, President Reagan began the fight to repeal Title X and the federal government soon began funding abstinence-only-until-(heterosexual)-marriage (AOUM) education. Despite the use of often gender-neutral language, AOUM frequently focuses on the harms of female but not male "promiscuity" [4]. It appears that the timing of the backlash to CSE and the subsequent push to focus on women's chastity through AOUM began once women began to gain sexual freedoms previously only afforded to their male peers.

Passage of the Adolescent Family Life Act in 1981 and Congressional funding for AOUM programs through the Clinton-era 1996 Personal Responsibility and Work Opportunity Reform Act (a welfare reform act) aided in the advancement of AOUM education and served to highlight the intersection of race and gender in AOUM. It appears that the inclusion of AOUM funding within a welfare reform act was intended to discourage poor women of color from having children out of wedlock [4,5].

Although funding for AOUM continued to increase (e.g., through the 2002 Community Based Abstinence Education program), increased national awareness of the risks of HIV/AIDs resulted in school-based education, which included the use of condoms, though abstinence was still the preferred method of disease prevention [2]. Finally, federal funding for AOUM decreased and funding for CSE increased during President Obama's time in office; however, President Trump's proposed 2018 budget included substantial funding for AOUM. In total, it is estimated that close to $2 billion has been spent in federal funding for AOUM since the 1990s [6]. Currently, only 30 states and the District of Columbia require school-based sex education (most include HIV education) while an additional 9 states require HIV education. The majority of states require that abstinence be stressed and that the importance of sex only within the context of marriage be highlighted [7].

Reproductive education in the United States

In addition to the general ineffectiveness of AOUM in preventing unintended pregnancies and STIs [8,9], no structured system (either AOUM or CSE) exists in the United States and internationally to provide comprehensive reproductive education to all individuals who want to conceive, whether married or otherwise. The primary educational focus on not conceiving or developing an STI, leaves many individuals without the reproductive or fertility knowledge needed to effectively conceive when family building is desired. Although education regarding how to conceive may not be appropriate for young children, emerging and young adults, many of whom plan to have children would benefit from such knowledge.

Institutions of higher learning

College campuses around the world provide a unique opportunity to provide both comprehensive sex and reproductive education to young adults who often report little understanding of reproduction [10–12]. However, not all young adults go to college and little evidence exists that colleges provide comprehensive reproductive/fertility knowledge to all students. Thus even after graduation from college it remains likely that most people will have significant deficits in knowledge related to reproduction and fertility.

Faith-based organizations

Another potential source of reproductive education are the national and international religious and faith-based organizations (FBOs) who may promote AOUM among congregants and would appear to have an interest in its members marrying and having children. Some argue that AOUM has at its core religious ideology as proponents of AOUM often define abstinence in terms of morality (e.g., chastity, purity) rather than in behavioral or health-related terms [9]. Indeed, many FBOs include a focus on the importance of chastity but do not provide traditional sex education either AOUM or CSE. However, some FBOs may provide education about HIV/AIDS prevention [13], some may provide limited reproductive knowledge during premarital counseling [14,15], and some may provide more extensive education regarding procreation to married heterosexual adults [16]. FBOs commonly provide procreative education to married heterosexual individuals in developing countries although the education is likely limited by the religious beliefs (e.g., opposition to birth control, sex outside of marriage, etc.) of those providing the education [17].

Parents

It is likely that most individuals in the United States and internationally do not receive comprehensive reproductive/fertility education through school, religion, or other sources. Although a young adult's parents could be seen as a source of both sex and reproductive/fertility knowledge, it is likely that parents who have been exposed to the United States, and other international similarly situated, educational and religious systems have not received adequate education to properly teach their children. Further, research shows that minor and adult children rarely speak with their parents about such topics due to embarrassment or fear of repercussions [18,19].

Healthcare providers

In the United States and other countries, healthcare providers appear to be the most common source of reproductive education. However, even those who can readily access and afford appropriate medical care may not receive such education. Research unfortunately shows that time and reimbursement issues as well as the failure of healthcare professionals to routinely and proactively provide such education raises the concern that little and likely disparate dissemination of reproductive/fertility education is occurring [10]. Further, the dissemination of reproductive/fertility education is also hampered by the fact that not all healthcare providers appear to have received the necessary reproductive education to properly counsel patients about conceiving [10,20–22].

Social networks and social media

Without proper education from any reputable source and potentially due to experiences of discrimination, many young and older adults (and teenagers) turn to social media and to the peers in their social networks for information about sex and reproduction. Although online technologies are increasingly being used to disseminate research-driven information on sex and reproduction (see, e.g., refs. [18,23–25]), it is unclear if the social media sources accessed by those looking for information about sex or reproduction are factual in nature [26–28].

The disparate effects of sex/reproductive education

LGBTQ individuals

Regardless of where one receives their education about sex and/or reproduction/fertility, it appears clear that certain groups of individuals are likely to receive less education and education which is biased in nature. This is particularly true for LGBTQ individuals as historically sex and reproductive education (both academic and religious) have focused on heterosexual cisgender individuals' sexuality [5,7,29,30]. Some US states, for example, not only exclude consideration of LGBTQ individuals' needs but also require the inclusion of negative information about homosexuality [7]. The exclusionary and/or hostile nature of sexual and reproductive education in the United States toward LGBTQ individuals not only impairs LGBTQ individual's understanding of sex and reproduction but also contributes to homophobia, transphobia, and thereby increased risk of discrimination and/or harassment [5]. Similar to their heterosexual cisgender peers, LGBTQ individuals frequently report a desire for children [31–33]. That many LGBTQ individuals do not think that children are something they should hope for suggests that the exclusion of LGBTQ individuals from conversations about sex and reproduction may negatively shape their beliefs about family building and their competence or appropriateness as parents [31–34].

Sex disparities

Historically AOUM had as a primary focus women's chastity and virginity with often a reinforcement of gendered double standards related to sexual activity. This early gendered message about sex has resulted in men being celebrated for their sexual prowess while women who fail to follow the expected model of chastity until marriage are deemed "sluts" and are shamed. Further, in AOUM, male testosterone is used to naturalize men's desire for sex while women's hormones (including testosterone) are not used to educate them about their sexual desire but rather are often primarily discussed with regard to women's hormones supporting their ability to have children. Sex education then has served to reinforce gender stereotypes of men as assertive and active participants in their sex lives and lives in general while women are seen as either victims of sexual abuse (with some evidence of victim blaming) or as passive caregivers waiting to meet the right heterosexual partner with whom to build a family [35–37].

The sex disparities evident in sex and reproductive education unfortunately continue into adulthood. As adults, women are frequently encouraged to have annual medical appointments for gynecological care and screening whereas men are less commonly encouraged to have yearly urologic screenings. This results in the likelihood that more women than men will have somewhat regular contact with medical professionals who could educate them about sex and fertility. It is unclear if routine provision of reproductive information occurs; it appears more typical that women receive such information only when they, rather than the healthcare professional, raise the topic [28]. What is clear is that men commonly report lower reproductive knowledge than women [12].

Racial minoritized groups

A primary focus of Title X enacted in 1970 was the provision of access to contraceptives to low-income women. This was supported both by those who supported reduced disparities in access to contraceptives but also by those concerned about the "excess fertility of poor urban (read Black)" women. Subsequently, the 1996 Personal Responsibility and Work Opportunity Reform Act appears to have been enacted in part to control birth outside of wedlock and included stereotypes of Black pregnant teenagers on welfare [4]. Stereotypes of non-White women and men's hypersexual appetites (and hyperfertility) are unfortunately common and AOUM education programs (often taught by White educators) further these stereotypes [36,37]. For example, in one AOUM program, an example is provided of a young girl named LaWanda. She is described as lonely with feelings of abandonment by her father and who when approached by a popular male student (Calvin), decides to have sex with him and is open to a possible pregnancy. Calvin on the other hand, abandons her. This example is particularly notable as LaWanda (whose name was likely chosen to indicate she is Black or at least not White) is one of the few teenagers who agrees to have sex and as all other examples in the AOUM education include teenagers with distinctly White sounding names [4]. Finally, given the long history of medical abuses enacted on Black and brown women's and men's bodies, mistrust of the medical system could lead to interaction with and therefore reduced education by medical providers [38].

Differently abled groups

Individuals with intellectual and/or physical disabilities appear likely to be excluded from traditional school-based sex education. Some students will not receive sex education at all when they are not included in traditional education settings, whereas others will be unlikely to see examples of students similar to them included in AOUM materials. Additionally, many differently abled individuals report that their healthcare providers also do not provide them with needed sexual health information. The failure to discuss the sexual needs and experiences of these youth and young adults is at least in part due to stereotypes related to the appropriateness of such individuals' engagement in sexual behaviors and stereotyped view of these individuals supposedly reduced sexual needs and desires. However, research not surprisingly shows that differently abled individuals do indeed desire sexual relationships and the ability to have children [39–41]. Without formal sex or reproductive education, many differently abled individuals turn to their peers and social media both of which may not be able to provide reliable or needed information [41].

The dangers of poor sex/reproductive education

Reproductive knowledge

Failure to provide routine education related to how to conceive results in limits of reproductive knowledge. Research on reproductive knowledge unfortunately confirms a lack of such education globally and also highlights that some patient populations are differentially disadvantaged by the lack of structured reproductive education [11,12,21,42,43]. For example, one study of fertility knowledge among infertility patients found that individuals who were heterosexual, White or Asian, and/or were from higher socioeconomic background had greater fertility knowledge than patients from other demographic backgrounds [42]. Men have also been found to have less accurate reproductive knowledge than women [12]. Although it is comforting to know that a single consultation with a reproductive endocrinologist, or a college course on preconception have been shown to improve fertility knowledge, access to such education is limited by financial and other resources [10,42].

The limited nature of reproductive knowledge has likely led to beliefs regarding reproduction being driven by informal education from individuals in one's social networks or via online sources [42,44]. It also appears likely that the limited provision of education about reproduction has led to mass belief in multiple harmful myths about reproduction. There are a host of reproductive myths but several include the myth that it is easier to conceive at any age and with any heterosexual partner than is true, that if it is not easy to conceive it is the woman's fault (e.g., because she is too stressed), and that miscarriage is rare and if it occurs it is likely the woman's fault [12,45–47]. As with other studies, research confirms that individuals who identify as non-White or who are from lower socioeconomic groups may be more likely to believe reproductive myths [48] or may have greater risk of unrealistic expectations regarding chances of conceiving [42]. The lack of reproductive/fertility education has also likely resulted in individuals/couples not knowing how to best time intercourse to conceive or not conceive [43]. Belief in the ease of reproduction and women's alleged culpability should it not be easy to conceive has contributed to the shaming and silencing of women and couples regarding their difficulties conceiving as well as disparate use of fertility treatments due to stigma related to infertility and reproductive loss [38,45].

The differential exposure to and belief in reproductive myths, and the greater likelihood of even less reproductive education given to men versus women, could also pose a multitude of problems for couples who are trying to conceive but only one partner has received accurate education about how fertility works. It is not uncommon, for example, for couples pursuing fertility treatment to report increased relationship distress and for differences in men and women's beliefs about infertility to affect marital distress [49]. Although research has not fully explored the cause of marital distress in diverse infertility patient populations, it is reasonable to assume that differences in beliefs about how fertility works may result in undue blame or efforts to pressure a partner into altering their lifestyle to conform to reproductive myths (e.g., restrictive diets, coercion to quit a stressful job, etc.) that could influence the experience of distress.

Infertility

Clearly, the lack of reproductive/fertility education and the belief in reproductive myths have the ability to increase the risk of infertility and childlessness. Patients who do not understand the importance of age; the equal contribution of male factor infertility in conception; the role of STIs, obesity, and substance use in fertility; optimal times for intercourse; and truths rather than myths of reproduction may intentionally delay childbearing or unintentionally delay childbearing by engaging in long periods of attempts to conceive without awareness of their impaired chances of success [50]. Any delays in conception result in patients attempting to conceive at older ages and thus increased risk of infertility [51].

The risk of infertility may be greater for patients who receive poorer education regarding reproduction as those receiving worse education may delay reproduction for longer periods or may attempt conception without medical intervention for longer periods of time. Unfortunately, research has identified the presence of decreased reproductive/fertility knowledge in individuals from diverse racial/ethnic groups, socioeconomic statuses, and sexes experiencing infertility [47,52]. Research by Missmer et al. [38] also appears to confirm disparities related to delay of fertility care finding that non-White women and women from lower socioeconomic groups may delay treatment longer that their wealthier White peers. No research has yet directly examined the role of racism or sexism in delayed conception. However, disparate and racially stereotyped sex and reproductive education and the lack of reproductive education given to men likely contribute to this problem as fertility knowledge has been shown to affect family planning; comprehensive reproductive/fertility education has been shown to reduce delays in family building [50]. Further, it is accepted that infertility is associated with increased risk of anxiety and depression, thus disparate reproductive education would reasonably be associated with increased risk of psychological distress.

Violence/discrimination/harassment/hostility toward women, racial/ethnic minority group members, gender nonconforming, nonheterosexual, and/or differently abled individuals

Underlying sexism and differential education of women and men increases the risk of violence against all women. The early education of boys about the role of women as passive sexual recipients to be conquered and as sexually vulnerable to the hypersexual and uncontrollable whims (e.g., "boys will be boys") of the male sex as well as the primary providers of care for men's offspring reinforces the historical subjugation of women. Educational messages presented to women indicate that they are required to be chaste and with no sexual desires lest they be otherwise labeled whores or worse yet, wind up as the often-cited stereotypical poor teenager unable to succeed in the world as they are burdened with their offspring. Ableist, homophobic, and transphobic content included in sex and reproductive education (as well as the lack of relevant education provided to these individuals) send the message that these individuals should not or are not deserving of conceiving or parenting. Racist stereotypes in sex/reproductive education and systemic racism in healthcare and other systems, falsely suggest that certain groups of individuals should always be open to sexual advances and/or should have no problems conceiving. These messages also serve to "other" (i.e., viewing people dissimilar to oneself as inferior) non-White, gender nonconforming, differently abled, and nonheterosexual individuals, which increases the risk of targeted harassment and/or violence (e.g., hate crimes, hate speech, sexual assault/harassment, etc.) [53–58].

The intersection of infertility and intimate partner violence

Physical, sexual, and/or psychological violence committed by an intimate partner is unfortunately common. Although women are the primary targets of intimate partner violence (IPV) and men are the primary perpetrators of such violence, men too can be victims of such abusive behaviors and women can be the aggressors. Stressors such as infertility and infertility treatment have frequently been shown to increase the risk of IPV (including reproductive coercion). Further, differential risk for IPV among those struggling to conceive has been identified with greater risks of IPV among women in lower socioeconomic groups [59]. Thus disparities in the provision of comprehensive sex and reproductive/fertility education, particularly disparities in education of women and men, and the resulting differences in understanding (and misunderstanding) the causes of infertility (e.g., "infertility is the woman's fault") place all women at risk of IPV and disproportionally place women who identify as being from lower socioeconomic groups at even higher risk.

Sexual dysfunction, the forgotten education

In addition to not teaching how sex should be performed to maximize pleasure or reproduction, no structured education is provided in the United States (and many other countries) regarding sexual dysfunction. The predominant focus of many education systems is on avoidance of all sex until married. It excludes discussion of how to maximize the benefits of recreational or procreational sex as well as avoids the topic of sex dysfunction despite the prevalence of sexual dysfunction worldwide [60,61]. As a result, not only is procreational and recreational sex often a taboo subject, but difficulties associated with sexual function in general are also not frequently discussed. Similar to research showing that patients and not their doctors are often the first to raise concerns about fertility, it appears that medical professionals may also not raise the topic of sexual dysfunction despite patient preferences otherwise [62].

Research also confirms that although sexual dysfunction is rarely the cause of infertility; infertility and prolonged infertility treatment are associated with increased risk of sexual dysfunction [63–67]. Further, sex dysfunction is associated with risk of domestic violence [68]. Thus failure to appropriately educate the general population about reproduction and sexual dysfunction not only may result in reduced treatment-seeking behaviors but also in increased risk of IPV.

Future directions

It is clear that there are a host of serious and disparate consequences of inadequate sex and reproductive education. Although the provision of honest, judgment-free, and inclusive information regarding sex and reproduction/fertility may result in some increases in anxiety [11], this anxiety likely pales in comparison to the psychological distress faced by individuals and couples who may not have struggled to conceive had they known the truth about how to conceive. Further, the provision of such comprehensive inclusive education also may serve to decrease (though not eliminate) the risk of violent or otherwise hostile attitudes and behaviors toward women and/or individuals who identify as transgender or gender nonconforming, homosexual, racially minoritized, differently abled, and other groups. Given that not all individuals will receive such comprehensive and inclusive education through school, FBOs, parents, healthcare professionals, or the internet; efforts to equally provide such information must be multifactorial in nature.

First and foremost, changes should be made to remove discriminatory and stereotyped language in state/government run sex education. Additionally, honest information about how conception functionally works should be provided beginning in adolescence. This may serve to reduce unintended pregnancies and would be unlikely to increase intended teenage pregnancies as even in the absence of such education, teenagers who desire to conceive would likely continue engagement in unprotected intercourse until conception occurred. These proposed changes to sex/reproductive education will likely be hampered however by pressures from religious and other ideological groups with a vested interested in the dominance of their views of morality. As a result, preconception courses could be required or at least offered at the collegiate level, though again, the taboos related to discussion of sex and religious mores about discussion of sex in schools will likely result in many schools not being able to provide such education.

Avenues to provide comprehensive value-free education outside of formal education systems may reduce interference by outside forces. Such strategies could include the creation and free dissemination of research-driven apps on cellular phones [69], though not everyone will be able to afford a cellular phone or be comfortable in accessing such applications. Another educational strategy could include required (yearly) documented proactive comprehensive education by medical professionals providing care to reproductive-aged patients. This is similar to the concept of required documented counseling by medical professionals regarding fertility preservation options for newly diagnosed cancer patients of reproductive age [70]. This medical counseling should also include the re-education of older generations (parents of reproductively aged children) on an annual basis to reduce the risk that parents may share unsupported sex/reproductive beliefs with their children as well as provide an opportunity for older individuals to discuss their own sex-related concerns. However, given the large number of medical systems operated by religious entities, mandatory value-free recreational and procreational counseling may also be difficult to achieve [71]. Therefore medical professionals should also partner with communities who are less likely or able to seek medical care or who do not have access to value-free care to provide comprehensive sex/reproductive education. It is only through a multipronged approach that the probability that all individuals will receive accurate, nonjudgmental, inclusive information about sex, reproduction, and sex dysfunction.

References

[1] Clarke CW. The American Social Hygiene Association. Public Health Rep 1955;70(4):421−7.
[2] Huber VJ, Firmin MW. A history of sex education in the United States since 1900. Int J Educ Reform 2014;23(1):25−51.
[3] Carter JB. Birds, bees, and venereal disease: toward an intellectual history of sex education. J Hist Sex 2001;10(2):213−49.
[4] Ehrlich JS. From birth control to sex control: unruly young women and the origins of the national abstinence-only mandate. Can Bull Med Hist 2013;30(1):77−99.
[5] Elia JP, Eliason MJ. Dangerous omissions: abstinence-only-until-marriage school-based sexuality education and the betrayal of LGBTQ youth. Am J Sex Educ 2010;5(1):17−35.
[6] Fox AM, Himmelstein G, Khalid H, Howell EA. Funding for abstinence-only education and adolescent pregnancy prevention: does state ideology affect outcomes? Am J Public Health 2019;109(3):497−504.
[7] Guttmacher Institute. Sex and HIV education. Available from: <https://www.guttmacher.org/state-policy/explore/sex-and-hiv-education>; 2020.
[8] Stanger-Hall KF, Hall DW. Abstinence-only education and teen pregnancy rates: why we need comprehensive sex education in the United States. PLoS One 2011;6(10):e24658.
[9] Santelli JS, Kantor LM, Grilo SA, Speizer IS, Lindberg LD, Heitel J, et al. Abstinence-only-until-marriage: an updated review of United States policies and programs and their impact. J Adolesc Health 2017;61(3):273−80.
[10] Delgado C. Pregnancy 101: a call for reproductive and prenatal health education in college. Matern Child Health J 2013;17(2):240−7.
[11] Boivin J, Koert E, Harris T, O'Shea L, Perryman A, Parker K, et al. An experimental evaluation of the benefits and costs of providing fertility information to adolescents and emerging adults. Hum Reprod 2018;33(7):1247−53.
[12] Pedro J, Brandao T, Schmidt L, Costa ME, Martins MV. What do people know about fertility? A systematic review on fertility awareness and its associated factors. Upsala J Med Sci 2018;123(2):71−81.
[13] Moore E, Berkley-Patton J, Bohn A, Hawes S, Bowe-Thompson C. Beliefs about sex and parent-child-church sex communication among church-based African American youth. J Relig Health 2015;54(5):1810−25.
[14] Slater LM, Cummings, Aholou TM. What you don't know may kill you: The importance of including sexual health in premarital counseling. Fam J Alex Va 2009;17(3):236−40.
[15] Aholou TM, Gale JE, Slater LM. African American clergy share perspectives on addressing sexual health and HIV prevention in premarital counseling: a pilot study. J Relig Health 2011;50(2):330−47.
[16] Boonstra HD. Matter of faith: support for comprehensive sex education among faith-based organizations. Guttmacher Policy Rev 2008;11(1):17−22.
[17] Barden-O'Fallon J. Availability of family planning services and quality of counseling by faith-based organizations: a three country comparative analysis. Reprod Health 2017;14(1):57.
[18] Jones K, Williams J, Sipsma H, Patil C. Adolescent and emerging adults' evaluation of a Facebook site providing sexual health education. Public Health Nurs 2019;36(1):11−17.
[19] Wilson EK, Dalberth BT, Koo HP, Gard JC. Parents' perspectives on talking to preteenage children about sex. Perspect Sex Reprod Health 2010;42(1):56−63.
[20] Yu L, Peterson B, Inhorn MC, Boehm JK, Patrizio P. Knowledge, attitudes, and intentions toward fertility awareness and oocyte cryopreservation among obstetrics and gynecology resident physicians. Hum Reprod 2016;31(2):403−11.
[21] Ikhena-Abel DE, Confino R, Shah NJ, Lawson AK, Klock SC, Robins JC, et al. Is employer coverage of elective egg freezing coercive?: a survey of medical students' knowledge, intentions, and attitudes towards elective egg freezing and employer coverage. J Assist Reprod Genet 2017;34(8):1035−41.
[22] Kudesia R, Chernyak E, McAvey B. Low fertility awareness in United States reproductive-aged women and medical trainees: creation and validation of the Fertility & Infertility Treatment Knowledge Score (FIT-KS). Fertil Steril 2017;108(4):711−17.
[23] Maeda E, Boivin J, Toyokawa S, Murata K, Saito H. Two-year follow-up of a randomized controlled trial: knowledge and reproductive outcome after online fertility education. Hum Reprod 2018;33(11):2035−42.
[24] Widman L, Nesi J, Kamke K, Choukas-Bradley S, Stewart JL. Technology-based interventions to reduce sexually transmitted infections and unintended pregnancy among youth. J Adolesc Health 2018;62(6):651−60.
[25] Steinke J, Root-Bowman M, Estabrook S, Levine DS, Kantor LM. Meeting the needs of sexual and gender minority youth: formative research on potential digital health interventions. J Adolesc Health 2017;60(5):541−8.
[26] Gonzalez-Ortega E, Vicario-Molina I, Martinez JL, Orgaz B. The Internet as a source of sexual information in a sample of Spanish adolescents: associations with sexual behavior. Sex Res Soc Policy 2015;12(4):290−300.
[27] Simon L, Daneback K. Adolescents' use of the internet for sex education: a thematic and critical review of the literature. Int J Sex Health 2013;25(4):305−19.
[28] Almeida-Santos T, Melo C, Macedo A, Moura-Ramos M. Are women and men well informed about fertility? Childbearing intentions, fertility knowledge and information-gathering sources in Portugal. Reprod Health 2017;14(1):91.

[29] Sondag KA, Johnson AG, Parrish ME. School sex education: teachers' and young adults' perceptions of relevance for LGBT students. J LGBT Youth 2020.

[30] Tabaac AR, Haneuse S, Johns M, Tan ASL, Austin SB, Potter J, et al. Sexual and reproductive health information: disparities across sexual orientation groups in two cohorts of us women. Sex Res Soc Policy 2020.

[31] Bergman K, Rubio RJ, Green R, Padron E. Gay men who become fathers via surrogacy: the transition to parenthood. J GLBT Family Stud 2010;6:111−41.

[32] Tornello SL, Bos H. Parenting intentions among transgender individuals. LGBT Health 2017;4(2):115−20.

[33] Tate DP, Patterson CJ, Levy AJ. Predictors of parenting intentions among childless lesbian, gay, and heterosexual adults. J Fam Psychol 2019;33(2):194−202.

[34] Murphy DA. The desire for parenthood: gay men choosing to become parents through surrogacy. J Fam Issues 2013;34:1104−24.

[35] Lamb S, Graling K, Lustig K. Stereotypes in four current AOUM sexuality education curricula: good girls, good boys, and the new gender equality. Am J Sex Educ 2011;6(4):370−80.

[36] Froyum CM. Making 'good girls': sexual agency in the sexuality education of low-income black girls. Cult Health Sex 2010;12(1):59−72.

[37] Garcia L. 'Now why do you want to know about that?': heteronormativity, sexism, and racism in the sexual (mis)education of Latina youth. Gend Soc 2009;23(4):520−41.

[38] Missmer SA, Seifer DB, Jain T. Cultural factors contributing to health care disparities among patients with infertility in Midwestern United States. Fertil Steril 2011;95(6):1943−9.

[39] Grove L, Morrison-Beedy D, Kirby R, Hess J. The birds, bees, and special needs: making evidence-based sex education accessible for adolescents with intellectual disabilities. Sex Disabil 2018;36(4):313−29.

[40] Bahner J. Cripping sex education: lessons learned from a programme aimed at young people with mobility impairments. Sex Educ 2018;18(6):640−54.

[41] Secor-Turner M, McMorris BJ, Scal P. Improving the sexual health of young people with mobility impairments: challenges and recommendations. J Pediatr Health Care 2017;31(5):578−87.

[42] Childress KJ, Lawson AK, Ghant MS, Mendoza G, Cardozo ER, Confino E, et al. First contact: the intersection of demographics, knowledge, and appraisal of treatment at the initial infertility visit. Fertil Steril 2015;104(1):180−7.

[43] Ayoola AB, Zandee GL, Adams YJ. Women's knowledge of ovulation, the menstrual cycle, and its associated reproductive changes. Birth 2016;43(3):255−62.

[44] Cheung NK, Coffey A, Woods C, de Costa C. Natural fertility, infertility and the role of medically assisted reproduction: the knowledge amongst women of reproductive age in North Queensland. Aust N Z J Obstet Gynaecol 2019;59(1):140−6.

[45] Lawson AK. Psychological stress and fertility. In: Stevenson EL, Hershberger PE, editors. Fertility and assisted reproductive technology (ART): theory, research, policy and practice for healthcare practitioners. New York: Springer Publishing Company; 2019, p. 65−86.

[46] Bardos J, Hercz D, Friedenthal J, Missmer SA, Williams Z. A national survey on public perceptions of miscarriage. Obstet Gynecol 2015;125(6):1313−20.

[47] Koert E, Harrison C, Bunting L, Gladwyn-Khan M, Boivin J. Causal explanations for lack of pregnancy applying the common sense model of illness representation to the fertility context. Psychol Health 2018;33(10):1284−301.

[48] Negris O, Lawson AK, Brown D, Warren C, Galic I, Bozen A, et al. Emotional stress and reproduction: what do fertility patients believe? J Assist Reprod Genet 2021;38(4):877−87.

[49] Peterson BD, Newton CR, Rosen KH. Examining congruence between partners' perceived infertility-related stress and its relationship to marital adjustment and depression in infertile couples. Fam Process 2003;42(1):59−70.

[50] Williamson LE, Lawson KL, Downe PJ, Pierson RA. Informed reproductive decision-making: the impact of providing fertility information on fertility knowledge and intentions to delay childbearing. J Obstet Gynaecol Can 2014;36(5):400−5.

[51] Hourvitz A, Machtinger R, Maman E, Baum M, Dor J, Levron J. Assisted reproduction in women over 40 years of age: how old is too old? Reprod Biomed Online 2009;19(4):599−603.

[52] Hoffman JR, Delaney MA, Valdes CT, Herrera D, Washington SL, Aghajanova L, et al. Disparities in fertility knowledge among women from low and high resource settings presenting for fertility care in two United States metropolitan centers. Fertil Res Pract 2020;6:15.

[53] Fitzgerald LF, Drasgow F, Hulin CL, Gelfand MJ, Magley VJ. Antecedents and consequences of sexual harassment in organizations: a test of an integrated model. J Appl Psychol 1997;82(4):578−89.

[54] Espelage DL, Basile KC, De La Rue L, Hamburger ME. Longitudinal associations among bullying, homophobic teasing, and sexual violence perpetration among middle school students. J Interpers Violence 2015;30(14):2541−61.

[55] Cowan G, Heiple B, Marquez C, Khatchadourian D, McNevin M. Heterosexuals' attitudes toward hate crimes and hate speech against gays and lesbians: old-fashioned and modern heterosexism. J Homosex 2005;49(2):67−82.

[56] Gover AR, Harper SB, Langton L. Anti-Asian hate crime during the COVID-19 pandemic: exploring the reproduction of inequality. Am J Crim Justice 2020;45:647−67.

[57] Mekawi Y, Bresin K, Hunter CD. White fear, dehumanization, and low empathy: Lethal combinations for shooting biases. Cultur Divers Ethnic Minor Psychol 2016;22(3):322−32.

[58] Forbes GB, Adams-Curtis LE, Pakalka AH, White KB. Dating aggression, sexual coercion, and aggression-supporting attitudes among college men as a function of participation in aggressive high school sports. Violence Against Women 2006;12(5):441−55.

[59] Barishansky S, Shapiro P, Pavone ME, Lawson AK. Intimate partner violence screening during infertility treatment. Fertility and Sterility Dialogue 2020. Available from: https://www.fertstertdialog.com/posts/58702-barishansky-consider-this.

[60] Kingsberg SA, Woodard T. Female sexual dysfunction: focus on low desire. Obstet Gynecol 2015;125(2):477−86.

[61] Lotti F, Maggi M. Sexual dysfunction and male infertility. Nat Rev Urol 2018;15(5):287−307.

[62] Nusbaum MR, Helton MR, Ray N. The changing nature of women's sexual health concerns through the midlife years. Maturitas. 2004;49(4):283−91.

[63] Keskin U, Coksuer H, Gungor S, Ercan CM, Karasahin KE, Baser I. Differences in prevalence of sexual dysfunction between primary and secondary infertile women. Fertil Steril 2011;96(5):1213−17.

References

[64] Song SH, Kim DS, Yoon TK, Hong JY, Shim SH. Sexual function and stress level of male partners of infertile couples during the fertile period. BJU Int 2016;117(1):173–6.

[65] Wincze JP. Psychosocial aspects of ejaculatory dysfunction and male reproduction. Fertil Steril 2015;104(5):1089–94.

[66] Bechoua S, Hamamah S, Scalici E. Male infertility: an obstacle to sexuality? Andrology 2016;4(3):395–403.

[67] Wischmann TH. Sexual disorders in infertile couples. J Sex Med 2010;7(5):1868–76.

[68] Metz ME, Epstein N. Assessing the role of relationship conflict in sexual dysfunction. J Sex Marital Ther 2002;28(2):139–64.

[69] Ford EA, Roman SD, McLaughlin EA, Beckett EL, Sutherland JM. The association between reproductive health smartphone applications and fertility knowledge of Australian women. BMC Womens Health 2020;20(1):45.

[70] Lawson AK, Klock SC, Pavone ME, Hirshfeld-Cytron J, Smith KN, Kazer RR. Psychological counseling of female fertility preservation patients. J Psychosoc Oncol 2015;33(4):333–53.

[71] Drake C, Jarlenski M, Zhang Y, Polsky D. Market share of United States catholic hospitals and associated geographic network access to reproductive health services. JAMA Netw Open 2020;3(1):e1920053.

Index

Note: Page numbers followed by "*f*" and "*t*" refer to figures and tables, respectively.

A

Abstinence-only-until-(heterosexual)-marriage (AOUM) education, 265
Acquired situational delayed ejaculation, 89–90
Acupuncture, 219, 230
Adolescent Family Life Act, 265–266
Adoption, 128
Alcohol abuse, 36–37
Ambivalent-insecure attachment style, 175
American Academy of Pediatrics (AAP), 16
American Association of Sex Educators, Counselors and Therapists (AASECT), 12
American Society for Reproductive Medicine (ASRM), 24, 126
American Society of Clinical Oncology (ASCO), 109
American Urological Association (AUA) Guidelines, 26
Anabolic-induced hypogonadism, 28
Anabolic steroids, 27–28
Anatomy and Physiology (AP), 14
Androgens, 100
Anejaculation (AE), 28, 77–78
Animalcules, 8
Antegrade ejaculation, 34
Antimullerian hormone (AMH), 95, 154
Antipsychotics, 61, 69
Anxiety, 46–47
Archaeologic record, 4
Aromatase inhibitors, 160
Arterial insufficiency, 60
Ashwagandha (Withania Somnifera), 222
Assisted reproductive technology (ART), 25–26, 126, 129–131, 142, 207, 238–239
  treatment, 47, 49, 192
Atherosclerosis, 60, 97–98
At-home insemination, 128–129
Attachment theory, 175
Avanafil, 64, 64*f*, 200
Avoidant-insecure attachment style, 175
Azoospermia, 30

B

Baby-making, 184–185
Beck Depression Inventory total score, 49
Behavioral techniques, 87
Biologic parenthood, methods for, 164*t*
Birth control, creation of, 238
Black, indigenous, and people of color (BIPOC) cancer survivors, 113
Body mass index (BMI), 37
Bulbourethral artery, 58–59

C

Cancer, 35
Cancer survivors, reproductive and sexual health (RSH) concerns for
  cancer's impact on sexual health, 106–107
  impact of cancer treatment on fertility, 105–106
  managing reproductive and sexual health concerns after cancer, 107–112
    clinical guidelines for fertility consultation and preservation, 109
    clinical guidelines for sexual health after cancer, 110–111
    improving partner communication about reproductive and sexual health concerns, 111–112
    improving patient-provider communication, 108–109
    management of infertility risk, 109–110
    management of men's sexual health problems, 111
    management of women's sexual health problems, 111
  reproductive concerns after cancer, 106
  special considerations, 112–113
    assumptions about sexual health, 112
    black, indigenous, and people of color (BIPOC) cancer survivors, 113
    LGBTQ+ cancer survivors, 112–113
    older adult cancer survivors, 113
Catholicism, 241, 250
Cavernosal innervations, loss of, 60–61
Cavernous arteries, 58–59
Cessation of menses, 154
Chemotherapy, 29
Chest feeding, 167–168
Childbirth, 134–135
Chinese medical theory, 229–230
Chinese medicine practitioners, 214
Chong Mai (Penetrating vessel), 218
Christian infertility, navigating, 250–251
Christianity, origin of, 238–239
Chronic renal failure, 60
Chronic stress, 191
Cisplatin-based chemotherapy, 106
Clitorodynia, 228
Clomiphene citrate, 65
Collaboration of religion, with treatment, 256–258
Communication, 185
Commuting to work, 209
Comprehensive school-based sex education, 265
Comprehensive Sex Education (CSE), 12–13
Comprehensive sexuality education programs, 14
Comprehensive value-free education, 270–271
Comstock Act of 1873, 11
Congenital bilateral absence of the vas deferens (CBAVD), 26
Conjugated equine estrogen (CEE), 97
Consent and Healthy Relationships (CHR), 14
Cordyceps (Dong Chong Xia Cao), 221–222
Coregulation, 177
Couple communication, 111–112
Cryopreservation, 251
Cryptorchidism, 35–36
Cupping, 220
Cyclic guanylate monophosphate (cGMP), 59
Cynomorium songaricum (Suo yang), 221
Cystic fibrosis (CF), 31
Cystic fibrosis transmembrane conductance regulator (CFTR) gene, 31
Cystic fibrosis transmembrane conductance regulator/congenital bilateral absence of vas deferens, 31

D

Daddy Boot Camp, 134–135
Dai channel (Belt vessel), 219
Delayed ejaculation (DE), 77, 83–85, 226
  etiological factors in, 85–86
  treatment of, 86–88
Detumescence, 59
Dhat syndrome, 86
Diabetes mellitus (DM), 33–34, 94
Diagnostic and Statistical Manual of Mental Disorders (DSM-5), 173
Differently abled groups, 159
Discriminatory legislation, 152
Donated sperm, 247
Donor IVF cycle, 129–130
Donor sperm, 30–31
  couples using, 131–132
  psychological consultation for patients using, 131–132

Donor sperm (*Continued*)
  psychological preparation for lesbians working with known sperm donor, 132–133
Dorsal penile artery, 58–59
DSM-V diagnostic guidelines, 84
Dual energy x-ray absorption (DEXA) scan, 96–97
Du channel (Governing vessel), 219
Dyspareunia, 227–228
Dysphoria, 162

E

Early-childhood attachment relationships, 175
Early ejaculators, edging practice for, 227
Early menopause (EM), 93–104
  comorbidities associated with, 96–97
  primary ovarian insufficiency
    diagnosis of, 96–97
    etiologies of, 93–95
    treatment of, 97–101
      choice of HT, 98–99
      contraceptive needs, 99
      emotional health, 101
      fertility, 99–100
      future of POI treatment, 101
      hormone therapy, 97–98
      sexual health, 100–101
Earth element, 218
Eastern medicine, 220
Edging practice for early ejaculators, 227
Education, reproduction, and sexual function, 265–274
  future directions, 270–271
  poor sex/reproductive education, dangers of, 268–270
    infertility, 269
    intersection of infertility and intimate partner violence, 269–270
    reproductive knowledge, 268–269
    violence/discrimination/harassment/hostility toward women, 269–270
  reproductive education in the United States, 266–267
    faith-based organizations, 266
    healthcare providers, 266–267
    institutions of higher learning, 266
    parents, 266
    social networks and social media, 267
  sex/reproductive education, disparate effects of, 267–268
    differently abled groups, 268
    LGBTQ individuals, 267
    racial minoritized groups, 267–268
    sex disparities, 267
  sexual dysfunction, 270
Egg donor, 145
Egg retrieval, 145
Eight extraordinary channels, 217
Ejaculatory dysfunction, 77, 226
  intravaginal, 226–227
Ejaculatory dysfunction and infertility, 77–92

acquired situational delayed ejaculation (case study), 89–90
case study, 82–83
delayed ejaculation, 83–85
  etiological factors in, 85–86
  treatment of, 86–88
lifelong, situational delayed ejaculation (case study), 88–89
premature ejaculation and infertility, 80
premature or rapid ejaculation, 78–79
retrograde ejaculation and anejaculation, 77–78
treatment for premature or rapid ejaculation, 80–82
Electroacupuncture (EA), 219
Electroejaculation (EEJ), 28, 34, 69–70, 70f, 78
Embryo cryopreservation, 157, 159, 162
Embryo donation, 248
Emergent modes of reproduction, 210–211
Enriching Communication Skills for Health Professionals in Oncofertility (ECHO) training program, 109
Erectile dysfunction, 57–76, 107, 191–192, 223
  assisted reproductive techniques, 69
    natural cycle intrauterine insemination with ejaculated sperm, 69
  diagnosis of, 223–224
  causes of, 60–63
    hormonal, 61–62
    lifestyle, 63
    medication-induced, 61
    neurologic, 60–61
    psychological or situational anxiety–related, 63
    vascular, 60
  historical and anatomical overview of, 57–59
    anatomy, 58–59
    history, prevalence, and incidence, 57–58
  infertility and relationship with, 59–60
  sperm retrieval/ICSI, 69–71
  traditional Chinese medicine treatment of, 224–225
  treating underlying problem, 68–69
  treatment of, 63–68, 224–225
    counseling, 65
    hormonal replacement, 65
    MUSE (intraurethral therapy), 67–68
    penile implant, 68
    penile injection therapy, 66–67
    phosphodiesterase 5 inhibitors, 64–65
    vacuum erection device (VED), 67
  treatment of infertility, 68
Erectile process, 60
Estradiol, 97, 155
Estrogen, 97
Estrogen-progestin combination therapy, 98
Estrogen therapy, 98
European Society for Human Reproduction and Embryology guidelines, 95–97
European Union Agency for Fundamental Rights Survey, 152
Exogenous testosterone, 27, 65

Expert interviews, 207

F

Faith-based organizations (FBOs), 152–153
Family and Medical Leave Act (FMLA), 136
Family balancing, 25
Female orgasm disorder (FOD), 48
Female problems, treatment plans for, 230–231
Female sexual function, 45–56
  case, 45–46
  female sexual function disorders leading to infertility, 49–50
  infertility leading to female sexual dysfunction, 48–49
  psychological distress and, 48
  psychological effects of infertility in women, 46–48
  referral, consultation, and treatment, 50–54
    infertility counseling, 52–53
    pharmacological and medical treatment, 53–54
    sex therapy, 51–52
  treatment outcomes, 50
Female Sexual Function Index (FSFI), 191–192
Female sexual interest/arousal disorder, 195
Female sexual issues, 227
  causes of, 228f
Female sexual pain, 229–230
Femininity, 12
Feminizing hormone therapy, 155
Fertile window, 193–194
Fertility, 222–223
Fertility awareness (FA), 14
Fertility consultation, 110–111
Fertility decisions, 206
Fertility Dost, 207
Fertility Dost WhatsApp, 208
Fertility preservation (FP), 16
Fertility preservation options
  for transgender men, 157–159
  for transgender men and nonbinary individuals assigned female at birth, 158t
  for transgender women, 160–163
  for transgender women and nonbinary individuals assigned male at birth, 161t
Fertility preservation outcomes
  for transgender men, 159–160
  for transgender women, 163–164
Fertility preservation utilization, 110–111
Fertility treatment, cost of, 130–131
Financial burden, 25–26
Finasteride, 29
Fire element, 218
Five-element system, 217
FMR1 gene, 94
Follicle stimulating hormone (FSH), 26–27, 61–62, 145
Formal fertility treatment, 130
Future of Sex Education (FOSE), 14
Fu Xing Zhu's Gynecology, 216–217

G

Gay couples, 145
Gay men, 141–148
  broader societal implications of gay men having children, 146–147
  evolving landscape of fertility treatments for, 143–144
  family building for, 144
  hoping of a family, 142–143
  process of gestational surrogacy pregnancy, 144–146
  progress in acceptance and law for, 141–142
  sexualizing gestational-surrogacy process for, 146
Gender-affirming hormones, 153, 155
Gender-affirming surgery, 153
Gender dysphoria, 36, 149–150
Gender Identity and Expression (GI), 14
Gender identity disorder, 149
Generative vitality, 7
Genetics, 94
Genitourinary (GU) system, 33
Gestational surrogacy, 142
Glucocorticoids, 191
Gonadotropin-releasing hormone (GnRH), 26–27, 61–62
Gonorrhea, 10
Grief, 174
Grief counseling, 53

H

Healthcare providers, 108, 112
Heart and Estrogen/Progestin Replacement Study (HERS), 97
Heart energy, 218
Hegemonic status to heterosexuality, 243
Herba Cistanche (Rou Cong-Rong), 222
Herbal medicine, 220
  and erectile dysfunction, 225–226
Heterosexuals, 144
High-wage information technology workers, 206
High-wage labor markets, 211
History gathering, 179t
Homosexuality, 147
Hormonal antiandrogens, 61
Hormonal causes of male infertility, 26–28
  anabolic steroids, 27–28
  iatrogenic testosterone replacement, 26–27
Hormonal replacement for men with ED, 65
Horny Goat Weed (Epimedium yin yang huo), 221
Human menopausal gonadotropins, 145
Human sexuality, 17
Hypoactive sexual desire disorder (HSDD), 49–50, 195
Hypogastric nerve plexus, 33
Hypogonadism, 27
Hypogonadotropic hypogonadism, 62, 65
Hypothalamic–pituitary–adrenal (HPA) axis, 26
Hypothalamic–pituitary–gonadal (HPG) axis, 62f, 191

I

Iatrogenic cavernosal nerve injury, 60–61
Iatrogenic testosterone replacement, 26–27
Idiosyncratic masturbatory style, 85
Implications and recommendations, 254–255
Improvised explosive device (IED), 180–181
Infertility, 23, 46, 173, 192, 269
  intersection of, 269–270
  psychological impact of, 192–193
  in Qur'an, 251–252
Infertility and sexuality, in couple
  marital implications, 196–197
Infertility and sexuality, in men
  clinical implications, 194
  psychosocial implications, 194–195
Infertility and sexuality, in women
  clinical implications, 195–196
  psychosocial implications, 196
Infertility counseling, 52–53
Infertility diagnosis, 200
Infertility-related stress, on sexuality, 193–197
Internalized homophobia, 136
International Classification of Diseases and Related Health Problems (ICD-11), 79, 84–85
International Society for Sexual Medicine (ISSM), 79
International Society for the Study of Vulvovaginal Disease (ISSVD), 228
Interpersonal Violence (IV), 14
Intimate partner violence (IPV), 269–270
Intracavernosal medications, 66
Intracavernosal therapy, injection procedure for, 66f
Intracytoplasmic sperm injection (ICSI), 29, 34, 69
Intrauterine insemination (IUI), 45, 165
Intravaginal ejaculatory dysfunction, case on, 226–227
Intravaginal ejaculatory latency time (IELT), 79
In vitro fertilization (IVF), 45, 142, 205
In vitro maturation (IVM), 99–100
Islam, origin of, 239

J

Jewish Orthodox couple, 246
Jing, 214–215
Job security anxieties, 209
Judaism, origin of, 238
Judeo-Christian perspectives on infertility and assisted reproduction, 244–249
  infertility in the Old Testament, 244–245
  navigating Jewish infertility, 246–249
Judeo-Christian views of homosexuality and status, 242–244
Judeo-Christian views on sexuality and sex, 239–242

K

Kidney energy, 217–218
Klinefelter syndrome (KS), 26, 29–30
Known sperm donor, 132–133, 136
Kung Fu Method, 215

L

Lactua serriola, 5–6
Legal and cultural evolution, 127
Lemba Lady, 5
Lesbians pursuing parenthood, 123–140
  adoption, 128
  assisted reproductive technology, 129–131
  at-home insemination, 128–129
  fertility clinic experience for, 133–134
  historical context, 125–127
  legal considerations, 136–137
  policies, procedures, and practices to support, 137–138
    recommendations for clinics and programs, 138
    recommendations for individual providers, 137
  postpartum phase, 135–136
  pregnancy and childbirth, 134–135
  preparing for pregnancy, 127
  psychological consultation for patients using donor sperm, 131–132
  psychological preparation for lesbians working with known sperm donor, 132–133
LGBTQ+ cancer survivors, 112–113
LGBTQ community, 143–144, 147
LGBTQ individuals, 267
Lichen sclerosus, 230
Lifelong, situational delayed ejaculation (case study), 88–89
Lifestyle issues, 36–37
Liver energy, 218
Liver Qi stagnation, 230
Longer-term therapeutic, 53
Low serum testosterone, 65
Lung energy, 218
Luteinizing hormone (LH), 26–27, 61–62

M

Magic pill, 29
Male deer exercise, 225
Male ejaculatory problems, treatment of, 77
Male factor infertility, 65
Male infertility, 5–6, 195
  anatomic, 31–33
    testicular cancer and retroperitoneal lymph node dissection, 33
    varicocele, 32–33
    vasectomy and vasectomy reversal, 31–32
  conceptualizing, 23–24
  financial burden, 25–26
  genetic, 29–31
    cystic fibrosis transmembrane conductance regulator/congenital bilateral absence of vas deferens, 31
    Klinefelter syndrome (KS), 29–30
    Y chromosome, 30–31
  hormonal causes, 26–28
    anabolic steroids, 27–28
    iatrogenic testosterone replacement, 26–27
  lifestyle issues, 36–37
  medications, 28–29

Male infertility (Continued)
  patient and partner perceptions of reproductive health and conception, 24–25
  perception of duration of trying/infertility, 25
  specific conditions, 26–33
  specific medical conditions, 33–36
    cancer, 35
    diabetes mellitus (DM), 33–34
    pediatric conditions and transitional care, 35–36
    spinal cord injury (SCI), 34–35
    transgender fertility issues, 36
Male sexuality, symbols of, 4
Male sexual problems, 223–227
  case studies, 225
  diagnosis of erectile dysfunction in, 223–224
  erectile dysfunction, 223
  treatment of erectile dysfunction, 224–225
Male virility, 5–6
Marital intervention, 198–199
Marriage counselors works with IT couples, 210
Masculinity, 12
Massachusetts Male Aging Study (MMAS), 57–58
Medicalization of reproduction, 189–204
  consultation, referral, and treatment options, 198–200
    clinical intervention, 200
    marital intervention, 198–199
    prevention of sexual dysfunction in infertile couples, 200
    psychosocial intervention, 199
    sex therapy, 199
  general stress and sexual dysfunction, in men and women, 191–192
  infertility, 192
  infertility and sexuality in men
    clinical implications, 194
    psychosocial implications, 194–195
  infertility and sexuality in the couple—marital implications, 196–197
  infertility and sexuality in women
    clinical implications, 195–196
    psychosocial implications, 196
  infertility-related stress on sexuality and pregnancy, 197–198
  psychological impact of infertility, 192–193
Medical screening, 146
Medical testosterone, 27
Medications for male infertility, 28–29
Medieval period, 237–238
Menopausal FSH, 95
Menopause, 93
Menstruation, 3–4
Mental health professionals, 54
Mental health providers, 132
Mental health treatments, 48
Metabolic syndrome, 60
Metal element, 218

Microcosmic orbit breathing, 222
Microtesticular sperm extraction (microTESE), 29
Minority Stress Model, 244
Modern antibiotics, 28
Modern Orthodox, 243
Modern reproductive health, 9–14
Monoamine oxidase inhibitors, 61
Moxabustion, 220
Mugwort, 231
Multiple sclerosis, 60–61
MUSE (intraurethral therapy), 67–68
Muslim infertility, navigating
  Shi'a Muslims, 253–254
  Sunni Muslims, 252–253
Myasthenia gravis, 94

N
National Health and Social Life Survey, 57–58
National Institute on Alcohol Abuse and Alcoholism (SAMHSA), 36–37
National Sexuality Education Standards (NSES), 14
National Survey of Family Growth, 14
National Transgender Discrimination Survey, 151
Natural cycle intrauterine insemination (IUI), 69
Negative religious coping methods, 255
Nerve damage, 111
Neural signaling pathways, 59
New Testament, 238–239
  infertility in, 249–250
Nitric oxide (NO), 59
Nitrofurantoin, 28
Nonobstructive azoospermia, 69
Norepinephrine, 59

O
Obstructive azoospermia, 69
Old Testament, 238–240, 243
  infertility in, 244–245
Oligozoospermia, 30
Oncofertility Consortium, 109
Oncology healthcare professionals, 113
Oocyte cryopreservation, 157, 159
Oocyte maturation techniques, 157
Open communication, 111–112
Open testis sperm extraction, 70f
Orgasmic disorders, 195
Orthodox Judaism, 241, 243, 248
Osteoporosis, 96–97
Ovarian aging, 93, 102
Ovarian reserve, 93
Ovarian tissue cryopreservation, 157–158
Ovist, 8

P
Pain and anxiolytic medications, 61
Papaverine (Trimix), 66
Partner communication, 111–112
Passionate Marriage, 216
Patient Protection and Affordable Care Act (ACA), 16

Pediatric conditions and transitional care, 35–36
  spina bifida, 35
  undescended testicles, 35–36
Penile erections, 64
Penile implant, 68
Penile injection therapy, 66–67
Penile rehabilitation postprostatectomy, 67
Penis, anatomy of, 58, 58f
Permission, Limited Information, Specific Suggestion, Intensive Therapy (PLISSIT) model, 109
Personal distress, 84
Pharmacological and medical treatment, for infertile women, 53–54
Phentolamine, 66
Phosphodiesterase 5 inhibitors (PDE5), 63–65, 111, 162
Physical therapist (PT), 231–232
Polycystic ovarian syndrome (PCOS), 154, 196, 208, 216
Polyvagal theory, 176
Poor sex/reproductive education, dangers of, 268–270
  infertility, 269
  intersection of infertility and intimate partner violence, 269–270
  reproductive knowledge, 268–269
  violence/discrimination/harassment/hostility toward women, 269–270
Positive religious coping methods, 255
Postpartum period, 167–168
Postpartum phase, 135–136
Posttraumatic growth, 177
Practicing homosexuals, 142
Pre-Cana, 242
Pregnancy, 134–135
Pregnancy, transgender men seeking, 166–168
  experience of pregnancy loss, 166–167
  intrapartum care, 167
  postpartum experience, 167–168
  preconception and antepartum experience, 166
Pregnancy rates, 143
Preimplantation genetic diagnosis (PGD), 31
Preimplantation genetic screening (PGS), 29–30
Preimplantation genetic testing (PGT), 145
Preimplantation genetic testing for aneuploidy (PGT-A), 248
Premature ejaculation (PE), 77, 225, 227
Premature ejaculation and infertility, 80
Premature ejaculation and traditional Chinese medicine, 227
Premature or rapid ejaculation, 78–79
  treatment for, 80–82
Primary ovarian insufficiency (POI), 93
  diagnosis of, 96–97
  etiologies of, 93–97
  hormone therapy options for, 99t
Procreation, 239–240, 243, 247
Professional autonomy, 152
Progestin therapy, 98
Prolactin, 61

Index

Prolonged estradiol exposure, 155
Prostaglandin E1 (alprostadil), 66–67
Prostate cancer, 107
Protective ambivalence, 181
Psychiatric and pain medications, 61
Psychoeducation, 183, 199
Psychoeducational counseling, 53
Psychogenic erections, 59
Psychological complications, 87–88
Psychological consultation, 132
Psychological distress and female sexual function, 48
Psychological effects of infertility in women, 46–48
Psychological trauma theory, 174–176
  trauma impacting attachment, 175
  trauma response theory, 175–176
Psychosocial intervention, 199
Puberty and Adolescent Sexual Development (PD), 14
Public school sex education, 265

Q
Qi, 215–216
Q-tip test, 228, 231

R
Racial minority groups, 159
Radical prostatectomy, 67
Ramapethicus, 3
Reciprocal IVF, 129–130
Recovery medication, 28
Reflexogenic erections, 59
Relationship needs, 208–210
Religious coping, 255
Religious rituals, 255
Ren channel (Conception vessel), 218
Reproduction, emergents of, 210–211
Reproductive-aged breast cancer survivors, 112
Reproductive-aged cancer survivors, 105
Reproductive function, in males, 68
Reproductive knowledge, 160–163
Reproductive story, 175
Reproductive trauma, 175
Retrograde ejaculation (RE), 33–34, 77–78
Retroperitoneal lymph node dissection (RPLND), 33
Rheumatoid arthritis, 94
Ripple effect, 174

S
Safe sex, 13
Same-sex male couples, 144–145
Same-sex parenting, 136
Screening tools, 108f
Second-parent adoption, 136
Secure attachment style, 175
Selective serotonin reuptake inhibitors (SSRIs), 50, 61, 81, 194
Self-regulation, 177
Semen analysis, 24–25
Semen parameters, 32–34
Sensory stimulation, 59
Serum testosterone, 26

Sex, 174, 237–238
Sex, religion, and infertility, 237–262
  collaboration of religion with treatment, 256–258
  historical overview of, 237–239
    assisted reproductive technology, 239
    infertility in the New Testament, 249–250
    Judeo-Christian perspectives on infertility and assisted reproduction, 244–249
    Judeo-Christian views of homosexuality and status, 242–244
    Judeo-Christian views on sexuality and sex, 239–242
    origin of Christianity, 238–239
    origin of Islam, 239
    origin of Judaism, 238
    sex, 237–238
  implications and recommendations, 254–255
  infertility in the Qur'an, 251–252
  navigating Christian infertility, 250–251
  navigating Muslim infertility
    Shi'a Muslims, 253–254
    Sunni Muslims, 252–253
Sex disparities, 157–158
Sex drive, 220–221
Sex drive and reproduction in traditional Chinese medicine, 220–222
Sex education, 9–10, 12
  in schools, 265
Sex educational programs, 11
Sex educators, 12
"Sex positive" approaches, 13
Sex/reproductive education, disparate effects of, 267–268
  differently abled groups, 268
  LGBTQ individuals, 267
  racial minoritized groups, 267–268
  sex disparities, 267
Sex selection, 248
Sex therapy, 51–52, 199
Sexual and intimacy concerns, 106–107
Sexual and reproductive health (SRH), 3
Sexual and reproductive health knowledge, 3–20
  early historical evidence, 4–5
  evolution of modern reproductive health and sex education in United States, 9–14
  fertility awareness and acquisition, 14–17
  interventions to improve fertility awareness, knowledge, and access to care, 17
  prehistory of, 3–4
  recorded history, 5–6
  science and fertility, 6–9
Sexual arousal, 59
Sexual aversion disorders, 195
Sexual desire, 48, 50–52, 111
Sexual desire disorders, 195
Sexual disruption, 50, 52, 54
Sexual dysfunction (SD), 48–49, 59, 163–164, 189–194
  etiology of, 191–192
Sexual function, 52
Sexual health, 13–14
Sexual health problems, for women after cancer, 107t
Sexual interaction, human, 9
Sexual intercourse, 3–4, 112
Sexual intimacy, 205, 207–208, 211
Sexuality, 222–223, 242
Sexuality Information and Education Council of the United States (SIECUS), 12, 14
Sexually transmitted infections (STIs), 265
Sexual Orientation and Identity (SO), 14
Sexual pain disorders, 195
Sexual status examination, 51
Sexual stimulation, 64
Sexual transmission of infection, 10
Shared IVF, 129–130
Sharia law, 239
Shattered assumption theory, 174–175
Shi'a Muslims, 253–254
Shen, 216
Sildenafil, 64, 64f, 200
Single-embryo transfer, 145
Situational anxiety, 65
Social infertility, 239
Social media, 155
Social networks, 155
Social support, 135
Sociocultural norms, 63
Sperm, 63–64
Spermatogenesis, 31, 162
Sperm cryopreservation, 161–162
Spermist, 8
Sperm motility, 71
Sperm parameters, 155, 163
Spina bifida, 35
Spinal cord injury (SCI), 34–35
Spiritual cognitive dissonance (SCD), 244
Spleen energy, 218
Squeeze technique, 80–81
Standard postmenopausal hormone therapy, 98–99
Stigmatization, 136
Stress, 189, 222–223
Structural interventions, 17
Substance Abuse and Mental Health Services Administration (SAMSHA), 178
Sumerian texts and seals, 5
Sunni Muslims, 252–253
Superficial penile arterial supply, 58–59
Surgical sperm retrieval (SSR), 78
Surrogacy, 165–166, 251, 253–254
Syphilis, 10
Systemic lupus erythematosus, 94

T
Tadalafil, 64, 64f, 200
Terminology, clarifying, 125
Testicular cancer, 33, 107
Testicular cancer and retroperitoneal lymph node dissection, 33
Testicular sperm extraction (TESE), 246–247
Testicular tissue cryopreservation, 162–163
Testicular varicocele, 32–33

Testis sperm retrieval techniques, 70–71
Testosterone, 100, 154
Testosterone deficiency, 26–27
Testosterone-induced amenorrhea, 154
Tetracyclines, 28
Therapeutic interventions and techniques, 53t
Thyroid hormone, dysfunction of, 62
Time demands of work, 209
Title X program, 13
Title X Public Health Service Act, 13
Tobacco use, 36
Traditional Chinese Medicine (TCM), 213–236
   diagnosis according to, 217
   Eastern medicine, 220
   edging practice for early ejaculators, 227
   eight extraordinary vessels, fertility, and sexuality, 218–219
   ejaculatory dysfunction (ED), 226
   female sexual issues, 227
      causes of, 228f
   five elements, fertility, and sexuality, 217–218
   herbal medicine and erectile dysfunction, 225–226
   intravaginal ejaculatory dysfunction, case on, 226–227
   lichen sclerosus and, 230
   low sex drive and trauma (case study), 222
      microcosmic orbit breathing, 222
   male deer exercise, 225
   male sexual problems and, 223–227
      case studies, 225
      diagnosis of erectile dysfunction in, 223–224
      erectile dysfunction, 223
      treatment of erectile dysfunction, 224–225
   modalities used in, 219–220
      acupuncture, 219
      cupping, 220
      electroacupuncture (EA), 219
      herbal medicine, 220
      moxabustion, 220
   premature ejaculation and, 227
   research on TCM and female sexual pain, 228–229
   sex drive and reproduction in, 220–222
   stress, fertility, sexuality, and, 222–223
   stress, infertility, and sexuality, 223
   texts on gynecology, sexuality, and fertility, 216–217
   three treasures, 214–216
      Jing, 223
      Qi, 215–216
      Shen, 216
   treatment plans, for female problems, 230–231
      vaginal streaming, 231
Transgender and nonbinary individuals, parenting in, 149–172
   barriers to parenting, 152–153
   demographics of transgender parenting, 150–151
   fertility care, 164–166
   fertility preservation, 155–157
   fertility preservation options for transgender men, 157–159
      embryo cryopreservation, 159
      oocyte cryopreservation, 159
      ovarian tissue cryopreservation, 157–158
   fertility preservation options for transgender women, 160–163
      embryo cryopreservation, 162
      sperm cryopreservation, 161–162
      testicular tissue cryopreservation, 162–163
   fertility preservation outcomes for transgender men, 159–160
   fertility preservation outcomes for transgender women, 163–164
   healthcare barriers, 151–152
   impact of gender-affirming care on reproductive function, 153–155
      feminizing hormones and fertility, 155
      masculinizing hormones and fertility, 153–154
   impact of parenting on children, 168
   impact of parenting on gender identity and quality of life, 169
   pregnancy, 166–168
      experience of pregnancy loss, 166–167
      intrapartum care, 167
      postpartum experience, 167–168
      preconception and antepartum experience, 166
   transgender parenting desires, 151
Transgender fertility issues, 36
Transgender individuals, 151–152
Transsexualism, 149
Trauma, 173
   assessment, 178–184
      feedback, 182–184
      partner 1 history gathering, 180–181
      partner 2 history gathering, 181–182
      special considerations, 184
      understanding the problem, 178–180
   clinical considerations, 184–185
   providing foundation for growth, 177–178
   psychological trauma theory, 174–176
      trauma impacting attachment, 175
      trauma response theory, 175–176
   and relationships, 176–177
   and sexual relationship, 173–174
      grief at the core of trauma and infertility, 174
Trauma recovery, 174, 177
Trauma response theory, 175–176
Travel for work, 209
Treatment plans for female problems, 230–231
Tricyclic antidepressants, 61
Tumescence, 59
Turner syndrome, 94, 96, 100–101

U

UK Fertility Education Initiative (FEI), 17
Ultra-Orthodox, 243
Undescended testicles, 35–36
Unintended infertility, 205–212
   defining, 206
   emergent modes of reproduction, 210–211
   marriage counselors works with IT couples, 210
   meeting with couples undergoing fertility assistance, 207
   workplace demands and relationship needs, 208–210
United Methodist Church (UMC), 241–242
United States, reproductive education in, 151
   faith-based organizations, 266
   healthcare providers, 153–154
   institutions of higher learning, 151–152
   parents, 153–155
   social networks and social media, 267

V

Vacuum erection device (VED), 67
Vaginismus, 49, 53–54, 195, 227–228, 231–232
Vardenafil, 64, 64f, 200
Varicocele, 26, 32–33
Vascular corpora cavernosa, 58
Vascular corpus spongiosum, 58
Vasectomy, 26, 31–32
Vasectomy reversal, 31–32
Vestibulodynia, 228
V-steam, 231
Vulnerability, 177
Vulvodynia, 227–228

W

Water element, 217–218
Western cultural traditions, 125–126
Women's Health Initiative (WHI) hormone trial, 97–98
Wood element, 218
Workplace demands, 208–210
World Health Organization (WHO), 13

Y

Y chromosome, 30–31
Yin and Yang Qiao vessels (vessels of one's stance), 219
Yin Wei and Yang Wei (linking vessels), 219

Printed in the United States
by Baker & Taylor Publisher Services

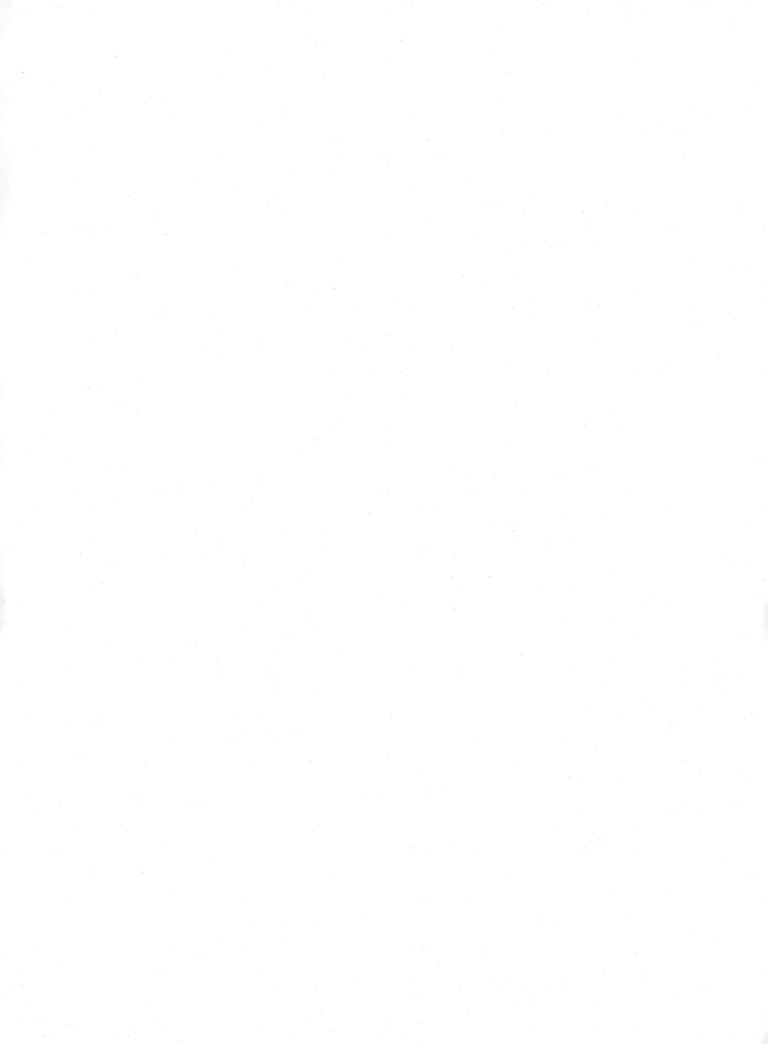